Craig's

RESTORATIVE DENTAL MATERIALS

Craig's RESTORATIVE DENTAL MATERIALS

FIFTEENTH EDITION

EDITED BY

Carmem Pfeifer, DDS, PhD
Weight Professor of Restorative Dentistry
Division Head, Biomaterial and Biomedical Sciences
School of Dentistry
Oregon Health & Science University
Portland, Oregon

Jack Ferracane, PhD
Professor and Chair
Department of Oral Rehabilitation and Biosciences
School of Dentistry
Oregon Health & Science University
Portland, Oregon

Ronald Sakaguchi, DDS, PhD, MS, MBA
Dean
School of Dentistry
Oregon Health & Science University
Portland, Oregon

ELSEVIER

Elsevier
3251 Riverport Lane
St. Louis, Missouri 63043

CRAIG'S RESTORATIVE DENTAL MATERIALS, FIFTEENTH EDITION

ISBN: 978-0-323-88276-7

Senior Content Strategists: Kelly Skelton, Lauren Boyle
Senior Content Development Specialist: Suddha S. Sen
Publishing Services Manager: Deepthi Unni
Project Manager: Manchu Mohan
Design Direction: Ryan Cook

Printed in India
Last digit is the print number: 9 8 7 6 5 4 3 2 1

To the many mentors, mentees, and colleagues
with whom we have collaborated

Contributors

Hongseok An, DDS, MSD, FACP
Associate Professor
Department of Oral Rehabilitation and Biosciences
Oregon Health & Science University
Portland, Oregon

Despoina Bompolaki, DDS, MS, FACP
Associate Professor
Director
Clinical Restorative Dentistry
Department of Oral Rehabilitation and Biosciences
Oregon Health & Science University
Portland, Oregon

Roberto R. Braga, DDS, PhD
Full Professor
Department of Biomaterials and Oral Biology
School of Dentistry
University of São Paulo
São Paulo, Brazil

Juliana Branco da Costa, DDS, MS
Professor
Division Head of Restorative Dentistry
Department of Oral Rehabilitation and Biosciences
Oregon Health & Science University
Portland, Oregon

Jack Ferracane, PhD
Professor and Chair
Department of Oral Rehabilitation and Biosciences
Oregon Health & Science University
Portland, Oregon

Jason Alan Griggs, PhD, FADM
Professor
Department of Biomedical Materials Science
Associate Dean for Research
School of Dentistry
University of Mississippi Medical Center
Jackson, Mississippi

Robert J. Kelly, DDS
Professor
Department of Reconstructive Sciences
University of Connecticut Health Center
Farmington, Connecticut

Justin Merritt, PhD
Professor
Department of Oral Rehabilitation and Biosciences
Oregon Health & Science University
Portland, Oregon

John C. Mitchell, PhD
Professor and Associate Dean
College of Dental Medicine-Arizona
Midwestern University
Glendale, Arizona
Professor and Associate Dean
College of Dental Medicine-Illinois
Midwestern University
Downers Grove, Illinois

Carmem Pfeifer, DDS, PhD
Professor
Division Head
Department of Biomaterial and Biomedical Sciences
Oregon Health & Science University
Portland, Oregon

Ronald Sakaguchi, DDS, PhD, MBA
Dean
Office of the Dean
Oregon Health & Science University
Portland, Oregon

Danielle P. Wingrove, DDS, EdD
Assistant Professor
Department of Endodontics
University of Utah School of Dentistry
Salt Lake City, Utah

Yu Zhang, PhD
Professor
Department of Preventive and Restorative Sciences
School of Dental Medicine
University of Pennsylvania
Philadelphia, Pennsylvania

Preface

The 15th edition of this classic textbook has been extensively updated to include many recent developments in dental biomaterials science and new materials for clinical use. The sequencing of the materials has also been streamlined. The book continues to be designed for predoctoral dental students and also provides an excellent update of dental biomaterials science and clinical applications of restorative materials for students in graduate programs and residencies.

Dr. Carmem S. Pfeifer takes on the lead editor role from Dr. Ronald L. Sakaguchi, who has served in that capacity for the 13th and 14th editions and now serves as coeditor. Dr. Pfeifer is professor and division head of Biomaterial and Biomedical Sciences, Department of Oral Rehabilitation and Biosciences at the School of Dentistry, Oregon Health & Science University (OHSU), with a joint appointment in the Department of Biomedical Engineering, School of Medicine, in Portland, Oregon. She earned her DDS and PhD in Dental Materials Sciences from the University of São Paulo, Brazil.

Dr. Sakaguchi serves as Dean of the School of Dentistry at OHSU. He earned a BS in cybernetics from the University of California Los Angeles (UCLA), a DDS from Northwestern University, an MS in prosthodontics from the University of Minnesota, a PhD in biomaterials and biomechanics from Thames Polytechnic (London, England; now the University of Greenwich), and an MBA in entrepreneurship from Babson College.

Dr. Jack L. Ferracane returns as coeditor of the 15th edition. Dr. Ferracane serves as professor and chair of the Department of Oral Rehabilitation and Biosciences at the School of Dentistry (OHSU) in Portland, Oregon. He earned a BS in biology from the University of Illinois and an MS and a PhD in biological materials from Northwestern University.

We thank our many chapter authors for their effort and expertise in revising the text from the previous edition: Dr. Hongseok An, Dr. Juliana Branco da Costa, and Dr. Justin Merritt from Oregon Health & Science University; Dr. Roberto R. Braga from the University of São Paulo; Dr. Jason Alan Griggs from the University of Mississippi; Dr. John C. Mitchell from Midwestern University; Dr. Danielle P. Wingrove from the University of Utah; and Dr. Yu Zhang from the University of Pennsylvania.

The organization of the 15th edition was updated so that each chapter focuses on a specific class of materials. The chapter on testing of dental materials and biomechanics is now provided as online content only. One new chapter dedicated to dental adhesives was created (Chapter 7), encompassing the new adhesive technologies. The chapter on dental composites (Chapter 8) has been extensively revised to include newer technology in photopolymerization. Chapter 13, on technology, has also seen a major update, with a focus not only on CAD-CAM but also on additive manufacturing technologies applied to dentistry.

An enhanced ebook version, included with every new print purchase, is available for this textbook. Included is the majority of the procedural, or materials handling, content that was in the previous editions. In addition, newly produced interactive videos for the most common procedures in dentistry are available at http://ebooks.health.elsevier.com/. The Evolve Resources website, available for instructors at http://evolve.elsevier.com/Pfeifer/restorative/, includes an image collection and PowerPoint lecture slides to supplement the print version of the book.

Carmem Pfeifer
Jack Ferracane
Ronald Sakaguchi

Acknowledgments

We are deeply grateful to Lauren Boyle and Kelly Skelton, Senior Content Strategists at Elsevier, for guidance in the initial planning and approval of the project; to Suddha Satwa Sen, Senior Developmental Editor at Elsevier, for the many suggestions and support throughout the design process and writing of the manuscript.

Thanks also to many others at Elsevier for their behind-the-scenes work and contributions to the book.

Lastly, we thank our colleagues in our respective institutions for the many informal chats and suggestions offered and our families who put up with us being at our computers late in the evenings and on many weekends. It truly does take a community to create a work like this textbook, and we thank you all.

Carmem Pfeifer
Jack Ferracane
Ronald Sakaguchi

Contents

1

Role and Significance of Restorative Dental Materials

RONALD SAKAGUCHI

CHAPTER OUTLINE

Developments in materials science, tissue engineering, regenerative dentistry, imaging and subtractive computer-aided design/computer-aided manufacturing (CAD/CAM), and additive (3D printing) manufacturing have dramatically changed the way we look at the replacement of components of the human anatomy. The replacement of tooth structure lost to disease, wear, and injury continues to be a large part of general dental practice. Restorative dental materials are the foundation for the replacement of tooth structure.

Form and function are important considerations in the replacement of lost tooth structure. Although tooth form and appearance are aspects most easily recognized, the function of the teeth and supporting tissues contributes greatly to the quality of life. The links between oral and general health are well known. Proper function of the elements of the oral cavity, including the teeth and soft tissues, is needed for eating, speaking, swallowing, proper breathing, and smiling.

Restorative dental materials make the reconstruction of the dental hard tissues possible. In many areas, the development of dental materials has progressed more rapidly than for other anatomical prostheses. Because of their long-term success, patients often expect dental prostheses to outperform the natural materials and structures they replace. The application of materials science is unique in dentistry because of the complexity of the oral cavity, which includes bacteria, high forces, ever-changing pH, and a warm, fluid environment. The oral cavity is considered to be the harshest environment for a material in the body. In addition, when dental materials are placed directly into tooth cavities as restorative materials, there are very specific requirements for manipulation of the material. Knowledge of materials science and biomechanics is very important when choosing materials for specific dental applications and when designing the best solution for restoration of tooth structure and replacement of teeth.

A review of the history of dentistry may be found on the book's website at http://evolve.elsevier.com/sakaguchi/restorative.

Scope of Materials Covered in Restorative Dentistry

Restorative dental materials include representatives from the broad classes of materials: metals, polymers, ceramics, and composites. Dental materials include such items as resin composites, ceramics, cement, glass ionomers, metals, gypsum materials, impression materials, denture base resins, casting investments, dental amalgams, and other materials used in restorative procedures. The requirements for material characteristics and performance range from high flexibility required by impression materials to high stiffness required in crowns and fixed dental prostheses. Materials for dental implants require integration with bone. Some materials are cast to achieve excellent adaptation to existing tooth structures, whereas others are machined under digital control to produce very reproducible dimensions and structured geometries. When describing these materials, physical and chemical characteristics are often used as criteria for comparison. To understand how a material works, we study its chemical structure, its physical and mechanical characteristics, and its manipulation to result in the best performance.

Most restorative materials are characterized by physical, chemical, and mechanical parameters that are derived from test data. Improvements in these characteristics might be shown in laboratory studies, but the real test is the material's performance in function in the mouth and the ability of the material to be manipulated properly by the dental team. In many cases, errors and variations in handling and manipulation can negate the improvements in physical, chemical, and mechanical properties. Therefore it is very important for the dental team to understand how to manipulate dental materials appropriately.

A Systems Approach to Restorative Materials

The practice of clinical dentistry requires a complete understanding of the various clinical techniques and a solid foundation of knowledge of the biological, chemical, and physical principles of human anatomy and function. It is important to understand the "how" and "why" associated with the function of natural and synthetic dental materials. The best patient outcomes will be achieved when a systems approach is used to assess the chemical, physical, and mechanical aspects of dental materials and oral function, together with the physiological, structural, and other biological properties of the tissues that support the restorative and rehabilitative constructs. This integrative approach, when combined with the best available scientific evidence, clinician experience, patient preferences, and patient modifiers, results in the best patient-centered care.

Application of Various Sciences

In the chapters that follow, fundamental characteristics of materials are presented, along with numerous practical examples of how the basic principles relate to clinical applications. Test procedures and fabrication techniques are discussed briefly but not emphasized. Many of the details of manipulation are found on the book's website at http://evolve.elsevier.com/sakaguchi/restorative.

Knowledge and application of fundamental principles of materials and mechanics are essential for the design and optimal prognosis of restorations. For example, the prognosis of long-span fixed dental prostheses, or bridges, is dependent on the stiffness and fracture resistance of the materials. When considering aesthetics, the hardness of the material is an important property because it influences the ability to polish the material. Some materials release fluoride when exposed to saliva, which might be beneficial in high-caries-risk patients. When selecting a ceramic for CAD-CAM fabrication of an all-ceramic crown, the machining and wear characteristics of the ceramic are important. For implants, surface texture, coating, and geometry are critical considerations for bone and soft tissue adaptation. These are just a few examples of the many interactions between the clinical performance of dental materials and fundamental scientific principles.

Future Developments in Biomaterials

The 2021 Global Burden of Disease Study reported that among the 371 diseases and injuries assessed, oral disorders were the most prevalent Level 3 diseases: dental caries in permanent teeth (#1), periodontal diseases (#8), dental caries in deciduous teeth (#14), and edentulism (#20) (GBD 2021 Diseases and Injuries Collaborators 2021). These oral diseases and conditions affect about 3.69 billion people worldwide.

In the United States, about 50% of adults aged 20 to 64 have lost at least one permanent tooth to an accident, periodontal disease, a failed root canal, or tooth decay. In adults aged 65 and older, 13% have lost all of their natural teeth. That number is twice as large for adults aged 75 and over (18%) than for adults aged 65 to 74 (9%) (CDC/NCHS, National Health and Nutrition Examination Survey). For children aged 5 to 19 years, 13% have untreated dental caries. For adults aged 20 to 44, that number is 26%.

The demand for restorative care continues to be high, although there are many inequities in the dental care available to and utilized by marginalized populations. For some populations, there has been a shift from removable prostheses to implant-supported, fixed prostheses. For single-tooth loss, implants enable restoration of single crowns rather than multiunit, longer-span restorations. Research into implant coatings, surface textures, graded properties, alternative materials, and new geometries will continue to grow. These advances will improve the viability of implants, with enhancements to bone and soft tissue health.

Dental and orofacial aesthetics will continue to be a focus for some consumers, which will promote the development and sales of tooth-whitening systems, Botox, and aesthetic restorations. A more natural-looking appearance with character is preferred by many over a uniform, dazzling white dentition, which was the trend of the last decade. There will be more demand for materials that mimic natural dentition and provide the same depth of color and optical characteristics as natural teeth.

With the aging of the population, exposed root surfaces, dry mouth, and worn dentitions will be more common. These are challenging conditions to restore, and materials will need to function in an environment with reduced salivary flow and atypical salivary pH and chemistry. This population will be managing multiple chronic illnesses with many medications and will have limitations in maintaining adequate oral home care. Restorative materials will be challenged in this difficult environment.

Advances in tissue regeneration are accelerating. Our understanding of the oral microbiome is expanding. Biofabrication and 3D bioprinting methods are creating new and more natural structures and materials. This is a very exciting time for materials research, and clinicians will have much to look forward to in the near future as this body of research develops new materials for expanded clinical applications.

Bibliography

Centers for Disease Control and Prevention and National Center for Health Statistics. *National Health and Nutrition Examination Study.* 2021–2022. https://wwwn.cdc.gov/nchs/nhanes/continuousnhanes/default.aspx?BeginYear=2021.

Choi CK, Breckenridge MT, Chen CS. Engineered materials and the cellular microenvironment: a strengthening interface between cell biology and bioengineering. *Trends Cell Biol.* 2010;20(12):705–714.

Denry I, Kelly JR. Emerging ceramic-based materials for dentistry. *J Dent Res.* 2014;93(12):1235–1242.

Horowitz RA, Coelho PG. Endosseous implant: the journey and the future. *Compend Contin Educ Dent.* 2010;31(7):545–547.

Jones JR, Boccaccini AR. Editorial: a forecast of the future for biomaterials. *J Mater Sci Mater Med.* 2006;17:963–964.

Murray CJL. The Global Burden of Disease Study at 30 years. *Nat Med.* 2022;28:2019–2026. https://doi.org/10.1038/s41591-022-01990-1.

Nakamura M, Iwanaga S, Henmi C, Arai K, Nishiyama Y. Biomatrices and biomaterials for future developments of bioprinting and biofabrication. *Biofabrication.* 2010;2(1):014110.

Rekow ED, Fox CH, Watson T, Petersen PE. Future innovation and research in dental restorative materials. *Adv Dent Res.* 2013;25(1):2–7.

Tabak LA. Looking forward, guest editorial. *JADA.* 2023;154(1):1–2.

U.S. Department of Health and Human Services, Centers for Disease Control and Prevention (CDC) and National Center for Health Statistics (NCHS). *Health, United States*; 2021. https://www.cdc.gov/nchs/data/hus/hus20-21.pdf.

U.S. Department of Health and Human Services. *Oral Health in America: A Report of the Surgeon General—Executive Summary.* Rockville, MD: U.S. Department of Health and Human Services, National Institute of Dental and Craniofacial Research, National Institutes of Health; 2000.

2

The Oral Environment

JUSTIN MERRITT

CHAPTER OUTLINE

The tooth contains three specialized calcified tissues: enamel, dentin, and cementum (Fig. 2.1). Enamel is unique in that it is the most highly calcified tissue in the body and contains the least organic content of any of these tissues. Enamel provides the hard outer covering of the crown that allows efficient mastication. Dentin and cementum, like bone, are vital, hydrated, biological composite structures formed mainly of a collagen type I matrix reinforced with the calcium phosphate mineral called *apatite*. Dentin forms the bulk of the tooth and is joined to the enamel at the dentin–enamel junction (DEJ). The dentin of the tooth root is covered by cementum, which provides a connection of the tooth to the alveolar bone via the periodontal ligament. Although the structure of these tissues is often described in dental texts, their properties are often discussed only superficially. However, these properties are important with regard to the interrelationships of the factors that contribute to the performance necessary for the optimum function of these tissues.

In restorative dentistry, we are interested in providing preventive treatments that will maintain tissue integrity and replace damaged tissues with materials that ideally mimic the natural appearance and performance of those tissues when necessary. Thus knowledge of the structure and properties of these tissues is desirable both as a yardstick to measure the properties and performance of restorative materials and as a guide to the development of materials that will mimic their structure and function. In addition, many applications, such as dental bonding, require us to attach synthetic materials to the calcified tissues, and these procedures rely on detailed knowledge of the composition, structure, and properties of the adhesive tissue substrates.

Enamel

Fig. 2.1 shows a schematic diagram of a posterior tooth sectioned to reveal the enamel and dentin components. Enamel forms the hard outer shell of the crown and, as the most highly calcified tissue, is well suited to resisting wear due to mastication.

Enamel is formed by ameloblasts starting at the DEJ and proceeding outward to the tooth surface. The ameloblasts exchange signals with odontoblasts located on the other side of the DEJ at the start of the enamel and dentin formation, and the odontoblasts move inward from the DEJ as the ameloblasts move outward to form the enamel of the crown. Most of the enamel organic matrix, which is composed of amelogenins and enamelins, is resorbed during tooth maturation to leave a calcified tissue that is largely composed of minerals and a sparse organic matrix. The structural arrangement of enamel forms keyhole-shaped structures known as *enamel prisms* or *rods* that are about 5 μm across, as seen in Fig. 2.2.

The overall composition of enamel is about 96% mineral by weight, with 1% lipid and protein and the remainder being water. The organic portion and water probably play important roles in tooth function and pathology, and it is often more useful to describe the composition on a volume basis. On that basis, we see that organic components make up about 3% and water 12% of the structure. The mineral is formed and grows into very long crystals of hexagonal shape about 40 nm across; these crystals have yet to be synthetically duplicated. There is some evidence that the crystals may span the entire enamel thickness, but this is difficult to prove because most preparation procedures lead to fracture of the individual crystallites. It appears that they are at least thousands of nanometers long. If this is true, then enamel crystals provide an extraordinary "aspect" ratio (length-to-width ratio) for a nanoscale material, and they are very different from the much smaller dentin crystals. The crystals are packed into enamel prisms or rods that are about 5 μm across, as shown in Fig. 2.2. These prisms are revealed easily by acid etching, extending in a closely packed array from the DEJ to the enamel surface and lying roughly perpendicular to the DEJ, except in cuspal areas where the rods twist and cross, known as *decussation*, which may increase fracture resistance. About 100 crystals of the mineral are needed to span the diameter of a prism, and the long axes of the crystals tend to align themselves along the prism axes, as seen in Fig. 2.2.

The crystals near the periphery of each prism deviate somewhat from the long axis toward the interface between prisms. The deviation in the tail of the prism is even greater. The individual crystals

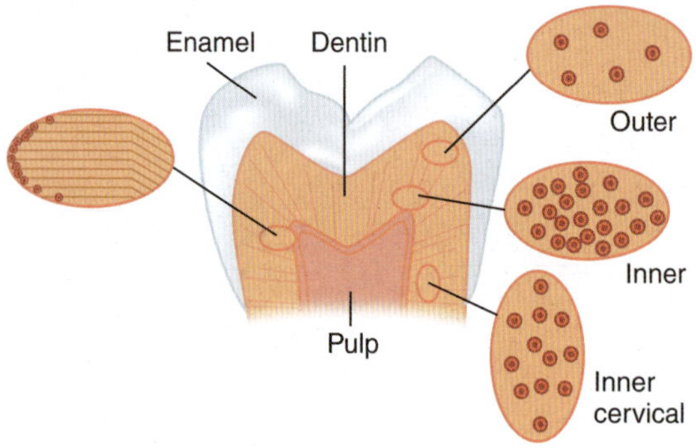

• **Fig. 2.1** Schematic diagram of a tooth cut longitudinally to expose the enamel, dentin, and the pulp chamber. On the *right* side are illustrations of dentin tubules as viewed from the top, which show the variation in the tubule number with location. On the *left* is an illustration of the change in direction of the primary dentin tubules as secondary dentin is formed. (From Marshall SJ, Balooch M, Breunig T, et al. Human dentin and the dentin-resin adhesive interface. *Acta Mater*. 1998;46:2529–2539).

within a prism are also coated with a thin layer of lipid and/or protein that plays important roles in mineralization, although much remains to be learned about the details. Recent work suggests that this protein coat may lead to increased toughness of the enamel. The interfaces between prisms, or interrod enamel, contain the main organic components of the structure and act as passageways for water and ionic movement. These areas, also known as *prism sheaths*, are of vital importance in etching processes associated with bonding and other demineralization processes, such as caries.

Etching of enamel with acids such as phosphoric acid, commonly used in enamel bonding, eliminates smear layers associated with cavity preparation, dissolves persisting layers of prismless enamel in deciduous teeth, and differentially dissolves enamel crystals in each prism. The pattern of etched enamel is categorized as type 1 (preferential prism core etching; Fig. 2.2A), type 2 (preferential prism periphery etching; Fig. 2.3C), and type 3 (mixed or uniform). Sometimes these patterns appear side by side on the same tooth surface (Fig. 2.3E). No differences in micromechanical bond strength of the different etching patterns have been established. In a standard cavity preparation for a composite, the orientation of the enamel surfaces being etched could be perpendicular to enamel prisms (perimeter of the cavity outline), oblique, cross section of the prisms (beveled occlusal or proximal margins), and axial walls of the prisms (cavity preparation walls). During the early stages of etching, when only a small amount of enamel crystal dissolution occurs, it may be difficult or impossible to detect the extent of the process. However, as the etching pattern begins to develop, the surface etched with phosphoric acid develops a frosty appearance (Fig. 2.3B), which has been used as the

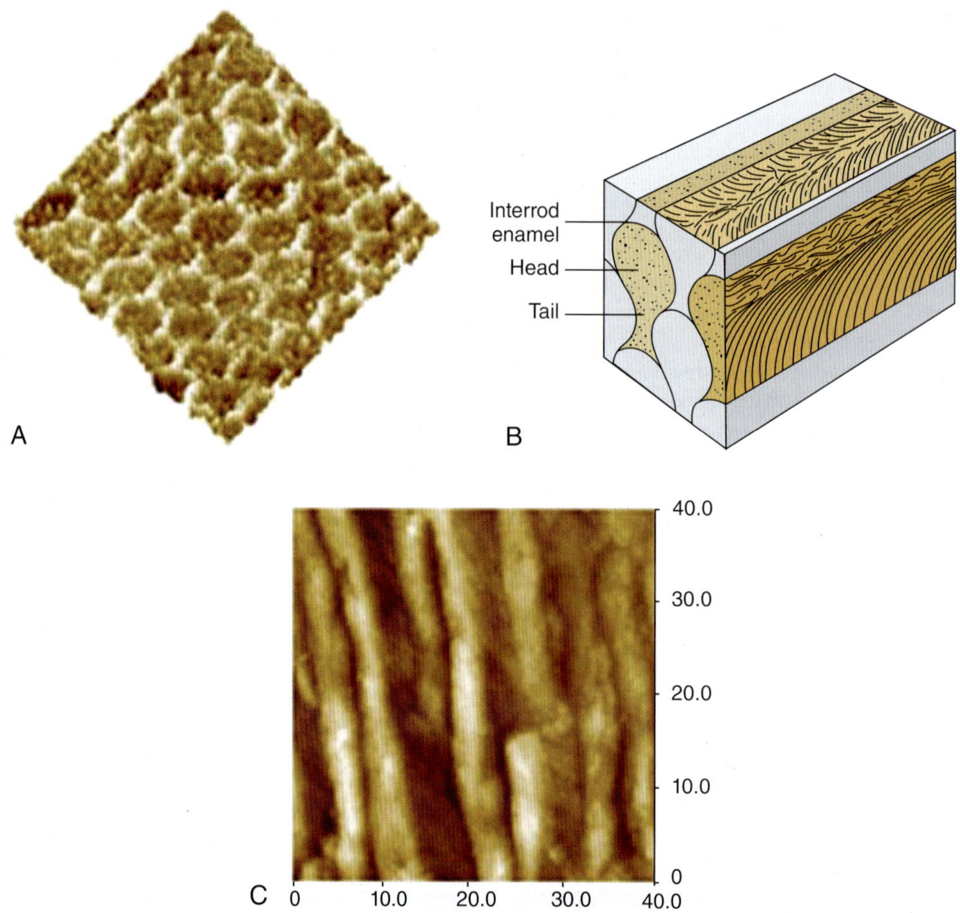

• **Fig. 2.2** Enamel microstructure. (A) Atomic force microscopy images showing prism cross sections. (B) Schematic diagram of keyhole-shaped enamel prisms or rods about 5 μm in diameter. (C) Atomic force microscopy images showing the axes of the prisms. Crystallite orientation deviates in the interrod and tail area and the organic content increases in the interrod area. (Modified from Habelitz S, Marshall SJ, Marshall GW, et al. Mechanical properties of human dental enamel on the nanometer scale. *Arch Oral Biol*. 2001;46:173–183.)

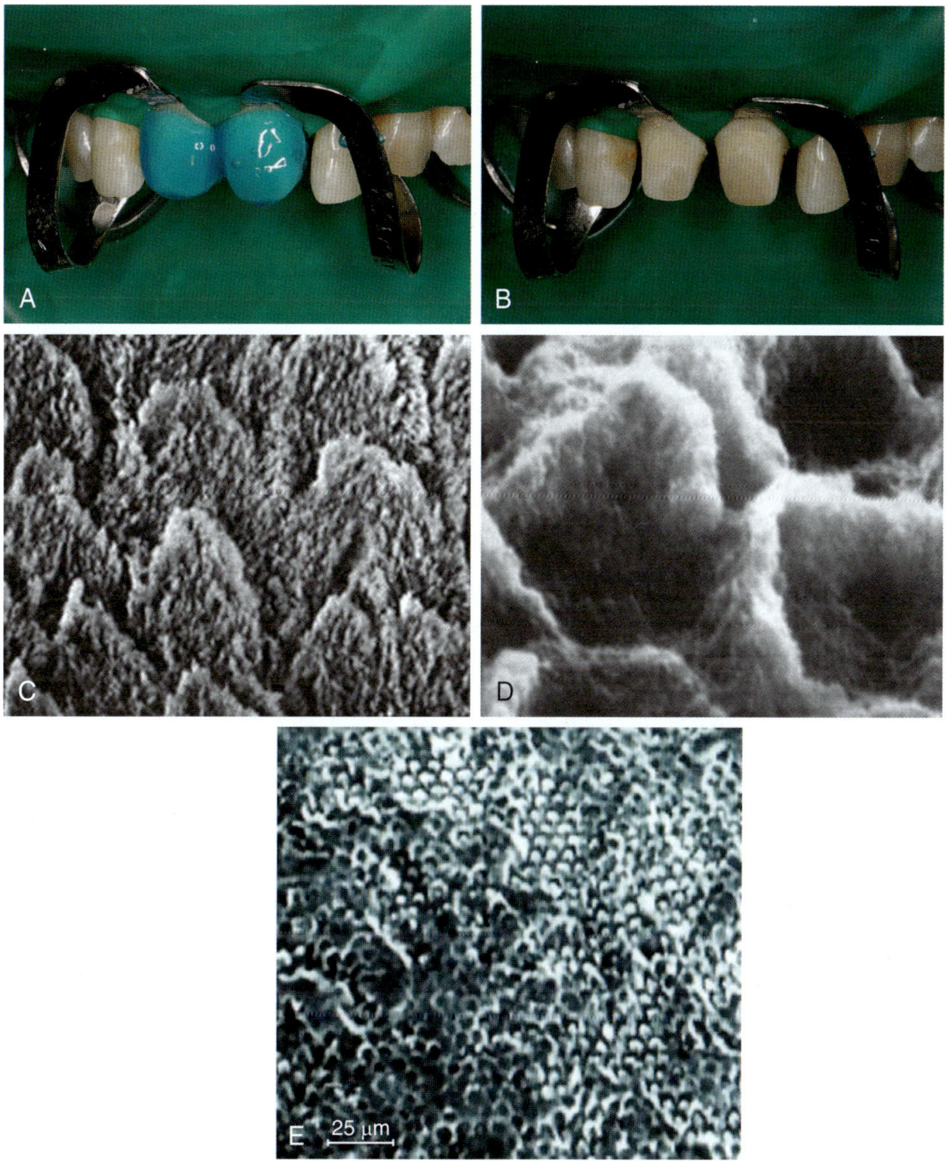

• **Fig. 2.3** Etching enamel. (A) Gel etchant dispensed on the enamel portion of the preparation. (B) Frosty appearance after etching, rinsing, and drying. (C) Magnified view of etch pattern with preferential prism periphery etch (type 1). (D) Bonding agent revealed after dissolving enamel. (E) Mixed etch patterns showing type 1 (light prisms with dark periphery) and type 2 (dark cores with light periphery) etching on the same surface. (C and D, After Marshall GW, Olson LM, Lee CV. SEM Investigation of the variability of enamel surfaces after simulated clinical acid etching for pit and fissure sealants. *J Dent Res*. 1975;54:1222–1231; E, After Marshall GW, Olson LM, Lee CV. SEM investigation of the variability of enamel surfaces after simulated clinical acid etching for pit and fissure sealants. *J Dent Res*. 1975;54:1222–1231; E, from Marshall GW, Marshall SJ, Bayne SC. Restorative dental materials: scanning electron microscopy and x-ray microanalysis. *Scanning Microsc*. 1988;2:2007–2028.)

traditional clinical indicator for sufficient etching. This roughened surface provides the substrate for infiltration of bonding agents that can be polymerized after penetration of the etched enamel structure so that they form micromechanical bonds to the enamel when polymerized. With weaker acids in most self-etching bonding agents, this frosty appearance typically cannot be detected.

There are two other important structural variations of enamel. Near the DEJ, the enamel prism structure is not as well developed in the very first enamel formed, so that the enamel very close to the DEJ may appear aprismatic or without the prism-like structure. Similarly, at the completion of the enamel surface, the ameloblasts degenerate and leave a featureless layer called *prismless enamel* on the outer surface of the crown. This layer is more often observed in deciduous teeth and is often worn off in permanent teeth. However, if present, this causes some difficulty in creating an effective etching pattern and may require roughening of the surface or additional etching treatments. The outer surface of the enamel is of great clinical significance because it is the surface subjected to daily wear and undergoes repeated cycles of demineralization and remineralization. As a result of these cycles, the composition of the enamel crystals may change, for example, as a result of exposure to fluoride. Thus the properties of the enamel might be expected

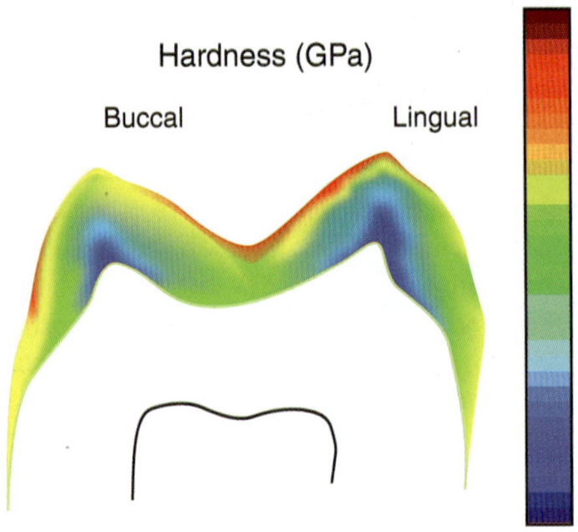

• **Fig. 2.4** Nanoindentation mapping of the mechanical properties of human molar tooth enamel. (From Cuy JL, Mann AB, Livi KJ, et al. Nanoindentation mapping of the mechanical properties of human molar tooth enamel. *Arch Oral Biol*. 2002;47(4):281–291.)

to vary from the external to the internal surface. Such variations, including a thin surface veneer of fluoride-rich apatite crystals, create differences in the enamel properties within the enamel. Enamel is usually harder at the occlusal and cuspal areas and less hard nearer the DEJ. Fig. 2.4 shows an example of the difference in hardness.

The Mineral

The mineral of all calcified tissues is a highly defective relative of the mineral hydroxyapatite (HA). The biological apatites of calcified tissues are different from the ideal HA structure in that the defects and chemical substitutions generally make them weaker and more soluble in acids. HA has the simple formula $Ca_{10}(PO_4)_6(OH)_2$, with an ideal molar ratio of calcium to phosphorus (Ca/P) of 1.67 and a hexagonal crystal structure. The apatite of enamel and dentin has a much more variable composition that depends on its formative history and other chemical exposures during maturity. Thus the mineral in enamel and dentin is a calcium-deficient, carbonate-rich, and highly substituted form related to HA. Metal ions such as magnesium (Mg) and sodium (Na) may substitute for calcium, whereas carbonate substitutes for the phosphate and hydroxyl groups. These substitutions distort the structure and make it more soluble. Perhaps the most beneficial substitution is the fluorine (F) ion, which substitutes for the hydroxyl group (OH) in the formula and makes the structure stronger and less soluble. Complete substitution of F for (OH) in HA yields fluorapatite mineral, $Ca_{10}(PO_4)_6(F)_2$, which is much less soluble than HA or the defective apatite of calcified tissues. It is worth noting that HA has attracted considerable attention as an implantable calcified tissue replacement. It has the advantage of being a purified and stronger form of the natural mineral and releases no harmful agents during biological degradation. Its major shortcoming is that it is extremely brittle and sensitive to porosity or defects, and therefore it fractures easily in load-bearing applications.

The approximate carbonate contents of the enamel and dentin apatites are significantly different, about 3% and 5% carbonate, respectively. In addition, the dentin apatite crystals are much smaller than the enamel crystals. This means that the dentin crystals present a higher surface area for attacking acids, and contain many more defects per unit volume, and thus exhibit considerably higher solubility than enamel crystals. Finally, as discussed further in the following section, the dentin mineral occupies only about 50% of the dentin structure, so there is not as much apatite in the dentin as there is in the enamel. All of these factors multiply the susceptibility of dentin to acid attack and provide insight into the rapid spread of caries when it penetrates the DEJ.

Dentin

Dentin is a complex, hydrated biological composite structure that forms the bulk of the tooth. Furthermore, dentin is modified by physiological, aging, and disease processes that result in different forms of dentin. These altered forms of dentin may be the precise forms that are most important in restorative dentistry. Some of the recognized variations include primary, secondary, reparative or tertiary, sclerotic, transparent, carious, demineralized, remineralized, and hypermineralized. These terms reflect alterations in the fundamental components of the structure as defined by changes in their arrangement, interrelationships, or chemistry. A number of these may have important implications for our ability to develop long-lasting adhesion or bonds to dentin.

Primary dentin is formed during tooth development. Its volume and conformation, reflecting tooth form, vary with the size and shape of the tooth. Dentin is composed of about 50 volume percent (vol%) carbonate-rich, calcium-deficient apatite; 30 vol% organic matter, which is largely type I collagen; and about 20 vol% fluid, which is similar to plasma. Other noncollagenous proteins are thought to be involved in dentin mineralization and other functions, such as controlling crystallite size and orientation. The role of noncollagenous proteins in biomineralization, or simpler molecules that can mimic some of their functions, may lead to dentin remineralization methods, and is the subject of ongoing research efforts. The major components are distributed into distinctive morphological features to form a vital and complex hydrated composite in which the morphology varies with location and undergoes alterations with age or disease. The tubules, one distinct and important feature of dentin, represent the tracks taken by the odontoblastic cells from the DEJ or cementum at the root to the pulp chamber and appear as tunnels piercing the dentin structure (Fig. 2.5). The tubules converge on

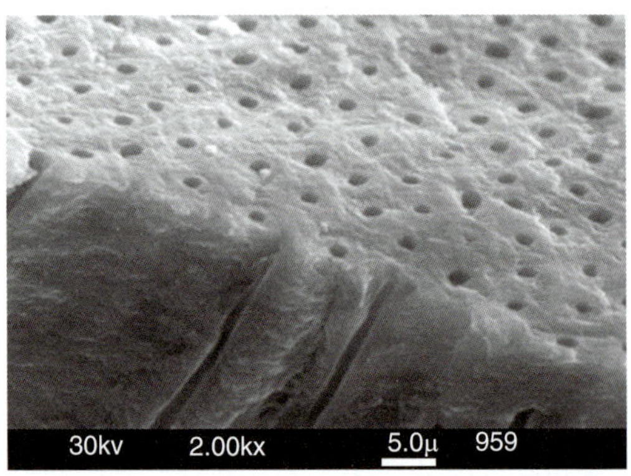

• **Fig. 2.5** Scanning electron microscopy image of normal dentin showing its unique structure as seen from two directions. At the *top* is a view of the tubules, each of which is surrounded by peritubular dentin. Tubules lie between the dentin–enamel junction and converge on the pulp chamber. The perpendicular surface at the bottom shows a fracture surface revealing some of the tubules as they form tunnel-like pathways toward the pulp. The tubule lumen normally contains fluid and processes of the odontoblastic cells. (From Marshall GW. Dentin: microstructure and characterization. *Quintessence Int*. 1993;24:606–617.)

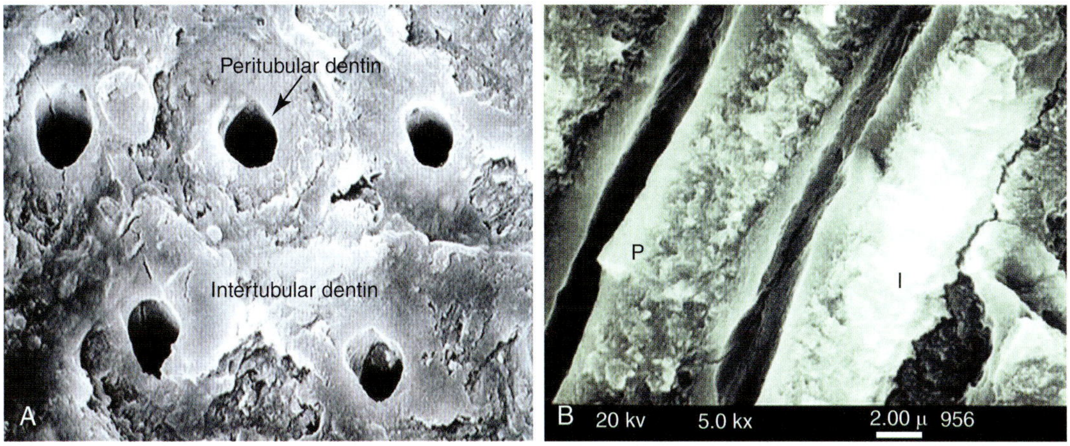

• **Fig. 2.6** Fracture surface of the dentin. (A) Viewed from the occlusal direction. (B) Viewed longitudinally. Peritubular (*P*; also called *intratubular*) dentin forms a cuff or lining around each tubule. The tubules are separated by intertubular dentin *(I)*. (Courtesy G.W. Marshall.)

the pulp chamber, and therefore tubule density and orientation vary from location to location (see Fig. 2.1). Tubule number density is lowest at the DEJ and highest at the predentin surface at the junction to the pulp chamber, where the odontoblastic cell bodies lie in a closely packed array. Lower tubule densities are found in the root. The contents of the tubules include odontoblast processes as well as fluid. The extent of the odontoblast process is still uncertain, but evidence is mounting that it extends all the way to the DEJ. For most of its course, the tubule lumen is lined by a highly mineralized cuff of peritubular dentin approximately 0.5 to 1 μm thick (Fig. 2.6). Because the peritubular dentin forms after the tubule lumen has formed, some argue that it may be more properly termed *intratubular dentin*, and it contains mostly apatite crystals with little organic matrix. A number of studies have concluded that the peritubular dentin does not contain collagen, and therefore might be considered a separate calcified tissue. The tubules are separated by intertubular dentin composed of a matrix of type I collagen reinforced by apatite (see Figs. 2.5 and 2.6). This arrangement means that the amount of intertubular dentin varies with location. The apatite crystals are much smaller (approximately 5 × 30 × 100 nm) than the apatite found in enamel and contain about 5% carbonate. The small crystallite size, heterogeneous structure, and higher carbonate content lead to the greater dissolution susceptibility, as described earlier.

Estimates of the size of tubules, the thickness of the peritubular region, and the amount of intertubular dentin have been reported in a number of studies. Calculations for occlusal dentin as a function of position from these data show that the percentage tubule area and diameter vary from about 22% and 2.5 μm near the pulp to 1% and 0.8 μm at the DEJ, respectively. Intertubular matrix area varies from 12% at the predentin to 96% near the DEJ, whereas peritubular dentin ranges from over 60% down to 3% at the DEJ. Tubule densities are compared in Table 2.1 based on work by various investigators. It is clear that the structural components will vary considerably over their course and necessarily result in location-dependent variations in morphology, distribution of the structural elements, and other important properties, such as permeability, moisture content, and available surface area for bonding. They may also affect bond strength, hardness, and other properties.

Because the odontoblasts come to rest just inside the dentin and line the walls of the pulp chamber after tooth formation, the dentin–pulp complex can be considered a vital tissue. This is different from mature enamel, which is acellular. Over time, secondary dentin forms, and the pulp chamber gradually becomes smaller. The border between primary and secondary dentin is usually marked by a change in orientation of the dentin tubules. Furthermore, the odontoblasts react to form tertiary dentin in response to insults, such as caries or tooth preparation, and this form of dentin is often less well organized than the primary or secondary dentin.

TABLE 2.1 Comparison of Mean Numerical Density of Tubules in Occlusal Dentin

Outer Dentin	Middle Dentin	Inner Dentin
15,000/mm^2	35,000/mm^2	65,000/mm^2
20,000/mm^2	35,000/mm^2	43,000/mm^2
24,500/mm^2	40,400/mm^2	51,100/mm^2
18,000/mm^2	39,000/mm^2	52,000/mm^2

From data reported in Marshall GW. Dentin: microstructure and characterization. *Quintessence Int.* 1993;24:606–617.

Early enamel carious lesions may be reversed by remineralization treatments. However, effective remineralization treatments are not yet available for dentin, and therefore the current standard of care dictates surgical intervention to remove highly damaged tissue with subsequent restoration as needed. Thus it is important to understand altered forms of dentin and the effects of such clinical interventions.

When dentin is cut or abraded by dental instruments, a smear layer develops and covers the surface, obscuring the underlying structure (Fig. 2.7). The bur cutting marks are shown in Fig. 2.7A and at higher magnification in Fig. 2.7B. Fig. 2.7C shows the smear layer thickness from the side and the development of smear plugs as the cut dentin debris is pushed into the dentin tubule lumen. The advantages and disadvantages of the smear layer have been extensively discussed for several decades. It reduces permeability and therefore aids in maintaining a drier field, and it reduces infiltration of noxious agents into the tubules and perhaps the pulp. However, it is now generally accepted that it is a hindrance to dentin bonding procedures and therefore is normally removed or modified by some form of acid conditioning.

Acid etching or conditioning allows for the removal of the smear layer and alteration of the superficial dentin, opening

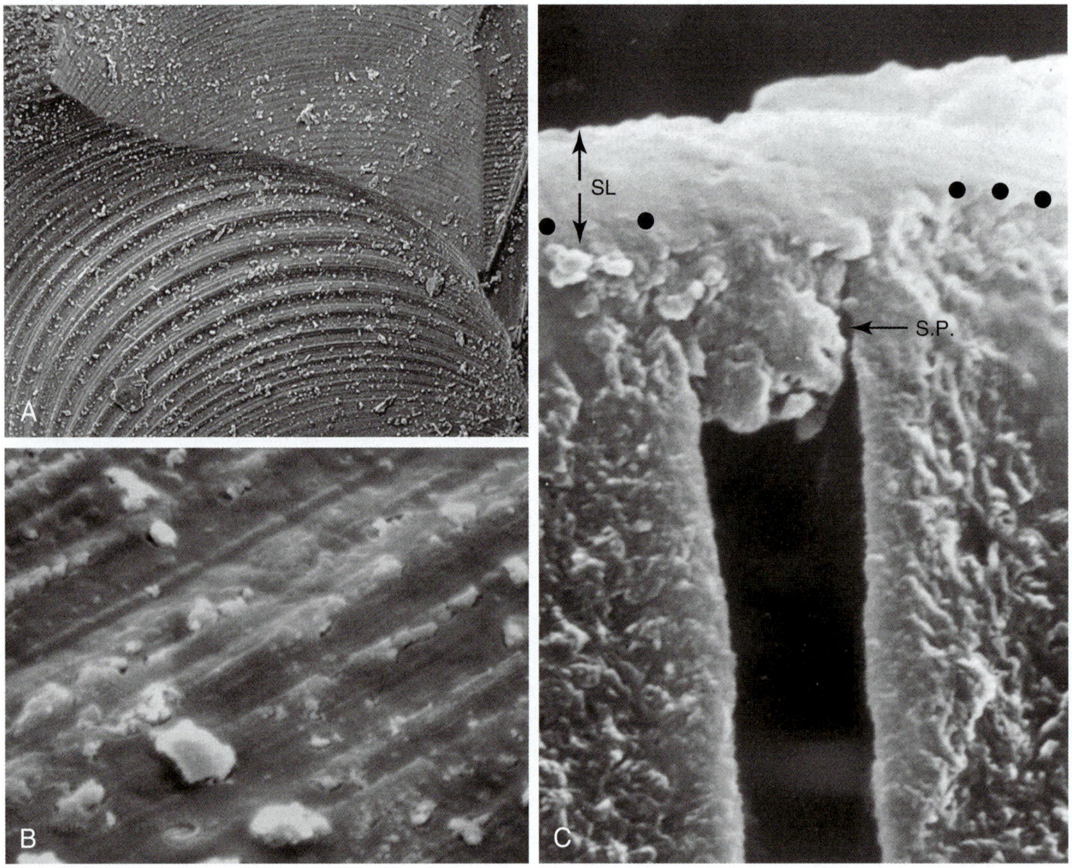

• **Fig. 2.7** Smear layer formation. (A) Bur marks on dentin preparation. (B) Higher magnification showing smear layer surface and cutting debris. (C) Section showing smear layer *(SL)* and smear plugs *(SP)*. (A and B, from Marshall GW, Marshall SJ, Bayne SC. Restorative dental materials: scanning electron microscopy and x-ray microanalysis. *Scanning Microsc*. 1988;2:2007–2028; C, from Pashley DH, Tao L, Boyd L, et al. Scanning electron microscopy of the substructure of smear layers in human dentine. *Arch Oral Biol*. 1988;33(4):265–270.)

channels for infiltration by bonding agents. Fig. 2.8 shows what happens in such an etching treatment. The tubule lumens widen as the peritubular dentin is preferentially removed because it is mostly mineral with sparse protein. The widened lumens form a funnel shape that is not very retentive.

Fig. 2.9 shows these effects in a slightly different way. Unetched dentin in Fig. 2.9A *(top)* has small tubules and peritubular dentin, which is removed from the treated dentin at the exposed surface after etching *(bottom)*. The two-dimensional network of collagen type I fibers is shown after treatment in Fig. 2.9A. Fig. 2.9B shows progressive demineralization of a dentin collagen fibril in which the external minerals and proteins are slowly removed to reveal the typical banded pattern of type I collagen. In Fig. 2.9C, this pattern is seen at high magnification of the treated dentin shown in Fig. 2.9A.

If the demineralized dentin is dried, the remaining dentin matrix shrinks, and the collagen fibrils become matted and difficult to penetrate by the liquid bonding agents used in restorative procedures. This is shown in Fig. 2.10, which compares demineralized and dried dentin with demineralized and hydrated dentin.

Most restorative procedures involve dentin that has been altered in some way. Common alterations include formation of carious lesions that form various zones and include transparent dentin that forms under the caries-infected dentin layer. Transparent dentin results when the dentin tubules become filled with minerals, which changes the refractive index of the tubules and produces a translucent or transparent zone.

Fig. 2.11 shows a section through a tooth with a carious lesion, which has been stained to reveal its zones. The gray zone under the stained and severely demineralized dentin is the transparent layer (Fig. 2.11A). Fig. 2.11B shows the transparent dentin in which most of the tubule lumens are filled with minerals. After etching, as shown in Fig. 2.11C, the peritubular dentin is etched away, but the tubules retain plugs of the precipitated mineral, which is more resistant to etching. This resistance to etching makes bonding more difficult.

Several other forms of transparent dentin are formed as a result of different processes. A second form of transparent dentin results from bruxism. An additional form of transparent dentin results from aging as the root dentin gradually becomes transparent. In addition, noncarious cervical lesions, often called *abfraction* or *notch* lesions, form at the enamel–cementum or enamel–dentin junction, usually on facial or buccal surfaces. Their etiology is not clear at this point; their formation has been attributed to abrasion, tooth flexure, and erosion, and most likely some combination of these processes. Nonetheless, these lesions occur with increasing frequency with age, and the exposed dentin becomes transparent as the tubules are filled. Fig. 2.12 shows examples of transparent dentin in which the tubule lumens are completely filled.

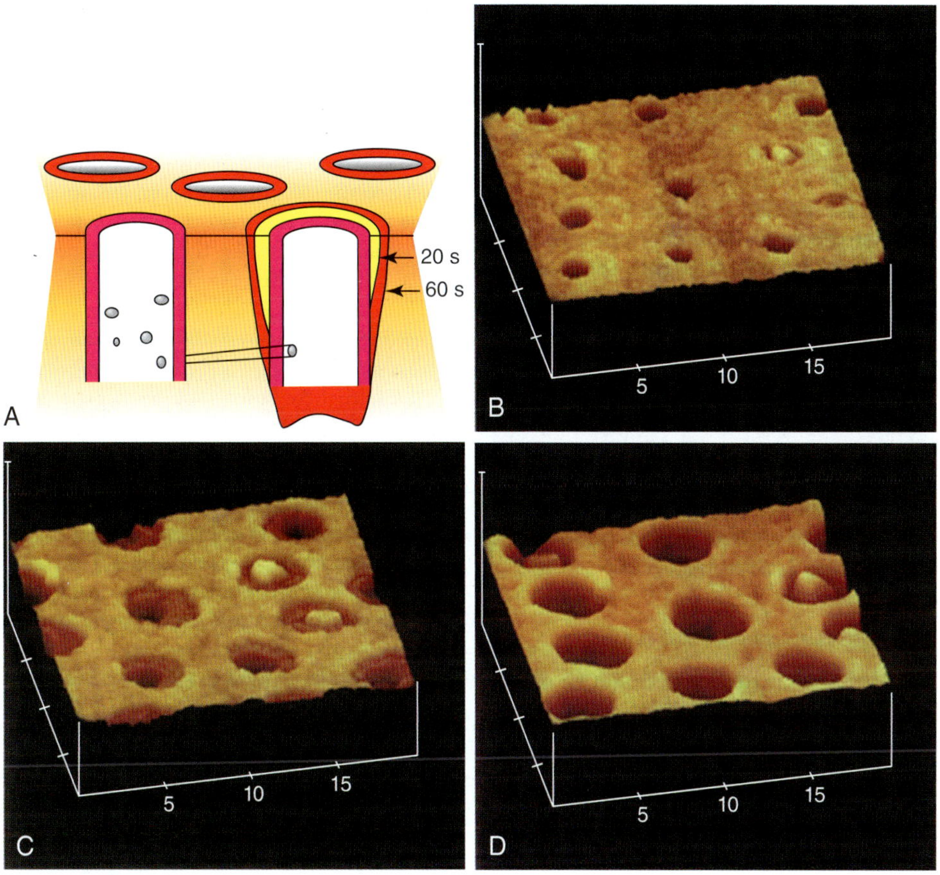

• **Fig. 2.8** Stages of dentin demineralization. (A) Schematic showing progressive stages of dentin demineralization. (B–D) Atomic force microscopy images showing stages of etching. The etching leads to wider lumens once the peritubular dentin is dissolved and funnel-shaped openings are formed. (B–D, from Marshall GW. Dentin: microstructure and characterization. *Quintessence Int*. 1993;24:606–617.)

The properties of the transparent dentin may differ from one to another depending on the processes that lead to the deposit of the mineral in the tubules. Several studies have shown that elastic properties of the intertubular dentin are not altered by aging, although the structure may become more susceptible to fracture. Similarly, arrested caries will contain transparent dentin, which has often been called *sclerotic dentin*, a term that implies it may be harder than normal dentin. However, other studies have shown that the elastic properties of the intertubular dentin may actually be unaltered or lower than normal dentin.

Physical and Mechanical Properties

The marked variations in the structural elements of dentin when located within the tooth imply that the properties of dentin will vary considerably with location. That is, variable structure leads to variable properties.

Because one major function of tooth structure is to resist deformation without fracture, it is useful to have knowledge of the forces that are experienced by teeth during mastication. Measurements have given values on cusp tips of about 77 kg distributed over the cusp tip area of 0.039 cm^2, suggesting a stress of about 200 MPa.

Difficulties in Testing

In Table 2.2, values are presented for some important properties of enamel and dentin. The wide spread of values reported in the literature is remarkable. Some of the reasons for these discrepancies should be appreciated and considered in practice or when reading the literature.

First, human teeth are small, which can create difficulties in obtaining and holding specimens for standard mechanical tests, such as tensile, compressive, or shear tests. When testing bonded teeth, the problem is even more complicated, and special tests have been developed to obtain insights into these properties. From the previous discussion of structural variations, it is also evident that testing such small heterogeneous specimens can lead to high variability.

Another problem is the great variation in structure in both tissues. Enamel prisms are aligned generally perpendicular to the DEJ, whereas dentin tubules change their number density with depth as they course toward the pulp chamber. Consequently, it can be challenging to prepare a uniform sample for testing with the structures running all in one direction. In addition, properties generally vary with direction and location, and the material is not isotropic; therefore a single value can only reveal an average value for the material at best.

Storage and time elapsed since extraction are also important considerations. Properties that exist in situ are of greatest interest. Clearly, this condition is almost impossible to achieve in most routine testing, so changes that have occurred as a result of storage conditions prior to testing must be considered. It is also important to consider biological hazards because extracted teeth must be treated as potentially infectious. How does one sterilize the teeth

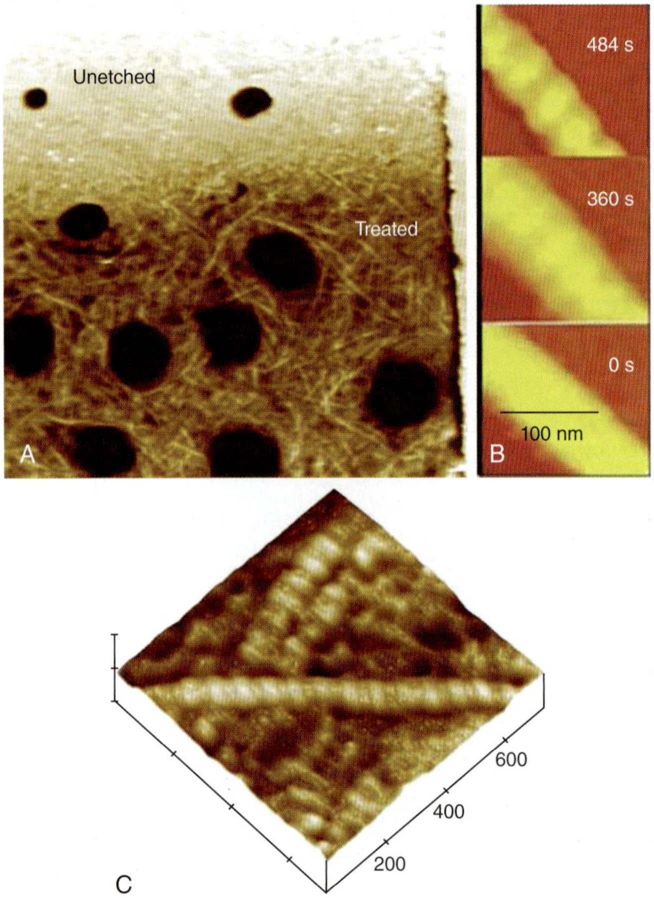

• **Fig. 2.9** Etching of dentin removes mineral from the intertubular dentin matrix leaving a collagen-rich layer and widening the dentin tubule orifices. (A) After etching, the tubule lumens are enlarged and the collagen network surrounding the tubules can be seen after further treatment. (B) Isolated dentin collagen fiber is slowly demineralized revealing the typical 67-nm repeat pattern of type I collagen. (C) High-magnification view of collagen fibers is shown in (A). (A and C, from Marshall GW, Yucel N, Balooch M, et al. Sodium hypochlorite alterations of dentin and dentin collagen. *Surf Sci*. 2001;491:444–455; B, modified from Balooch M, Habelitz S, Kinney JH, et al. Mechanical properties of mineralized collagen fibrils as influenced by demineralization. *J Struct Biol*. 2008;162:404–410.)

without altering their properties? The high heat used in autoclaving undoubtedly denatures proteins within teeth and is therefore highly inappropriate for dentin. It might impact enamel as well.

Finally, the fluid content of these tissues must be considered. Moisture is a vital component of both tissues and in vivo conditions cannot be replicated if the tissues have been desiccated (see Fig. 2.10). This becomes a critically important consideration when bonding to these tissues, as is discussed further in Chapter 7. In contrast to the importance of this issue, there is the issue of convenience. It is much more difficult to test the tissues in a fully hydrated condition than in a dry condition. All of these factors and a number of others, such as testing temperature, will influence the results and contribute to a spread in the values reported for the measured properties.

Despite these limitations, some generalizations about the properties of these tissues are useful (see Table 2.1). Root dentin is generally weaker and softer than coronal dentin. Enamel also appears to vary in its properties, with cuspal enamel being stronger and harder than other areas, presumably as an adaptation to masticatory forces. Dentin is less stiff than enamel (i.e., it has a lower elastic modulus) but has higher fracture toughness. This may be counterintuitive, but it will become clearer when these terms are defined in Chapter 4. In addition, dentin is viscoelastic, meaning its mechanical deformation characteristics are time dependent, and its elastic recovery is not instantaneous. Thus dentin may be sensitive to how rapidly it is deformed or strained, a phenomenon called *strain rate sensitivity*. Strain rate sensitivity is characteristic of polymeric materials; the collagen matrix imparts this property to tissues such as dentin. Under normal circumstances, ceramic materials do not exhibit this characteristic in their mechanical properties and are typically stiff, brittle, and fracture elastically (i.e., without permanent deformation). Pure HA shows this typical brittle characteristic, but when formed in enamel, it exhibits greater toughness (see Chapter 4), though it remains slightly less tough than dentin. This higher toughness of enamel versus pure HA is associated with the microstructure and the small protein component of enamel.

The Dentin–Enamel Junction

The DEJ is much more than the boundary between enamel and dentin. Because enamel is very hard and dentin is softer but

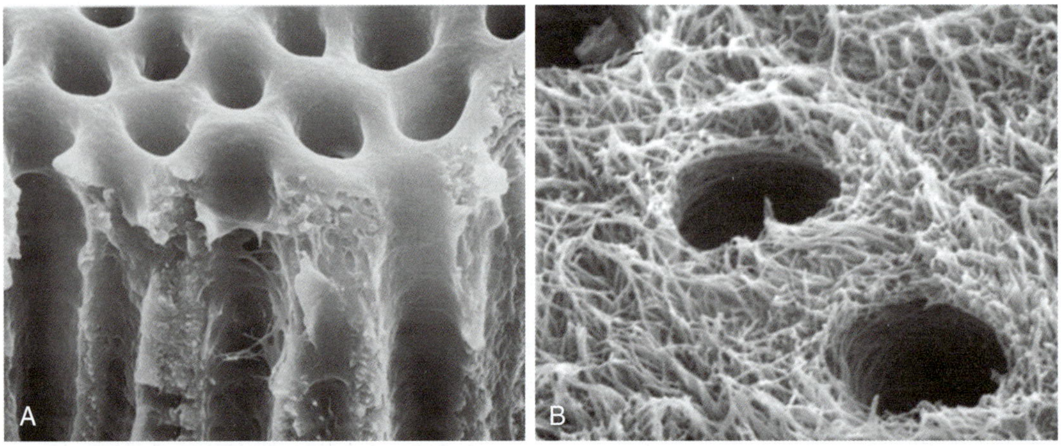

• **Fig. 2.10** Demineralized dentin is sensitive to moisture and shrinks on drying. (A) Demineralized dentin undergoes shrinkage when air dried, forming a collapsed layer of collagen that is difficult to infiltrate with resin-bonding agents. (B) When kept moist, the collagen network is open and can be penetrated by bonding agents. (From Marshall GW, Marshall SJ, Kinney JH, et al. The dentin substrate: structure and properties related to bonding. *J Dent*. 1997;25:441–458.)

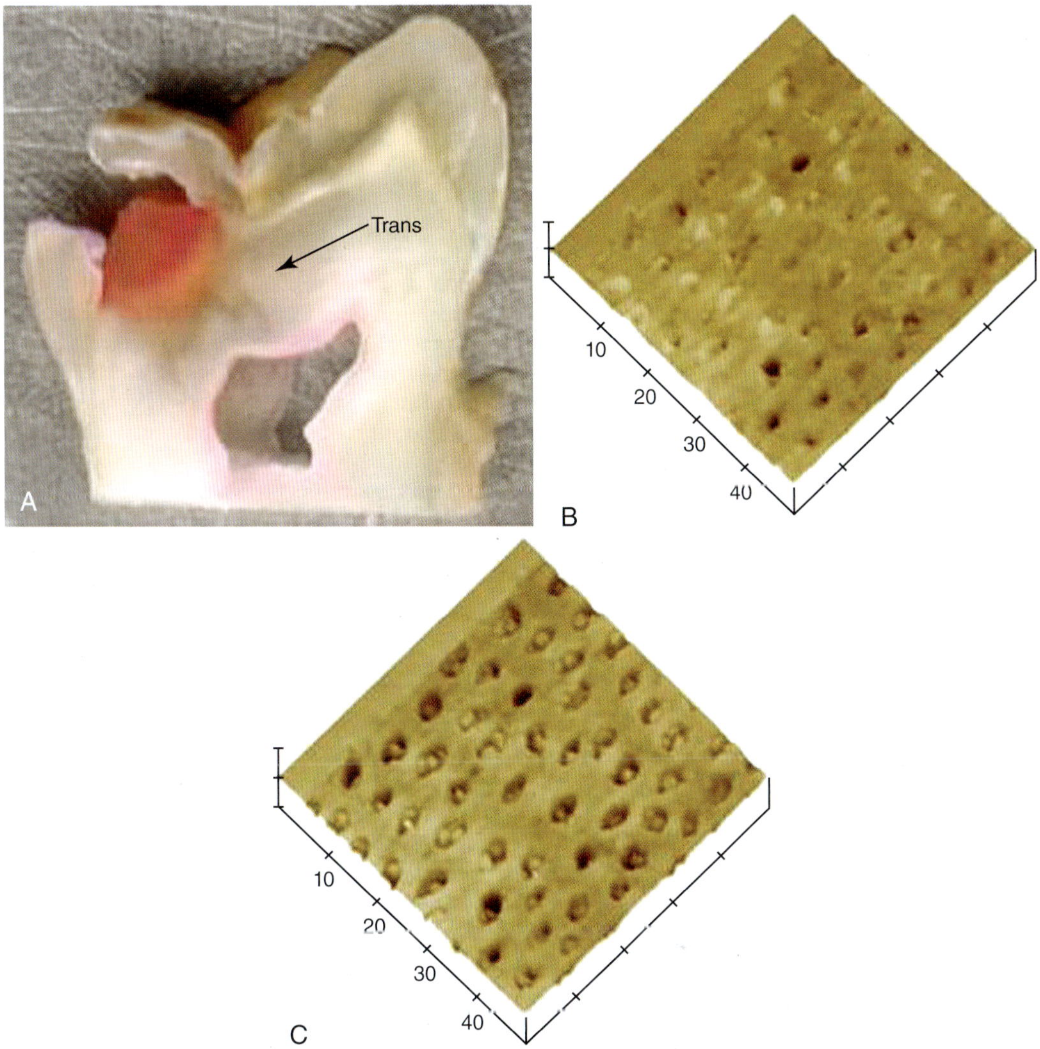

• **Fig. 2.11** Transparent dentin associated with carious lesions. (A) Carious lesion showing dentin carious zones revealed by staining, including the grayish transparent zone. (B) Atomic force microscopy of carious transparent dentin before etching. (C) After etching, the tubule lumens remain filled even as the peritubular dentin is etched away. (A, from Zheng L, Hilton JF, Habelitz S, et al. Dentin caries activity status related to hardness and elasticity. *Eur J Oral Sci*. 2003;111(3):243–252; B and C, from Marshall GW, Chang JY, Gansky SA, et al. Demineralization of caries-affected transparent dentin by citric acid: an atomic force microscopy study. *Dent Mater*. 2001;17:45–52.)

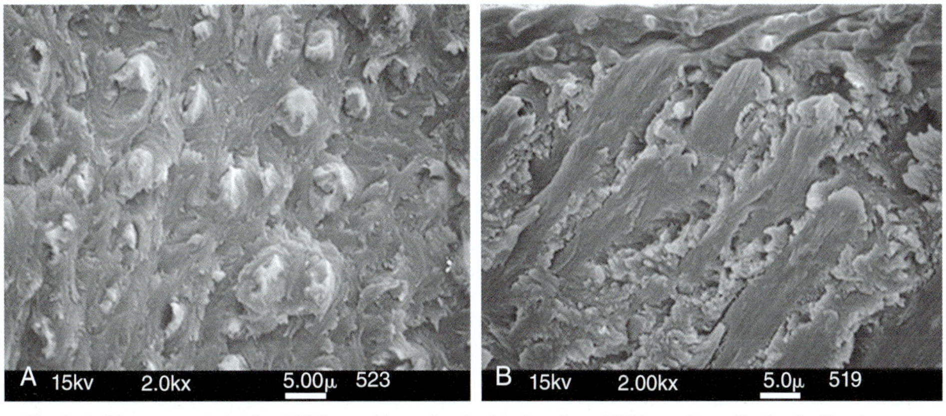

• **Fig. 2.12** Transparent dentin. (A) Viewed from the facial direction. (B) Viewed longitudinally. The transparent dentin results from filling of the tubules with mineral deposits that alter the optical properties of the tooth. (Courtesy G.W. Marshall.)

TABLE 2.2 Properties of Enamel and Dentin

Property	Enamel	Dentin
Density (g/cm^3)	2.96	2.1
Compressive		
Modulus of elasticity (GPa)	60–120	18–24
Proportional limit (MPa)	70–353	100–190
Strength (MPa)	94–450	230–370
Tensile		
Modulus of elasticity (GPa)		11–19
Strength (MPa)	8–35	30–65
Shear strength (MPa)	90	138
Flexural strength (MPa)	60–90	245–280
Hardness (GPa)	3–6	0.13–0.51

tougher, they need to be joined together to provide a biomechanically compatible system. Joining such dissimilar materials is a challenge, and it is not completely clear how nature has accomplished this. However, the DEJ not only joins these two tissues but also appears to resist cracks in the enamel from penetrating into dentin, cracks that would lead to tooth fracture, as shown in Fig. 2.13A. Many such cracks exist in the enamel but do not seem to propagate into the dentin. If the DEJ is intact, it is unusual to have tooth fracture, except in response to severe trauma. In Fig. 2.13B, microhardness indentations have been placed to drive cracks toward the DEJ *(orange)*. The crack stops at or just beyond the interface. This image also shows that the DEJ is scalloped, with its concavity directed toward the enamel. This means that most cracks approach the DEJ at an angle, and this may lead to the arrest of many of the cracks. The scalloped structure actually has three levels: scallops, microscallops within the scallops, and a finer structure. Fig. 2.13C–D shows images of larger scallops in molars (~24 µm across) and smaller scallops (~15 µm across) in anterior teeth after the removal of the enamel. Mathematical (finite element) models suggest that the scallops reduce stress concentrations at the interface, but it is not known whether the larger scallop size in posterior teeth is an adaptation to higher masticatory loads or a developmental variation. In Fig. 2.13E, the crystals of dentin are almost in contact with those of the enamel, so that the anatomical DEJ is said to be optically thin. However, measurements of property variations across the DEJ show that this is a graded interface with properties varying from those of the enamel to the adjacent mantle dentin over a considerable distance. This gradient, which is due in part to the scalloped nature of the DEJ, makes the functional width of the DEJ much larger than its anatomical appearance and further reduces stresses. In addition, although collagen is generally absent from enamel, collagen fibers cross the DEJ from dentin into enamel to further integrate the two tissues. Recent work suggests that other proteins that could be remnants of the basement membrane at the DEJ may include collagen types IV and VII and perhaps other proteins that could help stabilize the DEJ structure and contribute to its fracture resistance.

The enamel, dentin, and DEJ are highly complex structures that have varied physical and chemical properties. Their ability to work together to resist mechanical forces is critical for the survival of the tooth. In addition, they are constantly exposed to chemical insults within the oral environment. The main concern for teeth is their exposure to acids, including those present within imbibed foods and drinks, but especially from organic acids produced by the resident oral microbiome. Under certain conditions, the oral microbiota can form destructive biofilms that promote extensive demineralization of otherwise sound tooth structure, ultimately leading to caries lesions that require surgical interventions with dental restorative materials.

Oral Biofilms and Oral Health

Biofilms are complex, surface-adherent, spatially organized microbial communities encased within a hydrated matrix composed primarily of polysaccharides and extracellular DNA (eDNA), as well as various proteins and lipids. The biofilm matrix is typically referred to as extracellular polymeric substance (EPS). Oral biofilms that form on the surfaces of teeth and restorative biomaterials are also known as *dental plaque*. The microbes found within oral biofilms are directly derived from the oral microbiome, which includes both oral biofilm species as well as numerous additional organisms that normally reside on various mucosal surfaces of the oral cavity. The human oral microbiome is primarily composed of a diverse collection of bacterial species, but it is worth noting that fungi, protozoans, and viruses are all typically found in the oral microbiome as well. The overall microbial diversity in the oral cavity is second only to that in the human colon, with >700 different oral microbial species possible, making the oral cavity one of the most ecologically diverse environments of the entire human mucosa. The microbial communities present within dental plaque are highly dynamic, being subject to major compositional changes in response to both host genetics and behaviors. In oral health, the oral biofilm is primarily composed of commensal organisms that exhibit low pathogenic potential. Such a biofilm is sometimes referred to as eubiotic. In contrast, an oral biofilm enriched for pathogenic species is referred to as dysbiotic. The two most common dysbiotic oral diseases are caries and periodontitis. When the human diet is rich in fermentable carbohydrates, this can lead to the development of a dysbiotic oral biofilm containing an overabundance of cariogenic organisms (capable of producing or promoting caries). Such organisms tend to be both acidogenic (acid-producing) and aciduric (acid-tolerant) and can be found among certain species of *Streptococcus*, *Lactobacillus*, and even fungal *Candida* species. In addition, long-term oral biofilm accumulation can lead to mucosal inflammation and trigger a dysbiotic remodeling of oral biofilm ecology to favor the growth of highly inflammatory, tissue-invasive, proteolytic species associated with periodontal disease and periimplantitis (inflammation of the soft and hard tissues surrounding an implant). Dysbiotic diseases of the oral cavity exhibit a polymicrobial etiology, meaning there are no specific pathogens singularly responsible for diseases like caries and periodontitis; rather, disease results from the development of pathogenic synergistic *communities* containing multiple organisms. Thus oral disease susceptibility is a direct reflection of the underlying microbial ecology in the oral cavity.

Early Oral Biofilm Development on Enamel

Oral biofilm formation on tooth surfaces occurs through a highly reproducible and sequential process. The first step begins with the formation of a proteinaceous conditioning film on the tooth surface known as the salivary pellicle (also referred to as the acquired enamel pellicle). The salivary pellicle contains a diverse assortment of adsorbed phosphoproteins and glycoproteins derived from saliva, as well as adsorbed bacterial proteins derived from the oral

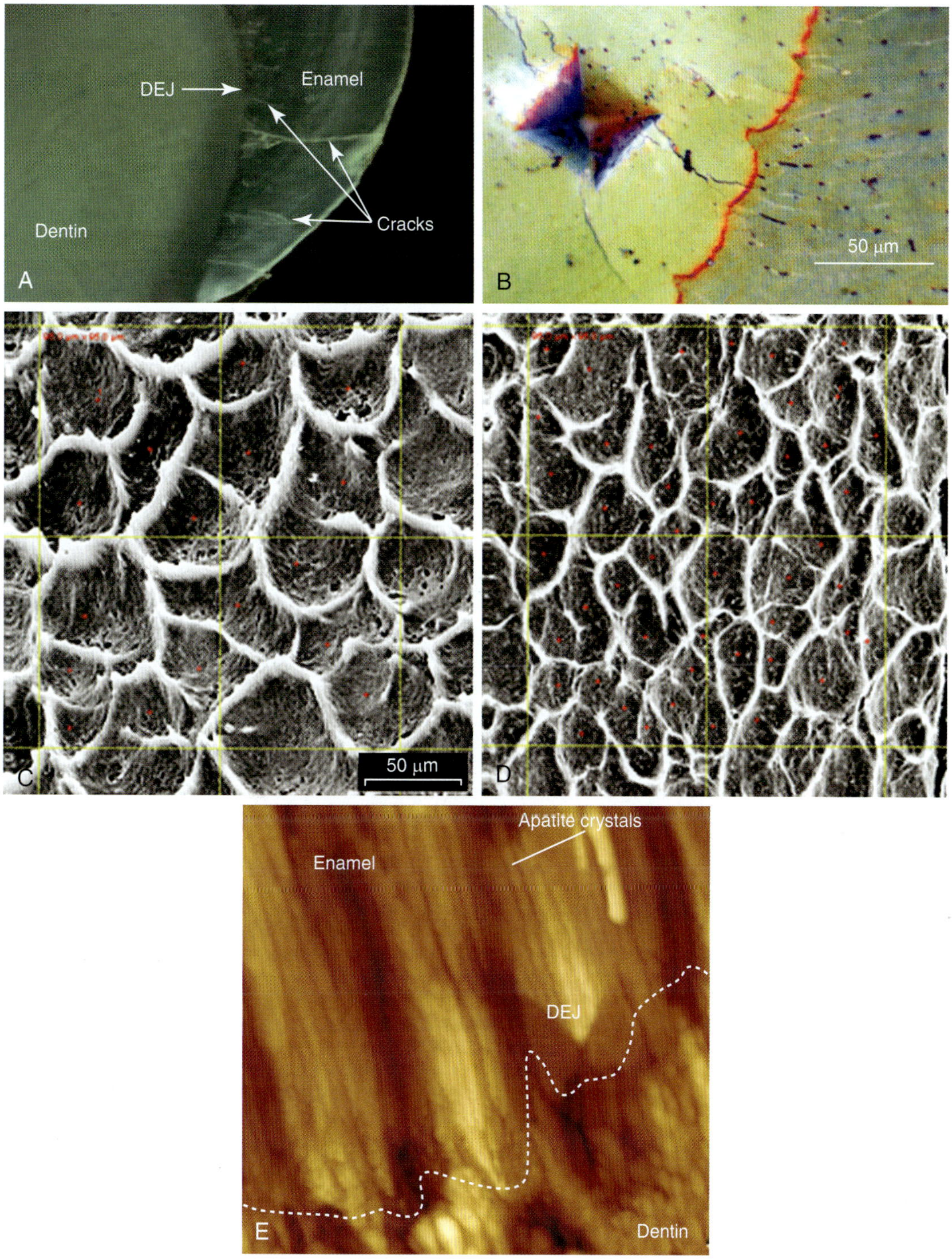

• **Fig. 2.13** Cracks in enamel appear to stop at the dentin–enamel junction (DEJ). (A) Low-magnification view of cracks in enamel. (B) Indentation-generated cracks stop near or at the scalloped DEJ *(orange)*. (C) Large scallops in molars. (D) Smaller scallops in anterior teeth. (E) Crystals of the enamel are nearly in contact with dentin crystals at the DEJ forming an optically thin, but functionally wide union. (A, C–E, from Marshall SJ, Balooch M, Habelitz S, et al. The dentin-enamel junction—a natural, multilevel interface. *J Eur Ceram Soc*. 2003;23:2897–2904; B, from Imbeni V, Kruzic JJ, Marshall GW, et al. The dentin-enamel junction and the fracture of human teeth. *Nat Mater*. 2005;4:229–232.)

microbiome. Salivary pellicle formation on the teeth occurs rapidly and spontaneously as a consequence of saliva exposure. The pellicle layer is normally stably attached to the teeth and generally survives tooth brushing but can be removed during professional cleaning. However, it reforms within minutes upon saliva exposure. The pellicle layer is quite thin, typically ranging from hundreds of nanometers to about 1 μm in thickness. The proper formation of a salivary pellicle is critical for maintaining the integrity of teeth as both a lubricating layer protecting from mastication-induced tooth wear as well as a mediator of tooth remineralization. The

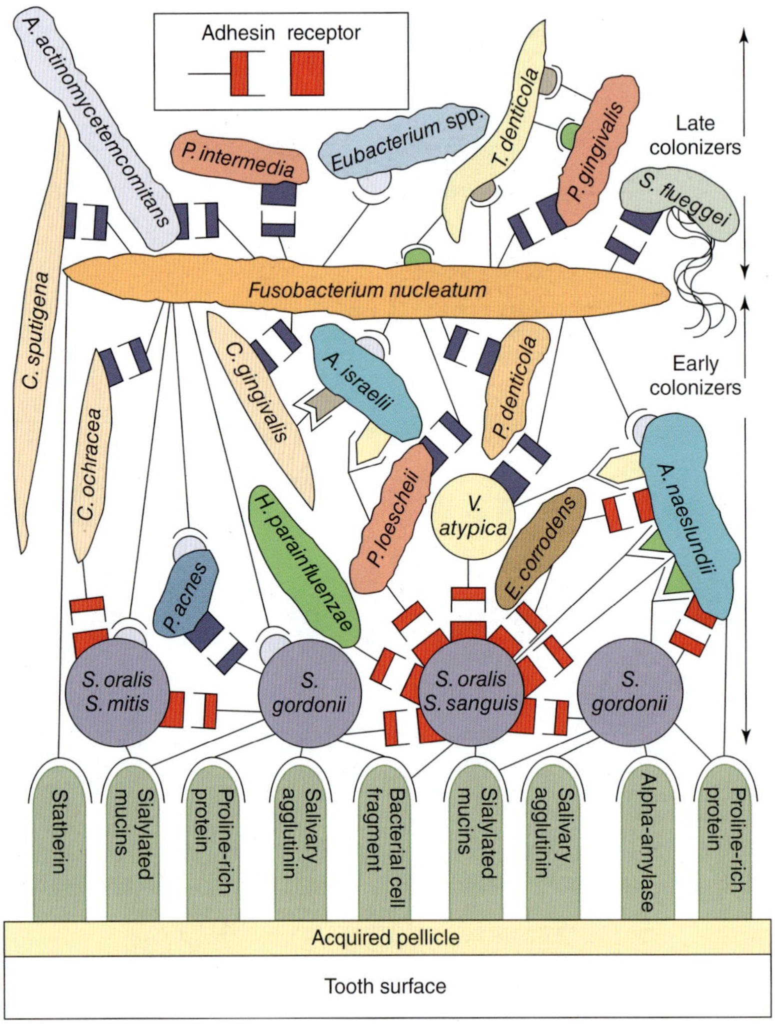

• **Fig. 2.14** Spatiotemporal model of oral bacterial colonization, showing recognition of salivary pellicle receptors by early colonizing bacteria and coaggregations between early colonizers, fusobacteria, and late colonizers of the tooth surface. Starting at the bottom, primary colonizers bind via adhesins *(round-tipped black line symbols)* to complementary receptors *(blue-green vertical round-topped columns)* in the salivary pellicle coating the tooth surface. Secondary colonizers bind to previously bound bacteria. Sequential binding results in the appearance of nascent surfaces that bridge with the next coaggregating partner cell. The bacterial strains shown are *Aggregatibacter actinomycetemcomitans, Actinomyces israelii, Actinomyces naeslundii, Capnocytophaga gingivalis, Capnocytophaga ochracea, Capnocytophaga sputigena, Eikenella corrodens, Eubacterium* spp., *Fusobacterium nucleatum, Haemophilus parainfluenzae, Porphyromonas gingivalis, Prevotella denticola, Prevotella intermedia, Prevotella loescheii, Propionibacterium acnes, Selenomonas flueggei, Streptococcus gordonii, Streptococcus mitis, Streptococcus oralis, Streptococcus sanguinis, Treponema* spp., and *Veillonella atypica*. (From Kolenbrander PE, Andersen RN, Blehert DS, et al. Communication among oral bacteria. *Microbiol Mol Biol Rev*. 2002;66(3):486–505.)

salivary pellicle also serves as the initial attachment substrate during oral biofilm development. A distinct subset of species from the oral microbiome produces cell surface receptors that bind to different proteins found in the salivary pellicle, allowing free-floating (planktonic) organisms to attach to uncolonized sites and initiate biofilm formation. These "pioneer colonizers" primarily comprise oral *Streptococcus* species and, to a lesser extent, *Actinomyces* (Fig. 2.14). The ability to bind to nonshedding surfaces, such as enamel, gives oral streptococci a tremendous colonization advantage over most other microbiome species. This also explains observations from clinical studies that have revealed streptococci to constitute 60% to 90% of the initial bacterial flora found on newly colonized enamel. Subsequent growth and cell division of the pellicle-attached organisms yield microcolonies that begin producing biofilm EPS to protect and house the developing community. Because the pioneer colonizers are almost exclusively oxygen-tolerant facultative anaerobes, their metabolic activity within the biofilm community eventually depletes the local oxygen concentration, subsequently creating an increasingly anaerobic environment within the developing biofilm that supports the growth of later colonizing obligate anaerobic species, including those often associated with gingivitis and periodontitis.

Oral Biofilm Maturation

Interactions among human oral bacteria are pivotal for the maturation and ecological diversification of developing oral biofilm communities. Of particular importance are genetically encoded coaggregation interactions (receptor/ligand-mediated adherence between genetically distinct cell types), which allow many later colonizing organisms to join the established biofilm communities initiated by the pioneer colonizers (see Fig. 2.14). In the first 4 hours of biofilm formation, Gram-positive cocci from the Mitis group of streptococci predominate. Even after 8 hours of growth, the majority of the bacterial population remains largely coccoid, but the appearance of rod-shaped organisms can also be observed. By 24 to 48 hours, thick deposits of cells with various morphologies can be detected, including coccoid, coccobacillary, rod-shaped, and filamentous bacteria. Within 4 days of biofilm growth, there is a major increase in the proportion of Gram-negative obligate anaerobes, with various *Prevotella* species and *Fusobacterium nucleatum* being particularly abundant. The latter organism is especially noteworthy due to its unique ability to coaggregate with an exceptionally wide variety of both Gram-positive and Gram-negative bacteria (Fig. 2.14). This ability is believed to play a pivotal role in the maturation of oral biofilms because it creates an extensive network of coaggregation bridges with both early and late colonizers, which results in increased mechanical stability of the biofilm as well as much greater microbial diversity within the community. Consequently, *F. nucleatum* is often referred to as a "bridge species." As the biofilm reaches maturity, all of the major bacterial morphotypes can be identified in the community, while the community composition skews in favor of Gram-negative obligate anaerobes. These ecological shifts in the microbial composition of the oral biofilm are important because they correlate with the development of gingivitis (inflammation of gingival tissues), which can subsequently lead to the further development of periodontitis.

Oral Biofilm Development on Restorative and Implant Materials

Though biofilms accumulate on restorative, orthodontic, endodontic, and implant biomaterials, the remainder of this section will specifically focus on biofilms that accumulate on the surfaces of restorative and implant materials. The precise mechanisms of bacterial adhesion and biofilm formation on dental materials have yet to be fully elucidated, but it is evident that it is a complex process analogous to that described for enamel surfaces. In vitro studies have demonstrated that the adhesion of salivary proteins and bacteria at small distances (5–100 nm) from the surfaces of biomaterials is influenced by a combination of Lifshitz–van der Waals forces, electrostatic interactions, and acid-base bonding. Other properties, such as substrate hydrophobicity, surface free energy, surface charge, and surface roughness, have been commonly investigated in vitro for their correlation to the number of adhering bacteria. Many of the aforementioned surface properties are described in later chapters.

The role of surface roughness in biofilm formation has been the subject of a number of detailed investigations. Smooth surfaces have been shown in vivo to support less biofilm development than rough surfaces. Similarly, hydrophobic supragingival surfaces develop less biofilm in vivo over a 9-day period compared to more hydrophilic surfaces. Conversely, an increase in the mean surface roughness parameter (R_a) above a threshold value of 0.2 μm or an increase in surface free energy were both found to result in more biofilm accumulation on dental materials. When both of those surface properties interact, surface roughness was observed to exert the more dominant effect upon biofilm accumulation. The creation of a rough restoration surface caused by abrasion, erosion, air polishing/ultrasonic instrumentation, or a lack of polishing after the fabrication of a restoration has been associated with enhanced biofilm formation.

Surfaces having a low surface energy were observed to retain the smallest amount of adherent biofilm because of the lower binding forces between bacteria and substrata, even after several days of exposure in the oral cavity. Reciprocally, the higher surface energy of many restorative materials compared with that of the tooth surface could result in a greater tendency for the surface and margins of the restoration to accumulate debris, saliva, and bacteria. This may partially account for the relatively high incidence of secondary (recurrent) carious lesions seen in enamel at the margins of resin composite and amalgam restorations. Salivary pellicle formation has also been shown to exert a masking effect on certain surface characteristics of biomaterials, which is an especially important consideration when developing novel bioactive dental materials.

Interactions of Oral Biofilms With Common Restorative Materials

Investigations of oral biofilms on restorative materials can generally be divided into in vivo, in situ, and in vitro studies, with the latter comprising both monospecies and multispecies investigations. Biofilms that are formed on restorative materials can vary in thickness and viability. In vivo and in situ studies of biofilm formation on dental materials have produced inconsistent results thus far. Therefore there is no widely accepted consensus regarding biofilm accumulation on commonly employed dental materials. Studies suggest that the levels of specific cariogenic organisms like *Streptococcus mutans* are higher in biofilms adjacent to posterior resin restorations compared to amalgam or glass ionomer restorations. Furthermore, the formation of cariogenic oral biofilms is associated with an increase in the surface roughness of resin composites, degradation of the material due to acid production by cariogenic organisms, hydrolysis of the resin matrix, and a decrease in microhardness of the restoration surface. Esterases of salivary and bacterial origin have also been implicated as sources of methacrylate resin degradation. In addition, it has been theorized that planktonic bacteria can enter gaps at the adhesive interface between the restorative material and the tooth, leading to secondary caries and pulp pathology. By contrast, trace amounts of unpolymerized resin, resin monomers, and the products of resin biodegradation, such as 2,2-bis[4(2,3-hydroxypropoxy) phenyl]propane (BisHPPP), triethylene glycol monomethacrylate (TEGMA), triethylene glycol (TEG), and methacrylic acid (MA), have been shown to modulate the growth of oral bacteria in the vicinity of resin restorations. All of these factors likely create a damaging positive feedback cycle of bacteria-surface interaction that further increases surface roughness and encourages additional bacterial attachment to the surface, thereby placing the adjacent enamel at a greater risk for secondary caries.

Like other restorative materials, glass ionomer and resin-modified glass ionomer biomaterials support oral biofilm formation, and bacterial metabolism on these materials can increase their surface roughness. Fluoride-releasing materials and glass ionomers (compomers in particular) can neutralize acids produced by biofilm bacteria. Released fluoride ions can also provide cariostatic benefits and have been demonstrated to interfere with bacterial metabolism in vitro. Presumably, the volume of saliva present in the oral cavity is too large for glass ionomer and resin-modified glass ionomer restorations to provide oral cavity-wide antibacterial protection via fluoride release. However, it could still be theoretically sufficient to minimize demineralization of the tooth structure directly adjacent to these restorations. In addition, glass ionomer materials can be recharged by daily exposure to fluoride-containing dentifrices, thereby compensating for the significant decrease in fluoride release that occurs over time. Interestingly, clinical studies have yet to clearly demonstrate that fluoride-releasing restorative materials significantly reduce the incidence of secondary caries compared to fluoride-free biomaterials. Thus the actual clinical efficacy of these materials remains an open question.

Bacterial adhesion to casting alloys and dental amalgams has received limited attention in recent years, as the use of dental amalgam is being phased down in response to global concerns about mercury (Hg) in the environment. However, biofilms formed on amalgam are reported to have low viability, which could be attributed to the presence of the Hg(II) form of mercury in dental amalgam. Interestingly, amalgam restorations have been shown to bolster the levels of Hg-resistant bacteria in vitro and in vivo. Resistance to antibiotics, particularly tetracycline, was observed to be concurrent with Hg resistance in oral bacteria. It is worth noting that Hg-resistant bacteria were also found in children without amalgam fillings or previous exposure to amalgam. Like amalgams, biofilms formed on gold-based casting alloys are also reported to be of low viability, possibly because of the bacteriostatic effect of elements in the gold alloy.

Information regarding the morphology of biofilms formed on ceramic restorations is limited, although it is generally accepted that ceramic crowns accumulate less biofilm than the adjacent tooth structure. However, the recent in vitro demonstration of increased surface roughness of zirconia surfaces following the use of hand and ultrasonic scaling instruments suggests that dental prophylaxis procedures could potentially result in increased biofilm accumulation on zirconia restorations.

Interactions Oral Biofilms With Denture and Implant Materials

Biofilms that adhere to denture base resins contain an abundance of fungal *Candida* species. However, initial adhesion to the denture base by pioneer colonizing bacteria like streptococci might be required to occur before *Candida* species can attach and form biofilms. For example, bacteria have been observed to attach to dentures within hours, whereas *Candida* species are only detected after multiple days. Furthermore, *Candida* species have been demonstrated to adhere to specific cell wall proteins of streptococci. Denture biofilms have been commonly associated with denture stomatitis (chronic inflammation of the oral mucosa) in both elderly and immunocompromised patients. The removal of biofilms from dentures typically requires mechanical and/or chemical means due to the avid adherence of biofilms to denture base resins.

The accumulation of biofilms on both titanium and titanium alloy dental implants has received significant attention due to the central role of biofilm formation in determining the success of an implant. The sequence of microbial colonization and biofilm formation on dental implants has been shown to be similar to that of teeth but differs in early colonization patterns. Several in vivo studies have confirmed that a reduction in mean R_a of implant materials below the threshold value of 0.2 μm has no major effect on adhesion, colonization, or microbial composition. Compared with polished titanium surfaces, titanium implant surfaces that were modified with titanium nitride (TiN) showed significantly less bacterial adhesion and biofilm formation in vivo, thereby potentially minimizing biofilm accumulation and subsequent periimplantitis. Other contributing factors, such as the hydrophobicity, surface chemistry, and surface free energy of the implant material, have been found to play critical roles in bacterial adhesion to dental implant materials. In addition, the surface characteristics of the bacteria, the design of the implant and abutment, and the microgap between the implant and abutment have all been demonstrated to influence microbial colonization of dental implants.

Caries Prevention

The most common reason for the replacement of dental restorations is secondary caries at the gingival tooth-restoration margin. It has been estimated that 50% to 80% of resin restorations are replaced annually in the United States alone. The cost of replacing restorations is estimated to be in the billions of dollars worldwide, and the number and cost of replacing restorations are increasing annually. Although bacteriological studies of secondary caries indicate that its etiology is similar to that of primary caries, the mechanisms by which secondary caries occur remain an active area of investigation.

The removal of tenaciously adherent oral biofilms from hard surfaces is crucial for the prevention of oral dysbiotic diseases and is most effectively accomplished by mechanical brushing with dentifrice, especially within interproximal regions and around posterior teeth. The use of adjunctive chemical agents can further improve clinical efficacy. Although tooth brushing has been suggested to increase the surface roughness of restorations over time due to the process of wear, mechanical removal has been shown to be more efficacious than chemical intervention alone. This is likely because biofilm-embedded bacteria are typically highly resistant to environmental insults, which in the oral cavity include the host immune response, antibiotics, and other antibacterial agents. Furthermore, most antimicrobial agents have been benchmarked using planktonic bacteria, which are killed by substantially lower concentrations of antimicrobials than biofilm bacteria. In some cases, this difference in susceptibility has been shown to reach several orders of magnitude. Long-term chemical control of biofilms has also been discouraged due to concerns about inducing antimicrobial resistance following prolonged usage. In addition, it is now widely accepted that the microbiota should not be completely eliminated due to its many important health-protective benefits. The preferred approach is to establish and/or maintain a favorable microbial ecology that prevents oral disease.

Bibliography

Arola D, Bajaj D, Ivancik J, et al. Fatigue of biomaterials: hard tissues. *Int J Fatigue*. 2010;32(9):1400–1412.

Bajaj D, Arola D. Role of prism decussation on fatigue crack growth and fracture of human enamel. *Acta Biomater*. 2009;5(8):3045.

Balooch M, Habelitz S, Kinney JH, et al. Mechanical properties of mineralized collagen fibrils as influenced by demineralization. *J Struct Biol*. 2008;162:404–410.

Brauer D, Marshall GW, Marshall SJ. Variation in DEJ scallop size with tooth type. *J Dent*. 2010;38:597–601.

Burwell AK, Thula-Mata T, Gower LB, et al. Functional remineralization of dentin lesions using polymer-induced liquid-precursor process. *PLoS One*. 2012;7(6):e38852.

Cuy JL, Mann AB, Livi KJ, et al. Nanoindentation mapping of the mechanical properties of human molar tooth enamel. *Arch Oral Biol*. 2002;47(4):281–291.

Fosse G, Saele PK, Eide R. Numerical density and distributional pattern of dentin tubules. *Acta Odontol Scand*. 1992;50:201–210.

Garberoglio R, Brannstrom M. Scanning electron microscopic investigation of human dentinal tubules. *Arch Oral Biol.* 1976;21:355–362.

Gower LB. Biomimetic model systems for investigating the amorphous precursor pathway and its role in biomineralization. *Chem Rev.* 2008;108:4551–4627.

Habelitz S. Materials engineering by ameloblasts (critical review). *J Dent Res.* 2015;94(6):759–767.

Habelitz S, Marshall SJ, Marshall GW, et al. Mechanical properties of human dental enamel on the nanometer scale. *Arch Oral Biol.* 2001;46:173–183.

Habelitz S, Rodriguez BJ, Marshall SJ, et al. Peritubular dentin lacks piezoelectricity. *J Dent Res.* 2007;86:908–911.

Imbeni V, Kruzic JJ, Marshall GW, et al. The dentin-enamel junction and the fracture of human teeth. *Nat Mater.* 2005;4:229–232.

Kolenbrander PE, Palmer Jr RJ, Rickard AH, Jakubovics NS, Chalmers NI, Diaz PI. Bacterial interactions and successions during plaque development. *Periodontol 2000.* 2006;42:47–79. https://doi.org/10.1111/j.1600-0757.2006.00187.x.

Marshall GW. Dentin: microstructure and characterization. *Quintessence Int.* 1993;24:606–617.

Marshall GW, Chang JY, Gansky SA, et al. Demineralization of caries-affected transparent dentin by citric acid: an atomic force microscopy study. *Dent Mater.* 2001;17:45–52.

Marshall GW, Habelitz S, Gallagher R, et al. Nanomechanical properties of hydrated carious human dentin. *J Dent Res.* 2001;80:1768–1771.

Marshall GW, Marshall SJ, Bayne SC. Restorative dental materials: scanning electron microscopy and x-ray microanalysis. *Scanning Microsc.* 1988;2:2007–2028.

Marshall GW, Marshall SJ, Kinney JH, et al. The dentin substrate: structure and properties related to bonding. *J Dent.* 1997;25:441–458.

Marshall GW, Olson LM, Lee CV. SEM investigation of the variability of enamel surfaces after simulated clinical acid etching for pit and fissure sealants. *J Dent Res.* 1975;54:1222–1231.

Marshall GW, Yucel N, Balooch M, et al. Sodium hypochlorite alterations of dentin and dentin collagen. *Surf Sci.* 2001;491:444–455.

Marshall SJ, Balooch M, Breunig T, et al. Human dentin and the dentin-resin adhesive interface. *Acta Mater.* 1998;46:2529–2539.

Marshall SJ, Balooch M, Habelitz S, et al. The dentin-enamel junction—a natural, multilevel interface. *J Eur Ceram Soc.* 2003;23:2897–2904.

McGuire JD, Gorski JP, Dusevich V, Wang Y, Walker MP. Type IV collagen is a novel DEJ biomarker that is reduced by radiotherapy. *J Dent Res.* 2014;93(10):1028–1034.

McGuire JD, Walker MP, Dusevich V, Wang Y, Gorski JP. Enamel organic matrix: potential structural role in enamel and relationship to residual basement membrane constituents at the dentin–enamel junction. *Connect Tissue Res.* 2014;55(Suppl 1):33–37.

Nazari A, Bajaj D, Zhang D, et al. Aging and the reduction in fracture toughness of human dentin. *J Mech Behav Biomed Mater.* 2009;2(5):550–559.

Olsson S, Olio G, Adamczak E. The structure of dentin surfaces exposed for bond strength measurements. *Scand J Dent Res.* 1993;101:180–184.

Pashley DH. Dentin: a dynamic substrate—a review. *Scanning Microsc.* 1989;3:161–176.

Pashley DH, Tao L, Boyd L, et al. Scanning electron microscopy of the substructure of smear layers in human dentine. *Arch Oral Biol.* 1988;33(4):265–270.

Shimizu D, Macho GA. Functional significance of the microstructural detail of the primate dentino-enamel junction: a possible example of exaptation. *J Hum Evol.* 2007;52(1):103–111.

Zheng L, Hilton JF, Habelitz S, et al. Dentin caries activity status related to hardness and elasticity. *Eur J Oral Sci.* 2003;111(3):243–252.

Oral Biofilms

Bernardo M, Luis H, Martin MD, et al. Survival and reasons for failure of amalgam versus composite posterior restorations placed in a randomized clinical trial. *J Am Dent Assoc.* 2007;138(6):775–783.

Bollen CM, Lambrechts P, Quirynen M. Comparison of surface roughness of oral hard materials to the threshold surface roughness for bacterial plaque retention: a review of the literature. *Dent Mater.* 1997;13(4):258–269.

Busscher HJ, Rinastiti M, Siswomihardjo W, et al. Biofilm formation on dental restorative and implant materials. *J Dent Res.* 2010;89(7):657–665.

Drummond J. Degradation, fatigue, and failure of resin dental composite materials. *J Dent Res.* 2008;87(8):710–719.

Ferracane JL. Resin-based composite performance: are there some things we can't predict? *Dent Mater.* 2013;29(1):51–58.

Hannig C, Hannig M. The oral cavity—a key system to understand substratum-dependent bioadhesion on solid surfaces in man. *Clin Oral Investig.* 2009;13(2):123–139.

Jakubovics NS. Intermicrobial interactions as a driver for community composition and stratification of oral biofilms. *J Mol Biol.* 2015;427(23):3662–3675.

Khalichi P, Singh J, Cvitkovitch DG, et al. The influence of triethylene glycol derived from dental composite resins on the regulation of *Streptococcus mutans* gene expression. *Biomaterials.* 2009;30(4):452–459.

Kolenbrander PE, Andersen RN, Blehert DS, et al. Communication among oral bacteria. *Microbiol Mol Biol Rev.* 2002;66(3):486–505.

Kolenbrander PE, Palmer Jr RJ, Rickard AH, et al. Bacterial interactions and successions during plaque development. *Periodontol 2000.* 2006;42:47–79.

Mjör IA. Clinical diagnosis of recurrent caries. *J Am Dent Assoc.* 2005;136(10):1426–1433.

Quirynen M, Bollen CM, Papaioannou W, et al. The influence of titanium abutment surface roughness on plaque accumulation and gingivitis: short-term observations. *Int J Oral Maxillofac Implants.* 1996;11(2):169–178.

Ready D, Qureshi F, Bedi R, et al. Oral bacteria resistant to mercury and to antibiotics are present in children with no previous exposure to amalgam restorative materials. *FEMS Microbiol Lett.* 2003;223(1):107–111.

Spencer P, Ye Q, Misra A, et al. Proteins, pathogens, and failure at the composite–tooth interface. *J Dent Res.* 2014;93(12):1243–1249.

Subramani K, Jung RE, Molenberg A, et al. Biofilm on dental implants: a review of the literature. *Int J Oral Maxillofac Implants.* 2009;24(4):616–626.

Teughels W, Van Assche N, Sliepen I, et al. Effect of material characteristics and/or surface topography on biofilm development. *Clin Oral Implants Res.* 2006;17(Suppl 2):68–81.

von Fraunhofer JA, Loewy ZG. Factors involved in microbial colonization of oral prostheses. *Gen Dent.* 2009;57(2):136–143 quiz 44–45.

Wiegand A, Buchalla W, Attin T. Review on fluoride-releasing restorative materials–fluoride release and uptake characteristics, antibacterial activity and influence on caries formation. *Dent Mater.* 2007;23(3):343–362.

3

Materials-Centered Treatment Design

JACK FERRACANE

CHAPTER OUTLINE

This section presents two concepts in dental treatment design: evidence-based dentistry and materials-centered design. Both concepts are used to develop rational treatment plans that consider the patient's needs and preferences, and materials characteristics appropriate for those needs.

Evidence-Based Dentistry

The American Dental Association (ADA) has defined *evidence-based dentistry* as "an approach to oral healthcare that requires the judicious integration of systematic assessments of clinically relevant scientific evidence, relating to the patient's oral and medical condition and history, with the dentist's clinical expertise and the patient's treatment needs and preferences." This approach is patient-centered and tailored to the patient's needs and preferences. All three elements are used in the decision-making process for patient care (Fig. 3.1).

Patient Evidence

Patient needs, conditions, and preferences are considered throughout the diagnostic and treatment planning process. *Observation* of patient needs and medical/dental history occurs first. In this phase, performance of prior and existing restorations, in terms of success or failure, should be noted. This is often a good indicator of conditions in the oral environment and the prognosis of success of similar materials in this environment. The patient's facial profile and orofacial musculature are good indicators of potential occlusal forces. Wear patterns on occlusal surfaces are indicators of bruxing, clenching, occlusal forces, and mandibular movements. Cervical abfractions may indicate heavy occlusal contact accompanied by bruxing or occlusal interferences and possibly in association with aggressive tooth brushing and acidic conditions. Erosion on anterior teeth typically suggests elevated levels of dietary acids, and generalized wear without occlusal trauma could involve a systemic disorder such as gastroesophageal reflux disease (GERD). Any of these conditions would compromise the longevity of restorative therapy. Unusually harsh environments require careful restoration design and selection of materials, sometimes different from the norm.

Restorative material options then need to be considered with the problems and needs of the patient. The integration of patient data and material characteristics forms a more comprehensive plan for treatment.

Scientific Evidence

When searching for scientific evidence, the best available evidence, usually compiled from a review of the scientific literature, provides objective information to inform the clinician and patient. The highest level of validity is chosen to minimize bias. These studies are typically meta-analyses of randomized controlled trials (RCTs), systematic reviews, or individual RCTs. Lower levels of evidence are found in case studies, cohort studies, and case reports. Laboratory studies are listed as "other evidence" because a clinical correlation can be made only as an extrapolation of the laboratory data. The listing of bench or laboratory research as "other evidence" should not be construed as meaning that bench research is not valid or useful. The hierarchy of evidence as presented for evidence-based data (EBD) is based on human clinical trials, for which laboratory tests are, at best, only a simulation.

Because new material developments that are enhancements to existing products are not required to undergo clinical testing by the Food and Drug Administration (FDA), published laboratory or in vitro studies are often the only forms of scientific evidence available for specific materials. This does not mean that no evidence is available. However, the clinician must recognize the limitations of these data, despite their scientific validity, when translating them to the clinical situation and making treatment decisions for a patient (Table 3.1).

Researchers in dental materials science have analyzed the correlation between one or two physical or mechanical properties of materials and clinical performance. Although it is possible to use laboratory tests to rank the clinical performance of different formulations of the same class of material, there is no one perfect predictor of clinical performance. This is logical, as clinical performance is a multifactorial process. In addition, differences in test configuration, specimen geometry, specimen processing, and environmental conditions make direct comparisons between laboratory tests difficult. However, understanding these tests and the

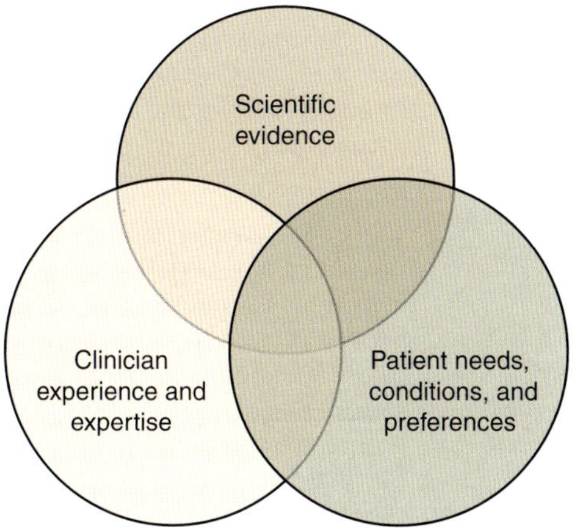

• **Fig. 3.1** The elements of evidence-based dentistry.

information they produce can provide guidance for the selection of a material for a specific situation. Tests and the properties they assess are discussed in supplemental online material.

Planning for Dental Treatment

Every patient is unique, including the patient's oral environment and general physiology. This provides a unique set of circumstances and challenges for implementing successful material choices in a treatment plan. In the next section, we present a rationale for selecting materials based on the treatment design approach proposed by Spear and Kokich. They advocate a treatment planning process that starts with an assessment of overall aesthetics and proceeds to consider function, structure, and biology in that order. Decisions made at every stage directly affect the following stages. Treatment begins with the acute problems and then progresses logically to facilitate a stepwise sequence that can be clearly defined and communicated among the clinicians involved in delivering care to the patient. Table 3.2 presents a summary of the approach with queries for each stage and relevant materials and properties to be considered.

An aesthetics appraisal analyzes the position of the midline and the length of the maxillary and mandibular incisors, which influence the position of the posterior occlusal plane, which in turn influences function. The aesthetics appraisal starts with an assessment of the position of the maxillary central incisors relative to the upper lip. If the incisal edge display is insufficient, lengthening of the incisal edges can be done surgically, by orthodontic treatment, or by restorative methods using dental materials. Most cultures would prefer materials that mimic natural dentition in color, texture, and reflectance. Ceramics and resin composites exhibit these properties. A number of options exist for these two classes of materials. Ceramics are discussed in Chapter 10. Resin composites are discussed in Chapter 8.

The next consideration in the aesthetics appraisal is position of the midline and inclination of the maxillary incisors. The labial surface characteristics and inclination influence the light reflectance of the incisors. Maximum light reflectance is achieved when the labial surface is perpendicular to the occlusal plane. Corrections to the midline and to the labial inclination can be done by orthodontics or restorative dentistry. Surface characteristics, light, reflection, and color are discussed in Chapter 4.

The next step assesses the maxillary posterior occlusal plane relative to an ideal position of the maxillary incisal edge. Corrections to the posterior occlusal plane can be achieved by surgery or restorative procedures. Materials for adjusting the posterior occlusion can be the same as for anterior restorations; however, the function of posterior teeth and occlusal relationships should be considered in the selection of materials. The wear of materials in contact, as well as the resistance to occlusal forces, are important considerations. Forces and wear are discussed in Chapter 4. Metals and alloys are discussed in Chapter 9.

TABLE 3.1 Assessing the Quality of Evidence

Study Quality	Diagnosis	Treatment/Prevention/Screening	Prognosis
Level 1: good-quality, patient-oriented evidence	Validated clinical decision rule SR/meta-analysis of high-quality studies High-quality diagnostic cohort study[a]	SR/meta-analysis or RCTs with consistent findings High-quality individual RCT[b] All-or-none study[c]	SR/meta-analysis of good-quality cohort studies Prospective cohort study with good follow-up
Level 2: limited-quality patient-oriented evidence	Unvalidated clinical decision rule SR/meta-analysis of lower-quality studies or studies with inconsistent findings Lower-quality diagnostic cohort study or diagnostic case-control study	SR/meta-analysis of lower-quality clinical trials or of studies with inconsistent findings Lower-quality clinical trial Cohort study Case-control study	SR/meta-analysis of lower-quality cohort studies or with inconsistent results Retrospective cohort study or prospective cohort study with poor follow-up Case-control study Case series
Level 3: other evidence	Consensus guidelines, extrapolations from bench research, usual practice, opinion, disease-oriented evidence (intermediate or physiologic outcomes only), or case series for studies of diagnosis, treatment, prevention, or screening		

RCT, Randomized controlled trial; *SR*, systematic review.

[a]High-quality diagnostic cohort study: cohort design, adequate size, adequate spectrum of patients, blinding, and a consistent, well-defined reference standard.

[b]High-quality RCT: allocation concealed, blinding if possible, intention-to-treat analysis, adequate statistical power, adequate follow-up (greater than 80%).

[c]In an all-or-none study, the treatment causes a dramatic change in outcomes, such as antibiotics for meningitis or surgery for appendicitis, which precludes study in a controlled trial.

From Newman MG, Weyant R, Hujoel P. JEBDP improves grading system and adopts strength of recommendation taxonomy grading (SORT) for guidelines and systematic reviews. *J Evid Based Dent Pract.* 2007;7:147–150.

TABLE 3.2 Decision Matrix for Selecting Dental Materials[a]

Assessment and Factors	Query	Relevant Properties and Dental Materials (Chapter No.)
Aesthetics: Maxillary		
Central incisors relative to upper lip	• Is the incisal edge display of the maxillary centrals sufficient?	Surface characteristics (4) Light, reflection, color (4) Resin composites (8) Ceramics (10) Adhesives and cements (7, 12)
Midline and inclination of incisors	• Does the maxillary midline need correction? • Does the inclination of the maxillary incisors need correction?	Surface characteristics (4) Light, reflection, color (4) Resin composites (8) Ceramics (10) Adhesives and cements (7, 12)
Posterior occlusal plane	• Does the maxillary posterior occlusal plane need correction? • Is sufficient tooth structure present? • What are the surface characteristics of the opposing dentition?	Forces and wear (4) Core buildup (8) Provisional materials (8) Resin composites (8) Adhesives and cements (7, 12) Metals and alloys (9) Ceramics (10)
Gingival levels	• Do gingival margins need correction?	Resin composites (8) Glass ionomers (8) Ceramics (10) Adhesives and cements (7, 12)
Aesthetics: Mandibular		
Same factors as for maxillary: Midline, inclination, posterior occlusal plane, and gingival levels		
Aesthetics and Function		
Missing teeth	• Are missing teeth in need of replacement? • Is a fixed or removable prosthesis preferred? • Should adjacent teeth be involved in the replacement? • What are the surface characteristics of the opposing dentition?	Forces, stress, and wear (4) Provisional materials (8) Adhesives and cements (7, 12) Denture materials (8) Metals and alloys (9) Ceramics (10) Impression materials (11) Casting materials (11) Implants (14)
Function		
Occlusion	• Does the occlusal relationship need correction? • What are the surface characteristics of the opposing dentition?	Forces, stress, and wear (4) Resin composites (8) Metals and alloys (9) Ceramics (10) Impression materials (11) Casting materials (11) Adhesives and cements (7, 12) Implants (14) Articulator
Structure		
Adequate tooth structure to support the planned restorations	• What are the types of restorations to be placed? • How will the restorations be retained?	Adhesives and cements (7, 12) Resin composites (8) Metals and Ceramics (9, 10) Acrylics (8)
Biologic		
Oral environment: enamel, dentin, pulp, and periodontal ligament	• Is acute disease present? • Are conditions in the oral environment favorable (e.g., saliva pH, salivary flow, oral hygiene, diet, supporting bone structure, pulp, occlusal habits)?	Oral environment (2) Forces, stress, and wear (4) Biocompatibility (4) Intermediary materials (6) Tissue engineering (15)

[a]This table augments the sequence and logic presented in the section "Planning for Dental Treatment" with factors, queries, and references to chapters in this textbook.

Gingival levels of the anterior teeth play a large role in aesthetics. Similarly, the appearance of the gingival margin of anterior restorations will influence their overall aesthetics. Ceramics can be used to fabricate restorations with an aesthetic gingival margin. The combination of ceramics and metal at the gingival margin, as in ceramic-metal restorations, can make the aesthetic gingival margin more difficult to achieve. Ceramic-metal materials are discussed in Chapters 9 and 10.

After completing the assessment and plan for the maxillary anterior and posterior teeth, the mandibular anterior and posterior teeth can be assessed and designed. Missing teeth can be restored by a fixed or removable dental prosthesis or a dental implant. The choice of dental material to replace parts of the tooth is based on an assessment of the overall structure of the tooth remaining to support the restoration. Materials for a fixed dental prosthesis include metals and ceramics. Removable prostheses or removable partial dentures can include these materials and polymers. Polymers for removable dentures are discussed in Chapter 8. Single or multiple missing teeth can be restored by dental implants that mimic the shape and position of the tooth root onto which restorations such as a crown or fixed dental prosthesis are secured. Implants are discussed in Chapter 14. Adhesives and cements for securing prostheses to tooth structure are discussed in Chapters 7 and 12.

The aesthetic plan is integrated with the functional occlusion by replicating the patient's dentition and occlusal relationships and then positioning these casts on an articulator. Materials for replicating dentition and oral tissues are called impression materials. These materials form a negative replica or mold of the tissues into which a rigid-setting material, often gypsum, is poured to make a positive replica of the oral tissues. Impression and casting materials are discussed in Chapter 11.

The biological assessment wraps up the diagnostics and planning. In this phase, the health of the supporting periodontal tissues, including the periodontal ligament, is evaluated, along with the conditions of the oral environment and the condition of the enamel, dentin, and pulp. If acute disease such as dental caries is present, intermediary materials can be used to stabilize the condition before definitive materials are used. Intermediary materials are discussed in Chapter 6. The oral environment is discussed in Chapter 2.

As mentioned at the start of this chapter, patient behaviors and preferences are also an important consideration. The patient may need instruction and coaching on the prevention and maintenance of dental treatment. Preventive materials are discussed in Chapter 6. The performance of prior dental treatment is evaluated. Reactions to materials used in prior restorations should be considered. Biocompatibility and tissue reactions are discussed in Chapter 4.

Refer to Table 3.2 for questions to consider in each stage of treatment design, along with relevant dental materials and properties. Chapter numbers are listed for the materials and properties for further information and review.

Bibliography

American Dental Association. Evidence-based databases. Accessed August 28, 2024. http://ada.org/resources/ada-library/evidence-based-databases.

Bader JD. Stumbling into the age of evidence. *Dent Clin North Am.* 2009;53(1):15.

Forrest JL. Introduction to the basics of evidence-based dentistry: concepts and skills. *J Evid Based Dent Pract.* 2009;9(3):108.

Forrest JL, Miller SA. Translating evidence-based decision making into practice: EBDM concepts and finding the evidence. *J Evid Based Dent Pract.* 2009;9(2):59.

Miller SA, Forrest JL. Translating evidence-based decision making into practice: appraising and applying the evidence. *J Evid Based Dent Pract.* 2009;9(4):164.

Newman MG, Weyant R, Hujoel P. JEBDP improves grading system and adopts strength of recommendation taxonomy grading (SORT) for guidelines and systematic reviews. *J Evid Based Dent Pract.* 2007;7:147–150.

Sakaguchi RL. Evidence-based dentistry: achieving a balance. *J Am Dent Assoc.* 2010;141(5):496–497.

Spear FM, Kokich VG. A multidisciplinary approach to esthetic dentistry. *Dent Clin N Am.* 2007;51:487.

Spear FM, Kokich VG, Mathews DP. Interdisciplinary management of anterior dental esthetics. *J Am Dent Assoc.* 2006;137:160.

4 Fundamentals of Materials Science

JACK FERRACANE

CHAPTER OUTLINE

Restorative dental materials are subjected to a very hostile environment in which pH, salivary flow, and mechanical loading fluctuate constantly and often rapidly. These challenges have required substantial research and development to provide products for the clinician. Much of this is possible through the application of fundamental concepts of materials science. The understanding of properties of polymers, ceramics, and metals is crucial to their selection and design of dental restorations.

No single property defines the quality of a material. Several properties, determined from standardized laboratory and clinical tests, are often used to describe quality. Clinical tests are expensive and inherently difficult to conduct, so laboratory tests are usually performed before clinical tests to provide standardized measures for comparing materials and guide the interpretation of clinical trials.

Standardization of laboratory tests is essential, however, to control quality and enable comparison of results between investigators. When possible, test specimens should mimic the size and shape of the structure in the clinical setting, using the same mixing and manipulating procedures as those used in routine clinical conditions.

Although standardized laboratory tests are useful to compare values of properties of different restorative materials (e.g., different brands), they are also essential to know the characteristics of the supporting hard and soft tissues. Many restorations fail clinically because of fracture or deformation. This is a material property issue. Some well-constructed restorations become unserviceable because the dentin or enamel fails. This is an interface or substrate failure. Consequently, when designing restorations and interpreting test results, it is important to remember that the success of the restoration depends not only on the physical qualities of the restorative material but also on the biophysical or physiological qualities of the supporting tissues.

The physical properties described in this chapter include mechanical properties, thermal properties, electrical and electromechanical properties, color, optical properties, and biocompatibility.

Mechanical Properties

In the oral environment, restorative materials are exposed to chemical, thermal, and mechanical challenges. These challenges can cause deformation of the material. The science that studies how biological materials interact and deform is called *biomechanics*. This section introduces concepts of elastic, plastic, and viscoelastic deformation and mechanical quantities, including force, stress, strain, strength, toughness, hardness, friction, and wear in terms of performance of materials in the oral environment.

Force

One body interacting with another generates force. Forces may be applied through actual contact of the bodies or at a distance (e.g., gravity). The result of an applied force on a body is translation or deformation of the body depending on whether the body is rigid or deformable and whether the body is constrained or not. If the body is constrained (i.e., does not move), the force causes the body to deform or change its shape. If the body is free of constraints, an applied force results in translation or movement.

A force is defined by three characteristics: point of application, magnitude, and direction of application. The International System of Units (SI) unit of force is the newton (N). One pound-force (lb-f) equals 4.4 newtons (N).

Occlusal Forces

Maximum occlusal forces range from 200 N to 3500 N. Occlusal forces between adult teeth are highest in the posterior region closest to the mandibular rotation axis and decrease from the molars to the incisors. Forces on the first and second molars vary from 400 N to 800 N. The average force on the premolars, canines, and incisors is about 300 N, 200 N, and 150 N, respectively. A somewhat nonlinear but definite increase in force from 235 N to 494 N occurs in growing children, with an average yearly increase of about 22 N.

Forces on Restorations

Patients with a partial removable denture generate occlusal forces in the range of 65 N to 235 N. For patients with a complete, tissue-supported removable denture, the average force on posterior teeth is about 100 N; the forces on the incisors average 40 N. Age and gender variations in the patient populations, as well as facial form and muscle definition, contribute to the large variation in force values. When designing restorations and selecting materials, it is important to consider the location in the arch, opposing dentition, and force-generating capacity of the patient. The success or failure of other restorations in the patient's mouth, as well as evidence of wear and cracks on existing teeth, should be an indication of how challenging those factors are to the dentition of that specific individual.

Stress

When a force acts on a constrained object, the object resists the force. This internal reaction is equal in magnitude and opposite in direction to the applied external force and is called *stress*, typically denoted as S or σ. Both the applied force and the internal resistance (stress) are distributed over an area of the object, so the stress in an object is defined as the *force per area*, or stress = force/area. Stress is difficult to measure directly, so the force and the area to which the force is applied are measured, and stress is calculated from the ratio of force per area. Therefore the unit of stress is the unit of force (N) divided by a unit of area and is commonly expressed in SI units as pascal ($1\ Pa = 1\ N/m^2 = 1\ MN/mm^2$). It is common to report stress in units of megapascals (MPa) or millions of pascals, $1\ MPa = 10^6\ Pa$.

Stress in a structure varies directly with the force and inversely with area, so the area over which the force acts is an important consideration. This is particularly true in dental restorations in which the areas over which the forces are applied often are extremely small. For example, cuspal areas of contact may have cross-sectional areas of only 0.16 to 0.016 cm^2.

Stresses of several hundred MPa occur in many types of restorations and of thousands of MPa when the contact area of a cusp or dental explorer is used to apply the force. This is one reason that premature contacts, in which small surface areas are supporting large occlusal forces, are so damaging. When equilibrating the occlusion, multiple simultaneous occlusal contacts are desirable. Distributing occlusal forces over larger surface areas reduces the local occlusal stress.

Types of Stress

A force can be applied from any angle or direction. Several forces often combine to develop complex stresses in a structure. It is rare for forces and stresses to be isolated to a single axis. Individually applied forces can be defined as axial, shear, bending, or torsional. These directional forces are illustrated in Fig. 4.1. All stresses, however, can be resolved into combinations of two basic types: axial and shear.

Tension results from two sets of forces directed away from each other in the same straight line or when one end is constrained and the other end is subjected to a force directed away from the constraint. *Compression* results from two sets of forces directed toward each other in the same straight line or when one surface is constrained and the other is subjected to a force directed toward and perpendicular to the constraint. *Shear* occurs from two sets of forces directed parallel to each other but not along the same straight line. *Torsion* results from the twisting of a body, and *bending* or *flexure* results from an applied bending moment. When tension is applied, the molecules making up the body resist being pulled apart. When compression is applied,

FORCE	DEFORMATION	
Axial, tension	Elongation	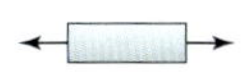
Axial, compression	Compression	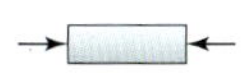
Shear	Shear	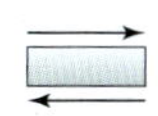
Twisting moment	Torsion	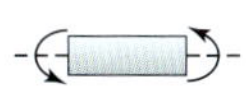
Bending moment	Bending	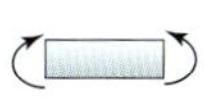

• **Fig. 4.1** Schematic of the different types of stresses and their corresponding deformations.

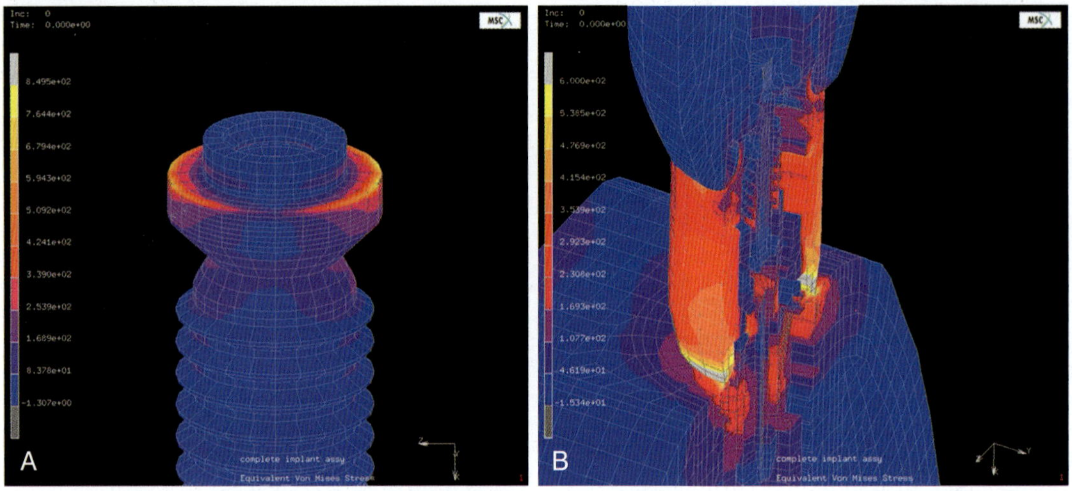

• **Fig. 4.2** Stress distribution in an implant-supported restoration. (A) Stresses on the shoulder of the implant body from an oblique occlusal load. (B) Stresses within the implant abutment and alveolar bone. (Courtesy Dr. Svenn Borgersen, Eagan, MN, and Dr. Ronald Sakaguchi).

they resist being forced more closely together. As a result of a shear stress application, one portion of the body must resist sliding past another. These resistances of a material to deformation represent the basic qualities of elasticity of solid bodies.

An example of the complexity and varying direction and magnitude of stresses in the oral cavity is shown in Fig. 4.2, in which a finite element model of a dental implant is loaded in compression. Fig. 4.2A shows the highest stresses in red and yellow on the shoulder of the implant resulting from occlusal forces. Fig. 4.2B shows the distribution of stresses in the implant abutment.

Strain

Each type of stress is capable of producing a corresponding deformation in a body (see Fig. 4.1). The deformation from a tensile force is an elongation in the axis of applied force, whereas a compressive force causes compression or shortening of the body in the axis of loading. Strain, ε, is described as the change in length ($\Delta L = L - L_o$) per original length (L_o) of the body when it is subjected to a load. The units of measurement (length/length) cancel in the calculation of strain, so strain is unitless.

$$\text{Strain}(\varepsilon) = \text{Deformation/Original length}$$
$$= (L - L_o)/L_o = \Delta L/L_o$$

If a load is applied to a wire with an original length of 2 mm, resulting in a new length of 2.02 mm, it has deformed 0.02 mm, and the strain is 0.02/2 = 0.01 or 1%. Strain is often reported as a percentage. Although the length units cancel in the calculation of strain, it is best to report the units with the final result to specify the scale of the measurement (m/m; mm/mm; μm/μm). The amount of strain will differ with each type of material and with the magnitude of the load applied. Note that regardless of the composition or nature of the material and regardless of the magnitude and type of load applied to the material, deformation and strain result with each stress application. Strain is an important consideration in dental restorative materials, such as orthodontic wires or implant screws, in which a large amount of strain can occur before failure. Wires can be bent and adjusted without fracturing. Strain is also important in impression materials, where the material needs to recover without permanent distortion when removing it from hard tissue retentive areas.

Stress-Strain Curves

If a bar of material is subjected to an applied force, *F,* the magnitude of the force and the resulting deformation (δ) can be measured. In another bar of the same material but different dimensions, the same applied force produces different force-deformation characteristics (Fig. 4.3A). However, if the applied force is normalized by the cross-sectional area *A* of the bar (stress), and the deformation is normalized by the original length of the bar (strain), the resulting stress-strain curve is independent of the geometry of the bar (Fig. 4.3B). It is therefore preferred that the stress-strain relations of an object be reported rather than the force-deformation characteristics. The stress-strain relationship of a dental material can be studied by measuring the load and deformation and then calculating the corresponding stress and strain.

When testing materials, loads should be applied at a uniform rate, and deformation should occur at a uniform rate. A typical universal testing machine can analyze materials in tension, compression, or shear. In the scheme illustrated in Fig. 4.4, a rod is clamped between two jaws, and a tensile force is applied. The load is measured with a force transducer, and the deformation is measured with an extensometer clamped over a specified length of the specimen. A plot of load versus deformation is produced, which can be converted to a plot of stress versus strain (Fig. 4.5) by the simple calculations described previously. By convention, strain is plotted on the x-axis as an independent variable because most tests are operated in strain control, where a constant strain is applied to the specimen, and the resulting force is measured as the dependent, or y-axis, variable.

In the calculation of stress, it is assumed that the cross-sectional area of the specimen remains constant during the test. Using this assumption, the stress-strain curve is called an *engineering stress-strain curve,* and stresses are calculated using the original cross-sectional area. When large loads are applied or the object is tested in tension, the cross-sectional area might change dramatically during testing. In that case, the true stress, calculated with the actual cross-sectional area in the denominator, is very different from the engineering stress, calculated with the original cross-sectional area. If the cross-sectional area decreases during the test, the true stress will be higher than the engineering stress because the denominator is smaller. In most mechanical tests, particularly those of small

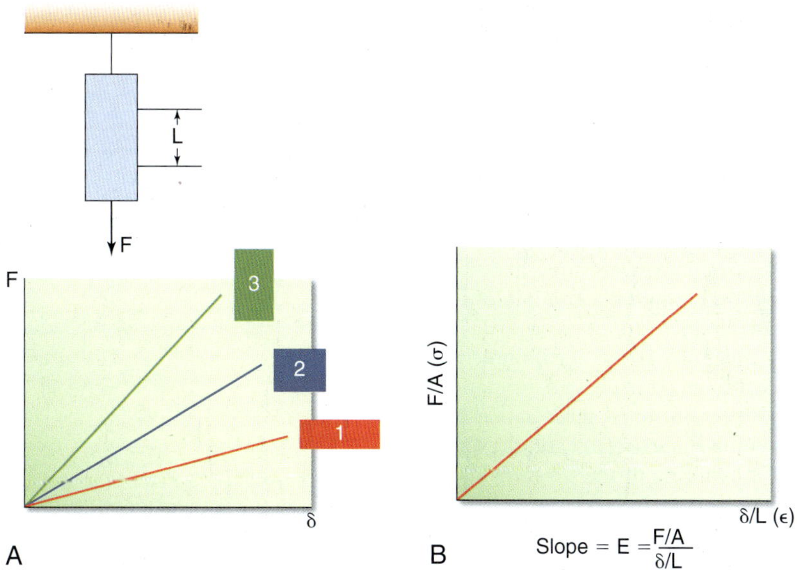

• **Fig. 4.3** Force-deformation characteristics. (A) Force-deformation characteristics for the same material but having different dimensions. (B) Stress-strain characteristics of the same group of bars. The stress-strain curve is independent of the geometry of the bar.

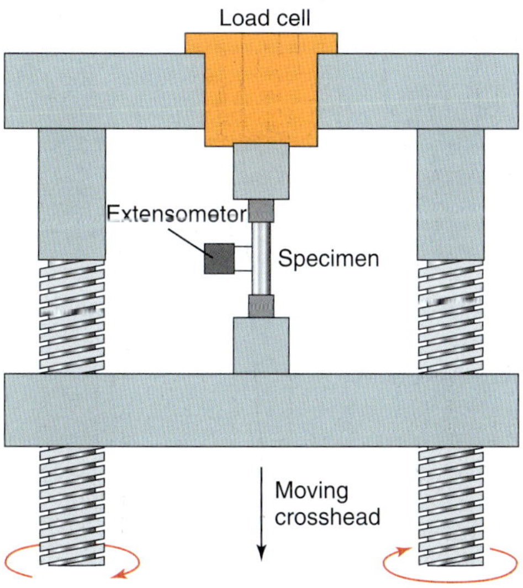

• **Fig. 4.4** Universal testing machine.

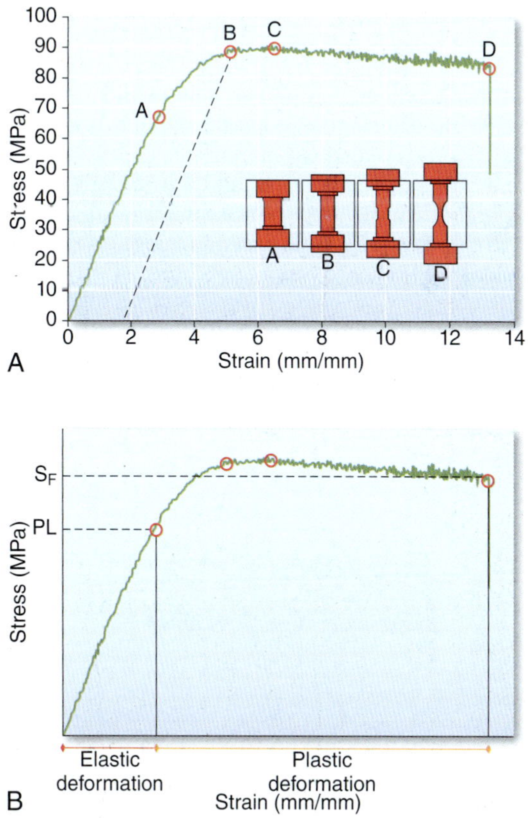

• **Fig. 4.5** Plotting stress-strain curves. (A) Stress-strain curve for a material subjected to tensile stress. Specimens illustrate amount of deformation at each point (*A–D*). (B) Elastic deformation is exhibited up to the proportional limit (*PL*) and plastic deformation is exhibited from PL to the failure point, where we register the stress at failure (S_F).

specimen dimensions, the original cross-sectional area is used for calculating stress because it is often very difficult to measure the cross-sectional area as it changes throughout the experiment. Engineering stress is used in the presentation of stress-strain curves obtained in tension in this chapter.

Proportional and Elastic Limits

A stress-strain curve for a hypothetical material subjected to increasing tensile stress until failure is shown in Fig. 4.5. As the stress is increased, the strain is increased. In the initial portion of the curve, from 0 to *A,* the stress is linearly proportional to the strain. As the strain is doubled, the stress is also doubled. After point *A*, the stress is no longer linearly proportional to the strain. Hence, the value of the stress at *A* is known as the *proportional limit* (S_{PL} or σ_{PL}), defined as the highest stress at which the stress-strain curve is a straight line; that is, stress is linearly proportional to strain. Below the proportional limit, no permanent deformation occurs in a structure. When the force is removed, the object will return to its original dimensions. Below the proportional limit, the material is elastic in nature.

The region of the stress-strain curve before the proportional limit is called the *elastic region.* When an object experiences a stress greater than the proportional limit, permanent or irreversible strain occurs. The region of the stress-strain curve beyond the proportional limit is called the *plastic region.* This characterization refers to linearly elastic materials such as many metals in which the relation between stress and strain is linear up to the proportional limit and nonlinear thereafter. There are exceptions to this general rule, however. Materials described as *superelastic* exhibit nonlinear elastic behavior; that is, their relationship between stress and strain in the elastic region does not follow a straight line, but removal of the load results in a return to zero strain.

The *elastic limit* (S_{EL} or σ_{EL}) is defined as the maximum stress that a material will withstand without permanent deformation. For linearly elastic materials, the proportional limit and elastic limit represent the same stress within the structure, and the terms are often used interchangeably in referring to the stress involved. An exception is when superelastic materials are considered. It is important to remember, however, that the two terms differ in fundamental concept; one deals with the proportionality of strain to stress in the structure, whereas the other describes the elastic behavior of the material. For the same material, values for proportional or elastic limits obtained in tension versus compression will differ.

The concepts of elastic and plastic behavior can be illustrated with a simple schematic model of the deformation of atoms in a solid under stress (Figs. 4.6 and 4.7). The atoms are shown in Fig. 4.6A, without stress, and in Fig. 4.6B, with a resulting stress that is below the value of the proportional limit. When the stress shown in (B) is removed, the atoms return to their positions shown in (A), indicating that the deformation was reversible. When the stress is greater than the proportional limit, the atoms move to a position as shown in Fig. 4.7B, and on removal of the stress, the atoms remain in this new position, indicating an irreversible, permanent deformation. When the stress is less than the proportional or elastic limit, the strain is reversible, whereas when the stress is greater than the proportional or elastic limit, there is an irreversible or permanent strain on the object.

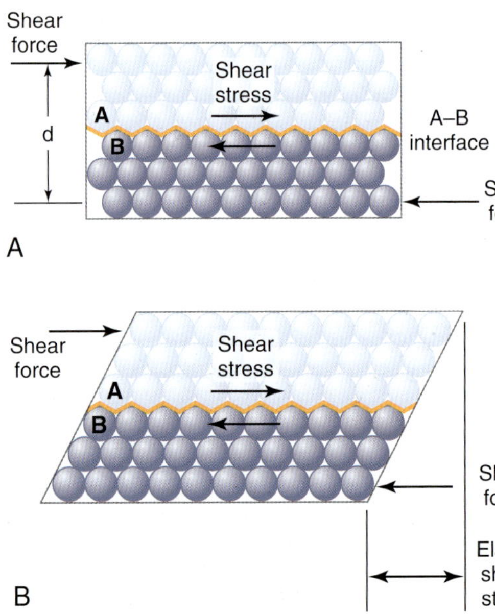

• **Fig. 4.6** Sketch of an atomic model showing atoms in original position (A) and after elastic deformation (B). (Modified from Anusavice KJ. *Phillips' Science of Dental Materials.* 11th ed. Saunders; 2003:79).

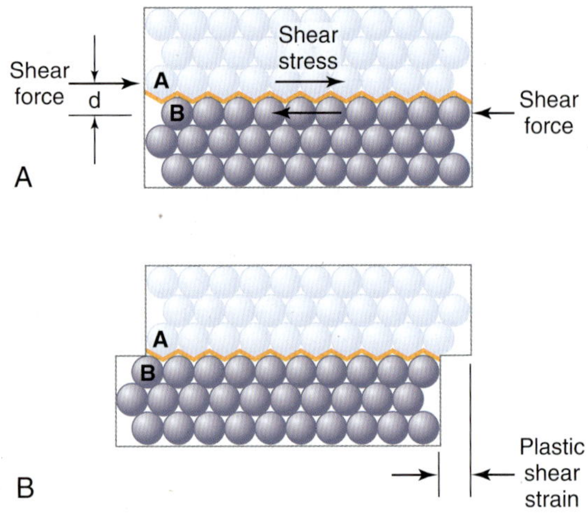

• **Fig. 4.7** Sketch of an atomic model showing atoms in original position (A) and after plastic deformation (B). (Modified from Anusavice KJ. *Phillips' Science of Dental Materials.* 11th ed. Saunders; 2003:79).

Yield Strength

It is often difficult to explicitly measure the proportional and elastic limits because the precise point of deviation of the stress-strain curve from linearity is difficult to determine. The *yield strength, yield stress,* or *yield point* (Y_S or σY) of a material is a property that can be determined readily and is often used to describe the stress at which the material begins to function in a plastic manner. At this point, a small, defined amount of permanent strain has occurred in the material. The yield strength is defined as the stress at which a material deforms plastically, and there is a defined amount of permanent strain. The amount of permanent strain is arbitrarily selected for the material being examined and may be indicated as 0.1%, 0.2%, or 0.5% (0.001, 0.002, or 0.005) permanent strain. The amount of permanent strain is referred to as the *percent offset.* Many specifications use 0.2% as a convention, but this depends on the plastic behavior of the material tested. For stiff materials with small elongation, the calculation of yield stress will include greater offsets than those materials with larger elongation or deformation.

The yield stress is determined by selecting the desired offset or strain on the x-axis and drawing a line parallel to the linear region of the stress-strain curve. The point at which the parallel line intersects the stress-strain curve is the yield stress. On the stress-strain curve shown in Fig. 4.5, for example, the yield strength is represented by the value *B.* This represents a stress of just under 90 MPa at a 0.25% offset. This yield stress is slightly higher than that for the proportional limit because it includes a specified amount of permanent deformation. Note that when a structure is permanently deformed, even to a small degree (such as the amount of deformation at the yield strength), it does not return completely to its original dimensions when the stress is removed. For this reason, the elastic limit and yield strength of a material are among its most important properties because they define the transition from elastic to plastic behavior.

Any dental restoration that is permanently deformed through the forces of mastication usually loses its functionality to some extent. For example, a fixed partial dental prosthesis (such as a three-unit prosthesis) that is permanently deformed by excessive occlusal forces would exhibit altered occlusal contacts. The restoration is permanently deformed because a stress equal to or greater than the yield strength was generated. It is important to remember that dysfunctional occlusal loading also changes the stresses placed on a restoration. A deformed restoration may therefore be subjected to greater stresses than originally intended because the occlusion that was distributed over a larger number of occlusal contacts may now be concentrated on a smaller number of contacts. Under these conditions, fracture does not occur if the material is able to plastically deform. However, this permanent change in shape represents a destructive example of deformation. Permanent deformation and stresses in excess of the elastic limit are desirable when shaping an orthodontic arch wire or adjusting a clasp on a removable partial denture. In these examples, the stress must exceed the yield strength to permanently bend or adapt the wire or clasp. Elastic deformation occurs as the wire or clasp engages and disengages a retentive region in the cervical area of the tooth. Retention is achieved through small-scale elastic deformation. This elastic or reversible deformation describes the function of elastic bands, clasps, o-rings, and implant screws.

Ultimate Strength

In Fig. 4.5 the test specimen exhibits a maximum stress at point *C*. The *ultimate tensile strength* or *stress* (*UTS*) is defined as the maximum stress that a material can withstand before failure in tension, whereas the *ultimate compressive strength* or *stress* (*UCS*) is the maximum stress a material can withstand in compression. The ultimate engineering stress is determined by dividing the maximum load in tension (or compression) by the original cross-sectional area of the test specimen. The ultimate tensile strength of the material in Fig. 4.5 is about 90 MPa, or just slightly above the yield strength in this particular case.

The ultimate strength of an alloy, as used in dentistry, specifies the maximum load and minimum cross-sectional area when designing a restoration. Note that an alloy that has been stressed to near the ultimate strength will be permanently deformed, so a restoration receiving that amount of stress during function would be useless. A safety margin should be incorporated into the design of the restoration and choice of material to ensure that the ultimate strength is not approached in normal function. The yield strength is often of greater importance than ultimate strength in design and material selection because it is an estimate of when a material will start to deform permanently.

Fracture Strength

In Fig. 4.5, the test specimen fractured at point *D*. The stress at which a brittle material fractures is called the *fracture strength* or *fracture stress* (SF or σF). Note that a material does not necessarily fracture at the point at which the maximum stress occurs. After a maximum tensile force is applied to some materials, the specimen begins to elongate excessively, resulting in "necking" or a reduction of cross-sectional area (see Fig. 4.5). The stress calculated from the force and the original cross-sectional area may decrease dramatically before final fracture occurs because of the reduction in cross-sectional area. Accordingly, the stress at the end of the curve is less than that at some intermediate point on the curve. Therefore, in materials that exhibit necking, the ultimate and fracture strengths are different. However, for the specific cases of many dental alloys and ceramics subjected to tension, the ultimate and fracture strengths (about 85 MPa in the example in Fig. 4.5) are similar, as shown later in this chapter. Note that the reduction in stress that is observed after the ultimate stress in materials that show necking is an artifact of using the original cross-sectional area in the calculation of stress. If the true cross-sectional area is used, the stress would increase.

Elongation

The deformation that results from the application of a tensile force is *elongation*. Elongation is extremely important because it gives an indication of the possible manipulation of an alloy. As may be observed from Fig. 4.5, the elongation of a material during a tensile test can be divided conveniently into two parts: (1) the increase in length of the specimen below the proportional limit (from 0 to *A*), which is not permanent and is proportional to the stress; and (2) the elongation beyond the proportional limit and up to the fracture strength (from *A* to *D*), which is permanent. The permanent deformation may be measured with an extensometer while the material is being tested and calculated from the stress-strain curve. Total elongation is commonly expressed as a percentage. The percent elongation is calculated as follows:

$$\text{Elongation} = \left(\frac{\text{Increase in length}}{\text{Original length}}\right) \times 100$$

Total elongation includes both the elastic elongation and the plastic elongation. Plastic elongation is usually the greatest of the two, except in materials that are quite brittle or those with very low stiffness. A material that exhibits a 20% total elongation at the time of fracture has increased in length by one-fifth of its original length. Such a material, as in many dental gold alloys, has a high value for plastic or permanent elongation and, in general, is a ductile type of alloy, whereas a material with only 1% elongation would possess little permanent elongation and be considered brittle.

An alloy that has a high value for total elongation can be bent permanently without danger of fracture. Clasps can be adjusted, orthodontic wires can be adapted, and crowns or inlays can be burnished if alloys with high values for elongation are used. Elongation and yield strength are generally related in many materials, including dental gold alloys, where, generally, the higher the yield strength, the lower the elongation.

Elastic Modulus

The measure of elasticity of a material is described by the term *elastic modulus*, also referred to as *modulus of elasticity* or *Young's modulus*, and denoted by the variable *E*. The word *modulus* means ratio and, in this case, the ratio of stress to strain. The elastic modulus represents the stiffness of a material within the elastic range. The elastic modulus can be determined from a stress-strain curve (see Fig. 4.5) by calculating the ratio of stress to strain or the slope of the linear region of the curve. The modulus is calculated from the following equation:

$$\text{Elastic modulus} = \text{Stress/Strain}$$

or

$$E = \sigma / \varepsilon$$

This equation is also known as Hooke's law. Because strain is unitless (length/length), the modulus has the same units as stress and is usually reported in MPa or GPa (1 GPa = 1000 MPa).

The elastic qualities of a material represent a fundamental property of the material. The interatomic or intermolecular forces

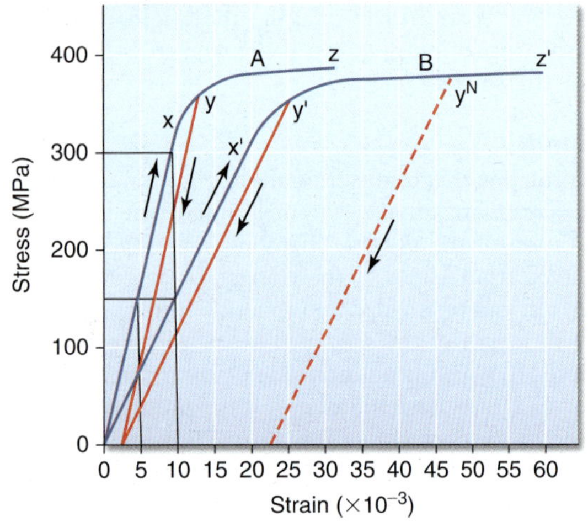

• **Fig. 4.8** Stress-strain curves of two hypothetical materials, A and B, subjected to tensile stress.

of the material are responsible for the property of elasticity (see Fig. 4.6). The stronger the basic attraction forces, the greater the values of the elastic modulus and the more rigid or stiff the material. Because this property is related to the attraction forces within the material, it is usually the same when the material is subjected to either tension or compression. The property is generally independent of any heat treatment or mechanical treatment that a metal or alloy has received but is quite dependent on the composition of the material.

The elastic modulus is determined by the slope of the elastic portion of the stress-strain curve, which is calculated by choosing any two stress and strain coordinates in the elastic or linear range. As an example, for the curve labeled A in Fig. 4.8, the slope can be calculated by choosing the following two coordinates:

$$\sigma_1 = 150\,\text{MPa}, \varepsilon_1 = 0.005$$

and

$$\sigma_2 = 300\,\text{MPa}, \varepsilon_2 = 0.010$$

The slope is therefore

$$(\sigma_2 - \sigma_1)/(\varepsilon_2 - \varepsilon_1) = (300 - 150)/(0.010 - 0.005)$$
$$30{,}000\,\text{MPa} = 30\,\text{GPa}$$

Stress-strain curves for two hypothetical materials, *A* and *B*, of different compositions are shown in Fig. 4.8. Inspection of the curves shows that for a given stress, *A* is elastically deformed less than *B*, with the result that the elastic modulus for *A* is greater than for *B*. This difference can be demonstrated numerically by calculating the elastic moduli for the two materials subjected to the same stress of 300 MPa. At a stress of 300 MPa, material *A* is strained to 0.01 (1%), and the elastic modulus is as follows:

$$E = 300\text{ MPa} / 0.010 = 30{,}000\text{ MPa} = 30\text{ GPa}$$

On the other hand, material *B* is strained to 0.02 (2%), or twice as much as material *A* for the same stress application. The equation for the elastic modulus for *B* is

$$E = 300\text{ MPa}/0.020 = 15{,}000\text{ MPa} = 15\text{ GPa}$$

TABLE 4.1 Elastic Modulus (GPa) of Selected Dental Materials

Material	Elastic Modulus (GPa)
Enamel	84
Dentin	17
Gold (type IV) alloy	90–95
Amalgam	28–59
Cobalt-chromium removable partial denture alloy	218–224
Feldspathic porcelain	69–70
Lithium disilicate ceramic	95
Zirconia ceramic	200
Resin composite	5–15
Poly (methyl methacrylate)	2.4
Silicone elastomer for maxillofacial prosthesis	0.002–0.003

The fact that material *A* has a steeper slope in the elastic range than material *B* means that a larger force is required to deform material *A* to a given amount than is required for material *B*. From the curves shown in Fig. 4.8, it can be seen that a stress of 300 MPa is required to deform *A* to the same amount elastically, to which *B* is deformed by a stress of 150 MPa. Therefore *A* is stiffer or more rigid than *B*. Conversely, *B* is more flexible than *A*. Materials such as elastomers and other polymers have low values for elastic modulus, whereas many metals and ceramics have much higher values, as shown in Table 4.1.

Poisson's Ratio

During axial loading in tension or compression, there is a simultaneous strain in the axial and transverse, or lateral, directions. Under tensile loading, as a material elongates in the direction of load, there is a reduction in cross section, known as *necking*. Under compressive loading, there is an increase in the cross section. Within the elastic range, the ratio of the lateral to the axial strain is called *Poisson's ratio* (ν). In tensile loading, Poisson's ratio indicates that the reduction in cross section is proportional to the elongation during the elastic deformation. The reduction in cross section continues until the material is fractured. Poisson's ratio is a unitless value because it is the ratio of two strains.

Most rigid materials, such as enamel, dentin, amalgam, and dental composite, exhibit a Poisson's ratio of about 0.3. Brittle substances such as hard gold alloys and dental amalgam show little permanent reduction in cross section during a tensile test. More ductile materials, such as soft gold alloys, which are high in gold content, show a higher degree of reduction in cross-sectional area and higher Poisson's ratios. Rubber has a Poisson's ratio of nearly 0.5. Cork exhibits little lateral expansion under compression and has a Poisson's ratio close to 0. This property has made cork a common material for sealing wine bottles.

Ductility and Malleability

Two significant properties of metals and alloys are ductility and malleability. The *ductility* of a material enables it to be drawn and shaped into wire by means of tension. When tensile forces are applied, the wire is formed by permanent deformation. The *malleability* of a material enables it to be hammered or rolled into thin sheets without fracturing. Malleability comes from the Latin *malleus* or hammer.

A high degree of elongation indicates good malleability and ductility, although some metals show some exceptions to this rule. The reduction in area in a specimen, together with the elongation at the breaking point, is, however, a good indication of the relative ductility of a metal or alloy.

Ductility is a property that has been related to the workability of a material in the mouth (e.g., ability to adjust the margins of a casting). Although ductility is important, the amount of force necessary to cause permanent deformation during the adjustment process (also referred to as "burnishing") must also be considered. A burnishing index has been used to rank the ease of burnishing alloys and is equal to the ductility (elongation) divided by the yield strength.

Gold and silver, which are still used in dentistry, are the most malleable and ductile of the metals, but other metals do not follow the same order for both malleability and ductility. In general, metals tend to be ductile, whereas ceramics tend to be brittle.

Resilience

Resilience is the resistance of a material to permanent deformation. It indicates the amount of energy necessary to deform the material to the proportional limit. Resilience is therefore measured by the area under the elastic portion of the stress-strain curve, as illustrated in Fig. 4.9A.

Resilience has particular importance in the evaluation of orthodontic wires. An example is the amount of work expected from a spring to move a tooth. The units of resilience are m·MN/m^3 (MN/m^2) or m·MPa/m (MPa). The amount of stress and strain at the proportional limit is also of interest because these factors determine the magnitude of the force that can be applied to the tooth and how far the tooth can move before the spring is no longer effective.

Toughness

Toughness, which is the resistance of a material to fracture, is an indication of the amount of energy necessary to cause fracture. The area under the *elastic* and *plastic* portions of a stress-strain curve, as shown in Fig. 4.9B, represents the toughness of a material. The units of toughness are the same as the units of resilience: m·MN/m^3 or m·MPa/m. Toughness represents the energy required to stress the material to the point of fracture. Note that a material can be tough by having a combination of high yield and ultimate strength and moderately high strain at rupture or by having moderately high yield and ultimate strength and a large strain at rupture. Brittle materials tend to have low toughness because little plastic deformation occurs before failure, thus the area under the elastic and plastic regions of the curve is not significantly different from the area under the elastic region alone.

Fracture Toughness

Concepts of fracture mechanics have been applied to a number of problems in dental materials. Fracture mechanics characterizes the behavior of materials with cracks or flaws. Flaws or cracks may arise naturally in a material or nucleate after a time in service. In either case, any defect generally weakens a material, and as a result, sudden fractures can arise at stresses below the yield stress. Sudden, catastrophic fractures typically occur in brittle materials that do not have the ability to plastically deform and redistribute stresses. The field of fracture mechanics analyzes the material behavior during these types of failures.

Two simple examples illustrate the significance of defects in the fracture of materials. Plates of glass or ceramic tiles are often scribed with a diamond or carbide instrument. The purpose of the scribe is to create a defect that propagates when additional stresses are introduced. Both are difficult to break without a scribed line or defect. If the same experiment is performed on a ductile material, the small surface notch has no effect on the force required to break the plate, and the ductile plate can be bent without fracturing (Fig. 4.10). For a brittle material such as glass, no local plastic deformation occurs with fracture, whereas for a ductile material, plastic deformation, such as the ability to bend, occurs without fracture. The ability to be plastically deformed without fracture, or the amount of energy required for fracture, is the *fracture toughness*.

In general, the larger a flaw, the lower the stress needed to cause fracture. This is because the stresses, which would normally be

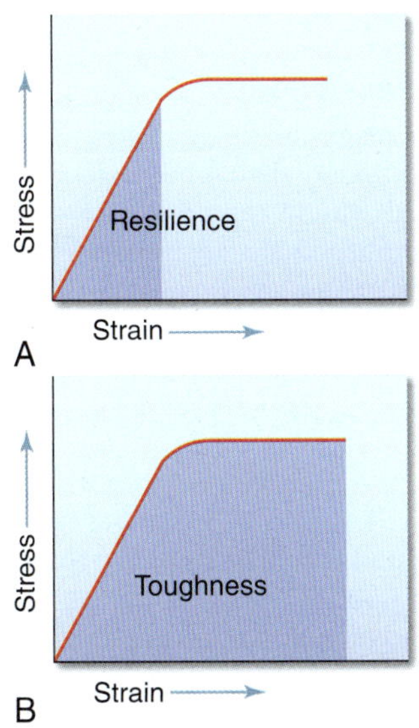

• **Fig. 4.9** Stress-strain curves showing (A) the area indicating the resilience and (B) the area representing the toughness of a material.

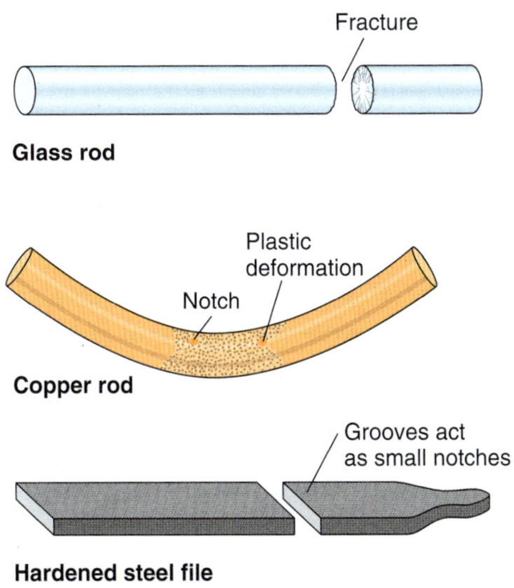

• **Fig. 4.10** Schematic of different types of deformation in brittle (glass, steel file) and ductile (copper) materials of the same diameter and having a notch of the same dimensions. (From Flinn RA, Trojan PK. *Engineering Materials and Their Applications*. Houghton Mifflin; 1981:535).

TABLE 4.2 Approximate Fracture Toughness (K_{IC}) of Selected Dental Materials

Material	K_{IC} (MN·m$^{-3/2}$)
Enamel	0.7–1.3
Dentin	3.1
Amalgam	1.3–1.6
Resin composite	1.0–2.0
Porcelain	0.9–1.0
Dental Ceramic	1.2–5.0

borne by a mass of material, are now concentrated at the tip of the flaw. The ability of a flaw to cause fracture depends on the fracture toughness of the material. Fracture toughness is a material property and is proportional to the energy consumed in plastic deformation.

Fracture toughness (K_{Ic}) has been measured for a number of important restorative materials, including amalgam, acrylic denture base materials, composites, ceramics, orthodontic brackets, cements, and human enamel and dentin. Typical values for composites, ceramics, enamel, and dentin are listed in Table 4.2.

The presence of fillers in polymers substantially increases fracture toughness. The mechanisms of toughening are presumed to be matrix-filler interactions, but these have not yet been established. Similarly, the addition of up to 50% by weight of zirconia to ceramic increases fracture toughness. As with other mechanical properties, aging or storage in a simulated oral environment or at elevated temperatures can decrease fracture toughness, but there is no agreement on this in the literature. Attempts to correlate fracture toughness with wear resistance have had mixed results. Fracture toughness is not a reliable predictor of the wear of restorative materials.

Properties and Stress-Strain Curves

The shape of a stress-strain curve and the magnitudes of the stress and strain allow the classification of materials with respect to their general properties. The idealized stress-strain curves in Fig. 4.11 represent materials with various combinations of physical properties. For example, materials *1* to *4* have high stiffness, materials *1, 2, 5,* and *6* have high strength, and materials *1, 3, 5,* and *7* have high ductility. If the only requirement for an application is stiffness, materials *1* to *4* are all satisfactory. However, if the requirements are both stiffness and strength, only materials *1* and *2* are acceptable. If the requirements are to also include ductility, the choice would be limited to material *1*. The properties of stiffness, strength, and ductility are independent, and materials may exhibit various combinations of these three properties.

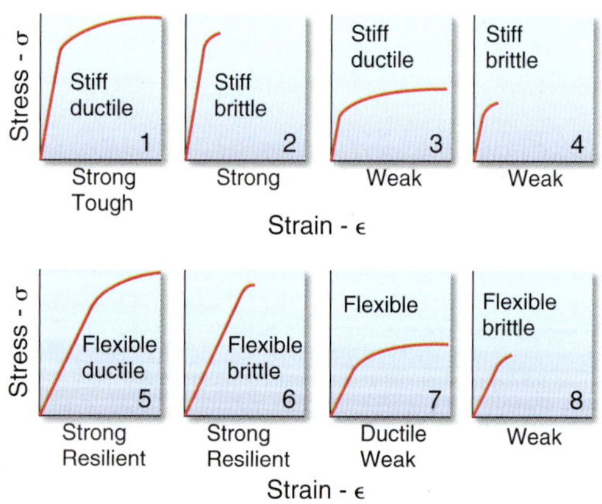

• **Fig. 4.11** Stress-strain curves for materials with various combinations of properties.

Tensile Properties of Brittle Materials

Many restorative materials, including dental amalgam, cements, ceramics, plaster, and stone, are much weaker in tension than in compression. This means cavity preparation design requirements for amalgams and ceramics, for example, are different than for ductile materials, such as metal alloys. One example is the amount of occlusal reduction necessary for ductile versus brittle materials. For brittle materials, such as ceramics, the occlusal reduction needs to be greater than for ductile materials, such as gold alloys. This is because ceramics require a larger cross-sectional area to present the same resistance as metals. Also, for that reason, the margins of preparation can be beveled for metal restorations but cannot be beveled for ceramic restorations.

Viscoelasticity

The mechanical properties of many dental materials, such as alginate, elastomeric impression materials, waxes, amalgam, polymers, bone, dentin, oral mucosa, and periodontal ligaments, depend on how fast they are loaded. For these materials, increasing the loading (strain) rate produces a different stress-strain curve with higher rates, giving higher values for the elastic modulus, proportional limit, and ultimate strength. Materials that have mechanical properties independent of loading rate are termed *elastic*. In these materials, strain occurs when the load is applied. Other materials exhibit a lag in response when a load is applied. This time lag is referred to as a *viscous response*. Materials that have mechanical properties dependent on loading rate and exhibit both elastic and viscous behavior are termed *viscoelastic*. These materials have characteristics of an elastic solid and a viscous fluid. The properties of an elastic solid were previously discussed in detail. Before viscoelastic materials and their properties are presented, fluid behavior and viscosity are reviewed in the following section.

Fluid Behavior and Viscosity

In addition to the many solid dental materials that exhibit some fluid characteristics, many dental materials, such as cements and impression materials, are in the fluid state when formed. Therefore fluid (viscous) phenomena are important. Viscosity (η) is the resistance of a fluid to flow and is equal to the shear stress divided by the shear strain rate, or

$$\eta = \tau / [d\varepsilon / dt]$$

When a cement or impression material sets, the viscosity increases, making it less viscous and more solidlike. The units of viscosity are poise, p (1 p = 0.1 Pa·s = 0.1 N·s/m^2), but often data are reported in centipoise, cp (100 cp = 1 p).

Rearranging the equation for viscosity, we see that fluid behavior can be described in terms of stress and strain, just like elastic solids.

$$\tau = \eta [d\varepsilon / dt]$$

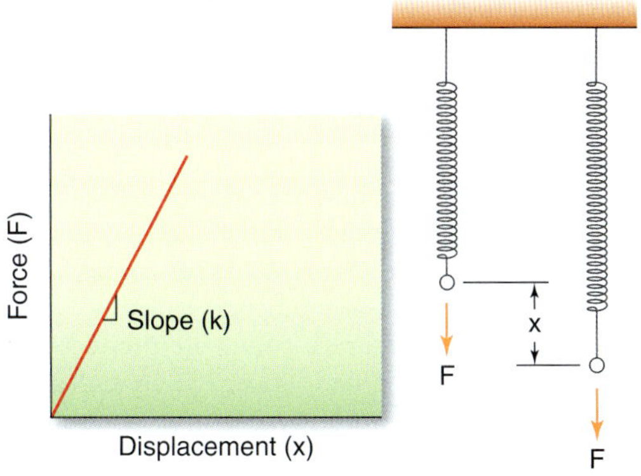

• **Fig. 4.12** Force versus displacement of a spring, which can be used to model the elastic response of a solid. (From Park JB. *Biomaterials Science and Engineering*. Plenum Press; 1984:26).

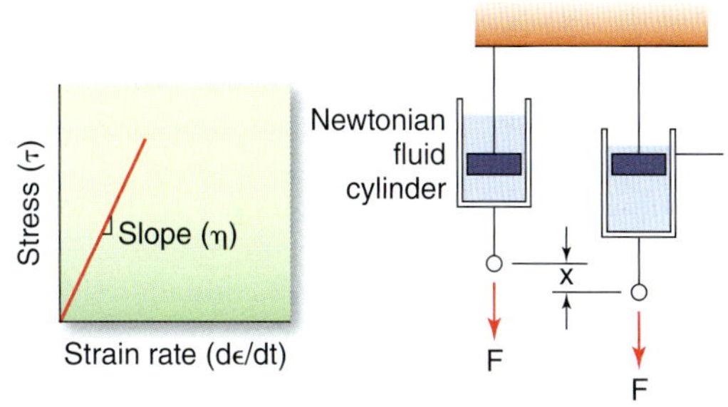

• **Fig. 4.13** Stress versus strain rate for a dashpot, which can be used to model the response of a viscous fluid. (From Park JB. *Biomaterials Science and Engineering*. Plenum Press; 1984:26).

In the case of an elastic solid, stress (σ) is proportional to strain (ε), with the constant of proportionality being the modulus of elasticity (*E*). The aforementioned equation indicates a similar situation for a viscous fluid, where the stress (shear) is proportional to the strain rate, and the constant of proportionality is the viscosity. The stress is therefore time dependent because it is a function of the strain rate or rate of loading. To better comprehend the concept of strain rate dependence, consider two limiting cases: rapid and slow deformation. A material pulled extremely fast ($dt \rightarrow 0$) results in an infinitely high stress, whereas a material pulled infinitesimally slow results in a stress of zero. This concept will be important in understanding stress relaxation and delayed gelation phenomena, explored later in this chapter. The behavior of elastic solids and viscous fluids can be understood by studying simple mechanical models. An elastic solid can be viewed as a spring (Fig. 4.12). When the spring is stretched by force, *F*, it displaces a distance, *x*. The applied force and resultant displacement are proportional, and the constant of proportionality is the spring constant, *k*. Therefore, according to Hooke's law,

$$F = kx$$

Note that this relation is equivalent to the equation presented in the Stress-Strain Curves section of this chapter:

$$\sigma = E\varepsilon$$

Also, note that the model of an elastic element does not involve time. The spring acts instantaneously when stretched. In other words, an elastic solid is independent of the loading rate.

A viscous fluid can be viewed as a dashpot or a piston moving through a viscous fluid (Fig. 4.13). When the fluid-filled cylinder is pulled, the rate of strain ($d\varepsilon/dt$) is proportional to the stress (τ), and the constant of proportionality is the viscosity of the fluid (π).

Although the viscosity of a fluid is proportional to the shear rate, the proportionality differs for different fluids. Fluids may be classified as Newtonian, pseudoplastic, or dilatant depending on how their viscosity varies with shear rate, as shown in Fig. 4.14. The viscosity of a Newtonian fluid is constant and independent of shear rate. Some dental cements and impression materials are Newtonian. The viscosity of a pseudoplastic fluid decreases with increasing shear rate. Monophase elastomeric impression materials are pseudoplastic. When subjected to low shear while an impression material is loaded in a tray in preparation for placing it into

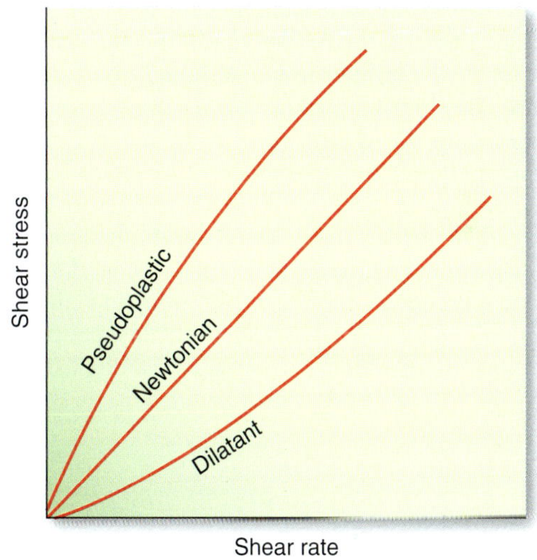

• **Fig. 4.14** Shear diagrams of Newtonian, pseudoplastic, and dilatant liquids. The viscosity is shown by the slope of the curve at a given shear rate.

the mouth, these impression materials have a high viscosity and stay in place without flowing. These materials, however, can also be used in a syringe because at the higher shear rates encountered as they pass through the syringe tip, the viscosity decreases by as much as tenfold. This characteristic is sometimes referred to as *thixotropy*, although that term actually describes the change in viscosity of a material with time. The tomato-based food condiment ketchup is also pseudoplastic, which makes it difficult to remove from a bottle. Shaking the bottle or rapping the side of the bottle increases its shear rate, decreases its viscosity, and improves its pourability. The viscosity of a dilatant fluid increases with increasing shear rate. Examples of dilatant fluids in dentistry include the fluid denture base resins.

Viscoelastic Materials

For viscoelastic materials, the strain rate can alter the stress-strain properties. The tear strength of alginate impression material, for example, is increased about four times when the rate of loading is increased from 2.5 cm/min to 25 cm/min. Alginate impressions should therefore be removed from the mouth quickly to improve their tear resistance. Another example of strain-rate dependence is the elastic modulus of dental amalgam, which is 21 GPa at slow rates of loading and 62 GPa at high rates of loading. A viscoelastic material therefore may have widely different mechanical properties depending on the rate of load application, and for these materials, it is particularly important to specify the loading rate with the test results.

Materials that have properties dependent on the strain rate are better characterized by relating stress or strain as a function of time. Two properties of importance to viscoelastic materials are stress relaxation and creep. *Stress relaxation* is the reduction in stress in a material subjected to constant strain, whereas *creep* is the increase in strain in a material under constant stress. Dynamic creep occurs when a material undergoes an increase in strain due to repeated loading.

As an example of stress relaxation, consider how the load-time curves at constant deformation are important in the evaluation of orthodontic elastic bands. The decrease in load (or force) with time for rubber and plastic bands of the same size at a constant extension of 95 mm is shown in Fig. 4.15. The initial force was much greater with the plastic band, but the decrease in force with time was much less for the rubber band. Therefore, plastic bands are useful for applying high forces, although the force decreases rapidly with time, whereas rubber bands apply lower forces, but the force decreases slowly with time in the mouth; rubber bands are therefore useful for applying more sustained loads.

The importance of creep can be seen by interpretation of the data in Fig. 4.16, which shows creep curves for low- and high-copper amalgam. For a given load at a given time, the low-copper amalgam has a greater strain. The implications and clinical importance of this are that the greater creep in the low-copper amalgam makes it more susceptible to strain accumulation and fracture, and also marginal breakdown, which can lead to secondary decay. The high creep behavior of low-copper amalgam contributed to its decline in popularity.

Creep Compliance

A creep curve yields insight into the relative elastic, viscous, and inelastic response of a viscoelastic material; such curves can be interpreted in terms of the molecular structure of the associated materials, which have structures that function as elastic, viscous, and inelastic elements. Creep recovery curves are produced from data collected during removal of a load (Fig. 4.17). In such a curve, after the load is removed, there is an instantaneous drop in strain and slower strain decay to some steady-state strain value, which may be nonzero. The instantaneous drop in strain represents the recovery of elastic strain. The slower recovery represents the anelastic strain, and the remaining permanent strain represents the viscous strain. A family of creep curves can be determined by using different loads. A more useful way of presenting these data is by calculating the creep compliance. *Creep compliance* (J_t) is defined as strain divided by stress at a given time. Once a creep curve is obtained, a corresponding creep compliance curve can be calculated. The creep compliance curve shown in Fig. 4.18 is characterized by the following equation:

$$J_t = J_0 + J_R + (t/\eta)$$

where J_0 is the instantaneous elastic compliance, J_R is the retarded elastic (inelastic) compliance, and t/η represents the

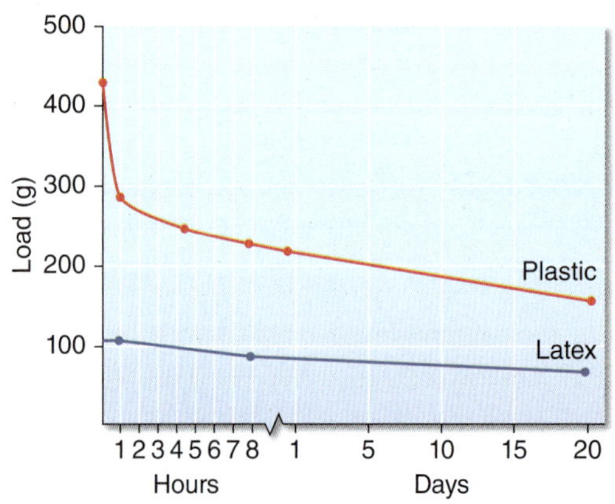

• **Fig. 4.15** Decrease in load of latex rubber and plastic bands as a function of time at a constant extension of 95 mm. (From Craig RG, ed. *Dental Materials: A Problem-Oriented Approach*. Mosby; 1978).

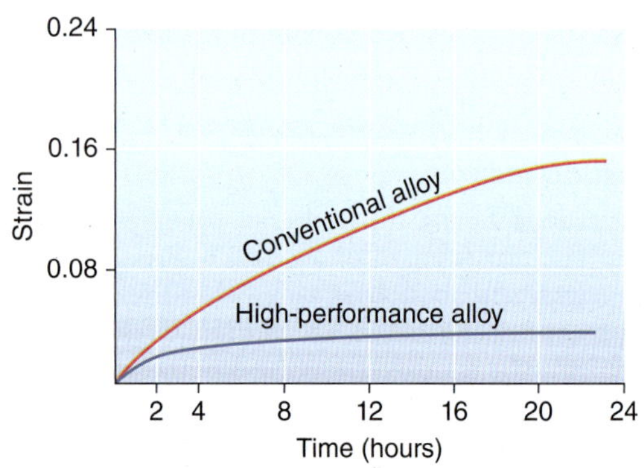

• **Fig. 4.16** Creep curves for conventional (low-copper) and high-performance (high-copper) amalgams. (From O'Brien WJ. *Dental Materials: Properties and Selection*. Quintessence; 1989:25).

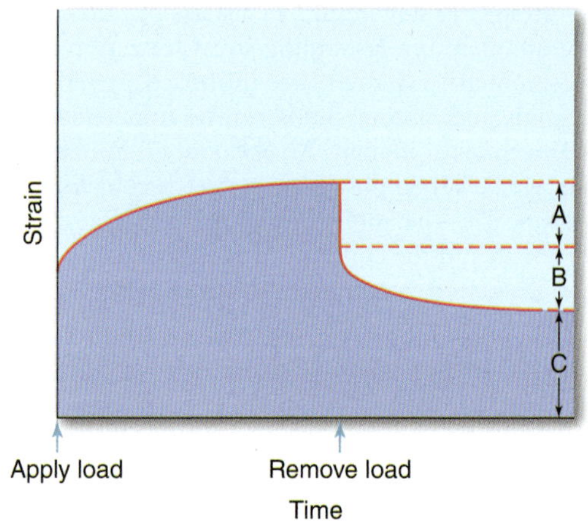

• **Fig. 4.17** Creep recovery curve showing (A) elastic, (B) anelastic, and (C) viscous strain.

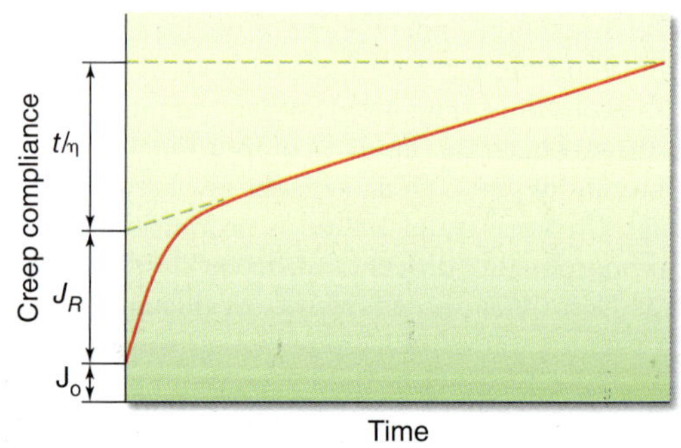

• **Fig. 4.18** Creep compliance versus time for a viscoelastic material. (Modified from Duran RL, Powers JM, Craig RG. Viscoelastic and dynamic properties of soft liners and tissue conditioners. *J Dent Res*. 1979;58(8):1801–1807).

viscous response at time t for a viscosity η. The strain associated with J_0 and J_R is completely recoverable after the load is removed; however, the strain associated with J_R is not recovered immediately but requires some finite time. The strain associated with t/η is not recovered and represents a permanent deformation. If a single creep compliance curve is calculated from a family of creep curves determined at different loads, the material is said to be linearly viscoelastic. In this case, the viscoelastic qualities can be described concisely by a single curve.

The creep compliance curve therefore permits an estimate of the relative amount of elastic, inelastic, and viscous behavior of a material. J_0 indicates the flexibility and initial recovery after deformation, J_R the amount of delayed recovery that can be expected, and t/η the magnitude of permanent deformation to be expected. Creep compliance curves for elastomeric impression materials are shown in Chapter 11.

Dynamic Mechanical Properties

Although static properties can often be related to the function of a material under dynamic conditions, there are limitations to using static properties to estimate the properties of materials subjected to dynamic loading. *Static testing* refers to continuous application of force at slow rates of loading, whereas *dynamic testing* involves cyclic loading or loading at high rates (*impact*). Dynamic methods, including a forced oscillation technique used to determine dynamic modulus and a torsion pendulum used for impact testing, have been used to study viscoelastic materials such as dental polymers. Ultrasonic techniques have been used to determine elastic constants of viscoelastic materials such as dentin. Impact testing has been applied primarily to brittle dental materials.

Dynamic Modulus

The *dynamic modulus* (E_D) is defined as the ratio of stress to strain for small cyclical deformations at a given frequency and at a particular point on the stress-strain curve. When measured in a dynamic oscillation instrument, the dynamic modulus is computed by

$$E_D = mqp^2$$

where m is the mass of the loading element, q is the height divided by twice the area of the cylindrical specimen, and p is the angular frequency of the vibrations.

In general, elastic modulus calculated from dynamic testing is higher than when calculated from static testing. For ideal elastic materials subjected to an oscillatory strain, the sinusoidal wave of the resultant stress matches perfectly the strain wave; it is said then that stress and strain are "in phase" (Fig. 4.19B) or that there is no energy lost to the environment because all the energy is used to provide a deformation. For liquids, the strain response lags the stress in time, that is, they are out of phase by the phase angle, δ (Fig. 4.19A). For Newtonian fluids (ideal liquids), the phase lag equals the greatest possible angle (δ = 90 degrees) between stress and strain waves for any given cycle. As discussed earlier, from the stress-strain curves, a complex modulus (E^*) can be calculated. The complex modulus therefore is the ratio of the stress amplitude to the strain amplitude and represents the stiffness of the material.

Most real materials subjected to oscillatory strain behave somewhere in between a perfectly elastic and perfectly plastic material, and in those cases, by resolving the complex modulus (E^*) into an "in-phase" elastic component (called *storage modulus*, or E') and an "out-of-phase" viscous component (called *loss modulus*, or E''), it is possible to gain insight into the elastic and viscous components, respectively (see Fig. 4.19A). They correlate according to the mathematical relationship shown in Fig. 4.19C, where $E' = E^*$ sin δ and $E'' = E^*$ cos δ. One useful concept that arises is the loss

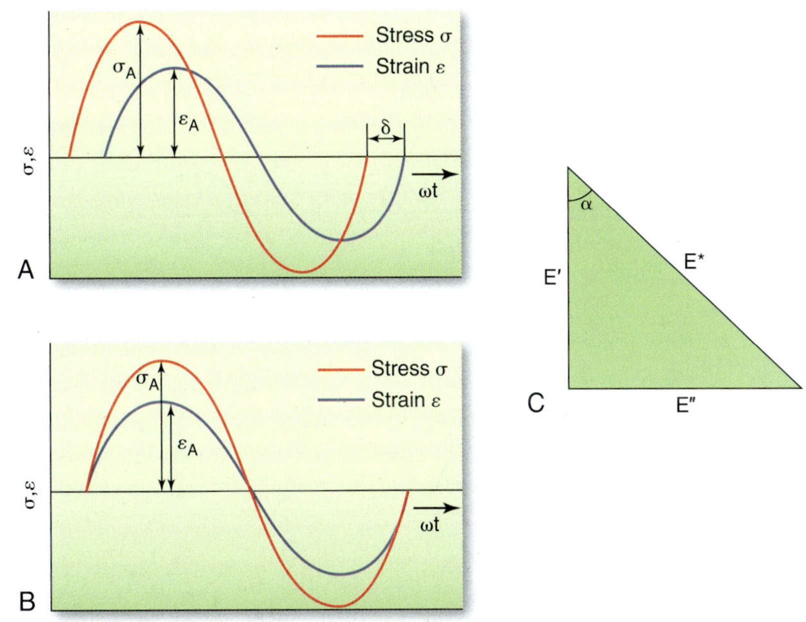

• **Fig. 4.19** Sinusoidal oscillation and response of (A) a liquid and (B) a purely elastic material; σ is the stress, ε is the strain, ωt is the frequency, and δ is the phase angle. (C) Mathematical correlation of complex *(E*)*, storage *(E')*, and loss *(E")* moduli.

TABLE 4.3 Values of Dynamic Modulus and Dynamic Resilience as a Function of Temperature for Some Dental Elastomers

Material	Temperature (°C)	Dynamic Modulus (MPa)	Dynamic Resilience (%)
Maxillofacial Materials			
Polyurethane	−15	5.98	15.0
	37	3.06	19.9
Polyvinylchloride	−15	12.2	6.0
	37	2.51	19.6
Silicone elastomer	−15	2.84	16.0
	37	2.36	23.2
Polyvinylacetate-Polyethylene Mouth Protector			
New	37	9.39	23.4
Worn	37	7.23	20.2

factor tan δ (calculated as $\tan \delta = E'/E''$). This relationship allows us to determine whether a material presents a predominantly elastic or viscous response when subjected to load while in service.

In conjunction with the dynamic modulus, values of internal friction and dynamic resilience can be determined. For example, cyclical stretching or compression of an elastomer results in irreversibly lost energy that is exhibited as heat. The internal friction of an elastomer is comparable with the viscosity of a liquid. The value of internal friction is necessary to calculate the *dynamic resilience*, which is the ratio of energy lost to energy expended.

The dynamic modulus and dynamic resilience of some dental elastomers are listed in Table 4.3. These properties are affected by temperature (−15°C to 37°C) for some maxillofacial elastomers. As shown in Table 4.3, the dynamic modulus decreases, and the dynamic resilience increases as the temperature increases. As a tangible example, the dynamic resilience of a polymer used for an athletic mouth protector is a measure of the ability of the material to absorb energy from a blow and thereby protect the oral structures.

Surface Mechanical Properties

In our discussion so far, we have introduced and discussed mechanical properties that are mainly dependent on the bulk characteristics of a material. In this section, mechanical properties that are more a function of the surface condition of a material are presented. In particular, the concepts of hardness, friction, and wear are summarized.

Hardness

Hardness may be broadly defined as the resistance to permanent surface indentation or penetration. Formulating a more rigorous definition of hardness is difficult because any test method will, at a microscopic level, involve complex surface morphologies and stresses in the test material, thereby involving a variety of qualities in any single hardness test. Despite this condition, the most common concept of hard and soft substances is their relative resistance to indentation. Hardness is therefore a measure of the resistance to plastic deformation and is measured as a force per unit area of indentation (Fig. 4.20).

Based on this definition of hardness, it is clear why this property is so important to dentistry. Hardness influences ease of

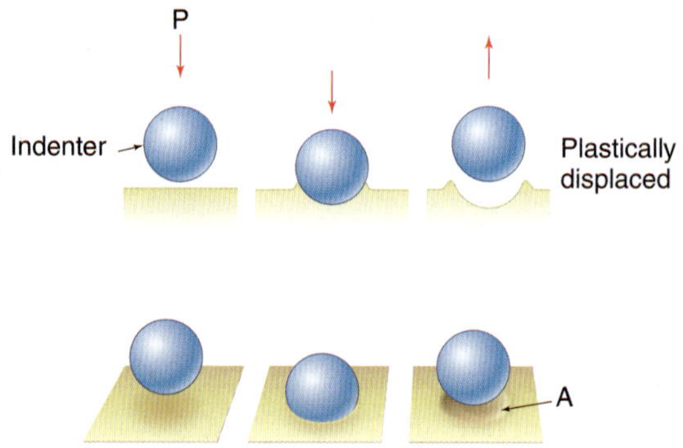

• **Fig. 4.20** Schematic representation of surface changes from indenter in Rockwell hardness test. *P*, Normal load; *A*, area of plastic deformation. (From Park JB. *Biomaterials Science and Engineering*. Plenum Press; 1984:18).

cutting, finishing, and polishing an object and its resistance to in-service scratching. Finishing or polishing a structure is important for aesthetic purposes, and, as discussed previously, scratches can compromise fatigue strength and lead to premature failure.

Some of the most common methods of testing the hardness of restorative materials are the Brinell, Knoop, Vickers, Rockwell, Barcol, and Shore A hardness tests. Each of these tests differs slightly in the indenter used and in the calculation of hardness. Each presents certain advantages and disadvantages. They have a common quality, however, in that each depends on the penetration of some relatively small, symmetrically shaped indenter into the surface of the material being tested. Based on size scale, tests such as Knoop and Vickers are typically referred to as microindentation methods. The size scale can become even more resolved with nanoindentation, where the size of the indent is on the nanoscale. The choice of a hardness test depends on the material of interest, the expected hardness range, and the desired degree of localization.

Friction

Friction is the resistance between contacting bodies when one moves relative to another (Fig. 4.21). A restraining force that resists movement is the (static) frictional force and results from

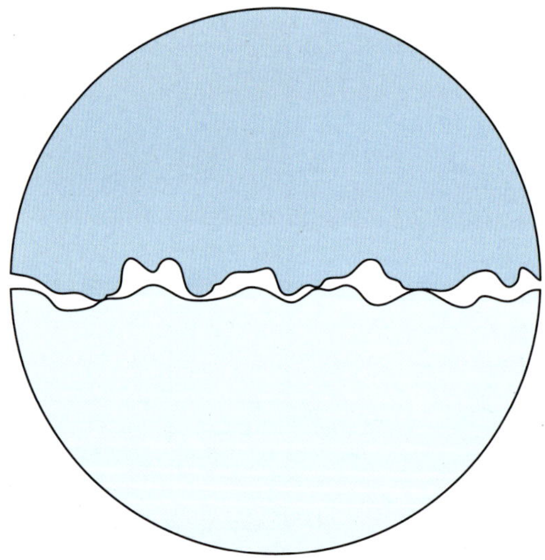

• **Fig. 4.21** Microscopic area of contact between two objects. The frictional force, which resists motion, is proportional to the normal force and the coefficient of friction.

the molecules of the two objects bonding where their surfaces are in close contact. The frictional force, F_s, is proportional to the normal force (F_n) between the surfaces and the (static) coefficient of friction (μ_s):

$$F_S = \mu_S F_N$$

The coefficient of friction varies between 0 and 1 and is a function of the two materials in contact, their composition, surface finish, and lubrication. Similar materials in contact have a greater coefficient of friction, and if a lubricating medium exists at the interface, the coefficient of friction is reduced.

Motion is possible when the applied force is greater than F_s. Once motion occurs, molecular bonds are made and broken, and microscopic pieces break off from the surfaces. With motion, a sliding or kinetic friction is produced, and the force of kinetic friction opposes the motion:

$$F_k = \mu_k F_N$$

Frictional behavior therefore arises from surfaces that, because of microroughness, have a small real contact area (see Fig. 4.21). These small surface areas result in high contact stresses, which lead to local yielding or permanent deformation. The resistance to shear failure of the junctions results in the frictional force. When static friction is overcome, and relative motion takes place, it is accompanied by the modification of the interface through kinetic friction and wear.

An example of the importance of friction in dentistry lies in the concept of sliding mechanics used in orthodontics. A known and controlled frictional force is required when an orthodontic wire is slid through a bracket. Combinations of different materials result in different frictional forces. Friction is also an important consideration when dissimilar restorative materials contact and slide against each other in the oral cavity, such as in protrusive or working movements of the mandible.

Wear

Wear is a loss of material resulting from removal and relocation of materials through the contact of two or more materials. When two solid materials are in contact, they touch only at the tips of their most protruding asperities (Fig. 4.22). Wear is usually undesirable, but under controlled conditions during finishing and polishing, controlled wear can be very useful.

Several factors make wear of biomaterials unique. Most important, wear can produce particles that can elicit an inflammatory response. The wear process can also produce shape changes in the object that can affect function. For example, wear of teeth and restorative materials is characterized by the loss of the original anatomical form of the material. Wear may result from mechanical, physiological, or pathological conditions. Normal mastication may cause attrition of tooth structure or materials. Bruxism is an example of a pathological form of wear in which clenching and grinding of teeth produce occlusal and incisal wear. Abrasive wear occurs when excessively abrasive toothpaste and hard toothbrush bristles are used when brushing teeth.

Wear is a function of a number of material and environmental factors, including the characteristics of wearing surfaces (i.e., inhomogeneity, crystal orientation, phases, and inclusions present); the microscopic contact; interaction between sliding surfaces (i.e., elevated stress, temperature, and flow at contact points, leading to localized yielding, melting, and hardening); lubrication;

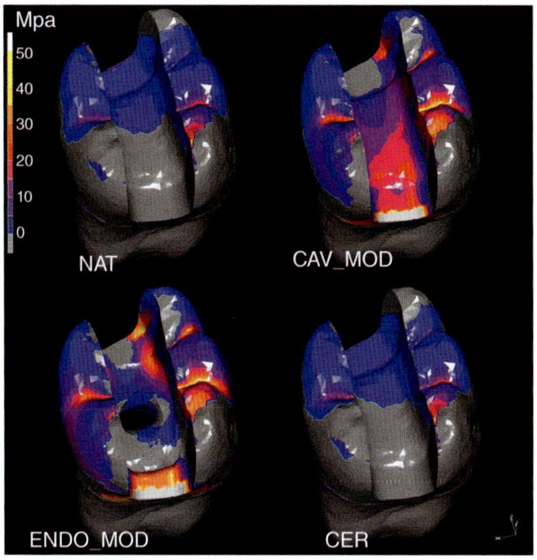

• **Fig. 4.22** Stress distribution in a finite element model of a molar with a 100-N occlusal load. (From Magne P. Efficient 3D finite element analysis of dental restorative procedures using micro-CT data. *Dent Mater.* 2007;23:539–548).

and different material combinations. In general, wear is a function of opposing materials and the interface between them. The presence of a lubricating film, such as saliva, separates surfaces during relative motion and reduces frictional forces and wear.

In general, there are four types of wear: (1) adhesive wear, (2) corrosive wear, (3) surface fatigue wear, and (4) abrasive wear. Adhesive wear is characterized by the formation and disruption of microjunctions. Microregions are pulled from one object and transferred to the other. Abrasive wear involves a harder material cutting or plowing into a softer material. There can be two types of abrasive wear: two- and three-body abrasive wear. This type of wear can be minimized if surfaces are smooth and hard and if third-party particles are kept off the surfaces. Corrosive wear is secondary to physical removal of a protective layer and is therefore related to the chemical activity of the wear surfaces. The sliding action of the surfaces accelerates corrosion. In surface fatigue wear, asperities or free particles with small areas of contact contribute to high localized stresses and produce surface or subsurface cracks. Particles break off under cyclic loading and sliding.

In general, metals are susceptible to adhesive, corrosive, and three-body wear, whereas polymers are susceptible to abrasive and fatigue wear.

The Colloidal State

The term *colloid* is used to describe a *state* of matter rather than a *kind* of matter. The main characteristic of colloidal materials is their high degree of microsegmentation. These fine particles also have certain physical properties, such as electrical charges and surface energies, that control the characteristics of the colloids. Particle size alone does not adequately define colloids.

Nature of Colloids

Substances are called *colloids* when they consist of two or more phases, with the units of at least one of the phases having a dimension slightly greater than simple molecular size. Although the range of size is somewhat arbitrary, it is usually recognized as being approximately 1 to 500 nm in maximum dimension. Thus colloidal systems can be fine dispersions, gels, films, emulsions, or foams. In other words, the colloidal state represents a highly dispersed system of fine particles of one phase in another, and a characteristic property of the dispersed phase is an enormous surface area. This is true whether a dispersed phase of oil droplets in an emulsion or a finely divided solid suspended in a liquid is considered. This increase in surface area gives rise to a corresponding increase in surface energy and surface reactions. Not only is the surface energy important, but the interface between the two phases also imparts important and characteristic properties to the system.

Except for a dispersion of a gas in a gas, which is a true solution, each of the three forms of matter—gas, liquid, and solid—may be dispersed as colloidal particles in the other and in itself as well. The dispersed phase, which may be in the form of a gas, liquid, or solid, may also exist in a variety of conditions. Some examples of these dispersed phases are (1) colloidal silica as a filler in resin composites, (2) colloidal silica in water to be mixed with high-strength dental stone to improve abrasion resistance, (3) droplets of oil in water used during steam sterilization to prevent rusting of dental instruments, (4) fillers used in elastomeric impression materials to control such properties as viscosity, and (5) agglomerates of detergent molecules in water that serve as wetting agents for wax patterns.

Typical Colloid Systems

The distinction between a sol and a gel is important because several of each are found in dental applications. A sol resembles a solution, but it is made up of colloidal particles dispersed in a liquid. When a sol is chilled or caused to react by the addition of suitable chemicals, it may be transformed into a gel. In the gel form, the system takes on a semisolid, or jellylike, quality.

The liquid phase of either a sol or a gel is usually water but may be some organic liquid, such as alcohol. Systems having water as one component are described as *hydrosols* or *hydrogels*. A more general term might be *hydrocolloid*, which is often used in dentistry to describe the alginate gels used as flexible impression materials. A general term to describe a system having an organic liquid as one component would be *organosol* or *organogel*.

Gels possess an entangled framework of solid colloidal particles in which liquid is trapped in the interstices and held by capillarity. Such a gel has some degree of rigidity, depending on the extent of the structural solids present. One example is the alginate hydrocolloid impression material.

Gels that are formed with water are hydrophilic (water-loving) in character and tend to imbibe large quantities of water if allowed to stand submerged. The imbibition is accompanied by swelling and a change in physical dimensions. In dry air, the gel loses water to the atmosphere, with an accompanying shrinkage. Such changes may be observed readily in alginate gels.

Diffusion Through Membranes and Osmotic Pressure

Osmotic pressure is the pressure developed by diffusion of a liquid or solvent through a membrane. The solvent passes from the dilute to the more concentrated solution through the membrane, separating the two solutions. The presence of dissolved material in a solvent lowers the escaping tendency of the solvent molecules; the greater the concentration, the more the escaping tendency is lowered. Accordingly, the solvent will diffuse or pass through a membrane to a region of greater concentration, thus diluting the concentration of the solution.

Osmotic pressure is a concept that has been used to explain the hypersensitivity of dentin. The change in pressure in carious, exposed dentin from contact with saliva or concentrated solutions causes diffusion throughout the structure that increases or decreases the pressure on the sensory system.

Just as diffusion through membranes is important, so is the diffusion from a substance of a given concentration to that of another concentration, which is important in many materials in dentistry. Salts and dyes diffuse through human dentin. Stains and discoloring agents diffuse through polymeric restorative materials. Diffusion of salts and acids through some cavity liners is a potential problem.

Adsorption, Absorption, and Sorption

In the adsorption process, a liquid or gas adheres to the surface of the solid or liquid firmly by the attachment of molecules, thus reducing their surface free energy. In a physical sense, if the two substances are alike, as, for example, two pieces of the same metal in the solid state pressed closely together, the mass is said to *cohere*. When a dissimilar substance, such as a gas or liquid, is in intimate contact with the surface of the solid, it is said to *adhere* to the surface. The process of adsorption or adhesion to the surface of a substance is important in the wetting process, in which the substance is coated or wetted with a foreign substance, such as a liquid. The degree to which saliva, for example, will wet or adhere to the enamel surface of a tooth depends on the tendency for surface adsorption. A substance that is readily wetted on the surface by water, as is glass or porcelain or tooth enamel, is considered to have adsorbed on its surface a layer of water molecules. When a wet, human enamel surface is desiccated, the first water to evaporate is bulk water, leaving physically and chemically adsorbed water. Considerable heat is required to remove physically adsorbed water, and even higher temperatures are needed to remove chemically adsorbed water. Thus any attempt to bond a restorative material to enamel must consider that adhesion will be to adsorbed water and not hydroxyapatite. High-energy surfaces such as metals will adsorb molecules more readily than low-energy surfaces such as waxes; oxides have intermediate surface energies.

The process of adsorption differs somewhat from the process of absorption. In the process of absorption, the substance absorbed penetrates into the solid material by a diffusion process, and the process is characterized by concentration of molecules at the surface.

In instances in which both adsorption and absorption are known to exist and it is not clear which process predominates, the whole process is known as *sorption*. In measurement of the moisture content of dental resins, the process is described as one of sorption of moisture by the resin.

Numerous examples of these processes are found in the use of various restorative dental materials. The process of absorption of water by alginate impression materials is particularly important to its stability. When the quantity of liquid absorbed into a substance is relatively large, there is likely to be an accompanying swelling of the absorbent.

Surface Tension and Wetting

Surface tension is measured in terms of force (dynes) per centimeter of the surface of liquid. In the case of water at 20°C, the value is 72.8 dynes/cm. At the same temperature, benzene has a value of 29 dynes/cm; alcohol, 22 dynes/cm; and ether, 17 dynes/cm. By contrast, mercury at 20°C has a surface tension of 465 dynes/cm. The values for each of these substances are influenced by factors such as temperature and purity. In general, there is a reduction in surface tension of all liquids as the temperature is increased. For example, the surface tension of water (in dynes/cm) is 76 at 0°C, 72 at 25°C, 68 at 50°C, and 59 at 100°C.

The surface tension of liquids is also reduced by the presence of impurities, some of which are exceedingly effective. Detergents, such as sodium lauryl sulfate, or the ingredients of soaps, including sodium stearate or sodium oleate, which have long hydrocarbon chains attached to hydrophilic groups (such as COONa), are particularly effective in reducing the surface tension of water.

These surface-active agents affect the surface tension by concentrating at the liquid-air interface or other interfaces or surfaces. As these molecules occupy surface positions in the water-air surface, they displace surface water molecules, thus reducing the cohesive force between water molecules over the surface area because the cohesion between water and surface-active agent is less than that between water and water. This effect is demonstrated in Fig. 4.23, which represents two drops placed on wax, one of which is water and the other water with detergent. The presence of the surface-active agent molecules in the surface layer reduces the pull on the surface molecules toward the liquid mass. This reduces the surface tension to increase wetting. The soap molecules are oriented so that the hydrophilic end is in the water, and the hydrophobic (hydrocarbon) end is oriented toward the wax or air.

The increased wettability of solids with liquids of reduced surface tension is important in numerous dental applications. The wetting power of a liquid is represented by its tendency to spread on the surface of the solid. When pouring a hydrophobic, polymeric impression material with plaster or stone (gypsum), the gypsum wets the impression to reproduce the details recorded in the impression. Hydrophobic impressions are not well wetted by gypsum, so a dilute solution of some wetting agent (such as 0.01% aerosol) is sprayed on the impression in small quantities to aid in the spreading of the gypsum. Without adequate wetting, the gypsum will not flow over the surface of the impression and replicate fine detail.

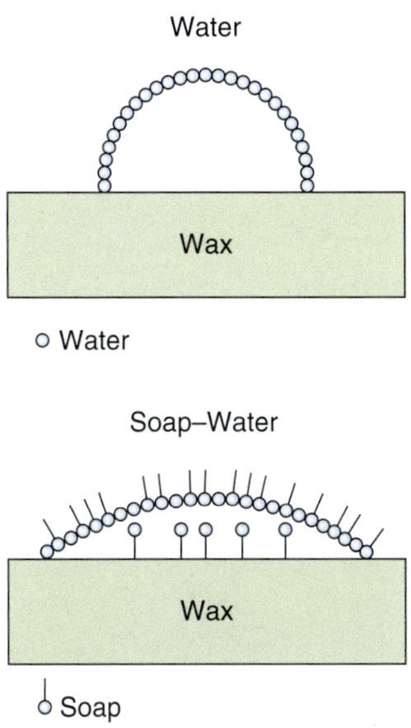

• **Fig. 4.23** Spreading of pure water *(top)* and water containing soap molecules on wax *(bottom)*.

Much can be learned about the spreading of liquids on solids, or the tendency for wetting surfaces, by measuring the angle of contact between the liquid and the solid surface. The angles of contact for different liquid droplets on a plane glass surface are illustrated in Fig. 4.24. The contact angle results from a balance of surface and interfacial energies. The greater the tendency to wet the surface, the lower the contact angle until complete wetting occurs at an angle equal to zero.

Contact angles of water and saliva in dental materials: The determination of contact angle is important in a number of clinically relevant situations. For example, the contact angle of water and saliva on complete denture plastics relates to the retention of the denture. The contact angle and the tendency of a drop of water to spread on paraffin wax and methyl methacrylate are shown for comparison in Fig. 4.25. The contact angle of saliva freshly applied to an acrylic surface is similar to the one formed by water.

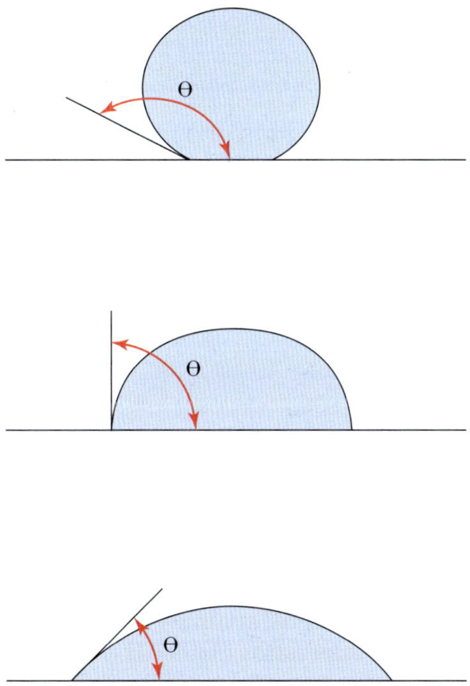

• **Fig. 4.24** Relation of contact angle to the spreading or wetting of a liquid on a solid.

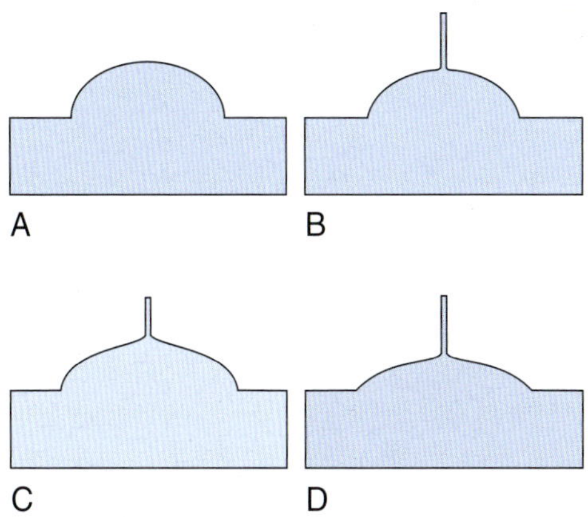

• **Fig. 4.25** Diagrams show the contact angle formed by a drop of water or saliva on wax and acrylic plastic. (A) Water on wax. (B) Water on plastic. (C) Fresh saliva on plastic. (D) Saliva after remaining in contact with plastic.

This angle drops if saliva is allowed to stand overnight in contact with the plastic material, which indicates that the surface wetting is somewhat improved. Table 4.4 gives contact angle values for water on selected materials.

Contact angles can also provide important information regarding the wettability of dental elastomeric materials, defining the ease of pouring a mix of dental stone and water to produce a model. The contact angles of water on various dental elastomeric impression materials are listed in Table 4.5, along with the castability of an impression of a very critical comb-like model. Surfactants can be added to the surface to artificially decrease the contact angle.

Contact angles between metals during casting, soldering, and amalgamation: The surface tension of metals is relatively high in comparison with that of other liquids because of the greater cohesive forces between the liquid metal atoms in the liquid-air surface compared to water. The surface tension of most metals, except mercury, cannot be measured at room temperature because of their high melting points. Typical values of a few metals are included in Table 4.6. This is important because it defines the ease of spreading the molten metal or alloy on the investment material surface during casting and determines the accuracy and reproduction of detail in the final restoration. The same applies to the spreading of molten flux on hot metal during melting or soldering operations. If the contact angle of the solder is too great, it will not penetrate into the fine detail of the structures to be joined, compromising adhesion.

TABLE 4.4 Contact Angles of Water on Solids at 27°C

Solid	Advancing Angle (degrees)
Acrylic polymer	74
Teflon	110
Glass	14
Amalgam	77
Composite filling material	51

Modified from O'Brien WJ. *Capillary Penetration of Liquids Between Dissimilar Solids*, Doctoral Thesis. University of Michigan; 1967:40.

TABLE 4.5 Wettability and Castability of Stone Models in Flexible Impression Materials

	Advancing Contact Angle of Water (degrees)	Castability of Water Mixes of High Strength Stone (%)
Addition silicone-hydrophobic	98	30
Addition silicone-hydrophilic	53	72

TABLE 4.6 Surface Tension of Metals

Metal	Temperature (°C)	Surface Tension (dynes/cm)
Lead	327	452
Mercury	20	465
Zinc	419	758
Copper	1131	1103
Gold	1120	1128

Adhesion

Surface Considerations

Atoms or molecules at the surfaces of solids or liquids differ greatly from those in the bulk of the solid or liquid, and neighboring atoms may be arranged anisotropically. In addition, some atoms or molecules may accumulate at the surface and thus cause unusual physical and chemical properties. These solid surfaces have atoms of higher energy than bulk atoms because of the absence of some neighboring atoms and thus readily adsorb ambient atoms or molecules. To produce a clean solid surface, one with less than 1% of an adsorbed monolayer, a vacuum of 10^{-9} Torr or 1.33×10^{-7} Pa is required to keep a surface clean for about an hour. At a vacuum of about 3×10^{-6} Torr, a newly cleaned surface would be coated with ambient atoms or molecules in only a few seconds. Therefore, all dental materials and dental surfaces would be covered with a layer of ambient atoms or molecules, and thus adhesives would bond to these adsorbed monolayers.

The energy involved in the adsorption of atoms or molecules onto the substrate may be at the level of a chemical reaction or chemisorption, or may be at the level of van der Waals reaction or physiosorption. The former is irreversible, whereas the latter is reversible.

Thus an important concept in surface chemistry is that critically important properties of a material may be more related to the chemistry of the surface layer and its composition than to the bulk properties. Such surface effects dominate the surface mechanical properties of adhesion and friction, the optical surface phenomena of the perception of color and texture, the tissue reaction to materials, the attachment of cells to materials, the wettability and capillarity of surfaces, the nucleation and growth of solids, and many other areas of crucial interest in biomaterials.

Dental applications of surface chemistry can be seen in the elements chosen in metal alloys. Stainless steel used mainly in orthodontics is 72% to 74% iron but has acceptable corrosion resistance in the mouth because the 18% chromium content forms an adherent oxide layer on the surface, which provides corrosion resistance. Titanium and its alloys, and noble alloys containing small amounts of indium and tin, have excellent biocompatibility properties as a result of oxides of titanium, indium, and tin on the surface.

Penetration Coefficient

The rate of penetration of a liquid into a crevice is an important aspect of capillary phenomena. An example is the penetration of a sealant into a fissure and the fine microscopic spaces created by etching of an enamel surface. The properties of the liquid affecting the rate of penetration may be related to the penetration coefficient (*PC*) where γ is the surface tension, η is the viscosity, and θ is the contact angle of the sealant on the enamel:

$$PC = \gamma \cos / 2\eta$$

The PCs for sealants have been shown to vary from 0.6 cm/s to 12 cm/s. Narrow occlusal fissures can be filled almost completely if the PC value is at least 1.30 cm/s, provided that no air bubbles

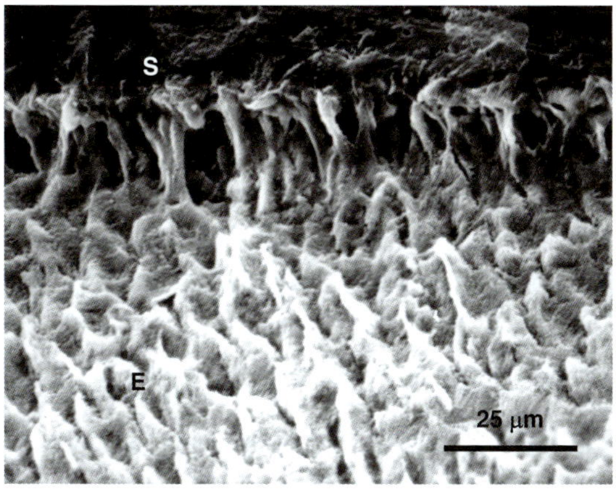

• **Fig. 4.26** Scanning electron micrograph of the interface of sealant *(S)* and enamel *(E)* showing sealant tags that had penetrated into the etched enamel surface. (From O'Brien WJ, Fan PL, Apostolidis A. Penetrativity of sealants and glazes. The effectiveness of a sealant depends on its ability to penetrate into fissures. *Oper Dent.* 1978;3(2):51–56).

trapped in the fissure are present. The same analysis applies to the penetration of pit and fissure sealants into the etched surface of the enamel to form polymer resin tags, as shown in Fig. 4.26.

Optical Properties

Color

The perception of color is the result of a physiological response to a physical stimulus. The sensation is a subjective experience, whereas the beam of light, which is the physical stimulus that produces the sensation, is entirely objective. The perceived color response results from either a reflected or a transmitted beam of white light or a portion of that beam. According to one of Grassmann's laws, the eye can distinguish differences in only three parameters of color. These parameters are dominant wavelength, luminous reflectance, and excitation purity.

The dominant wavelength (λ) of a color is the wavelength of a monochromatic light that, when mixed in suitable proportions with an achromatic color (gray), will match the color perceived. Light having short wavelengths (400 nm) is violet in color, and light having long wavelengths (700 nm) is red. Between these two wavelengths are those corresponding to blue, green, yellow, and orange light. This attribute of color perception is also known as *hue.*

Of all the visible colors and shades, there are only three primary colors: red, green, and blue (or violet). Any other color may be produced by the proper combination of these colors. For example, yellow light is a mixture of green and red lights.

The luminous reflectance of a color classifies an object as equivalent to a member of a series of achromatic, grayscale objects, ranging from black to white for light-diffusing objects and from black to perfectly clear and colorless for transmitting objects. A black standard is assigned a luminous reflectance of 0, whereas a white standard is assigned 100. This attribute of color perception is described as *value* in one visual system of color measurement.

The excitation purity or saturation of a color describes the degree of its difference from the achromatic color perception most resembling it. Numbers representing excitation purity range from 0 to 1. This attribute of color perception is also known as *chroma.*

Measurement of Color

The color of dental restorative materials is most commonly measured in reflected light using a color-measuring instrument or a visual method.

Color-Measuring Instrument

Curves of spectral reflectance versus wavelength can be obtained over the visible range (405 to 700 nm) with a recording spectrophotometer and integrating sphere. Typical curves for a resin composite before and after 300 hours of accelerated aging in a weathering chamber are shown in Fig. 4.27. From the reflectance values and tabulated color-matching functions, the tristimulus values (X, Y, Z) can be computed relative to a particular light source. These tristimulus values are related to the amounts of the three primary colors required to give, by additive mixture, a match with the color being considered. Typically, the tristimulus values are computed relative to the Commission Internationale de l'Eclairage (CIE) (International Commission on Illumination) light source, of which examples are D55, D65, and C. The ratios of each tristimulus value of a color to their sum are called the *chromaticity coordinates* (x, y, z). The dominant wavelength and excitation purity of a color can be determined by referring its chromaticity coordinates to a chromaticity diagram, such as the one shown in Fig. 4.28. The luminous reflectance is equal to the value of the second (Y) of the three tristimulus values.

A diagram of the CIE $L^*a^*b^*$ color space is shown in Fig. 4.29. The $L^*a^*b^*$ color space is characterized by uniform chromaticities. Value (black to white) is denoted as L^*, whereas chroma (a^*b^*) is denoted as red ($+a^*$), green ($-a^*$), yellow ($+b^*$), and blue ($-b^*$). Ranges of CIE $L^*a^*b^*$ values for bleaching shades of resin composites are listed in Table 4.7.

Differences between two colors can be determined from a color-difference formula. One such formula that relates to the Lab color space has the following form:

$$\Delta E_{ab}^*(L^*a^*b^*) = [(\Delta L^*)^2 + (\Delta a^*)^2 + (\Delta b^*)^2]^{1/2}$$

where L^*, a^*, and b^* depend on the tristimulus values of the specimen and of a perfectly white object. A value of ΔE^* of as low as 1 can be observed visually by half of the observers under

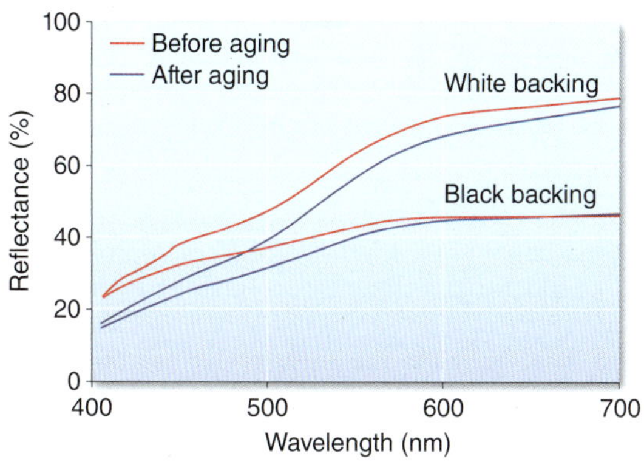

• **Fig. 4.27** Curves of spectral reflectance versus wavelength for a resin composite before and after exposure to conditions of accelerated aging. The specimen was exposed continuously for 300 hours to the radiation of a 2500-W xenon lamp and intermittently sprayed with water. The aging chamber was held at 43°C and 90% relative humidity. Spectral reflectance curves for translucent specimens often are obtained with both black and white backings.

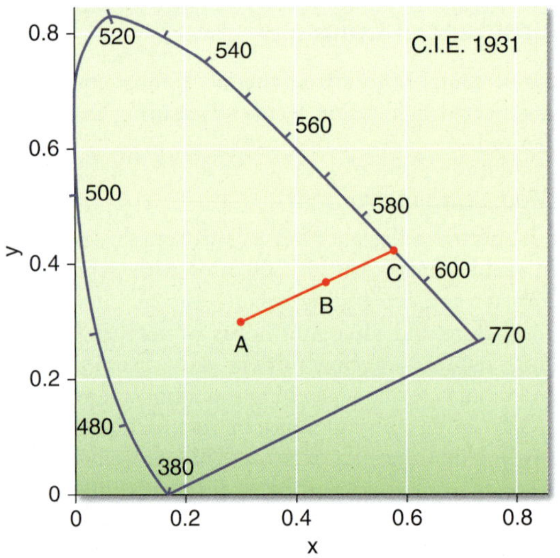

• **Fig. 4.28** Chromaticity diagram (*x, y*) according to the 1931 Internationale de l'Eclairage (CIE) Standard Observer and coordinate system. Values of dominant wavelength determine the spectrum locus. The excitation purity is the ratio of two lengths *(AB/AC)* on the chromaticity diagram, where *A* refers to the standard light source, and *B* refers to the color being considered. The point *C*, the intersection of line *AB* with the spectrum locus, is the dominant wavelength.

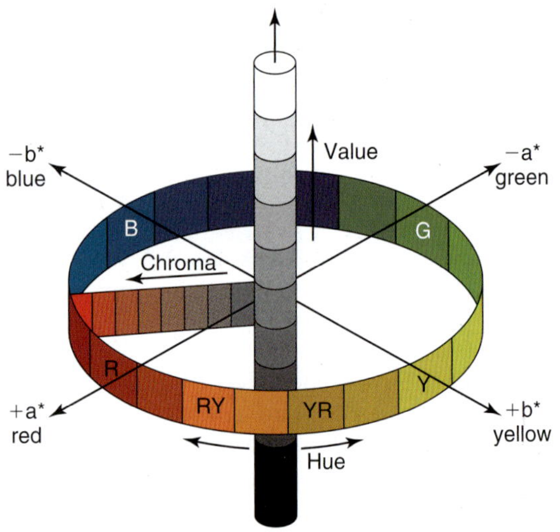

• **Fig. 4.29** Internationale de l'Eclairage (CIE) $L^*a^*b^*$ color arrangement. (From Seghi RR, Johnston WM, O'Brien WJ. Spectrophotometric analysis of color differences between porcelain systems. *J Prosthet Dent.* 1986;56:35–40).

TABLE 4.7 Ranges of CIE $L^*a^*b^*$ (D55, 10 degrees, CIE 1964) Values for Bleaching Shades of Resin Composites

Material	L*	a*	b*
Microhybrid composites	56.3 to 82.4	−0.4 to −3.8	−4.1 to 3.3
Microfilled composites	62.1 to 77.8	−1.9 to −2.8	−2.9 to 1.7
Control shade 1M1	62.9	−0.8	2.9
Control shade B1	58.2	−0.8	1.5

CIE, Internationale de l'Eclairage.
Modified from Paravina RD, Ontiveros JC, Powers JM. Accelerated aging effects on color and translucency of bleaching-shade composites. *J Esthet Restor Dent.* 2004;16:117–1126; discussion 126–127.

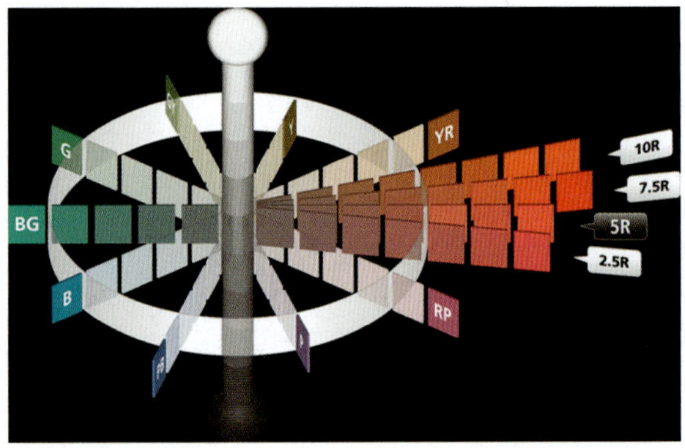

• **Fig. 4.30** Munsell scales of hue, value, and chroma in color space. (Image courtesy Munsell Color, Grand Rapids, MI).

standardized conditions. A value of ΔE^* of approximately 2 or below is considered the clinically acceptable threshold for color difference.

Several inaccuracies in the equation led to the development of a new, slightly more complicated equation, Delta E2000 (or CIEDE2000), which is now used in most of the current dental literature.

Visual Method

A popular system for the visual determination of color is the Munsell color system, the parameters of which are represented in three dimensions, as shown in Fig. 4.30. A large set of color tabs is used to determine the color. Value (lightness) is determined first by the selection of a tab that most nearly corresponds with the lightness or darkness of the color. Value ranges from white (10/) to black (0/). Chroma is determined next with tabs that are close to the measured value but are of increasing saturation of color. Chroma ranges from achromatic or gray (/0) to a highly saturated color (/18). The hue of the color is determined last by matching with color tabs of the value and chroma already determined. Hue is measured on a scale from 2.5 to 10 in increments of 2.5 for each of the 10 color families (red, R; yellow-red, YR; yellow, Y; green-yellow, GY; green, G; blue-green, BG; blue, B; purple-blue, PB; purple, P; red-purple, RP). For example, the color of the attached gingiva of a healthy patient has been measured as 5R 6/4 to indicate a hue of 5R, a value of 6, and a chroma of 4.

Two similar colors also can be compared in the Munsell color system by a color-difference formula such as the one derived by Nickerson:

$$I = (C/5)(2\Delta H) + 6\Delta V + 3\Delta C$$

where C is the average chroma and ΔH, ΔV, and ΔC are differences in hue, value, and chroma of the two colors. For example, if the color of the attached gingiva of a patient with periodontal disease was 2.5R 5/6, the color difference, I, between the diseased tissue and the aforementioned healthy tissue (5R 6/4) would be as follows:

$$I = (5/5)(2)(2.5) + (6)(1) + (3)(2) = 17$$

A trained observer can detect a color difference, I, equal to 5.

Surface Finish and Thickness

When white light shines on a solid, some of the light is directly reflected from the surface and remains white light. This light mixes with the light reflected from the body of the material and dilutes the color. As a result, an extremely rough surface appears lighter than a smooth surface of the same material. This problem is associated with unpolished or worn glass ionomer and resin composite restorations. For example, as the resin matrix of a composite wears away, the restoration appears lighter and less chromatic (grayer).

The thickness of a restoration can affect its appearance. For example, as the thickness of a composite restoration placed against a white background increases, the lightness and the excitation purity decrease. This is observed as an increase in opacity as the thickness increases.

Pigmentation

Aesthetic effects are sometimes produced in a restoration by incorporating colored pigments in nonmetallic materials, such as resin composites, denture acrylics, silicone maxillofacial materials, and dental ceramics. The perceived color results from the absorption of specific wavelengths of light by the pigments and the reflection of other wavelengths. Mercuric sulfide, or vermilion, is red because it absorbs all colors except red, and it reflects red. The mixing of pigments therefore involves the process of subtracting colors. For example, a green color may be obtained by mixing a pigment such as cadmium sulfide, which absorbs blue and violet, with ultramarine, which absorbs red, orange, and yellow. The only color reflected from such a mixture of pigments is green, which is the color observed.

Inorganic pigments are often preferred to organic dyes because the pigments are more permanent and durable in their color qualities. When colors are combined with the proper translucency, restorative materials can be made to closely match the surrounding tooth structure or soft tissue. To match tooth tissue, various shades of yellow and gray are blended into the white base material, and occasionally, some blue or green pigments are added. To match the pink gingival tissues, various blends of red and white are used, with occasional additions of blue, brown, and black in small quantities. The color and translucency of gingival tissues vary widely from patient to patient and from one area of the mouth to another.

Metamerism

Metameric colors are color stimuli of identical tristimulus values under a particular light source but with different spectral energy distributions. The spectral reflectance curves of two such pairs would be complicated, with perhaps three or more crossing points. Under some lights, the pairs would appear to match, but under other lights, they would be different (Fig. 4.31).

The quality and intensity of light are factors that must be controlled when matching colors in dental restorations. Because the light spectrum of incandescent lamps, fluorescent lamps, and the sun differ from each other, a color match between a restorative material and tooth structure in one lighting condition might not match in another. Whenever possible, shade matching should be done in conditions where most of the patient's activities will occur.

Fluorescence

Fluorescence is the emission of luminous energy by a material when a beam of light is shone on it. The wavelength of the emitted light usually is longer than that of the exciting radiation. Typically, blue or ultraviolet light produces fluorescent light that is in the visible range. Light from most fluorescent substances is emitted in a single, broad, well-shaped curve, the width and peak depending on the fluorescing substance.

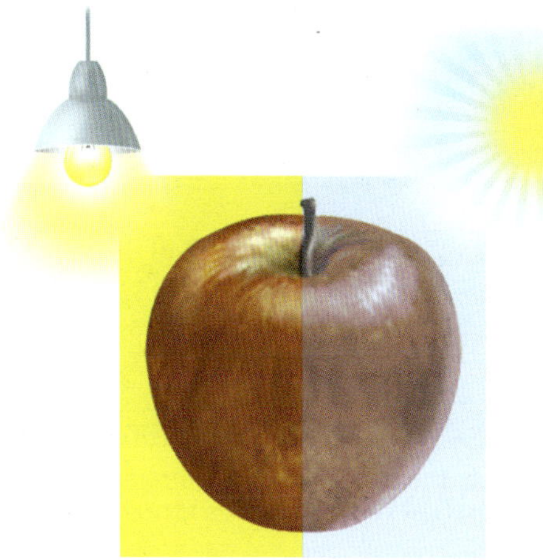

• **Fig. 4.31** Example of metamerism: the apple changes color depending on the light source used to illuminate it.

Sound human teeth emit fluorescent light when excited by ultraviolet radiation (365 nm), the fluorescence being polychromatic with the greatest intensity in the blue region (450 nm) of the spectrum. Some anterior restorative materials and dental porcelains are formulated with fluorescing agents to better reproduce the natural appearance of tooth structure.

Opacity, Translucency, Transparency, and Opalescence

The color of an object is modified not only by the intensity and shade of the pigment or coloring agent but also by the translucency or opacity of the object. Hard and soft tissues vary in their degree of opacity. Most exhibit some translucency. This is especially true of tooth enamel and the surrounding gingival tissues.

Opacity is a property of materials that prevents the passage of light. When all of the colors of the spectrum from a white light source, such as sunlight, are reflected from an object with the same intensity as received, the object appears white. When all the spectrum colors are absorbed equally, the object appears black. An opaque material may absorb some of the light and reflect the remainder. If, for example, red, orange, yellow, blue, and violet are absorbed, the material appears green in reflected white light.

Translucency is a property of substances that permits the passage of light but disperses the light so objects cannot be seen through the material. Some translucent materials used in dentistry are ceramics, resin composites, and acrylics.

Transparent materials allow the passage of light, so little distortion takes place, and objects may be clearly seen through them. Transparent substances such as glass may be colored if they absorb certain wavelengths and transmit others. For example, if a piece of glass absorbed all wavelengths except red, it would appear red by transmitted light. If a light beam containing no red wavelengths were shone on the glass, it would appear opaque because the remaining wavelengths would be absorbed.

Opalescent materials, such as dental enamel, are able to scatter shorter wavelengths of light. Under transmitted light, they appear brown/yellow, whereas shades of blue are perceptible under reflected light (Fig. 4.32). To produce highly aesthetic restorations

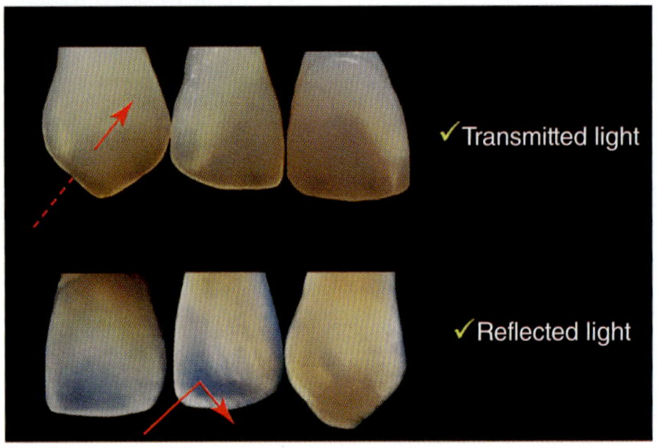

• **Fig. 4.32** Demonstration of opalescence in a ceramic restoration. The tooth appears brown under transmitted light and blue under reflected light.

that truly mimic the natural appearance of the tooth, materials with opalescent properties should be used. This has popularized the use of porcelain veneering materials, as well as direct restorative composites.

Index of Refraction

The index of refraction (n) for any substance is the ratio of the velocity of light in a vacuum (or air) to its velocity in the medium. When light enters a medium, it slows from its speed in air (300,000 km/s) and may change direction. For example, when a beam of light traveling in air strikes the surface of water at an oblique angle, the light rays are bent toward the normal. The *normal* is a line drawn perpendicular to the water surface at the point where the light contacts the water surface. If the light is traveling through water and contacts a water-air surface at an oblique angle, the beam of light is bent or refracted away from the normal. The index of refraction is a characteristic property of the substance (Table 4.8) and is used extensively for identification. One of the most important applications of refraction is the control of the refractive index of the dispersed and matrix phases in materials, such as resin composites and dental ceramics, designed to have the translucent appearance of tooth tissue. A perfect match in the refractive indices results in a transparent solid, whereas large differences result in opaque materials. Manufacturers can use this concept to create composite materials that are more opaque, which may be needed to block out underlying stains or discolorations or very translucent, like enamel, as depicted in Fig. 4.33.

TABLE 4.8 Index of Refraction (n) of Various Materials

Material	Index of Refraction
Feldspathic porcelain	1.504
Quartz	1.544
Synthetic hydroxyapatite	1.649
Tooth structure, enamel	1.655
Water	1.333

Optical Constants

As light interacts with an object, several phenomena can be observed. Incident light can be reflected, absorbed, scattered (or backscattered), or transmitted. These parameters can all be calculated to more objectively characterize the optical properties of the material (Fig. 4.34). Aesthetic dental materials such as ceramics, resin composites, and tooth structures are turbid, or intensely light-scattering, materials. In a turbid material, the intensity of incident light is diminished considerably when light passes through the specimen. These considerations are important not only for shade matching but also in situations where the restorative material is used to conceal imperfections in the tooth being restored, such as stains or other flaws. The optical properties of restorative materials are described by the Kubelka-Munk equations, which develop relations for monochromatic light between the reflection of an infinitely thick layer of a material and its absorption and scattering coefficients. These equations can be solved algebraically by hyperbolic functions derived by Kubelka.

Secondary optical constants (a and b) can be calculated as follows:

$$a = [R(B) - R(W) - R_B + R_W - R(B)R(W)R_B + R(B)R(W)R_W + R(B)R_BR_W - R(W)R_BR_W - R(W)R_BR_W] / \{2[R(B)R_W - R(W)RB]\}$$

and

$$b = (a^2 - 1)^{1/2}$$

where R_B is the reflectance of a dark backing (the black standard), R_W is the reflectance of a light backing (the white standard), R(B) is the light reflectance of a specimen with the dark backing, and R(W) is the light reflectance of the specimen with the light backing.

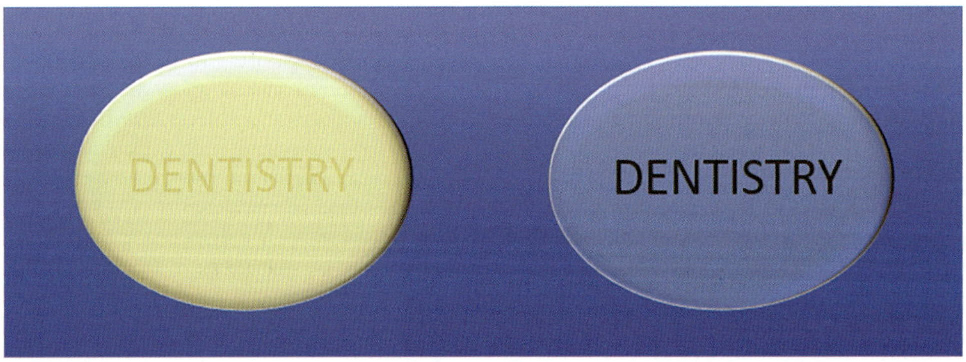

• **Fig. 4.33** Depiction of index of refraction difference between reinforcing fillers and polymer matrix in a dental composite—opacity from a poor match (*left*) and high translucency from an excellent match (*right*).

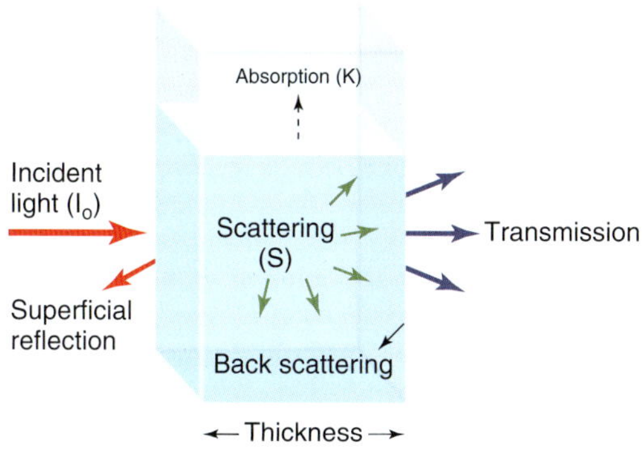

• **Fig. 4.34** Schematic of the possible interactions of light with a solid.

These equations are used under the assumptions that (1) the material is turbid, dull, and of constant finite thickness; (2) edges are neglected; (3) optical inhomogeneities are much smaller than the thickness of the specimen and are distributed uniformly; and (4) illumination is homogeneous and diffused.

In a very practical sense, the masking ability of restorative materials, that is, how well they can block out underlying colors/stains, depends on their optical constants and on their thickness.

Scattering Coefficient

The scattering coefficient is the fraction of incident light flux lost by reversal of direction in an elementary layer. The scattering coefficient, *S*, for a unit thickness of a material is defined as follows:

$$S = (1/bX)\,Arctgh[1 - a(R + R_g) + RR_g/b\,(R - R_g)],\ \text{mm}^{-1}$$

where *X* is the actual thickness of the specimen, *Ar ctgh* is an inverse hyperbolic cotangent, and *R* is the light reflectance of the specimen with the backing of reflectance, R_g.

The scattering coefficient varies with the wavelength of the incident light and the nature of the colorant layer, as shown in Fig. 4.35 for several shades of a resin composite. Composites with larger values of the scattering coefficient are more opaque.

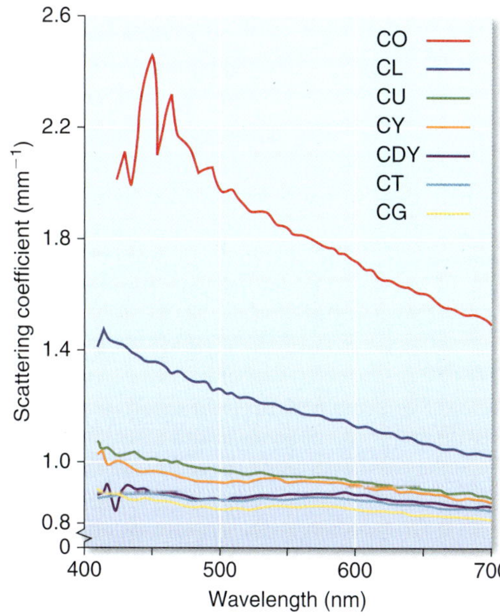

• **Fig. 4.35** Scattering coefficient versus wavelength for shades of a composite, *C*. Shades are *O*, opaque; *L*, light; *U*, universal; *Y*, yellow; *DY*, dark yellow; *T*, translucent; and *G*, gray. (From Yeh CL, Miyagawa Y, Powers JM. Optical properties of composites of selected shades. *J Dent Res*. 1982;61(6):797–801).

Absorption Coefficient

The absorption coefficient is the fraction of incident light flux lost by absorption in an elementary layer. The absorption coefficient, *K*, for a unit thickness of a material, is defined as follows:

$$K = S(a - 1),\ \text{mm}^{-1}$$

The absorption coefficient also varies with the wavelength of the incident light and the nature of the colorant layer, as shown in Fig. 4.36 for several shades of a resin composite. Composites with larger values of the absorption coefficient are more opaque and more intensely colored.

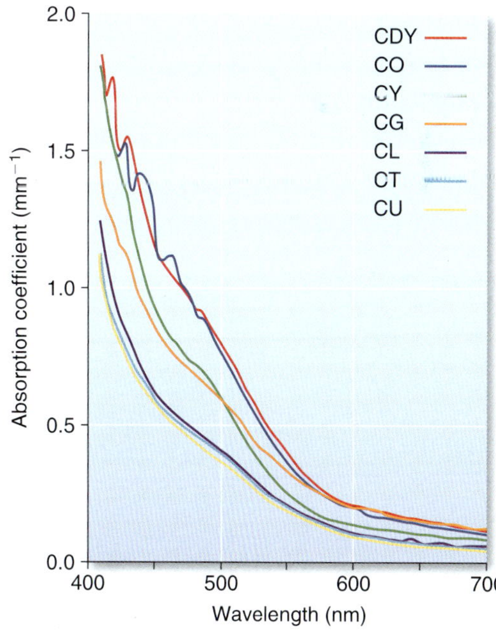

• **Fig. 4.36** Absorption coefficient versus wavelength for shades of a composite, *C*. Shades are *DY*, dark yellow; *O*, opaque; *Y*, yellow; *G*, gray; *L*, light; *T*, translucent; and *U*, universal. (From Yeh CL, Miyagawa Y, Powers JM. Optical properties of composites of selected shades. *J Dent Res*. 1982;61(6):797–801).

Light Reflectivity

The light reflectivity, *RI*, is the light reflectance of a material of infinite thickness and is defined as follows:

$$RI = a - b$$

This property also varies with the wavelength of the incident light and the nature of the colorant layer.

The light reflectivity can be used to calculate a thickness, *XI*, at which the reflectance of a material with an ideal black background would attain 99.9% of its light reflectivity. The infinite optical thickness, *XI*, is defined for monochromatic light as follows:

$$XI = \left(\frac{1}{bS}\right) \text{Arctgh}\left[\frac{1-0.999aRI}{0.999bRI}\right], \text{mm}$$

The variation of *XI* with wavelength is shown in Fig. 4.37 for a resin composite. It is interesting that composites are more opaque to blue than to red light, yet blue light is used to cure light-activated composites. The reason for this is that the photoinitiator molecule typically used in dental composites to begin the polymerization reaction is yellow and thus absorbs blue light most effectively (see Chapter 8).

Contrast Ratio

Once a, b, and *S* are obtained, the light reflectance, *R*, for a specimen of any thickness *(X)* in contact with a backing of any reflectance (R_g) can be calculated using the following formula:

$$R = \left[1 - R_g\left(a - \text{bctghbSX}\right)\right] / \left(a + \text{bctghbSX} - R_g\right)$$

An estimate of the opacity of a 1-mm-thick specimen can then be calculated from the contrast ratio *(C)* as follows:

$$C = R_0 / R$$

where R_0 is the computed light reflectance of the specimen with a black backing.

Typically, the brightness (Y) of light reflecting through a dental material, such as a composite or ceramic disk, is measured with the material placed on *top* of a black background and a white background, with the contrast ratio being the ratio between the two (Y_B/Y_W).

Translucency Parameter

Another measure of the ability of a translucent material to mask underlying colors is the translucency parameter. This parameter is calculated from the color coordinates, L*, a*, and b*, as measured over both white (W) and black (B) backgrounds, using the following equation:

$$TP = [(L_W^* - L_B^*)^2 + [(a_W^* - a_B^*)^2 + (b_W^* - b_B^*)^2]^{1/2}$$

Thermal Properties

Temperature

The temperature of a substance can be measured with a thermometer or a thermocouple. An important application of temperature assessment in dentistry is the measurement of heat during cavity preparation or during light activation of resin composites. Examples of the effect of heat generation by the handpiece while on rotation and coolants on temperature in tooth structure during cavity preparation are shown in Fig. 4.38. The temperature was measured by a thermocouple inserted into a small opening that extended into the dentoenamel junction. The tooth was then cut in the direction of the thermocouple, and the maximum temperature was recorded.

Transition Temperatures

The arrangement of atoms and molecules in materials is influenced by the temperature; as a result, thermal techniques are important in understanding the properties of dental materials.

Differential thermal analysis (DTA) has been applied to study the components of dental waxes. The DTA curve of a mixture of paraffin and carnauba wax is shown in Fig. 4.39. The thermogram was obtained when the difference in temperature between the wax and a standard was recorded under the same heating conditions in which thermocouples were used. The difference in temperature was recorded as a function of the temperature of the surroundings. A decrease in the value of ΔT indicated an endothermic process in the specimen. The endotherms at 31.5°C and 35°C are solid-solid transitions occurring in the paraffin wax as the result of a change of crystal structure. The endotherm at 52°C represents the solid-liquid transition of paraffin wax, whereas the endotherms at 68.7°C and 80.2°C result from the melting of carnauba wax. The heat of transition of the two solid-solid transitions is about 8 cal/g, and the melting transition of paraffin and carnauba wax is approximately 39 cal/g and 11 cal/g, respectively. These and other thermograms show that 25% carnauba wax added to paraffin wax

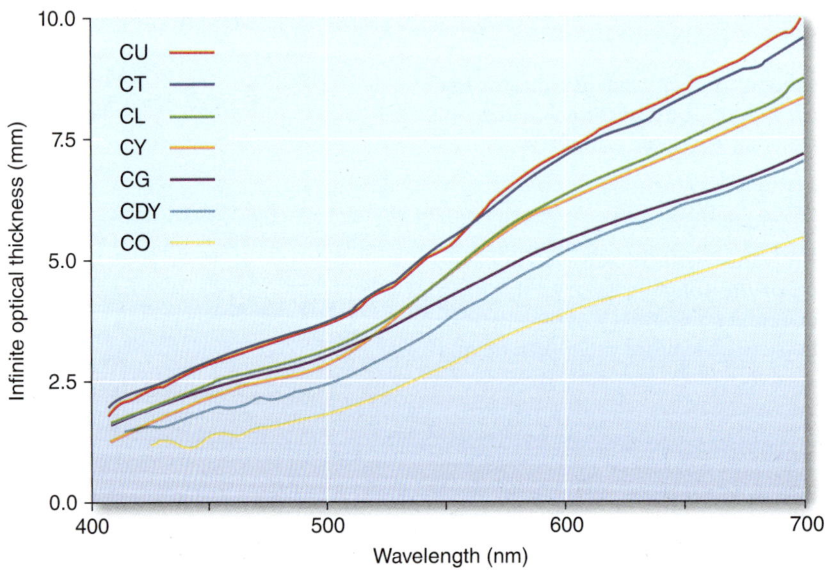

• **Fig. 4.37** Infinite optical thickness (XI) versus wavelength for shades of a composite, *C*. Shades are *U*, universal; *T*, translucent; *L*, light; *Y*, yellow; *G*, gray; *DY*, dark yellow; and *O*, opaque. (From Yeh CL, Miyagawa Y, Powers JM. Optical properties of composites of selected shades. *J Dent Res.* 1982;61(6):797–801).

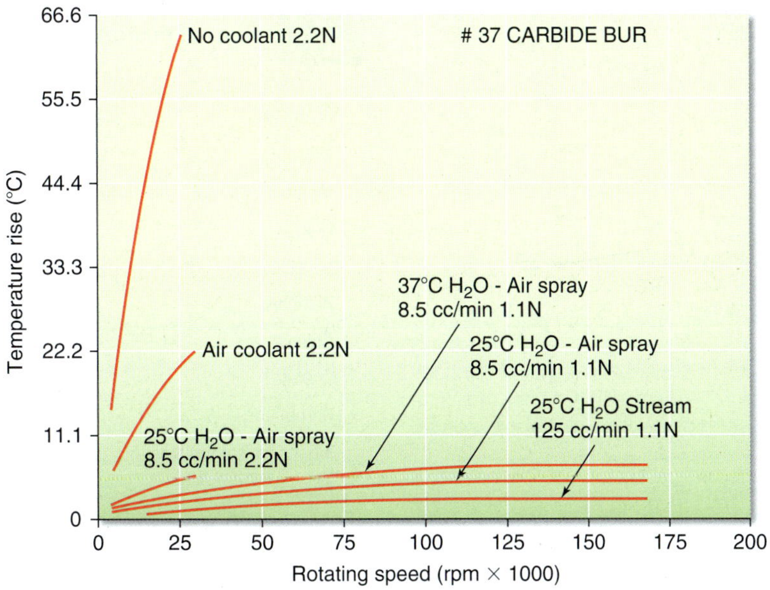

• **Fig. 4.38** Temperature rises developed by carbide burs during cutting of tooth tissue, operated at different speeds and with and without coolants. (Modified from Peyton FA. Effectiveness of water coolants with rotary cutting instruments. *J Am Dent Assoc.* 1958;56(5):664–675).

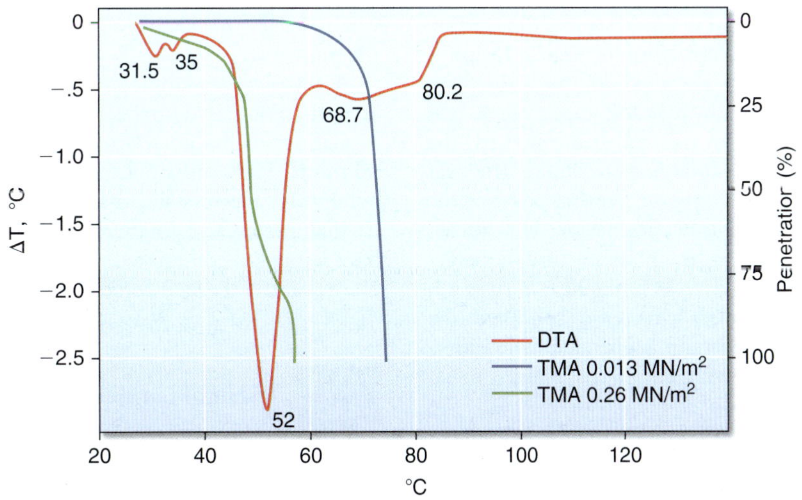

• **Fig. 4.39** Thermograms of a 75% paraffin and 25% carnauba wax mixture.

has no effect on the melting point of paraffin wax but increases the melting range by about 28°C.

Thermomechanical analysis (TMA) of the carnauba-paraffin wax mixture is also shown in Fig. 4.39. The percent penetration of the wax mixture by a cylindrical probe is shown for two stresses of 0.013 and 0.26 MPa. The penetration of the wax at the lower stress was controlled by the melting transition of the carnauba wax component, whereas the penetration at the higher stress was dominated by the solid-solid and solid-liquid transitions of the paraffin wax components. About 44% penetration, which is related to flow, occurred before the melting point of the paraffin wax was reached.

Other properties correlate with thermograms. The coefficient of thermal expansion of paraffin wax increases from about 300 × 10^{-6}/C to 1400 × 10^{-6}/C just before the solid-solid transition, and the flow increases greatly in this temperature range.

Dynamic mechanical analysis (DMA) of a dental polymer is shown in Fig. 4.40. A thin film of the copolymer was subjected to a sinusoidal tensile strain at a frequency of 11 Hz. As the temperature was increased, values of modulus of elasticity (E') and loss tangent (tan δ) were obtained. The glass transition temperature (T_g) is sometimes determined from the identification of the beginning of a rapid decrease in E' with temperature (−25°C in Fig. 4.40) but may also be identified as the temperature at which there is a peak in the tan δ curve (48°C in Fig. 4.40). The value of T_g identifies the temperature at which a glassy polymer transforms to a softer, rubbery state upon heating, which in turn relates to the increase in the number of degrees of freedom given to the molecules by the increased entropy. A lower value of T_g can result

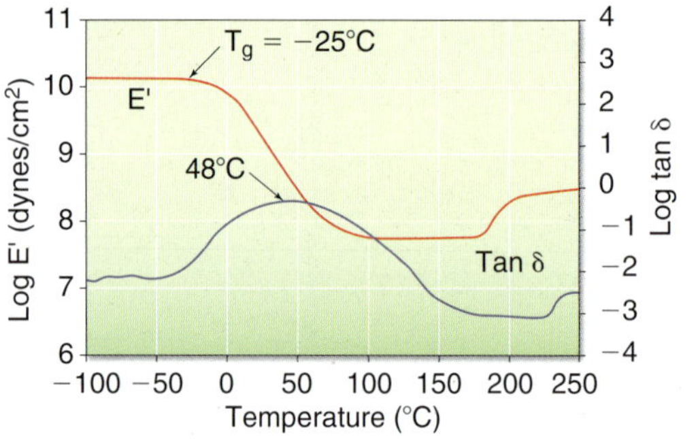

• **Fig. 4.40** Dynamic mechanical properties of a 75 wt% bisphenol A-glycidyl methacrylate (Bis-GMA)/25 wt% triethylene glycol dimethacrylate (TEGDM) copolymer. (From Wilson TW, Turner DT. Characterization of polydimethacrylates and their composites by dynamic mechanical analysis. *J Dent Res*. 1987;66:1032–1035).

from a lower degree of conversion of double bonds, less cross-linked, more flexible networks, or from saturation by water. As discussed later, the value of the coefficient of thermal expansion of a polymer changes at T_g.

Heat of Fusion

The heat of fusion, L, is the heat in calories, or joules, J, required to convert 1 g of a material from solid to liquid state at the melting temperature. The equation for the calculation of heat of fusion is $L = Q/m$, where Q is the total heat absorbed, and m is the mass of the substance melted. Therefore, in practical applications, it is apparent that the larger the mass of material being melted, the more heat is required to change the total mass to liquid. The heat of fusion is closely related to the melting or freezing point of the substance because when the change in state occurs, it is always necessary to apply additional heat to the mass to cause liquefaction, and as long as the mass remains molten, the heat of fusion is retained by the liquid. When the mass is frozen or solidified, the heat that was retained in the liquid state is liberated. The difference in energy content is necessary to maintain the kinetic molecular motion, which is characteristic of the liquid state.

The values for heat of fusion of some common substances (given in round numbers) are listed in Table 4.9. It may be seen that the values for heat of fusion of gold and the metals used for dental gold alloys (silver and copper) are below those of many other metals and compounds. This is true also for the specific heat of gold and its alloys.

Thermal Conductivity

The thermal conductivity, K, of a substance, is the quantity of heat in calories, or joules, per second passing through a body 1 cm thick with a cross section of 1 cm^2 when the temperature difference is 1°C. The units are cal/s/cm^2/(°C/cm). The conductivity of a material changes slightly as the surrounding temperature is altered, but generally, the difference resulting from temperature changes is much less than the difference that exists between different types of materials.

Several important applications of thermal conductivity exist in dental materials. For example, a large amalgam filling or gold crown in proximity to the pulp may cause the patient considerable discomfort when hot or cold foods produce temperature changes; this effect is mitigated when adequate tooth tissue remains, or cavity liners are placed between the tooth and filling for insulation. Cavity liners are relatively poor thermal conductors and insulate the pulp area.

A better understanding of the conductivities of various restorative materials is desirable to develop an appropriate degree of insulation for the pulp tissue, comparable with that in the natural tooth. The conductivity of certain dental materials is listed in Table 4.10. Nonmetallic materials have lower thermal conductivity than metals and are therefore good insulators. Dental cements have a thermal conductivity similar to that of dentin and enamel. Note that the thermal conductivity of a liner or base is important

TABLE 4.9 Heat of Fusion (*L*) of Some Materials

Materials	Temperature (°C)	Heat of Fusion (cal/g [J/g])
Metals		
Mercury	−39	3 [12]
Gold	1063	16 [67]
Silver	960	26 [109]
Platinum	1773	27 [113]
Copper	1083	49 [205]
Cobalt	1495	58 [242]
Chromium	1890	75 [314]
Aluminum compounds	660	94 [393]
Alcohol	−114	25 [104]
Paraffin	52	35 [146]
Beeswax	62	42 [176]
Glycerin	18	47 [196]
Ice	0	80 [334]

TABLE 4.10 Thermal Conductivity (*K*) of Various Materials

	THERMAL CONDUCTIVITY	
Material	cal/s/cm²/(°C/cm)	J/s/cm²(°C/cm)
Metals		
Silver	1.006	4.21
Copper	0.918	3.84
Gold	0.710	2.97
Platinum	0.167	0.698
Dental amalgam	0.055	0.23
Mercury	0.020	0.084
Nonmetals		
Gypsum	0.0031	0.013
Resin composite	0.0026	0.011
Porcelain	0.0025	0.010
Enamel	0.0022	0.0092
Dentin	0.0015	0.0063
Acrylic resin	0.0005	0.0021
Beeswax	0.00009	0.0004

in reducing the thermal transfer to the pulp and that the temperature difference across an insulator depends on the extent of the heating or cooling period and the magnitude of the temperature difference.

Specific Heat

The specific heat, *Cp*, of a substance is the quantity of heat needed to raise the temperature of 1 g of the substance by 1°C. Water is usually chosen as the standard substance and 1 g as the standard mass. The heat required to raise the temperature of 1 g of water from 15°C to 16°C is 1 cal, which is used as the basis for the definition of the heat unit. Most substances are more readily heated, gram for gram, than water.

Obviously, the total heat required to raise the temperature of a substance by 1°C depends on the total mass and the specific heat. For example, 100 g of water requires more calories than 50 g of water to raise the temperature by 1°C. Likewise, because of the difference in specific heat of water and alcohol, 100 g of water requires more heat than 100 g of alcohol to raise the temperature the same amount. In general, the specific heat of liquids is higher than those of solids. Some metals have specific heat values of less than 10% that of water.

During the melting and casting process, the specific heat of the metal or alloy is important because of the total amount of heat that must be applied to the mass to raise the temperature to the melting point. Fortunately, the specific heat of gold and the metals used in gold alloys is low, so prolonged heating is unnecessary. The specific heat of both enamel and dentin is higher than that of metals used for fillings, as shown in Table 4.11.

TABLE 4.11 Specific Heat (Cp) of Various Materials

Material	Specific Heat (cal/g/°C [J/g/°C])
Solids	
Gold	0.031 [0.13]
Platinum	0.032 [0.13]
Silver	0.056 [0.23]
Copper	0.092 [0.38]
Enamel	0.18 [0.75]
Quartz	0.19 [0.79]
Aluminum	0.21 [0.88]
Porcelain	0.26 [1.09]
Dentin	0.28 [1.17]
Acrylic resin	0.35 [1.46]
Liquids	
Water	1.000 [4.18]
Paraffin	0.69 [2.88]
Glycerin	0.58 [2.42]
Alcohol (ethyl)	0.547 [2.29]
Mercury	0.033 [0.14]

Thermal Diffusivity

The thermal diffusivity, Δ, is a measure of transient heat flow and is defined as the thermal conductivity, *K*, divided by the product of the specific heat, *Cp*, times the density, ρ:

$$\Delta = K/(Cp\rho)$$

The units of thermal diffusivity are mm^2/s.

The thermal diffusivity describes the rate at which a body with a nonuniform temperature approaches equilibrium. For a gold crown or a dental amalgam, the low specific heat combined with the high thermal conductivity creates a thermal shock more readily than a normal tooth structure does. For this reason, clinicians may consider placing a base of low thermal diffusivity material, specifically one such as glass ionomer cement that bonds to and seals the floor of the cavity preparation to protect the dental pulp from thermal and electrical shocks when there is little dentin thickness remaining between the pulp and a metallic restoration. Values of thermal diffusivity of some materials are listed in Table 4.12. These values may vary somewhat with composition of the particular restorative material.

As mentioned in the discussion of thermal conductivity, thickness of the material is important. A parameter governing lining efficiency *(Z)* is related to thickness *(T)* and thermal diffusivity (Δ) as follows:

$$Z = T/(\Delta)^{1/2}$$

Coefficient of Thermal Expansion

The change in length ($l_{final} - l_{original}$) per unit length of a material for a 1°C change in temperature is called the *linear coefficient of thermal expansion*, α, and is calculated as follows:

$$(l_{final} - l_{original})/[l_{original} \times (°C_{final} - °C_{original})] = \alpha$$

The units are represented by the notation /°C, and because the values are usually small, they are expressed in exponential form, such as 22×10^{-6}/°C. A less common practice is to report the change in parts per million (ppm), and the previous number would be expressed as 22 ppm.

The linear coefficients of thermal expansion for some materials important in restorative dentistry are given in Table 4.13. Although the coefficient is a material constant, it does not remain

TABLE 4.12 Thermal Diffusivity (Δ) of Various Materials

Material	Thermal Diffusivity (mm^2/s)
Pure gold (calculated)	119.0
Amalgam	9.6
Resin composite	0.675
Porcelain	0.64
Enamel	0.469
Glass ionomer cement	0.198
Dentin	0.183
Acrylic resin	0.123

TABLE 4.13 Linear Coefficient (α) of Thermal Expansion of Various Materials

Material	Coefficient (×10⁻⁶/°C)
Inlay waxes	350–450
Silicone impression material	210
Pit and fissure sealants	71–94
Acrylic resin	76.0
Mercury	60.6
Resin composites	14.5
Amalgam	22–28
Silver	19.2
Copper	16.8
Gold	14.4
Porcelain	12.0
Tooth (crown portion)	11.4
Glass ionomer (type 2)	10.2–11.4

constant over wide temperature ranges. For example, the linear coefficient of thermal expansion of a dental wax may have an average value of 300 × 10^{-6}/°C up to 40°C, whereas it may have an average value of 500 × 10^{-6}/°C from 40°C to 50°C. The coefficient of thermal expansion of a polymer changes as the polymer goes from a glassy state to a softer, rubbery material. This change in the coefficient corresponds to the glass transition temperature (T_g).

Either the linear or volumetric coefficient of thermal expansion may be measured, and for most materials that function as isotropic solids, the volumetric thermal coefficient may be considered to be three times the linear thermal coefficient.

Both linear expansion and volume expansion are important in restorative materials and processes. It is obvious that with a reduction of temperature or cooling, there is a contraction of the substance that is equal to the expansion that results from heating. Accordingly, tooth structure and restorative materials in the mouth will expand when warmed by hot foods and beverages but will contract when exposed to cold substances. Such expansions and contractions may break the marginal seal of a filling in the tooth, particularly if the difference between the coefficient of expansion of the tooth and the restorative material is large. The high coefficient of expansion of pattern waxes is an important factor in the construction of properly fitting restorations. The change in volume as a result of cooling is responsible for the shrinkage spots or surface cracks that often develop in gold alloy castings during solidification. Compensation for the contraction that occurs during the cooling of gold alloys must be made if accurate gold castings are to result. The values in Table 4.13 show that with comparable temperature changes, materials such as acrylic resin and amalgam expand more than tooth tissue, whereas ceramic expands less. The coefficient of inlay pattern wax is exceptionally high when compared with that of other materials.

Of particular importance in casting investments is the property of thermal expansion of three crystalline polymorphic forms of silica. As a principal ingredient in dental investments that are to be heated before a metal casting is made, the amount of expansion at various temperatures is critical and important. This quality of silica compounds in relation to use in casting investments was

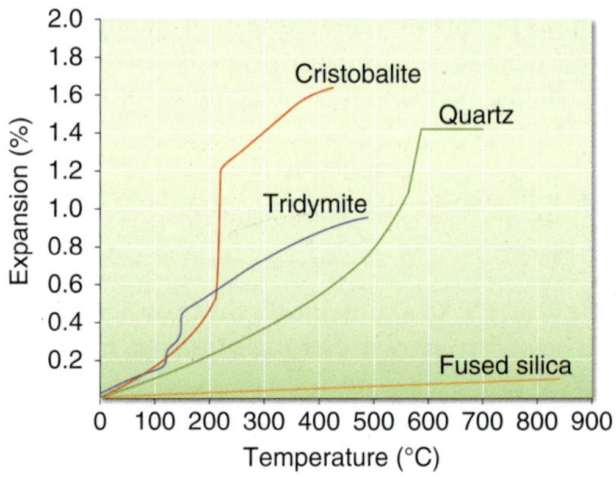

• **Fig. 4.41** Thermal expansion curves for four types of silica. (Modified from Volland RH, Paffenbarger GC. Cast gold inlay technic as worked out in the cooperative research at the National Bureau of standards and applied by a group of practicing dentists. *J Am Dent Assoc*. 1932;19(2):185–205).

described in 1932. Curves in Fig. 4.41 illustrate the relative percentage of thermal expansion of the four forms of silica at different temperatures below about 800°C. Of the crystalline forms, cristobalite shows the greatest expansion at the lowest temperature, and quartz requires a higher temperature to develop an equal amount of expansion as cristobalite. Fused silica has long been recognized as having an exceedingly low thermal expansion.

Electrical Properties

Electrical Conductivity and Resistivity

The ability of a material to conduct an electric current may be stated as either specific conductance or conductivity or, conversely, as the specific resistance or resistivity. *Resistivity* is the more common term. The resistance of a homogeneous conductor of uniform cross section at a constant temperature varies directly with the length and inversely with the cross-sectional area of the specimen, according to the equation

$$R = \rho l / A$$

where R is the resistance in ohms, ρ (rho) is the resistivity, l is the length, and A is the section area. The resistivity depends on the nature of the material. If a unit cube of 1-cm edge length is employed, the l and A are equal to unity, and in this case, $R = \rho$. The resistivity is expressed as ohm-centimeters, where R is in ohms, l is in centimeters, and A is in square centimeters.

The change in electrical resistance has been used to study the alteration in internal structure of various alloys as a result of heat treatment. An early investigation of the gold-copper alloy system by electrical conductivity methods revealed a change in internal crystal structure with an accompanying change in conductivity. The correlation of these conductivity studies with related changes in other properties established the fundamental basis of structural changes associated with heat-treatment operations on dental gold alloys.

Values for the resistivity of human tooth structure are shown in Table 4.14. Resistivity is important in the investigation of the pain perception threshold resulting from applied electrical stimuli and of displacement of fluid in teeth caused by ionic movements. The electrical resistance of normal and carious teeth has been observed to differ, with less resistance offered by the carious tissue. Sound

TABLE 4.14 Values of Resistivity (r) of Human Tooth Structure and Glass Ionomer Cement

Material	Resistivity (ohm·cm)
Human Enamel	
Bjorn (1946)	$2.9–3.6 \times 10^6$
Mumford (1967)	$2.6–6.9 \times 10^6$
Human Dentin	
Bjorn (1946)	$0.7–6.0 \times 10^4$
Mumford (1967)	$1.1–5.2 \times 10^4$
Dental Cement	
Glass ionomer	$0.8–2.5 \times 10^4$

TABLE 4.15 Dielectric Constant (ε_r) for Human Dentin and Glass Ionomer Cement

Material	Dielectric Constant
Human dentin	8.6
Glass ionomer	2 to 7×10^5

enamel is a relatively poor conductor of electricity, whereas dentin is somewhat better (see Table 4.14).

The conductivity of materials used to replace tooth tissue is of concern in restorative dentistry. The effectiveness of insulating cement bases and other nonmetallic restorative materials is not yet established. Several studies have measured the resistivity of dental cements (see Table 4.14). Glass ionomer cements are the most conductive of the cements and have values most similar to dentin.

Dielectric Constant

A material that provides electrical insulation is known as a *dielectric*. Values of the dielectric constant for human dentin and several dental cements are listed in Table 4.15. The dielectric constant of a dental cement generally decreases as the material hardens. This decrease reflects a change from a paste that is relatively ionic and polar to one that is less so. As shown by the high values of permittivity of glass ionomer cements in Table 4.15, these cements have a high ionic content and are quite polar compared with human dentin.

The problem of electrical insulation is made more complex by the presence of galvanic currents in the mouth, resulting from cells formed from metallic restorations. Recent studies indicate that a cement base does not effectively insulate the pulp from the electric current developed in a metallic restoration in the mouth. How much insulation is essential or how to effectively restore the tooth to its original status of equilibrium is currently not known.

Electromotive Force

Working with metals and alloys for dental restorations or with instruments that are susceptible to corrosion necessitates some understanding of the relative position of the metal in the electromotive force series. The electromotive series is a listing of electrode potentials of metals according to the order of their decreasing tendency to oxidize in solution. This serves as the basis for comparison of the tendency of metals to oxidize in air. Those metals with a large negative electrode potential are more resistant to tarnish than those with a high positive electrode potential. In general, the metals above copper in the series, such as aluminum, zinc, and nickel, tend to oxidize relatively easily, whereas those below copper, such as silver, platinum, and gold, resist oxidation. A list of oxidation-reduction potentials for some common corrosion reactions in water is given in Table 4.16. The values of electrode potential and the order of the series change when measured in a saline solution rather than water. The electrode potentials of some dental alloys measured in artificial saliva at 35°C are listed in Table 4.17.

Likewise, it is possible to determine from the electromotive force series that the reduction of the oxides of gold, platinum, and silver to pure metal can be accomplished more readily than with those metals that have a higher electromotive force value.

Galvanism

The presence of metallic restorations in the mouth may cause a phenomenon called *galvanic action* or galvanism. This results from a difference in potential between dissimilar fillings in opposing or adjacent teeth. These fillings, in conjunction with saliva or bone fluids such as electrolytes, make up an electric cell. When two opposing fillings contact each other, the cell is short-circuited, and if the flow of current occurs through the pulp, the patient

TABLE 4.16 Oxidation-Reduction Potentials for Corrosion Reactions in Water and Salt Water

Metal	Corrosion Reaction	In Water, Electrode Potential at 25°C (Volts vs. Normal Hydrogen Electrode)
Magnesium	$Mg \rightarrow Mg^{2+} + 2e$	+2.370
Aluminum	$Al \rightarrow Al^{3+} + 3e$	+1.662[a]
Zinc	$Zn \rightarrow Zn^{2+} + 2e$	+0.763
Chromium	$Cr \rightarrow Cr^{3+} + 3e$	+0.744
Iron	$Fe \rightarrow Fe^{2+} + 2e$	+0.440
Cobalt	$Co \rightarrow Co^{2+} + 2e$	+0.277
Nickel	$Ni \rightarrow Ni^{2+} + 2e$	+0.250
Tin	$Sn \rightarrow Sn^{2+} + 2e$	+0.136
Hydrogen	$H_2 \rightarrow 2H^+ + 2e$	0.000
Copper	$Cu \rightarrow Cu^{2+} + 2e$	−0.337
	$4(OH-) \rightarrow O_2 + 2H_2O + 4e$	−0.401
Mercury	$2Hg \rightarrow Hg_2^{2+} + 2e$	−0.788
Silver	$Ag \rightarrow Ag^+ + e$	−0.799
Palladium	$Pd \rightarrow Pd^{2+} + 2e$	−0.987
Platinum	$Pt \rightarrow Pt^{2+} + 2e$	−1.200
	$2H_2O \rightarrow O_2 + 4H^+ + 4e$	−1.229
Gold	$Au \rightarrow Au^{3+} + 3e$	−1.498

[a]A positive value indicates a strong tendency for the metal to go into solution. Higher positive values are more anodic, whereas higher negative values are more cathodic.

Modified from Flinn RA, Trojan PK. *Engineering Materials and Their Applications.* 4th ed. Houghton Mifflin; 1990.

TABLE 4.17 Galvanic Series of Some Dental Alloys in Artificial Saliva at 35°C

Material	Volts[a]
Hydrogen/H	0.000
Amalgam	
Conventional spherical	−0.023
Dispersed high-copper	−0.108
Nickel-chromium alloy	−0.126 to 0.240
Cobalt-chromium alloy	−0.292
Gold Alloy	
Au-Cu-Ag	−0.345
Au-Pt-Pd-Ag	−0.358 to −0.455

[a]High positive sign indicates a strong tendency for the metal to go into solution.

[a]Measured in Hanks' balanced salt solution at 30°C.

Modified from Arvidson K, Johansson EG. Galvanic series of some dental alloys. *Scand J Dent Res.* 1977;85:485–491.

experiences pain, and the more anodic restoration may corrode. A single filling plus the saliva and bone fluid may also constitute a cell of liquid junction type.

Studies have indicated that relatively large currents will flow through metallic fillings when they are brought into contact. The current rapidly falls off if the fillings are maintained in contact, probably as a result of the polarization of the cell. The magnitude of the voltage, however, is not of primary importance because indications support the fact that the sensitivity of the patient to the current has a greater influence on whether pain is felt. Although most patients feel pain at a value between 20 µamp and 50 µamp, some may feel pain at 10 µamp, whereas others do not experience it until 110 µamp is developed. This is a possible explanation for the fact that some patients are bothered by galvanic action and others are not, despite similar conditions in the mouth.

The galvanic currents developed from the contact of two metallic restorations depend on their composition and surface area. An alloy of stainless steel develops a higher current density than either gold or cobalt-chromium alloys when in contact with an amalgam restoration. As the size of the cathode (such as a gold alloy) increases relative to that of the anode (such as an amalgam), the current density may increase. The larger cathode, likewise, can enhance the corrosion of the smaller anode.

Electrochemical Corrosion

The corrosion and electrochemical behavior of restorative materials have received much interest in the study of multiphase systems, such as gold alloys and dental amalgam. Corrosion can cause surface pitting and discoloration, as well as marginal deterioration, especially for amalgam. Studies of corrosion of surgical stainless steel and stainless steel orthodontic brackets also have been reported. Corrosion of these alloys and others can result in decreased mechanical properties and the formation of corrosion products, which in some instances accumulate in the human organs. Corrosion can be affected by the environment, and certain metals such as cobalt and copper corrode more rapidly in a saline solution containing serum albumin and fibrinogen proteins.

Other Properties

Certain properties often are highly important in the selection and manipulation of materials for use either in the mouth or for laboratory applications. Five such properties are tarnish and discoloration, water sorption, solubility, disintegration, setting time, and shelf life.

Tarnish and Discoloration

Discoloration of a restorative material from any cause is a very troublesome quality. The tarnish of metal restorations from oxide, sulfide, or any other materials causing a surface reaction is a critical quality of metal restorations in the mouth and of laboratory and clinical instruments. The process of steam sterilization of surgical instruments has long presented a serious problem of tarnish and corrosion. Many nonmetallic materials, such as cements and composite restorations, have displayed a tendency to discolor in service because colored substances penetrate the materials and continue chemical reactions in the composites.

Various in vitro tests have been proposed to study tarnish, particularly that of crown, bridge, and partial denture alloys. Testing generally relies on controlled exposure of the alloy to a solution rich in sulfides, chlorides, and phosphates. Most recently, the discoloration of alloys exposed to such solutions has been evaluated by spectrophotometric methods to determine a color-difference parameter discussed earlier in this chapter.

Water Sorption

Water sorption of a material represents the amount of water adsorbed on the surface and absorbed into the body of the material during fabrication or while the restoration is in service. Water sorption of denture acrylic, for example, is measured gravimetrically in $\mu g/mm^3$ after 7 days in water. The tendency of plastic denture base materials to have a high degree of water sorption is the reason this quality was included in American National Standards Institute/American Dental Association (ANSI/ADA) specification No. 12 for this type of material. Usually, a serious warpage and dimensional change in the material are associated with a high percentage of water sorption. The tendency of alginate impression materials to imbibe water if allowed to remain immersed and then to change dimensions requires careful disinfection procedures and pouring within the manufacturer's recommended time.

Setting Time

Setting time characteristics are associated with the reaction rates and affect the practical applications of many materials in restorative dentistry. Materials such as cements, impression materials, dental plaster, stone, and casting investments depend on a critical reaction time and hardening rate for their successful application. From the practical standpoint of manipulation and successful application, the time required for a material to set or harden from a plastic or fluid state may be its most important quality. The setting time does not indicate the completion of the reaction, which may continue for much longer times. The time varies for different materials, depending on the particular application, but duplication of results from one lot to another or from one trade brand of material to another is highly desirable. The influence of manipulative procedures on the setting time of various types of materials is important to the dentist and the assistant.

Shelf Life

Shelf life is a term applied to the general deterioration and change in quality of materials during shipment and storage. The temperature, humidity, and time of storage, as well as the bulk of material involved and the type of storage container, are significant factors that vary greatly from one material to another. A material that has exceptionally good properties when first produced may be quite impractical if it deteriorates badly after a few days or weeks. These qualities are discussed in chapters dealing with gypsum materials and impression materials. Some studies of these qualities of various materials have been made in recent years, and through accelerated aging tests, improvements in quality can sometimes be made. Anesthetics, dental adhesives, and a few other products carry dates of expiration beyond which the product should not be expected to be serviceable. This practice assures the user that the material is not deteriorated because of age. Most materials that meet the requirements of the ADA specifications carry a date of production as a part of the serial number or as a separate notation.

Biocompatibility and Tissue Reaction to Biomaterials

Biocompatibility is formally defined as the ability of a material to elicit an appropriate biological response in a given application in the body. Inherent in this definition is the idea that a single material may not be biologically acceptable in all applications. For example, a material that is acceptable as a full cast crown may not be acceptable as a dental implant. Also implicit in this definition is an expectation for the biological performance of the material. For an implant in bone, the expectation is that the material will allow the bone to integrate with the implant. Thus an appropriate biological response for the implant is osseointegration. In a full cast crown, the expectation is that the material will not cause inflammation of pulpal or periodontal tissues, but osseointegration is not an expectation. Whether or not a material is biocompatible therefore depends on the physical function for which the material will be used and the biological response that will be required from it. Using this definition, it makes little sense to say that any given material is or is not biocompatible, and so how the material will be used must be defined before that can be assessed.

In that regard, biocompatibility is much like color. Color is a property of a material interacting with its environment (light), and the color of a material depends on the light source and the observer of the light. Similarly, biocompatibility is a property of a material interacting with its environment. The biological response will change if changes occur in the host, the application of the material, or the material itself.

In the development of any biomaterial, one must consider the strength, aesthetics, and functional aspects of the material, as well as its biocompatibility. Furthermore, demands for appropriate biological responses are increasing as materials are expected to perform more sophisticated functions in the body for longer time periods. Thus considerations of biocompatibility are important to manufacturers, practitioners, scientists, and patients. The field of biocompatibility is interdisciplinary and draws on knowledge from materials science, bioengineering, biochemistry, molecular biology, tissue engineering, and other fields.

Reactions of Pulp

Microleakage

There is evidence that restorative materials may not adequately bond to or seal enamel or dentin. In this case, bacteria, food debris, or saliva may be drawn into the gap between the restoration and the tooth by capillary action. This effect has been termed *microleakage*, and its influence on pulpal irritation has been extensively studied. Several early studies reported that various dental restorative materials irritated pulp tissue in animal tests. However, several other studies hypothesized that the products of microleakage, not the restorative materials, caused the irritation. Subsequently, numerous studies suggested that bacteria present under restorations and in dentinal tubules might be responsible for pulpal irritation. Other studies showed that bacteria or bacterial products such as lipopolysaccharides could cause pulp irritation within hours of being applied to dentin.

Finally, a classic animal study shed light on the roles of restorative materials and microleakage on pulpal irritation. Amalgam, composite, zinc phosphate cement, and silicate cement were used as restorative materials in class 5 cavity preparations in monkey teeth. The materials were placed directly on pulp tissues. Half of the restorations were surface sealed with zinc oxide eugenol (ZOE) cement. Although some irritation was evident in all restorations at 7 days, after 21 days, the sealed restorations showed less pulpal irritation than those not sealed, presumably because microleakage had been eliminated. Only zinc phosphate cement elicited a long-term inflammatory response. Furthermore, the sealed teeth exhibited a much higher rate of new dentin formation, termed *dentin bridging*, under the material. Only amalgam seemed to prevent bridging. This study suggests that microleakage plays a significant role in pulpal irritation but that the materials can also alter normal pulpal and dentinal repair.

Recently, the concept of *nanoleakage* has been put forward. Like microleakage, nanoleakage refers to the leakage of saliva, bacteria, or material components through the interface between a material and tooth structure. However, nanoleakage refers specifically to dentin bonding and may occur between mineralized dentin and a bonded material in the very small spaces of demineralized collagen matrix into which the bonded material did not penetrate. Thus nanoleakage can occur even when the overall bond between the material and dentin is intact. It is not known how significant a role nanoleakage plays in the biological response to materials, but it is suspected of contributing to the hydrolytic degradation of the dentin-material bond, leading ultimately to much more serious microleakage.

The full biological effects of restorative materials on the pulp are still not clear. Restorative materials may directly affect pulpal tissues or may play an auxiliary role by causing sublethal changes in pulpal cells that make them more susceptible to bacteria or neutrophils. It is clear, however, that the design of tests measuring pulpal irritation to *materials* must include provisions for eliminating bacteria, bacterial products, and other microleakage. Furthermore, the role of dentin in mitigating the effects of microleakage remains to be fully understood. Recent research has focused on the effects that resin components have on the ability of odontoblasts to form reparative dentin. Other research has established the rates at which these components traverse the dentin (see the following section on dentin bonding).

Although it is true that the majority of studies in this arena have in the past focused on the damaging effects of materials on the cells of the pulp and dentin, more recent evidence suggests that there are potentially beneficial effects that may derive from these interactions. Subtoxic exposure to certain dental materials, such as acid etchants, bonding resins, liners and bases, cements, and restorative materials, may solubilize molecules sequestered within the dentin during tooth development. These molecules include growth factors and other proteins and enzymes capable of stimulating existing odontoblasts or signaling undifferentiated cells to migrate to the site and begin the process of dentinal regeneration. These events may occur whether or not the material produces a sealed margin with the tooth and are likely moderated by the health of the tooth in terms of the level of inflammation and the presence of bacterial infection. The exciting aspect of acquiring this new knowledge is the potential to design dental materials capable of initiating the tooth repair process in a systematic rather than random way. This is discussed at greater length in Chapter 15, Tissue Engineering.

Dentin Bonding

Traditionally, bond strengths to enamel have been higher than those to dentin. Bonding to dentin has proved more difficult because of its composition (being both organic and inorganic), wetness, and lower mineral content. The wettability of demineralized dentin collagen matrix has also been problematic. Because the dentinal tubules and their resident odontoblasts are extensions of the pulp, bonding to dentin also involves biocompatibility issues.

After being cut, such as in cavity preparation, the dentin surface that remains is covered by a 1- to 2-μm layer of organic and inorganic debris. This layer has been named the *smear layer* (Fig. 4.42).

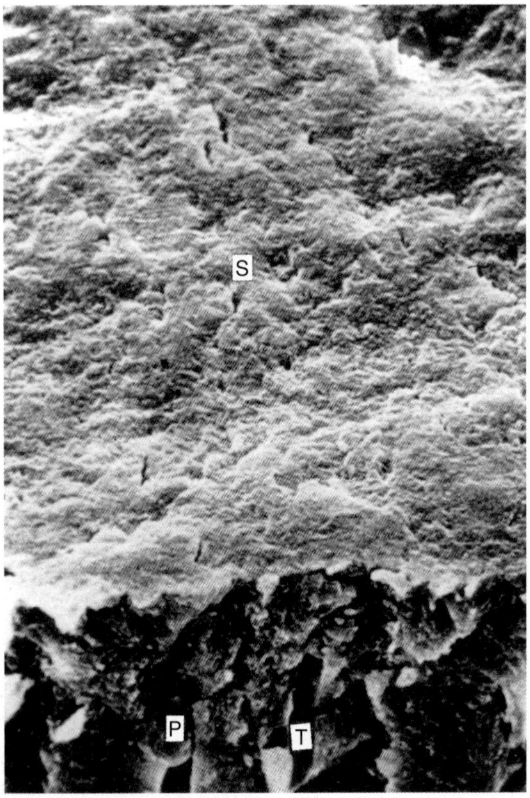

• **Fig. 4.42** **Scanning electron micrograph of cut dentin.** When a dentin surface is cut with a bur, a layer of debris called the *smear layer (S)*, remains on the surface. The smear layer consists of organic and inorganic debris that covers the dentinal surface and the tubules *(T)*. Often, the debris fills the distal part of the tubules in a smear plug *(P)*. (From Brännström M. *Dentin and Pulp in Restorative Dentistry*. Wolfe Medical Publications; 1982).

In addition to covering the surface of the dentin, the smear layer debris is also deposited into the tubules to form dentinal plugs. The smear layer and dentinal plugs, which appear impermeable when viewed by electron microscopy, reduce the flow of fluid (convective transport) significantly. However, research has shown that diffusion of molecules as large as albumin (66 kDa) will occur through the smear layer.

Numerous studies have shown that removing the smear layer improves the strength of the bond between dentin and restorative materials with contemporary dentin-bonding agents. A variety of agents have been used to remove the smear layer, including acids and chelating agents such as ethylenediaminetetraacetic acid (EDTA), sodium hypochlorite, and proteolytic enzymes. Removing the smear layer increases the wetness of the dentin and requires that the bonding agent be able to wet the dentin and displace dentinal fluid. The precise mechanism by which bonding occurs remains unclear. However, it appears that the most successful bonding agents are able to penetrate into the layer of collagen fibrils that remains after acid etching removes the mineral component. There, they create a *hybrid layer* of resin and collagen in intimate contact with dentin and dentinal tubules. The strength of the collagen itself has also been shown to be important to bond strengths.

From the standpoint of biocompatibility, the removal of the smear layer may pose a threat to the pulp for three reasons. First, its removal juxtaposes resin materials and dentin without a barrier and therefore increases the risk that these materials can diffuse and cause pulpal irritation. Second, the removal of the smear layer makes any microleakage more significant because a significant barrier to the diffusion of bacteria or bacterial products toward the pulp is removed. Third, the acids used to remove the smear layer are a potential source of irritation themselves. Nevertheless, removal of the smear layer is now a routine procedure because superior bond strengths are achieved.

Numerous acids, including phosphoric, hydrochloric, citric, and lactic acids, have been used to remove the smear layer. The effect of these acids on pulp tissues depends on a number of factors, including thickness of dentin between the restoration and the pulp, strength of the acid, and degree of etching. Most studies have shown that dentin is a very efficient buffer of protons and that most of the acid never reaches the pulp if sufficient dentin remains. A dentin thickness of 0.5 mm has proved adequate in this regard. Citric or lactic acids are not as well buffered, probably because these weak acids do not dissociate as efficiently. Usage tests that have studied the effects of acids have shown that phosphoric, pyruvic, and citric acids produce moderate pulpal inflammatory responses, but this resolves after 8 weeks. Recent research has shown that, in most cases, the penetration depth of acid into the dentin is less than 100 μm. However, the possibility of adverse effects of these acids cannot be ruled out because odontoblastic processes in the tubules may be affected even though the acids do not reach the pulp itself.

The more positive aspect of this dissolution of the dentin by acids used in dentin-bonding agents may be the release of potentially bioactive molecules entrapped during development. Significant research has shown that extracted dentin matrix proteins, which contain a large variety of phosphorylated and nonphosphorylated proteins, proteoglycans, metalloproteinases, and a variety of growth factors, may be released from intact dentin by basic and acidic chemicals, including acid etchants used in dental adhesives. Studies have shown that many of these molecules may serve as cell signaling agents to recruit undifferentiated cells or as direct stimulants to upregulate the production of extracellular matrix as a step in the process of dentin remineralization. The specific role of each of the molecules in this process is not currently known, nor is it known what the desirable concentration of a specific protein or combination of molecules is to produce optimal results. However, the fact that these naturally present molecules may be released by routine dental restorative procedures and serve as participants in the repair process provides an opportunity for the development and design of future materials.

Bonding Agents

There have been a number of studies on the biocompatibility of dentin-bonding systems. Many of these reagents are cytotoxic to cells in vitro if tested alone. However, when placed on dentin and rinsed with water between applications of subsequent reagents as prescribed by the manufacturer, cytotoxicity is reduced. Longer-term in vitro studies suggest, however, that components of the bonding agents may penetrate up to 0.5 mm of dentin and cause significant suppression of cellular metabolism for up to 4 weeks after application. This suggests that residual unbound constituents may cause adverse reactions.

Hydroxyethyl methacrylate (HEMA), a hydrophilic resin contained in several bonding systems, is at least 100 times less cytotoxic in tissue culture than bisphenol A-glycidyl methacrylate (Bis-GMA). Studies using long-term in vitro systems have shown, however, that adverse effects of resins occur at much lower concentrations (by a factor of 100 or more) when exposure times are increased to 4 to 6 weeks. Many cytotoxic effects of resin components are reduced significantly by the presence of a dentin barrier. However, if the dentin in the floor of the cavity preparation is thin (<0.1 mm), there is some evidence that HEMA is cytotoxic in vivo. Further, studies have shown that HEMA is capable of diffusing through the dentin, presumably via the dentinal tubules, even in opposition to an outward flow of fluid driven by normal pulpal pressure. What effect HEMA may then have on the pulp cells in situ is not known, but HEMA has been shown to stimulate the expression of growth factors in mouse odontoblast-like cells.

Other studies have established the in vitro cytotoxicity of most of the common resins in bonding agents, such as Bis-GMA, triethylene glycol dimethacrylate, and urethane dimethacrylate (UDMA). Combinations of HEMA and other resins found in dentin-bonding agents may act synergistically to cause cytotoxic effects in vitro. There have been very few clinical studies of the diffusion of hydrophilic and hydrophobic resin components through dentin. These studies indicated that some diffusion of these components occurs in vivo as well. Interestingly, there has been one report that some resin components enhance the growth of oral bacteria. If substantiated, this would cause concern about the ability of resin-based materials to increase plaque formation.

Finally, studies have also shown that the release of matrix metalloproteinases (MMPs) from dentin by virtue of its interaction with the acid components in dentin adhesives may cause degradation of the adhesive bond by enzymatic action on the exposed collagen within the hybrid layer. The application of an MMP inhibitor, such as chlorhexidine, has been shown to minimize this effect and has been recommended for maintaining the clinical durability of the dentin bond. However, the overall effect of chlorhexidine on pulp cells has yet to be determined.

Resin-Based Materials

Resin-based materials have been used as dental cements and restorative materials. Because they are a combination of organic and inorganic phases, these materials are called *resin composites.* In vitro, freshly set chemically cured and light-cured resins often cause moderate cytotoxic reactions in cultured cells over 24 to 72 hours of exposure, although several newer systems seem to have minimal toxicity. The cytotoxicity is significantly reduced 24 to 48 hours after setting and by the presence of a dentin barrier. Several studies have shown that some materials are persistently cytotoxic in vitro even up to 4 weeks, whereas others gradually improve, and a few newer systems show little toxicity even initially. In all cases, cytotoxicity is thought to be mediated by resin components released from the materials. Evidence indicates that the light-cured resins are less cytotoxic than chemically cured systems, but this effect is highly dependent on the curing efficiency of the light and the type of resin system. In vivo usage tests have been used to assess the biological response to resin composites. The pulpal inflammatory response to chemically and light-activated resin composites was low to moderate after 3 days when they were placed in cavities with approximately 0.5 mm of remaining dentin. Any reaction diminished as the postoperative periods increased to 5 to 8 weeks and was accompanied by an increase in reparative dentin (Fig. 4.43). With a protective liner or a bonding agent, the reaction of the pulp to resin composite materials is minimal. The longer-term effects of resins placed directly on pulpal tissue are not known but are suspected to be less favorable.

Amalgam and Casting Alloys

Biocompatibility of amalgam as a dental restorative material is thought to be determined largely by the corrosion products released while in service. Amalgam is a complex metallic material composed of multiple phases, and its corrosion, in turn, depends on the type of amalgam, whether it contains the tin-mercury γ_2 phase and its composition. In cell culture screening tests, free or nonreacted mercury from amalgam is toxic. With the addition of copper, amalgams become toxic to cells in culture, but low-copper amalgam that has been set for 24 hours does not inhibit cell growth.

Implantation tests show that traditional low-copper amalgams were well tolerated, but the more modern high-copper amalgams caused severe reactions when in direct contact with tissue. Unreacted mercury or copper leaching out from these high-copper

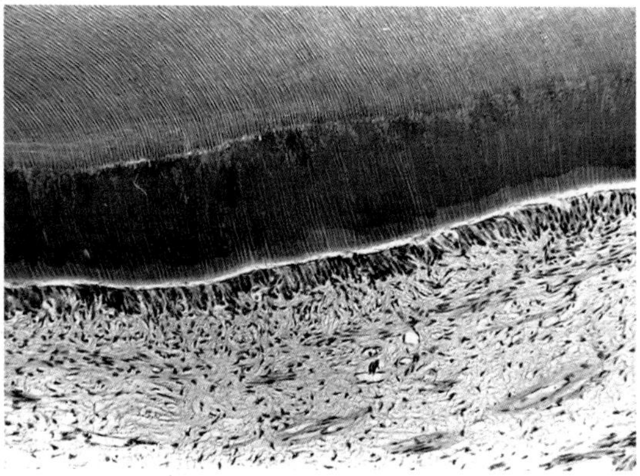

• **Fig. 4.43 Light micrograph of the dentinal and pulpal response to unlined composite at 5 to 8 weeks in a monkey.** The primary dentin is the lighter layer seen at the *top*. The tubules are evident. Secondary dentin is occurring *(the dark, wide middle layer),* and it is closely approximated by intact odontoblasts in the pulp. Few inflammatory cells are present. The response seen in this micrograph is indicative of a favorable response to the material. (Courtesy A.K. Avery, Ann Arbor, Michigan.)

alloys has usually been the constituent leading to adverse responses. An in vitro study of the effects of particulate amalgams and their individual phases on macrophages showed that all particles except γ_2 are effectively phagocytized by macrophages. Cell damage was seen in treated cultures exposed to particulate γ_1, the silver-mercury matrix phase of amalgams. In usage tests, the response of the pulp to amalgam in shallow cavities or in deeper but lined cavities is minimal, and amalgam rarely causes irreversible damage to the pulp. However, pain results from using amalgams in deep, unlined cavity preparations (0.5 mm or less remaining dentin), with an inflammatory response occurring after 3 days.

This pain may be related to the high thermal and electrical conductivity of the material, which is significantly mitigated by the presence of a barrier of remaining dentin or an insulating material. Thus in cavities with less than 0.5 mm to 1.0 mm of dentin remaining on the floor, a base should be placed on the floor of the cavity preparation for two reasons. First, the transfer of hot and cold stimuli, primarily from food and drink, through the amalgam may be substantial. Second, margins of newly placed amalgam restorations show significant microleakage. Marginal leakage of salivary and microbial products is probably enhanced by the natural daily thermal cycle in the oral cavity, which may expand and contract the marginal gap, leading to a percolation of fluids. Although long-term sealing of the margins occurs through the buildup of corrosion products, the timeframe over which this occurs is somewhat a function of the composition of the amalgam, being longer for the high-copper amalgams in use today.

Usage tests reported that after 3 days, the pulpal response to high-copper amalgams appears similar to that elicited by low-copper amalgams in deep, unlined cavities. At 5 weeks, they provoked only a slight pulpal response. At 8 weeks, the inflammatory response was reduced. Bacterial tests on the high-copper amalgam pellets have revealed little inhibitory effect on serotypes of *Streptococcus mutans*, thus suggesting that metallic elements were not released in amounts necessary to kill these microorganisms. Although the high-copper amalgams seem biologically acceptable in usage tests, liners are suggested for all deep cavities. Again, this may be related more to a need for thermal and electrical insulation than a concern over toxicity. Further, the diffusion of released metallic elements into the tooth structure produces discoloration and may be minimized by the presence of an intervening liner. There are also reports of inflammatory reactions of the dentin and pulp, similar to the reactions to many other restorative materials. Mercury has been found in the lysosomes of macrophages and fibroblasts in some patients with lesions.

Cast alloys have been used for single restorations, fixed partial dentures, ceramic-metal crowns, and removable partial dentures. The gold content in these alloys ranges from 0 wt% to 85 wt%. These alloys contain several other noble and nonnoble metals that may have an adverse effect on cells if they are released from the alloys. However, metal ions released from these materials are most likely in contact with gingival and mucosal tissues, whereas the pulp is more likely to be affected by the cement retaining the restoration.

Glass Ionomers

Glass ionomer has been used as a cement (luting agent), liner, base, and restorative material. Light-cured ionomer systems use HEMA or other monomers or oligomers as additives or as pendant chains on the polyacrylic acid main chain. In screening tests, freshly prepared ionomer is mildly cytotoxic, but this effect is reduced over time. The fluoride release from these materials, which may have some therapeutic value, has been implicated in this cytotoxicity in vitro. Some researchers have reported that certain systems are more cytotoxic than others, and though the reasons for this are not clear, presumably, it is related to the composition of the glasses used in the material, which may contain aluminum, calcium, manganese, zinc, strontium, and other metallic elements.

The overall pulpal biocompatibility of glass ionomer materials has been attributed to the weakly acidic nature of the polyacrylic acid, as well as to its high molecular weight. Thus polyacrylic acid is unable to diffuse through dentin due to its large size. In usage tests, the pulp reaction to these cements is mild, and histological studies show that any inflammatory infiltrate from ionomer is minimal or absent after 1 month. There have been several reports of pulpal hyperalgesia for short periods (days) after placing glass ionomers in cervical cavities. This effect is probably the result of increased dentin permeability after acid etching. In any case, glass ionomer has not been shown to be well tolerated when placed directly on living pulp tissue as a direct pulp-capping agent.

As previously discussed with dentin-bonding agents, acidic dental materials have the capacity for demineralizing dentin and therefore releasing bioactive molecules present within this tissue. Although this effect has not been shown specifically for glass ionomers to date, it seems reasonable to assume that it does occur clinically. In a recent study in nonhuman primates, dentin matrix proteins were shown to enhance the formation of reactionary dentin over exposed pulps, compared with calcium hydroxide or resin-modified glass ionomer. Although the response to resin-modified glass ionomer was less consistent than calcium hydroxide, in many cases, it did result in new dentin formation, even when directly exposed to the pulp. It is important to note that the natural tooth repair process producing reactionary dentin does occur, following an initial inflammatory reaction, under glass ionomer when the material is placed over an existing dentin surface. Thus it is possible that the repair process is again aided by the presence of the bioactive molecules released from the dentin by the mild demineralization produced by the material under these conditions.

Liners, Varnishes, and Non-resin Cements

Calcium hydroxide cavity liners come in many forms, typically as pastes with a very alkaline pH (>12). Resin-containing preparations also exist and are capable of light-activated polymerization. The high pH of calcium hydroxide in suspension leads to extreme cytotoxicity in screening tests. Calcium hydroxide cements containing resins cause mild-to-moderate cytotoxic effects in tissue culture in both the freshly set and long-term set conditions. Inhibition of cell metabolism is reversible in tissue culture by high levels of serum proteins, suggesting that protein binding or buffering in inflamed pulp tissue may play an important role in detoxifying these materials in vivo. The initial response after exposing pulp tissue to these highly alkaline aqueous pulp-capping agents is necrosis to a depth of 1 mm or more. The alkaline pH also helps coagulate any hemorrhagic exudate of the superficial pulp.

Shortly after necrosis occurs, neutrophils infiltrate into the subnecrotic zone. After 5 to 8 weeks, only a slight inflammatory response remains. Within weeks to months, however, the necrotic zone undergoes dystrophic calcification, which appears to be a stimulus for dentin bridge formation.

When resins are incorporated into the compound, these calcium hydroxide compounds become less irritating and are able to stimulate dentin bridge formation more quickly than the $Ca(OH)_2$ suspension alone. Significantly, this occurs with no zone of necrosis, and reparative dentin is laid down adjacent to

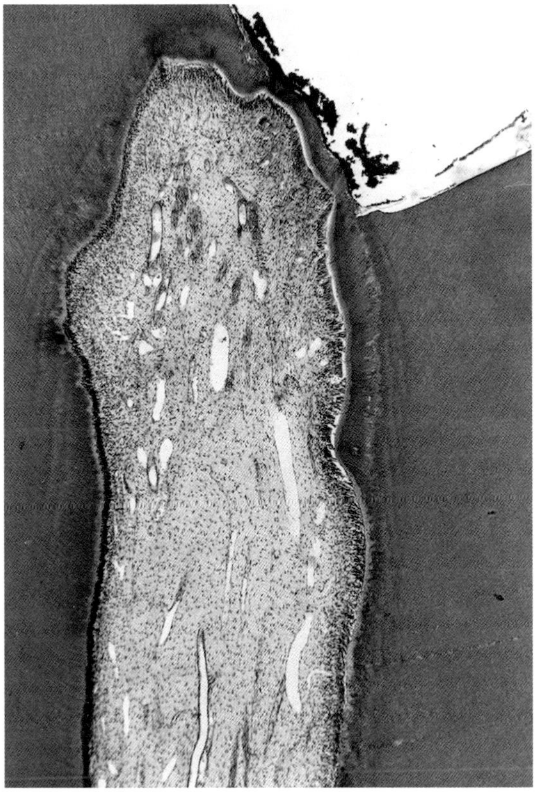

• **Fig. 4.44 Light micrograph of a dentin bridge that has formed between a material and the pulp in a monkey.** Initially, the pulp of the tooth was purposely exposed *(top right)* with a bur. The exposure was covered with a calcium hydroxide pulp-capping agent for 5 weeks before histological evaluation. A layer of secondary dentin has formed at the site of the pulp exposure, forming a dentin bridge. Some inflammatory cells are evident under the bridge, but the pulpal response is generally favorable. (Courtesy D.R. Heys, Ann Arbor, Michigan.)

the liner (Fig. 4.44). This indicates that replacement odontoblasts form the dentin bridge in contact with the liner. However, some of these materials evidently break down with time and create a gap between the restoration and the cavity wall. Resin-containing calcium hydroxide pulp-capping agents are the most effective liners now available for treating pulp exposures, and after treatment, the uninfected pulp undergoes a relatively uncomplicated wound-healing process.

Recent evidence suggests that calcium hydroxide placed on residual dentin in a tooth preparation may also have a stimulating effect on dentin remineralization through the solubilization of noncollagenous proteins, including growth factors such as transforming growth factor-beta-1 (TGF-β1), and glycosaminoglycans from the dentin. Mineral trioxide aggregate (MTA) has the same effect, and possibly to an even greater degree. This is perhaps not surprising because the main soluble component from MTA has been shown to be calcium hydroxide. Thus when placed in contact with dentin, these materials may cause the release of these bioactive molecules, which then serve as signaling agents to recruit undifferentiated cells to the wound site.

These cells may then differentiate into odontoblast-like cells that begin the process of dentin bridge formation described earlier. Evidence exists both in cell culture and in situ that pulp cells exposed to MTA undergo proliferation and migration, followed by differentiation to odontoblast-like cells. Further, studies have shown that MTA-derived products can stimulate osteoblast-like cells and fibroblasts to express proteins, such as osteonectin, osteocalcin, and osteopontin, which are involved with extracellular matrix formation and mineralization. Thus the mode of dentin bridge formation under materials such as calcium hydroxide and MTA may be more complex than simply a reaction to an elevated pH stimulus.

Numerous investigators have analyzed the effects of applying thin liners such as resin-based copal *varnishes* and polystyrenes under restorations. These materials are not generally used under resin-based materials because resin components dissolve the thin film of varnish. Because liners are used in such thin layers, they do not provide thermal insulation but initially isolate the dentinal tubule contents from the cavity preparation. They may also reduce the penetration of bacteria or chemical substances for a time. However, because of the thinness of the film and the formation of pinpoint holes, the integrity of these materials is not as reliable as that of other cavity liners applied at a greater thickness.

Zinc phosphate has been widely used as a cement for seating castings and fixing orthodontic bands and as a thermal insulating base under metallic dental restorations because the thermal conductivity of this cement is approximately equal to that of enamel and is considerably less than that of metals. In vitro screening tests indicate that zinc phosphate cement elicits strong-to-moderate cytotoxic reactions that decrease with time. Leaching of zinc ions and a low pH may explain these effects. The dilution of leached cement products by dentin filtration has been shown to protect the pulp from most of these cytotoxic effects. Focal necrosis, observed in implantation tests with zinc phosphate cements injected into rat pulp, confirms the cytotoxic effects of this cement when it contacts pulp tissue. In usage tests in deep cavity preparations, moderate-to-severe localized pulpal damage is produced within 3 days, probably because of the initial low pH (4.2 at 3 minutes). However, the pH of the set cement approaches neutrality after 48 hours. By 5 to 8 weeks, only mild chronic inflammation is present, and reparative dentin has usually formed. Because of the initially painful and damaging effects on the pulp by this cement when placed in deep cavity preparations, the placement of a protective layer of a dentin-bonding agent, ZOE, varnish, or calcium hydroxide, is recommended in preparations with minimal remaining dentin covering the pulp.

ZOE cements have been used in dentistry for many years. In vitro, eugenol from ZOE fixes cells, depresses cell respiration, and reduces nerve transmission with direct contact. Surprisingly, it is relatively innocuous in usage tests with class 5 cavity preparations. This is not contradictory for a number of reasons. The effects of eugenol are dose dependent and diffusion through dentin dilutes eugenol by several orders of magnitude. Thus, although the concentration of eugenol in the cavity preparations just below the ZOE has been reported to be 10^{-2} M (bactericidal), the concentration on the pulpal side of the dentin may be 10^{-4} M or less. This lower concentration reportedly suppresses nerve transmission and inhibits the synthesis of prostaglandins and leukotrienes (anti-inflammatory). In addition, and as described before, ZOE may form a temporary seal against bacterial invasion. In cavity preparations in primate teeth (usage tests), ZOE caused only a slight-to-moderate inflammatory reaction within the first week. This was reduced to a mild, chronic inflammatory reaction, with some reparative dentin formation (within 5–8 weeks) when cavities were deep. For this reason, it has been used as a negative control substance for comparison with restorative procedures in usage tests.

Bleaching Agents

The use of bleaching agents on vital teeth has become commonplace. These agents usually contain some form of peroxide (generally carbamide or hydrogen peroxide) in a gel that can be applied to the teeth either by a dentist or at home by a patient. The agents may be in contact with teeth for several minutes to several hours, depending on the formulation of the material. Home bleaching agents may be applied for weeks to even months in some cases. In vitro studies have shown that peroxides can rapidly (within minutes) traverse the dentin in sufficient concentrations to be cytotoxic. The cytotoxicity depends to a large extent on the concentration of the peroxide in the bleaching agent. Other studies have even shown that peroxides can rapidly penetrate intact enamel and reach the pulp in a few minutes. In vivo studies have demonstrated adverse pulpal effects from bleaching, and most reports agree that a legitimate concern exists about the long-term use of these products on vital teeth. In clinical studies, the occurrence of tooth sensitivity is very common with the use of these agents, although the cause of these reactions is not known. Bleaching agents will also chemically burn the gingiva if the agent is not sequestered adequately in the bleaching tray. This is not a problem with a properly constructed tray, but long-term, low-dose effects of peroxides on the gingival and periodontal tissues have not been completely elucidated.

Reaction of Other Oral Soft Tissues to Restorative Materials

Restorative materials may cause reactions in the oral soft tissues such as the gingiva. It is not clear how much of the in vivo cytotoxicity observed is caused by the restorative materials and how much is caused by-products of bacterial plaque that accumulate on teeth and restorations. In general, conditions that promote the retention of plaque, such as rough surfaces or open margins, increase inflammatory reactions around these materials. However, released products from restorative materials also contribute either directly or indirectly to this inflammation. This is particularly true in areas where the washing effects of saliva are minimal, such as in interproximal areas, in deep gingival pockets, or under removable appliances. Several studies have documented increased inflammation or recession of gingiva adjacent to restorations where plaque indices are low. In these studies, released products from materials could cause inflammation in the absence of plaque or could inhibit the formation of plaque and cause inflammation in the gingiva. In vitro research has shown that components from dental materials and plaque may synergize to enhance inflammatory reactions.

Cements exhibit some soft-tissue cytotoxicity in the freshly set state, but this decreases substantially over time. The buffering and protein-binding effects of saliva appear to mitigate these cytotoxic effects.

Resin composites in direct contact with fibroblasts are initially very cytotoxic in vitro. This cytotoxicity most likely results from unpolymerized components in the air-inhibited layer that leach out from the materials. Other in vitro studies, in which the composites were aged in artificial saliva for up to 6 weeks, have shown that toxicity diminishes with some materials but remains high for others. Some composites with non-Bis-GMA and non-UDMA matrices have significantly lower cytotoxicity in vitro, presumably because of lower amounts of leached components. Polished composites show markedly less cytotoxicity in vitro, although some materials are persistently toxic even in the polished state.

In the last decade, there has been significant controversy about the ability of bisphenol A and bisphenol A dimethacrylate to cause estrogen-like responses in vitro. These compounds are basic components of many commercial composites. However, there is no evidence that xenoestrogenic effects are a concern in vivo from any commercial resin. Relatively little is known about other in vivo effects of released components of composites on soft tissues, although the concerns are similar to those regarding denture base resin and soft liners (see later discussion in this section). There is some evidence that methacrylate-based composite components may cause significant rates of hypersensitivity, although few clinical trials exist.

Amalgams have been extensively used for 150 years. In spite of its substantial history, however, periodically, concern arises about the biocompatibility of amalgam. Allergic reactions to amalgam restorations are rare, although there are case reports of allergic contact dermatitis, gingivitis, stomatitis, and remote cutaneous reactions. Such responses usually disappear in a few days or, if not, on removal of the amalgam or with the use of a cavity liner. Other local or systemic effects from mercury contained in dental amalgam have not been demonstrated. No well-conducted scientific study has conclusively shown that dental amalgam, placed and used correctly, produces any ill effects. Despite this, a global consensus has been reached to phase down the use of mercury in all industries, dentistry included. Thus amalgam use continues to decline throughout the world, and this, in large part, is due to environmental concerns over mercury contamination in the air, water, and soil.

In patients with oral lesions near *amalgam* sites, positive patch tests have been reported. However, the appropriate patch test has still not been determined. Amalgam restorations carried into the gingival crevice may cause inflammation of the gingiva because of products of corrosion or bacterial plaque. Seven days after placing an amalgam, a few inflammatory cells appear in the gingival connective tissue, and hydropic degeneration of some epithelial cells may be seen. Some proliferation of epithelial cells into the connective tissue may also occur within 30 days, and chronic mononuclear cell infiltration of connective tissue is evident. Increased vascularity persists, with more epithelial cells invaginating into the connective tissue. Some of these changes may be a chronic response of the gingiva to the plaque on the margins of the amalgam. Nevertheless, corrosion products from amalgam cannot be ruled out at this time because implanted amalgams produce similar responses in connective tissues in animals. In addition, although copper enhances the physical properties of amalgam and is bactericidal, it is also toxic to host cells and causes severe tissue reactions in implantation tests.

There is literature that shows that amalgam and resin composites release cytotoxic materials that cause tissue responses, at least at sites of implantation. However, in general, implantation tests show that the material is fairly well tolerated in soft and hard tissues. For materials that are placed where they are rinsed in saliva, these cytotoxic agents are probably washed away before they harm the gingiva.

However, rough surfaces on these types of restorations have been associated with increased inflammation in vivo. Usage tests in which restorations were extended into the gingival crevice have shown that finished materials gave a much milder inflammatory response than unfinished materials. The detrimental effect of surface roughness has been attributed to the increased plaque retention on these surfaces. However, rough surfaces on alloy restorations have also been shown to cause increased cytotoxic effects in vitro, where plaque was absent. This and other in vitro studies would again suggest that the cytotoxic response to alloys may be associated with the release of elements from the alloys and that the increased surface area of a rough surface may enhance the release of these elements.

In another series of studies, low- and high-copper amalgam powders and various phases of amalgam were implanted subcutaneously in guinea pigs. After 1.5 to 3 months, fine secondary particles containing silver and tin were distributed throughout the lesions. These gave rise to macroscopic tattooing of the skin. Secondary material and small, degrading, primary particles from both types of amalgam were detected in the submandibular lymph nodes. Elevated mercury levels were detected in the blood, bile, kidneys, liver, spleen, and lungs, with the highest concentrations found in the renal cortex. In another study, primates received occlusal amalgam fillings or maxillary bone implants of amalgam for 1 year. Amalgam fillings cause the deposition of mercury in the spinal ganglia, anterior pituitary, adrenal, medulla, liver, kidneys, lungs, and intestinal lymph glands. Maxillary amalgam implants released mercury into the same organs, except for the liver, lungs, and intestinal lymph glands. Organs from control animals were devoid of precipitate. However, neither of these studies, nor any other, has demonstrated any changes in biochemical function of any of the laden organs.

Note that studies using powdered amalgam likely overestimate the amount of breakdown products and therefore biological response because the surface area of powders can be 5 to 10 times the surface area of a solid component. It must also be emphasized that any reaction to amalgam, whether in cell culture, local tissue response, or systemic response, does not necessarily imply a reaction to mercury. Such reactions could be in response to some other constituent of the amalgam or corrosion product. For example, in vitro cell culture testing that measured fibroblasts affected by various elements and phases of amalgams has shown that pure copper and zinc show greater cytotoxicity than pure silver and mercury. Pure tin has not been shown to be cytotoxic (Fig. 4.45). The γ_1 phase is moderately cytotoxic. Cytotoxicity is decreased by the addition of 1.5% and 5% tin (Fig. 4.46). However, the addition of 1.5% zinc to γ_1 containing 1.5% tin increases cytotoxicity to the same level as that of pure zinc. Whenever zinc is present, higher cytotoxicity is revealed. High-copper amalgams show the same cytotoxicity as a zinc-free, low-copper amalgam.

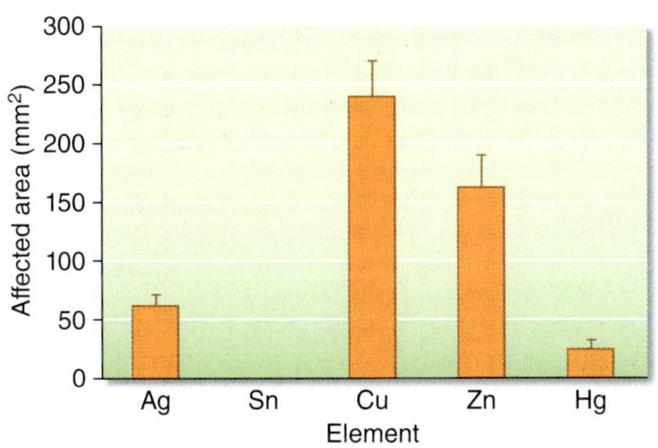

• **Fig. 4.45** Quantitative representation of the affected areas of fibroblasts reveals the magnitude of cytotoxicity of amalgam elements. Standard deviations are represented by vertical bars. *Ag*, Silver; *Cu*, copper; *Hg*, mercury; *Sn*, tin; *Zn*, zinc. (From Kaga M, Seale NS, Hanawa T, Ferracane JL, Waite DE, Okabe T. Cytotoxicity of amalgams, alloys, and their elements and phases. *Dent Mater*. 1991;7(1):68–72).

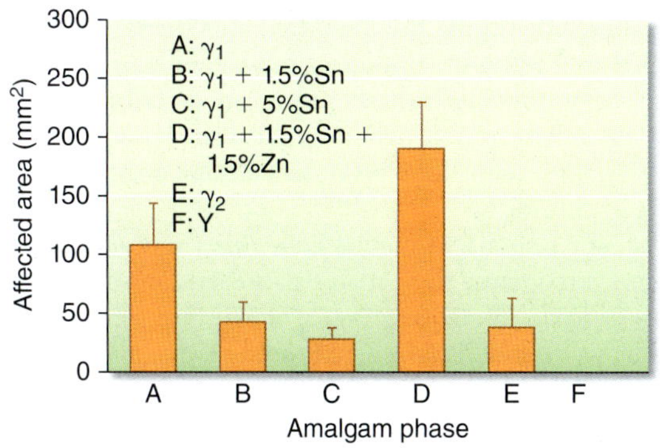

• **Fig. 4.46** Quantitative representation of the affected areas of fibroblasts reveals the magnitude of cytotoxicity of amalgam phases. Standard deviations are represented by vertical bars. (From Kaga M, Seale NS, Hanawa T, Ferracane JL, Waite DE, Okabe T. Cytotoxicity of amalgams, alloys, and their elements and phases. *Dent Mater*. 1991;7(1):68–72).

The addition of selenium does not reduce amalgam cytotoxicity, and excessive additions of selenium increase cytotoxicity. The cytotoxicity of amalgams decreases after 24 hours, possibly from the combined effects of surface oxidation and further amalgamation. The results of this study suggest that the major contributor to the cytotoxicity of amalgam alloy powders is probably copper, whereas that for amalgam is zinc.

Casting alloys have a long history of in vivo use with a generally good record of biocompatibility. Some questions about the biological liability of elemental release from many of the formulations developed in the past 10 years have arisen, but there is no clinical evidence that elemental release is a problem aside from hypersensitivity. Nickel allergy is a relatively common problem, occurring in 10% to 20% of females. It is a significant risk from nickel-based alloys because the release of nickel ions from these alloys is generally higher than for noble or high-noble alloys. Stainless steels, commonly used in preformed pediatric crowns and orthodontic appliances, also contain a significant concentration of Ni in their composition. Palladium sensitivity has also been a concern in some countries, although the incidence of true palladium allergy is one-third that of nickel allergy. While it has been clinically documented that patients with palladium allergy are virtually always allergic to nickel, the converse is not true.

Numerous in vitro studies have examined the effects of metal ions on cells in the gingival tissues, such as epithelial cells, fibroblasts, and macrophages. For the most part, the concentrations of metal ions required to cause problems with these cells in vitro are greater than those released from most casting alloys. However, some recent research has shown that extended exposures to low doses of metal ions may also have biological liabilities. This is noteworthy because the low-dose concentrations approach those known to be released from some alloys. The clinical significance of this research, however, is not known.

Denture base materials, especially methacrylates, have been associated with immune hypersensitivity reactions of gingiva and mucosa more than any other dental material. The greatest potential for hypersensitization is for dental and laboratory personnel who are exposed repeatedly to a variety of unreacted components. Hypersensitivity has been documented to the acrylic and diacrylic monomers, certain curing agents, antioxidants, amines, and formaldehyde. For patients, however, most of these materials have undergone the polymerization reaction, and the incidence of hypersensitization is quite low. Screening tests for sensitization potential include testing the unreacted ingredients, the polymeric substance after reaction, and oil, saline, or aqueous extracts of the polymer using the in vitro tests previously described. In addition to hypersensitivity, visible light-cured denture base resins and denture base resin sealants have been shown to be cytotoxic to epithelial cells in culture.

Soft-tissue responses to *soft denture liners* and *denture adhesives* are of concern because these materials are used in intimate contact with the gingiva. Plasticizers, incorporated into some materials to make them soft and flexible, are released in vivo and in vitro. Cell culture tests have shown that some of these materials are extremely cytotoxic and affect a number of cellular metabolic reactions. In animal tests, several of these materials have caused significant epithelial changes, presumably from the released plasticizers. In usage, the effects of the released plasticizers are probably often masked by the inflammation already present in the tissues onto which these materials are placed. Denture adhesives have been evaluated in vitro and show severe cytotoxic reactions. Several had substantial formaldehyde content. The adhesives also allowed significant microbial growth. Newer formulations that add antifungal or antibacterial agents have not yet been shown to be clinically effective.

Reaction of Bone and Soft Tissues to Implant Materials

Interest in the biocompatibility of implant materials has grown because the use of implants in clinical practice has increased dramatically. Successful dental implant materials either promote osseointegration or biointegration (see Dental and Orofacial Implants, Chapter 14).

Reactions to Ceramic Implant Materials

Ceramic materials may be conveniently divided into two groups: bioactive materials and nonbioactive ceramics. Most ceramic implant materials have very low toxic effects on tissues because they are already in an oxidized state and are highly corrosion resistant. As a group, not only are they minimally toxic, but they also are nonimmunogenic and noncarcinogenic. Nonbioactive ceramic materials generally invoke fibrous encapsulation when implanted, as mentioned earlier.

Reactions to Implant Metals and Alloys

Pure metals and alloys are the oldest type of oral implant materials. Initially, metallic implant materials were selected based on strength and ease of fabrication. Over time, however, biocompatibility with bone and soft tissue and the longevity of the implant have become more important. Although a variety of implant materials have previously been used (including stainless steel and chromium-cobalt-molybdenum), the only metallic dental implant materials in common use today are titanium-based alloys.

Titanium is a pure metal when initially cast. However, in less than a second, the surface forms a thin conformal layer of various titanium oxides. This oxide layer is corrosion resistant and allows bone to osseointegrate. A major disadvantage of this metal is that it is difficult to cast. It has been wrought into various forms, but this process introduces metallic impurities into the surface that may adversely affect bone cell response unless extreme care is taken during manufacturing. Titanium implants have been used with success as root forms to support a prosthesis. With frequent recall and good oral hygiene, implants have been maintained in healthy tissue for longer than three decades. Titanium-aluminum-vanadium alloys (Ti-6Al-4V) have been used successfully in this regard as well. This alloy is significantly stronger than commercially pure titanium, and has better fatigue resistance, but has the same desirable stiffness and thermal properties as the commercially pure (CP) metal. Although titanium and titanium alloy implants have corrosion rates that are markedly less than other metallic implants, they do release titanium into the body. Currently, there is no evidence that released titanium ions are a problem locally or systemically. However, questions remain about the liability of released aluminum and vanadium from alloys.

In soft tissue, the bond epithelium forms with titanium is morphologically similar to that formed with the tooth, but this interface has not been fully characterized. Connective tissue apparently does not bond to the titanium but does form a tight seal that seems to limit the ingress of bacteria and bacterial products. Techniques are being developed to limit down-growth of the epithelium and loss of bone height around the implant because this will ultimately cause implant failure. Periimplantitis is now a documented disease around implants and involves many of the same bacteria as periodontitis. The role of the implant material or its released components in the progression of periimplantitis is not known, but this disease is considered to be a major contributor to implant failure and the subject of much investigation.

Reactions to Resorbable Materials

With the survival of implanted materials for decades or more, the predominant thought began to shift in emphasis from achieving a benign (or tolerated) tissue response to instead producing bioactive materials that could elicit a controlled action and reaction in the physiological environment. Continuing in this vein was the development of resorbable biomaterials that exhibit clinically appropriate, controlled chemical breakdown and resorption. In these materials, the problem of a tissue-material interface is resolved because the materials provoke a physiologic response to replace the material with regenerated tissues. One of the earliest examples of these materials was the development of resorbable sutures. These materials were composed of a copolymer of polylactic acid (PLA) and polyglycolic acid (PGA). When implanted in the body, they undergo a hydrolytic decomposition into CO_2 and H_2O. By the mid-1980s, clinical use of resorbable polymeric sutures was commonplace. Resorbable fracture fixation plates and screws, guided tissue membranes, and controlled drug-release systems have rapidly followed. Although generally well tolerated by tissues in vivo, the resorbability of these materials depends on the volume of material implanted, and because these materials degrade into acidic by-products, the subsequent drop in pH in the surrounding tissues may invoke an inflammatory response. Other polymeric materials such as polycaprolactone and hyaluronan derivatives, as well as natural polymers such as crosslinked collagen, starch, and cellulose, are currently being investigated for their ability to resorb in vivo after serving their function as an implant.

Summary

The physical properties of oral restorations must adequately withstand the stresses of mastication. Several methods may be used to ensure proper performance of a restoration. With a constant force, the stress is inversely proportional to the contact area; therefore stresses may be reduced by increasing the area over which the force is distributed. In areas of high stress, materials having high elastic moduli and strength properties should be used if possible. If a weaker material has desirable properties, such as aesthetic qualities, one may minimize the stress by increasing the bulk of the material when possible or ensuring proper occlusion on the restoration.

Restorations and appliances should be designed so the resulting forces of mastication are distributed as uniformly as possible. In addition, sharp line angles, nonuniform areas, and notched, scratched, or pitted surfaces should be avoided to minimize stress concentrations. For example, joints between abutments and pontics of fixed partial dental prostheses should be properly radiused to distribute stress during function. Implant screws should not be scratched or notched when inserted.

Restorative materials are generally weaker in tension than in compression. Restorations should be designed to minimize areas of high tension. Material flaws can further contribute to areas prone to failure. Fatigue is also an important consideration. For example, repeated flexure of an improperly loaded implant-supported restoration can concentrate stresses in the abutment screw or implant body, leading to fatigue fracture.

The dentist is often concerned not so much with the fracture of an appliance as with the deflection that occurs when a force is applied. This is the case with a fixed partial dental prosthesis, which may be cast as a single unit or may consist of soldered units. As discussed earlier in this chapter, the deflection of a beam, or in this case, a fixed partial dental prosthesis, supported on each end with a concentrated load in the center, depends directly on the cube of the beam length and indirectly on the cube of the beam thickness. Doubling the length of the beam therefore increases the deflection by eight times. This also indicates that decreasing the thickness of the beam by one-half increases the deflection by eight times. If too much bulk were required to develop the stiffness desired, changing to a material with a higher elastic modulus, or stiffness, would be beneficial. If repeated failures occur, consider increasing the occlusogingival dimension of the proximal connectors, balancing the occlusion over a larger surface area, and narrowing the occlusal table.

These isolated examples of applied knowledge of biting forces and stresses in dental structures indicate why an understanding of this subject is necessary for the practicing dentist.

In summary, three interrelated factors are important in the long-term function of dental restorative materials: (1) material choice, (2) component geometry (e.g., to minimize stress concentrations), and (3) component design (e.g., to distribute stresses as uniformly as possible). It should be noted that failures can and do occur. In such instances, a failure analysis should be performed by answering several questions: (1) Why did it fail? (2) How did it fail? (3) Did the material or design fail? and (4) How can this failure be prevented in the future? Lastly, remember that dental material behavior depends on interrelated physical, chemical, optical, mechanical, thermal, electrical, and biological properties, and improvement of one specific property often leads to a reduction in another property.

Biocompatibility of a dental material depends on its composition, location, and interactions with the oral cavity. Metal, ceramic, and polymer materials elicit different biological responses because of differences in composition. Furthermore, diverse biological responses to these materials depend on whether they release their components and whether those components are toxic, immunogenic, or mutagenic at the released concentrations. The location of a material in the oral cavity partially determines its biocompatibility. Materials that are biocompatible in contact with the oral mucosal surface may cause adverse reactions if they are implanted beneath it. Materials that are toxic in direct contact with the pulp may be essentially innocuous if placed on dentin or enamel. Finally, interactions between the material and the body influence the biocompatibility of the material. A material's response to changes in pH, application of force, or the effect of biological fluids can alter its biocompatibility. Surface features, such as the roughness of a material, may promote or discourage the attachment of bacteria, host cells, or biological molecules. These effects also determine whether the material will promote plaque retention, integrate with bone, or adhere to dentin.

Bibliography

Mechanical Properties

Forces on Dental Structures

Anusavice KJ. *Phillips' Science of Dental Materials.* 11th ed. Saunders; 2003.

Bujtár P, Sándor GK, Bojtos A, Szucs A, Barabás J. Finite element analysis of the human mandible at 3 different stages of life. *Oral Surg Oral Med Oral Pathol Oral Radiol Endod.* 2010;110(3):301–309.

Castelo PM, Pereira LJ, Bonjardim LR, Gavião MB. Changes in bite force, masticatory muscle thickness, and facial morphology between primary and mixed dentition in preschool children with normal occlusion. *Ann Anat.* 2010;192(1):23–26.

Koolstra JH, van Euden TM. Application and validation of a three-dimensional mathematical model of the human masticatory system in vivo. *J Biomech.* 1992;25:175–187.

Korioth TW, Versluis A. Modeling the mechanical behavior of the jaws and their related structures by finite element (FE) analysis. *Crit Rev Oral Biol Med.* 1997;8:90–104.

Kuhlberg AJ, Priebe D. Testing force systems and biomechanics—measured tooth movements from differential moment closing loops. *Angle Orthod.* 2003;73:270–280.

Magne P, Versluis A, Douglas WH. Rationalization of incisor shape: experimental-numerical analysis. *J Prosthet Dent.* 1999;81:345–355.

Plesh O, Bishop B, McCall WD Jr. Kinematics of jaw movements during chewing at different frequencies. *J Biomech.* 1993;26:243–250.

Stress Analysis and Design of Dental Structures

Brunski JB. Biomechanical factors affecting the bone-dental implant interface. *Clin Mater.* 1992;10:153–201.

Hart RT, Hennebel VV, Thongpreda N, et al. Modeling the biomechanics of the mandible: a three-dimensional finite element study. *J Biomech.* 1992;25:261–286.

Ko CC, Kohn DH, Hollister SJ. Micromechanics of implant/tissue interfaces. *J Oral Implantol.* 1992;18:220–230.

Kohn DH. Overview of factors important in implant design. *J Oral Implantol.* 1992;18:204–219.

Korioth TW, Hannam AG. Deformation of the human mandible during simulated tooth clenching. *J Dent Res.* 1994;73:56–66.

Meredith N. A review of nondestructive test methods and their application to measure the stability and osseointegration of bone anchored endosseous implants. *Crit Rev Biomed Eng.* 1998;26:275–291.

Sakaguchi RL, Borgersen SE. Nonlinear finite element contact analysis of dental implant components. *Int J Oral Maxillofac Implants.* 1993;8:655–661.

Sakaguchi RL, Borgersen SE. Nonlinear contact analysis of preload in dental implant screws. *Int J Oral Maxillofac Implants.* 1995;10:295–302.

Sakaguchi RL, Brust EW, Cross M, DeLong R, Douglas WH. Independent movement of cusps during occlusal loading. *Dent Mater.* 1991;7:186–190.

Sakaguchi RL, Cross M, Douglas WH. A simple model of crack propagation in dental restorations. *Dent Mater.* 1992;8:131–136.

Tantbirojn D, Versluis A, Pintado MR, DeLong R, Douglas WH. Tooth deformation patterns in molars after composite restoration. *Dent Mater.* 2004;20:535–542.

General Biomechanics

Fung YC. *Biomechanics, Mechanical Properties of Living Tissues.* 2nd ed. Springer-Verlag; 1993.

Hayashi K, Kamiya A, Ono K. eds. *Biomechanics, Functional Adaptation and Remodeling.* Springer-Verlag; 1996.

Park JB, Lakes RS. *Biomaterials: An Introduction.* 3rd ed. Springer Science-Business Media; 2007.

Peterson DR, Bronzino JD. *Biomechanics: Principles and Applications.* 2nd ed. CRC Press; 2007.

Fracture Toughness

Baran GR, McCool JI, Paul D, Boberick K, Wunder S. Weibull models of fracture strengths and fatigue behavior of dental resins in flexure and shear. *J Biomed Mater Res.* 1998;43:226–233.

Flinn RA, Trojan PK. *Engineering Materials and Their Applications.* Houghton Mifflin; 1981.

Fujishima A, Ferracane JL. Comparison of four modes of fracture toughness testing for dental composites. *Dent Mater.* 1996;12:38–43.

Mecholsky JJ Jr. Fracture mechanics principles. *Dent Mater.* 1995;11:111–112.

Scherrer SS, Denry IL, Wiskott HW. Comparison of three fracture toughness testing techniques using a dental glass and a dental ceramic. *Dent Mater.* 1998;14:246–255.

Uctasli S, Harrington E, Wilson HJ. The fracture resistance of dental materials. *J Oral Rehabil.* 1995;22:877–886.

Shear Strength

Drummond JL, Sakaguchi RL, Racean DC, Wozny J, Steinberg AD. Testing mode and surface treatment effects on dentin bonding. *J Biomed Mater Res.* 1996;32:533–541.

Bending and Torsion

Magne P. Efficient 3D finite element analysis of dental restorative procedures using micro-CT data. *Dent Mater.* 2007;23:539–548.

Viscoelasticity

Craig RG, ed. *Dental Materials: A Problem-Oriented Approach.* Mosby–Year Book; 1978.

Duran RL, Powers JM, Craig RG. Viscoelastic and dynamic properties of soft liners and tissue conditioners. *J Dent Res.* 1979;58(8):1801–1807.

Lee JK, Choi JY, Lim BS, Lee YK, Sakaguchi RL. Change of properties during storage of a UDMA/TEGDMA dental resin. *J Biomed Mater Res B Appl Biomater.* 2004;68:216–221.

O'Brien WJ. *Dental Materials: Properties and Selection.* Quintessence; 1989.

Dynamic Properties

American Society for Testing and Materials. Impact resistance of plastics and electrical insulating material, D 256–92. *ASTM Standards 1993. vol. 8.01.* American Society for Testing and Materials; 1993.

Graessley WW. Linear viscoelasticity. In: *Polymeric Liquids and Networks: Dynamics and Rheology.* Taylor and Francis Group; 2008.

Rubinstein M, Colby RH. Networks and gelation. In: *Polymer Physics.* Oxford University Press; 2008.

Sakaguchi RL, Shah NC, Lim BS, Ferracane JL, Borgersen SE. Dynamic mechanical analysis of storage modulus development in light-activated polymer matrix composites. *Dent Mater.* 2002;18:197–202.

Properties of Composite Materials

Choi KK, Condon JR, Ferracane JL. The effects of adhesive thickness on polymerization contraction stress of composite. *J Dent Res.* 2000;79:812–817.

Condon JR, Ferracane JL. Reduction of composite contraction stress through non-bonded microfiller particles. *Dent Mater.* 1998;14:256–260.

Ferracane JL, Berge HX, Condon JR. In vitro aging of dental composites in water—effect of degree of conversion, filler volume, and filler/matrix coupling. *J Biomed Mater Res.* 1998;42:465–472.

Ferracane JL, Condon JR. In vitro evaluation of the marginal degradation of dental composites under simulated occlusal loading. *Dent Mater.* 1999;15:262–267.

Peutzfeldt A. Resin composites in dentistry: the monomer systems. *Eur J Oral Sci.* 1997;105:97–116.

Sakaguchi RL, Wiltbank BD, Murchison CF. Prediction of composite elastic modulus and polymerization shrinkage by computational micromechanics. *Dent Mater.* 2004;20:397–401.

Urabe I, Nakajima S, Sano H, Tagami J. Physical properties of the dentin-enamel junction region. *Am J Dent.* 2000;13:129–135.

Tear Strength and Tear Energy

American Society for Testing and Materials. Strength of conventional vulcanized rubber and thermoplastic elastomers, D 624–91. *ASTM Standards 1994. vol. 9.01.* American Society for Testing and Materials; 1994.

Hardness, Friction, and Wear

Abe Y, Sato Y, Akagawa Y, Ohkawa S. An in vitro study of high-strength resin posterior denture tooth wear. *Int J Prosthodont.* 1997;10:28–34.

Condon JR, Ferracane JL. Factors effecting dental composite wear in vitro. *J Biomed Mater Res.* 1997;38:303–313.

Condon JR, Ferracane JL. In vitro wear of composite with varied cure, filler level, and filler treatment. *J Dent Res.* 1997;76:1405–1411.

Ferracane JL, Mitchem JC, Condon JR, Todd R. Wear and marginal breakdown of composites with various degrees of cure. *J Dent Res.* 1997;76:1508–1516.

Hu X, Harrington E, Marquis PM, Shortall AC. The influence of cyclic loading on the wear of a dental composite. *Biomaterials.* 1999;20:907–912.

Hu X, Marquis PM, Shortall AC. Two-body in vitro wear study of some current dental composites and amalgams. *J Prosthet Dent.* 1999;82:214–220.

Koczorowski R, Wloch S. Evaluation of wear of selected prosthetic materials in contact with enamel and dentin. *J Prosthet Dent.* 1999;81:453–459.

Teoh SH, Ong LF, Yap AU, Hastings GW. Bruxing-type dental wear simulator for ranking of dental restorative materials. *J Biomed Mater Res.* 1998;43:175–183.

Turssi CP, De Moraes Purquerio B, Serra MC. Wear of dental resin composites: insights into underlying processes and assessment methods. A review. *J Biomed Mater Res B Appl Biomater.* 2003;65:280–285.

Xu HH, Smith DT, Jahanmir S, et al. Indentation damage and mechanical properties of human enamel and dentin. *J Dent Res.* 1998;77:472–480.

Yap AU, Ong LF, Teoh SH, Hastings GW. Comparative wear ranking of dental restoratives with the BIOMAT wear simulator. *J Oral Rehabil.* 1999;26:228–235.

Colloidal State, Surface Properties, Adhesion

Iler RK. *The Chemistry of Silica-Solubility, Polymerization, Colloid and Surface Properties, and Biochemistry.* John Wiley & Sons; 1979.

O'Brien WJ. *Capillary Penetration of Liquids Between Dissimilar Solids, Doctoral Thesis.* University of Michigan; 1967.

O'Brien WJ, Fan PL, Apostolidis A. Penetrativity of sealants and glazes. The effectiveness of a sealant depends on its ability to penetrate into fissures. *Oper Dent.* 1978;3(2):51–56.

Rosales JI, Marshall GW, Marshall SJ, et al. Acid-etching and hydration influence on dentin roughness and wettability. *J Dent Res.* 1999;78:1554–1559.

Somorjai GA. *Introduction to Surface Chemistry and Catalysis.* John Wiley & Sons; 1994.

van Meerbeek B, Williams G, Celis JP, et al. Assessment by mono-indentation of the hardness and elasticity of the resin-dentin bonding area. *J Dent Res.* 1993;72:1434–1442.

Willems G, Celis JP, Lambrechts P, Braem M, Vanherle G. Hardness and young's modulus determined by nanoindentation technique of filler particles of dental restorative materials compared with human enamel. *J Biomed Mater Res.* 1993;27:747–755.

Yoshida Y, van Meerbeek B, Nakayama Y, et al. Evidence of chemical bonding at biomaterial-hard tissue interfaces. *J Dent Res.* 2000;79:709–714.

Yoshida Y, van Meerbeek B, Snowwaert J, et al. A novel approach to AFM characterization of adhesive tooth-biomaterials interfaces. *J Biomed Mater Res.* 1999;47:85–90.

Color and Optical Properties

American Society for Testing and Materials. Specifying color by the Munsell system, D1535–D68 (1974). *ASTM Standards, 1975, Part 20.* American Society for Testing and Materials; 1975.

Cho MS, Yu B, Lee YK. Opalescence of all-ceramic core and veneer materials. *Dent Mater.* 2009;25:695–702.

Corciolani G, Vichi A, Louca C, Ferrari M. Influence of layering thickness on the color parameters of a ceramic system. *Dent Mater.* 2010;26:737–742.

Heffernan MJ, Aquilino SA, Diaz-Arnold AM, Haselton DR, Stansford CM, Vargas MA. Relative translucency of six all ceramics. Part I: core materials. *J Prosthet Dent.* 2000;88:4–9.

Heffernan MJ, Aquilino SA, Diaz-Arnold AM, Haselton DR, Stansford CM, Vargas MA. Relative translucency of six all ceramics. Part II: core and veneer materials. *J Prosthet Dent.* 2000;88:10–15.

Hyun HK, Christoferson CK, Pfeifer CS, Felix C, Ferracane JL. Effect of shade, opacity and layer thickness on light transmission through a nano-hybrid dental composite during curing. *J Esthet Restor Dent.* 2017;29:362–367.

Johnston WM, Ma T, Kienle BH. Translucency parameter of colorants for maxillofacial prostheses. *Int J Prosthodont.* 1995;8:79–86.

Judd DB, Wyszecki G. *Color in Business, Science, and Industry.* 3rd ed. John Wiley & Sons; 1975.

Kiat-Amnuay S, Lemon JC, Powers JM. Effects of opacifiers on color stability of pigmented maxillofacial silicone A-2186 subjected to artificial aging. *J Prosthodont.* 2002;11:109–116.

Kubelka P. New contributions to the optics of intensely light-scattering materials. Part I. *Opt Soc Am J.* 1948;38:448–457.

Lee Y-K, Lim B-S, Powers JM. Color changes of dental resin composites by a salivary enzyme. *J Biomed Mater Res.* 2004;70:66–72.

Noie F, O'Keefe KL, Powers JM. Color stability of resin cements after accelerated aging. *Int J Prosthodont.* 1995;8:51–55.

O'Keefe KL, Powers JM, Noie F. Effect of dissolution on color of extrinsic porcelain colorants. *Int J Prosthodont.* 1993;6:558–563.

Paravina RD, Ghinea R, Herrera LJ, et al. Color difference thresholds in dentistry. *J Esthet Restor Dent.* 2015;27(Suppl 1):S1–S9.

Paravina RD, Ontiveros JC, Powers JM. Curing-dependent changes in color and translucency parameter of composite bleach shades. *J Esthet Restor Dent.* 2002;14:158–166.

Paravina RD, Ontiveros JC, Powers JM. Accelerated aging effects on color and translucency of bleaching-shade composites. *J Esthet Restor Dent.* 2004;16:117–126 discussion 126–127.

Paravina RD, Powers JM, eds. *Esthetic Color Training in Dentistry.* Mosby; 2004.

Ragain JC, Johnston WM. Accuracy of Kubelka-Munk reflectance theory applied to human dentin and enamel. *J Dent Res.* 2001;80:449–452.

Seghi RR, Johnston WM, O'Brien WJ. Spectrophotometric analysis of color differences between porcelain systems. *J Prosthet Dent.* 1986;56:35–40.

Vichi A, Ferrari M, Davidson CL. Influence of ceramic and cement thickness on the masking of various types of opaque posts. *J Prosthet Dent.* 2000;83:412–417.

Yeh CL, Miyagawa Y, Powers JM. Color of selected shades of composites by reflection spectrophotometry. *J Dent Res.* 1982;61(1):1176–1179.

Thermal Properties

Antonucci JM, Toth EE. Extent of polymerization of dental resins by differential scanning calorimetry. *J Dent Res.* 1983;62:121–125.

Craig RG, Peyton FA. Thermal conductivity of tooth structure, dental cements, and amalgam. *J Dent Res.* 1961;40:411–418.

de Vree JH, Spierings TA, Plasschaert AJ. A simulation model for transient thermal analysis of restored teeth. *J Dent Res.* 1983;62:756–759.

Murayama T. *Dynamic Mechanical Analysis of Polymeric Materials.* Elsevier Science; 1978.

Peyton FA. Effectiveness of water coolants with rotary cutting instruments. *J Am Dent Assoc.* 1958;56(5):664–675.

Volland RH, Paffenbarger GC. Cast gold inlay technic as worked out in the cooperative research at the National Bureau of standards and applied by a group of practicing dentists. *J Am Dent Assoc.* 1932;19(2):185–205.

Wilson TW, Turner DT. Characterization of polydimethacrylates and their composites by dynamic mechanical analysis. *J Dent Res.* 1987;66:1032–1035.

Electrical and Electrochemical Properties

Arvidson K, Johansson EG. Galvanic series of some dental alloys. *Scand J Dent Res.* 1977;85:485–491.

Bergman M, Ginstrup O, Nilner K. Potential and polarization measurements in vivo of oral galvanism. *Scand J Dent Res.* 1978;86:135–145.

Fairhurst CW, Marek M, Butts MB, Okabe T. New information on high copper amalgam corrosion. *J Dent Res.* 1978;57:725–729.

Gjerdet NR, Brune D. Measurements of currents between dissimilar alloys in the oral cavity. *Scand J Dent Res.* 1977;85:500–502.

Holland RI. Galvanic currents between gold and amalgam. *Scand J Dent Res.* 1980;88:269–272.

Hörsted-Bindslev P, Vilkinis V, Sidlauskas A. Direct capping of human pulps with a dentin bonding system or with calcium hydroxide cement. *Oral Surg Oral Med Oral Pathol Oral Radiol Endod.* 2003;96(5):591–600.

Maijer R, Smith DC. Corrosion of orthodontic bracket bases. *Am J Orthod.* 1982;81:43–48.

Mohsen NM, Craig RG, Filisko FE. The effects of different additives on the dielectric relaxation and the dynamic mechanical properties of urethane dimethacrylate. *J Oral Rehabil.* 2000;27:250–268.

Mumford JM. Electrolytic action in the mouth and its relationship to pain. *J Dent Res.* 1957;36:632–640.

Mumford JM. Resistivity of human enamel and dentin. *Arch Oral Biol.* 1967;12:925–927.

Phillips LJ, Schnell RJ, Phillips RW. Measurement of the electric conductivity of dental cement. IV. Extracted human teeth; in vivo tests; summary. *J Dent Res.* 1955;34:839–848.

Tay WM, Braden M. Dielectric properties of glass ionomer cements. *J Dent Res.* 1981;60:1311–1314.

Other Properties

Raptis CM, Powers JM, Fan PL, Yu R. Staining of composite resins by cigarette smoke. *J Oral Rehabil.* 1982;9:367–371.

Biocompatibility

Abdul Razak AA. Mercury toxicity and its implications—a review of the literature. *Dent J Malays.* 1988;10:5–10.

Addy M, Martin MV. Systemic antimicrobials in the treatment of chronic periodontal diseases: a dilemma. *Oral Dis.* 2003;9:38–44.

al-Dawood A, Wennberg A. Biocompatibility of dentin bonding agents. *Endod Dent Traumatol.* 1993;9:1–7.

American Dental Association (ADA) Council on Scientific Affairs. Dental amalgam: update on safety concerns. *J Am Dent Assoc.* 1998;129: 494–503.

Aoba T, Fejerskov O. Dental fluorosis: chemistry and biology. *Crit Rev Oral Biol Med.* 2002;13:155–170.

Banerjee R, Nageswari K, Puniyani RR. Hematological aspects of biocompatibility—review article. *J Biomater Appl.* 1997;12:57–76.

Beltran-Aguilar ED, Goldstein JW, Lockwood SA. Fluoride varnishes. A review of their clinical use, cariostatic mechanism, efficacy and safety. *J Am Dent Assoc.* 2000;131:589–596.

Berkenstock OL. Issues concerning possible cobalt-chromium carcinogenicity: a literature review and discussion. *Contemp Orthop.* 1992;24:265–278.

Bouillaguet S, Ciucchi B, Holz J. Potential risks for pulpal irritation with contemporary adhesive restorations: an overview. *Acta Med Dent Helv.* 1996;1:235.

Brackett WW, Tay FR, Brackett MG, Dib A, Sword RJ, Pashley DH. The effect of chlorhexidine on dentin hybrid layers in vivo. *Oper Dent.* 2007;32:107–111.

Brannstrom M. *Dentin and Pulp in Restorative Dentistry.* Wolfe Medical Publications; 1982.

Brodin P. Neurotoxic and analgesic effects of root canal cements and pulp-protecting dental materials. *Endod Dent Traumatol.* 1988;4:1–11.

Brune D. Metal release from dental biomaterials. *Biomaterials.* 1986;7:163–175.

Carrilho MRO, Geraldeli S, Tay F, et al. In vivo preservation of the hybrid layer by chlorhexidine. *J Dent Res.* 2007;86:529–533.

Clarkson TW. The toxicology of mercury. *Crit Rev Clin Lab Sci.* 1997;34:369–403.

Cook SD, Dalton JE. Biocompatibility and biofunctionality of implanted materials. *Alpha Omegan.* 1992;85:41–47.

Cox CF, Hafez AA. Biocomposition and reaction of pulp tissues to restorative treatments. *Dent Clin North Am.* 2001;45:31–48; v.

Cox CF, Keall CL, Keall HJ, Ostro EO, Bergenholtz G. Biocompatibility of surface-sealed dental materials against exposed pulps. *J Prosthet Dent.* 1987;57:1–8.

Dahl JE, Pallesen U. Tooth bleaching—a critical review of the biological aspects. *Crit Rev Oral Biol Med.* 2003;14:292–304.

Duque C, Hebling J, Smith AJ, Giro EMA, Oliveira MF, de Souza Costa CA. Reactionary dentinogenesis after applying restorative materials and bioactive dentin matrix molecules as liners in deep cavities prepared in nonhuman primate teeth. *J Oral Rehabil.* 2006;33:452–461.

Eliades T, Athanasiou AE. In vivo aging of orthodontic alloys: implications for corrosion potential, nickel release, and biocompatibility. *Angle Orthod.* 2002;72:222–237.

Ferracane JL. Elution of leachable components from composites. *J Oral Rehabil.* 1994;21:441–452.

Ferracane JL, Cooper PR, Smith AJ. Can interaction of materials with the dentin-pulp complex contribute to dentin regeneration? *Odontology.* 2010;98:2–14.

Gerzina TM, Hume WR. Diffusion of monomers from bonding resin-resin composite combinations through dentine in vitro. *J Dent.* 1996;24:125–128.

Geurtsen W, Leyhausen G. Biological aspects of root canal filling materials—histocompatibility, cytotoxicity, and mutagenicity. *Clin Oral Investig.* 1997;1:5–11.

Geurtsen W, Leyhausen G. Chemical-biological interactions of the resin monomer triethyleneglycol-dimethacrylate (TEGDMA). *J Dent Res.* 2001;80(12):2046–2050.

Geurtsen W. Biocompatibility of resin-modified filling materials. *Crit Rev Oral Biol Med.* 2000;11:333–355.

Geurtsen W. Substances released from dental resin composites and glass ionomer cements. *Eur J Oral Sci.* 1998;106:687–695.

Glantz PO. Intraoral behaviour and biocompatibility of gold versus non precious alloys. *J Biol Buccale.* 1984;12:3–16.

Gochfeld M. Cases of mercury exposure, bioavailability, and absorption. *Ecotoxicol Environ Saf.* 2003;56:174–179.

Goldberg M. In vitro and in vivo studies on the toxicity of dental resin components: a review. *Clin Oral Investig.* 2008;12(1):1–8.

Goldberg M, Smith AJ. Cells and extracellular matrices of dentin and pulp: a biological basis for repair and tissue engineering. *Crit Rev Oral Biol Med.* 2004;15:13–27.

Graham L, Cooper PR, Cassidy N, Nor JE, Sloan AJ, Smith AJ. The effect of calcium hydroxide on solubilisation of bio-active dentin matrix components. *Biomater.* 2006;27:2865–2873.

Grimaudo NJ. Biocompatibility of nickel and cobalt dental alloys. *Gen Dent.* 2001;49:498–503; quiz 504–505.

Gross UM. Biocompatibility—the interaction of biomaterials and host response. *J Dent Educ.* 1988;52:798–803.

Hauman CH, Love RM. Biocompatibility of dental materials used in contemporary endodontic therapy: a review. Part 1. Intracanal drugs and substances. *Int Endod J.* 2003;36:75–85.

Hauman CH, Love RM. Biocompatibility of dental materials used in contemporary endodontic therapy: a review. Part 2. Root-canal-filling materials. *Int Endod J.* 2003;36:147–160.

Hayden J Jr. Considerations in applying to man the results of drug effects observed in laboratory animals. *J Am Dent Assoc.* 1977;95:777–786.

Haywood VB, Heymann HO. Nightguard vital bleaching: how safe is it? *Quint Int.* 1991;22:515–523.

Hensten-Pettersen A. Skin and mucosal reactions associated with dental materials. *Eur J Oral Sci.* 1998;106:707–712.

Horsted-Bindslev P. Amalgam toxicity—environmental and occupational hazards. *J Dent.* 2004;32:359–365.

Hubbard MJ. Calcium transport across the dental enamel epithelium. *Crit Rev Oral Biol Med.* 2000;11:437–466.

Hume WR, Gerzina TM. Bioavailability of components of resin-based materials which are applied to teeth. *Crit Rev Oral Biol Med.* 1996;7:172–179.

Hume WR, Massey WL. Keeping the pulp alive: the pharmacology and toxicology of agents applied to dentine. *Aust Dent J.* 1990;35:32–37.

Hume WR. A new technique for screening chemical toxicity to the pulp from dental restorative materials and procedures. *J Dent Res.* 1985;64:1322–1325.

International Standards Organization (ISO). *ISO 10993: Biological Evaluation of Medical Devices.* ISO; 1992.

International Standards Organization (ISO). *ISO 7405: Preclinical Evaluation of Biocompatibility of Medical Devices Used in Dentistry – Test Methods for Dental Materials.* ISO; 1997.

Jarup L. Hazards of heavy metal contamination. *Br Med Bull.* 2003;68:167–182.

Jontell M, Okiji T, Dahlgren U, Bergenholtz G. Immune defense mechanisms of the dental pulp. *Crit Rev Oral Biol Med.* 1998;9:179–200.

Jorge JH, Giampaolo ET, Machado AL, Vergani CE. Cytotoxicity of denture base acrylic resins: a literature review. *J Prosthet Dent.* 2003;90:190–193.

Kaga M, Seale NS, Hanawa T, Ferracane JL, Waite DE, Okabe T. Cytotoxicity of amalgams, alloys, and their elements and phases. *Dent Mater.* 1991;7(1):68–72.

Kuratate M, Yoshiba K, Shigetani Y, Yoshiba N, Ohshima H, Okiji T. Immunohistochemical analysis of nestin, osteopontin, and proliferating cells in the reparative process of exposed dental pulp capped with mineral trioxide aggregate. *J Endod.* 2008;34:970–974.

Leggat PA, Kedjarune U. Toxicity of methyl methacrylate in dentistry. *Int Dent J.* 2003;53:126–131.

Lemons J, Natiella J. Biomaterials, biocompatibility, and peri-implant considerations. *Dent Clin North Am.* 1986;30:3–23.

Lewis B. Formaldehyde in dentistry: a review for the millennium. *J Clin Pediatr Dent.* 1998;22:167–177.

Li Y. Peroxide-containing tooth whiteners: an update on safety. *Compend Contin Educ Dent Suppl.* 2000;28:S4–S9 ; quiz S48.

Mackert JR Jr, Bergland A. Mercury exposure from dental amalgam filling: absorbed dose and the potential for adverse health effects. *Crit Rev Oral Biol Med.* 1997;8:410–436.

Mackert JR Jr. Side-effects of dental ceramics. *Adv Dent Res.* 1992;6:90–93.

Mantellini MG, Botero T, Yaman P, Dennison JB, Hanks CT, Nör JE. Adhesive resin and the hydrophilic monomer HEMA induce VEGF expression on dental pulp cells and macrophages. *Dent Mater.* 2006;22:434–440.

Masuda-Murakami Y, Kobayashi M, Wang X, et al. Effects of mineral trioxide aggregate on the differentiation of rat dental pulp cells. *Acta Histochem.* 2010;112(5):452–458.

Marigo L, Vittorini Orgeas G, Piselli D, Saccomanno S, Rumi G. Pulpo-dentin protection: the biocompatibility of materials most commonly used in restorative work. A literature review. *Minerva Stomatol.* 1999;48:373–395.

Meryon SD. The influence of dentine on the in vitro cytotoxicity testing of dental restorative materials. *J Biomed Mater Res.* 1984;18:771–779.

Messer RL, Bishop S, Lucas LC. Effects of metallic ion toxicity on human gingival fibroblasts morphology. *Biomaterials.* 1999;20:1647–1657.

Mongkolnam P. The adverse effects of dental restorative materials—a review. *Aust Dent J.* 1992;37:360–367.

National institutes of health consensus development conference statement: dental implants. *J Am Dent Assoc.* 1988;117(3):509 , 511, 513. Erratum in: *J Dent Educ.* 1988;52(12):824.

Nicholson JW. Glass-ionomers in medicine and dentistry. *Proc Inst Mech Eng H.* 1998;212:121–126.

Pierce LH, Goodkind RJ. A status report of possible risks of base metal alloys and their components. *J Prosthet Dent.* 1989;62:234–238.
Pillai KS, Stanley VA. Implications of fluoride—an endless uncertainty. *J Environ Biol.* 2002;23:81–87.
Ratner BD. Replacing and renewing: synthetic materials, biomimetics, and tissue engineering in implant dentistry. *J Dent Educ.* 2001;65:1340–1347.
Rogers KD. Status of scrap (recyclable) dental amalgams as environmental health hazards or toxic substances. *J Am Dent Assoc.* 1989;119:159–166.
Santerre JP, Shajii L, Leung BW. Relation of dental composite formulations to their degradation and the release of hydrolyzed polymeric-resin-derived products. *Crit Rev Oral Biol Med.* 2001;12:136–151.
Schmalz G. The biocompatibility of non-amalgam dental filling materials. *Eur J Oral Sci.* 1998;106:696–706.
Schuurs AH. Reproductive toxicity of occupational mercury. A review of the literature. *J Dent.* 1999;27:249–256.
Shabalovskaya SA. On the nature of the biocompatibility and on medical applications of NiTi shape memory and superelastic alloys. *Biomed Mater Eng.* 1996;6:267–289.
Sidhu SK, Schmalz G. The biocompatibility of glass-ionomer cement materials. A status report for the American journal of dentistry. *Am J Dent.* 2001;14:387–396.
Smith AJ. Vitality of the dentin-pulp complex in health and disease: growth factors as key mediators. *J Dent Educ.* 2003;67:678–689.
Smith GE. Toxicity of fluoride-containing dental preparations: a review. *Sci Total Environ.* 1985;43:41–61.
Soderholm KJ, Mariotti A. Bis-GMA–based resins in dentistry: are they safe? *J Am Dent Assoc.* 1999;130:201–209.
Stanley HR. Effects of dental restorative materials: local and systemic responses reviewed. *J Am Dent Assoc.* 1993;124:76–80.
Stanley HR. Pulpal responses to ionomer cements—biological characteristics. *J Am Dent Assoc.* 1990;120:25–29.
Tomson PL, Grover LM, Lumley PJ, Sloan AJ, Smith AJ, Cooper PR. Dissolution of bio-active dentine matrix components by mineral trioxide aggregate. *J Dent.* 2007;35:636–642.
Veron MH, Couble ML. The biological effects of fluoride on tooth development: possible use of cell culture systems. *Int Dent J.* 1992;42:108–112.
Wahl MJ. Amalgam—resurrection and redemption. Part 2: the medical mythology of anti-amalgam. *Quint Int.* 2001;32:696–710.
Ward RA. Phagocytic cell function as an index of biocompatibility. *Nephrol Dial Transplant.* 1994;9:46–56.
Wataha JC, Hanks CT, Strawn SE, Fat JC. Cytotoxicity of components of resins and other dental restorative materials. *J Oral Rehabil.* 1994;21:453–462.
Wataha JC, Hanks CT. Biological effects of palladium and risk of using palladium in dental casting alloys. *J Oral Rehabil.* 1996;23:309–320.
Wataha JC. Biocompatibility of dental casting alloys: a review. *J Prosthet Dent.* 2000;83:223–234.
Wataha JC. Principles of biocompatibility for dental practitioners. *J Prosthet Dent.* 2001;86:203–209.
Watts A, Paterson RC. Initial biological testing of root canal sealing materials—a critical review. *J Dent.* 1992;20:259–265.
Whitford GM. The physiological and toxicological characteristics of fluoride. *J Dent Res.* 1990;69:539–549 discussion 556–557.
Williams DF. *Fundamental Aspects of Biocompatibility.* vol. 2. CRC Press; 1981.

5 General Classes of Biomaterials

JACK FERRACANE

CHAPTER OUTLINE

Dental biomaterials are generally categorized into four classes: metals, polymers, ceramics, and composites. The four classes are distinctly different from each other in terms of density, stiffness, translucency, processing method, application, and cost. One class, composites, is a combination of two or more classes that produce materials that can be engineered for specific applications. For some applications, such as intracoronal and extracoronal restorations, several classes offer suitable materials. For other applications, such as removable partial dental denture frameworks, one class is most appropriate. Requirements such as aesthetics, mechanical properties, biocompatibility, and cost may dictate the choice of material class. Restoration design and material class are always coordinated to achieve the best patient outcome.

This chapter is organized into four sections by the class of material. Fundamental concepts of each class are presented here. Additional detail is provided in other chapters when specific applications are discussed.

Metals and Alloys

Metals and alloys are used in almost all aspects of dental practice, including the dental laboratory, direct and indirect dental restorations, implants, and instruments used to prepare and clean teeth. Metals and alloys have optical, physical, chemical, thermal, and electrical properties that are unique among the basic types of materials and suitable for many dental applications. Metals provide strength, stiffness, fracture resistance, and longevity for long-term dental applications that are often not achievable with other classes of materials. Their major drawback is their lack of tooth-like aesthetics. Evidence in the scientific literature of clinical performance is the most extensive for this material class.

As a class, metals are ductile and malleable and therefore exhibit elastic and plastic behavior; they are good electrical and thermal conductors, are higher in density than other classes, exhibit good fracture resistance, are opaque, and can be polished to a luster. Metals may be cast, drawn into wires, or machined to create dental restorations and instruments.

Chemical and Atomic Structure of Metals

A metal is any element that ionizes positively in solution. As a group, metals constitute nearly two-thirds of the periodic table (Fig. 5.1). During ionization, metals release electrons. This ability to exist as free, positively charged, stable ions is a key factor in the behavior of metals and is responsible for many metallic properties that are important in dentistry. Another important group of elements shown in Fig. 5.1 are the metalloids, including boron, silicon, germanium, arsenic, antimony, tellurium, and polonium. Carbon is sometimes referred to as a metalloid but mostly as a nonmetal. Although metalloids do not always form free positive ions, their conductive and electronic properties make them important components of many dental alloys.

Atomic Structure

While it is possible to produce amorphous metals, at the atomic level, pure metals exist mostly as crystalline arrays (Fig. 5.2) that are continuous in three dimensions. In these arrays, the nuclei and core electrons occupy the atomic center, with the ionizable electrons floating freely among the atomic positions. The mobility of the valence electrons is responsible for many properties of metals, such as electrical and thermal conductivity. It is important to note that the positively charged atomic centers are held together by the electrons, and their positive charge is simultaneously neutralized by the negative electrons. Thus pure metals have no net charge.

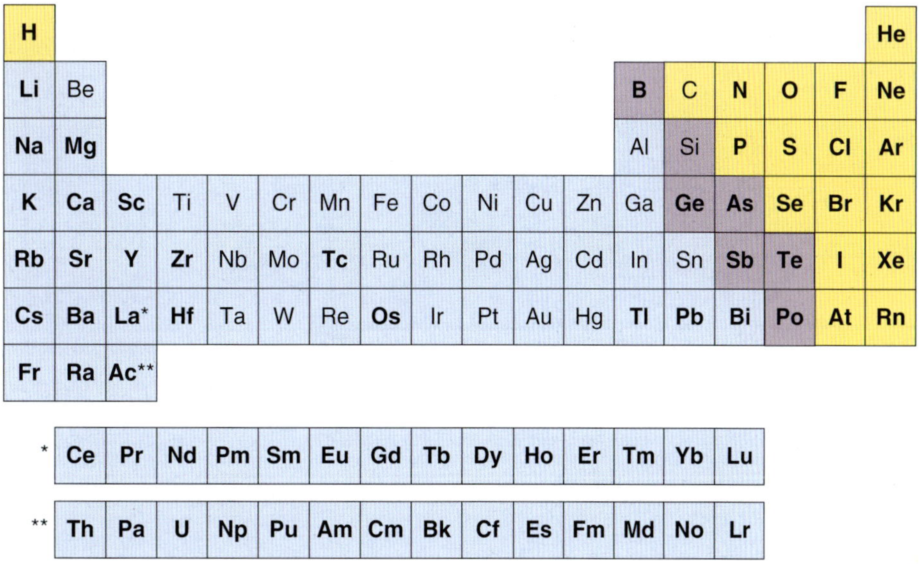

• **Fig. 5.1** Periodic table of elements. The periodic table of the elements can be subdivided into metals *(blue background)*, metalloids *(purple background)*, and nonmetals *(yellow background)*. Elements in nonbolded type are used in dental alloys or as pure metals. The metals are elements that ionize positively in solution and comprise the majority of elements in the periodic table. Note that not all elements are shown. Hydrogen is often included in group IA *(left column)* because it forms compounds with oxidation numbers of both +1 and −1. In addition, under very high pressures, hydrogen exhibits the properties of a metal. The *single asterisk* indicates the insertion point in the table for the lanthanide series of elements, whereas the *double asterisk* indicates the insertion point for the actinide series of elements.

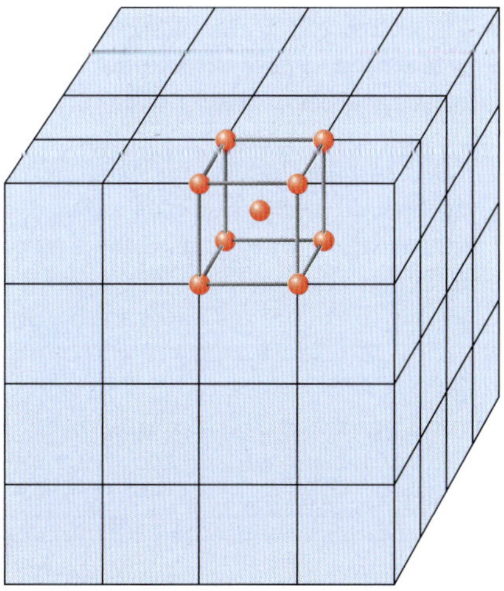

• **Fig. 5.2** A typical metallic crystal lattice, in this case, a body-centered cubic (BCC) lattice. Every lattice has a unit cell (*shown in bold*) that extends (repeats) in three dimensions for large distances. Electrons are only relatively loosely bound to atomic nuclei and core electrons. The nuclei occupy specific sites (*shown as dots in the unit cell*) in the lattice, whereas the electrons are relatively free to move about the lattice. In reality, the metal atoms are large enough to touch each other.

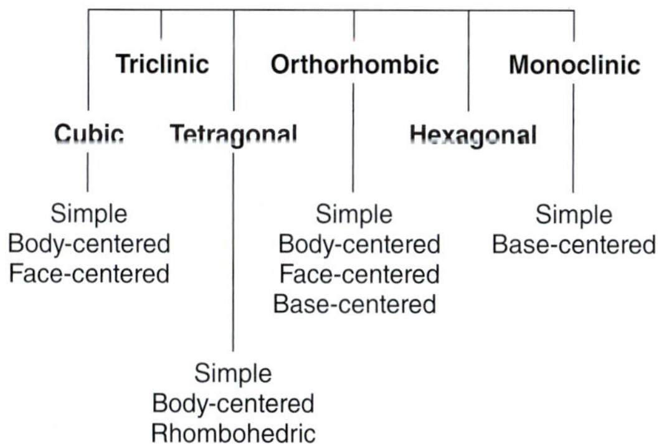

• **Fig. 5.3** Lattice structures. All metals occur in one of the lattice structures shown. There are six families of lattices, four of which can be subdivided. Each family is defined by the distances between vertices and the angles at the vertices. The body-centered cubic (BCC), face-centered cubic (FCC), and hexagonal lattices (*asterisks*) are the most common in dental alloys and pure metals.

The relationships between the atomic centers in a metallic crystalline array are not always uniform in all directions. The distances in the x, y (horizontal), and z (vertical) axes may be the same or different, and the angles between these axes may or may not be 90 degrees. In all, six crystal systems occur (Fig. 5.3), and they can be further divided into 14 crystalline arrays. Metallic nuclei may occur at the center of faces or vertices of the crystal. Within each array, the smallest repeating unit that captures all the relationships among atomic centers is called a *unit cell* (see Fig. 5.2). The unit cells for the most common arrays in dental metals are shown in Fig. 5.4. In the body-centered cubic (BCC) array, all angles are 90 degrees, and all atoms are equidistant from one another in the horizontal and vertical directions. Metallic atoms are located at the corners of the unit cell, and one atom is at the center of the unit cell (hence the name *BCC*). This is the crystal structure of iron and is common for many iron alloys.

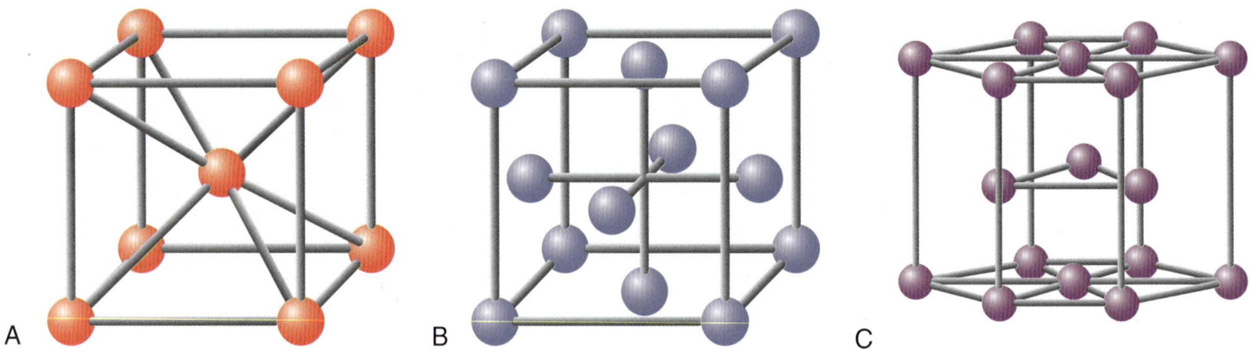

• **Fig. 5.4** The three most common crystal lattice unit cells in dental metals and alloys. (A) Body-centered cubic cell (BCC); (B) face-centered cubic (FCC) cell; and (C) hexagonal close-packed cell. The atoms (*circles*) in all three cases would be larger and touching each other. They were drawn smaller to make the structures easier to visualize.

The face-centered cubic (FCC) array has 90-degree angles and atomic centers that are equidistant horizontally and vertically (as does the BCC), but atoms are located in the centers of the faces with no atom in the center of the unit cell (hence the name *FCC*). Most pure metals and alloys of gold, palladium, cobalt, and nickel exhibit the FCC array. Titanium exhibits the more complex hexagonal close-pack array. In this array, the atoms are equidistant from each other in the horizontal plane but not in the vertical direction.

In a metallic crystal, the atomic centers are positively charged because the free valence electrons float in the crystal. Although we might expect the atomic centers to repel each other, the freely floating electrons bind the centers together and create a strong force between the atomic centers. This is known as the *metallic bond* and is a fundamentally important type of primary bond. The metallic bond is fundamentally different from other primary bonds, such as covalent bonds that occur in organic compounds and ionic bonds that occur in ceramics.

Physical Properties of Metals

All properties of metals result from the metallic crystal structure and metallic bonds. In general, metals have high densities that result from the efficient packing of atomic centers in the crystal lattice. Metals are electrically and thermally conductive because of the mobility of the valence electrons in the crystal lattice. The opacity and reflective nature of metals result from the ability of the valence electrons to absorb and emit light. Melting occurs as the metallic bond energy is overcome by the applied heat. Interestingly, the number of valence electrons per atomic center somewhat influences the melting point. As the number of valence electrons increases, the metallic bond develops some covalent character that contributes to higher melting points. This phenomenon occurs for iron (Fe^{3+}) and nickel (Ni^{2+}).

The corrosion properties of metals depend on the ability of atomic centers and electrons to be released in exchange for energy. The amount of energy required depends on the strength of the metallic force, which is related to the freedom of the valence electron, and the energy that the released ion can gain by solvating in solution. For metals such as sodium and potassium, the metallic bond is weaker because the valence electrons are loosely held, and the energy of solvation is high. These metals corrode into water with explosive energy release. For metals such as gold and platinum, the metallic bond is stronger; valence electrons are more tightly held, and solvation energies are relatively low. Thus gold and platinum are far less likely to corrode and are considered more stable. The corrosion of metals always involves oxidation and reduction. The released ion is oxidized because the electrons are given up, and the electrons (that cannot exist alone) are gained by some molecules in the solution (that are therefore reduced).

Because the distances between metal atoms in a crystal lattice may be different in the horizontal and vertical directions (see Fig. 5.4), properties such as conductivity of electricity and heat, magnetism, and strength may also vary by direction if a single crystal is observed. These directional properties of metals and metalloids have been exploited in the semiconductor industry to fabricate microchips for computers. However, in dentistry, a single crystal is rarely observed. Rather, a collection of randomly oriented crystals, each called a *grain*, generally make up a dental alloy. In this case, the directional properties are averaged across the material. In general, a fine-grained structure is desirable to encourage alloys with uniform properties in any direction. Nonuniformity of directional properties is termed *anisotropy*.

Like the physical properties, the mechanical properties of metals are also a result of the metallic crystal structure and metallic bonds. Metals generally have good ductility (ability to be drawn into a wire) and malleability (ability to be hammered into a thin sheet) relative to polymers and ceramics. To a large extent, these properties result from the ability of the atomic centers to slide against each other into new positions within the same crystal lattice. Because the metallic bonds are essentially nondirectional, such sliding is possible.

If the metallic crystals were perfect, calculations have shown that the force required to slide the atoms in the lattice would be hundreds of times greater than experiments indicate. Less force is necessary because the crystals are not perfect; they have flaws called *dislocations*. Dislocations allow the atomic centers to slide past each other one plane at a time (Fig. 5.5). Because movement can occur one plane at a time, the force required is much less than if the forces of all the planes have to be overcome simultaneously. An analogy is moving a large, heavy rug by forming a small fold or kink in the rug and pushing the fold from one end of the rug to the other. Dislocations are of several types, but all serve to allow the relatively easy deformation of metals. All methods for

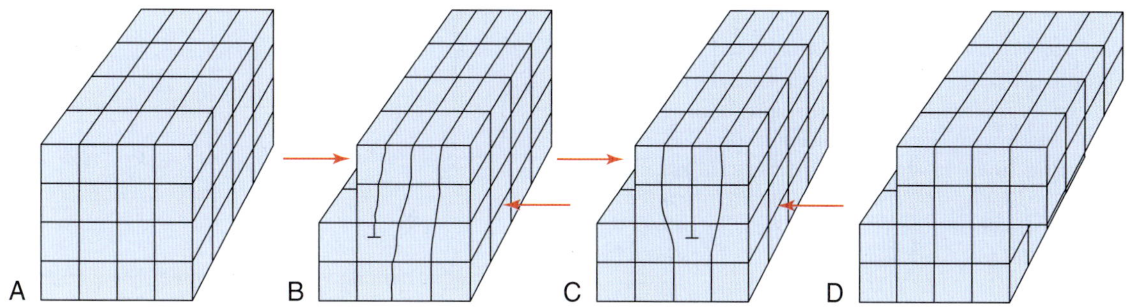

• **Fig. 5.5** Sketches representing a crystal and slip mechanisms resulting from movement of a dislocation. By the dislocation moving through the metal one plane at a time (A to B to C to D), far less energy is necessary to deform the metal. Furthermore, the movement occurs without fracture or failure of the crystal lattice.

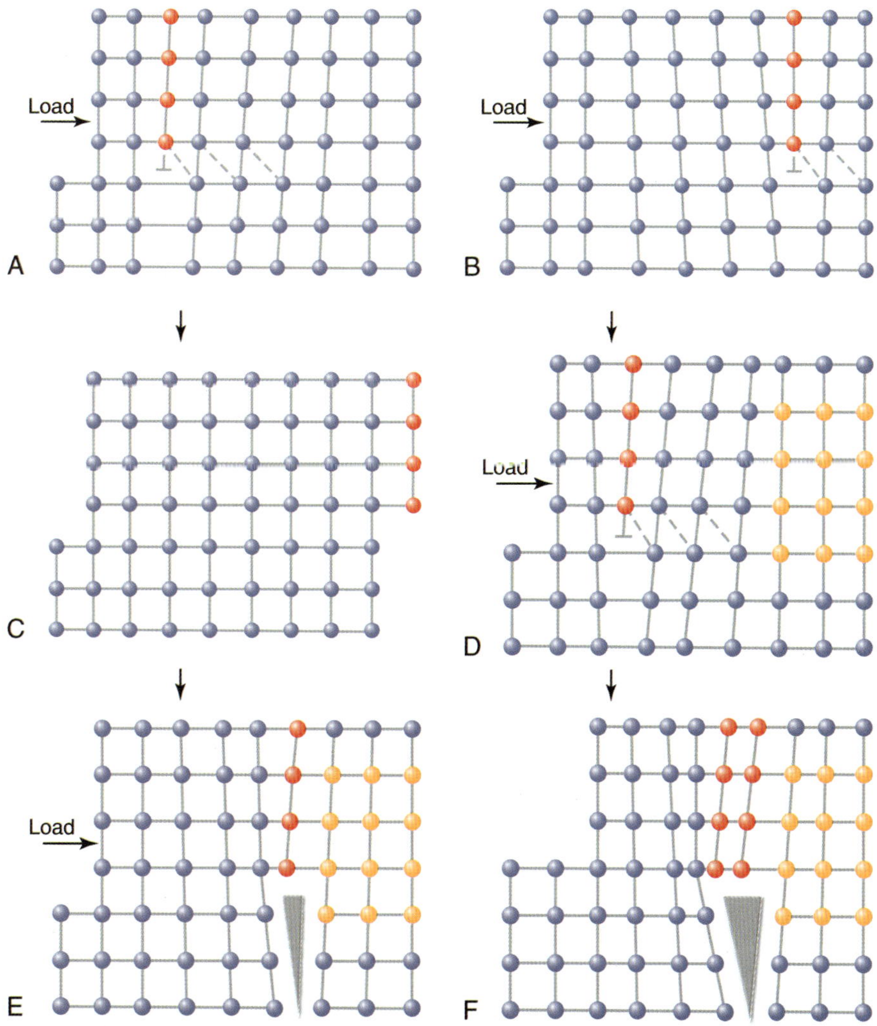

• **Fig. 5.6** Sketches showing plastic shearing with crack formation at the site of an impurity (*orange circles*). Without the impurity (A–C), the load forces the dislocations completely through the lattice without fracture (note the progression of *red circles* from *left* to *right*). However, when the impurity is present (D–F), it stops the progress of the dislocation. As other dislocations build up, the lattice below them cannot accommodate and a crack forms in the lattice (E). In (E and F), note the broken bonds between atoms. Once formed, a crack can grow rapidly and relatively easily and lead to catastrophic failure.

increasing the strength of metals act by impeding the movement of dislocations.

Metals fracture when the atomic centers cannot slide past one another freely. For example, this failure can happen when impurities block the flow of dislocations (Fig. 5.6). The inability of the dislocation to be moved through the solid results in the lattice rupturing locally. Once this small crack is started, it takes little force to propagate the crack through the lattice. An example illustrates this idea. Consider a plate of steel 15-cm wide and 6-mm thick. Suppose it has a 5-cm crack running into one side. The force required to make the crack run the remaining 10 cm would be about 1800 Newtons (N). Without the aid of the crack, 2.2 million Newtons (MN) would be required if the steel were the best commercial grade available. If the steel were a single, flawless crystal, 44 MN would be necessary! The fracture of metals depends heavily on dislocations and the local rupture of the crystal lattice.

Polymers

Polymers are commonly used for applications such as tooth restoratives, sealants, cements, orthodontic space maintainers and elastics, obturators for cleft palates, impressions, provisional restorations, root canal filling materials, denture bases, and athletic mouth protectors. In addition, polymers are typically one of the components of the fourth class of material, composites, which are discussed later in this chapter. As a class, polymers are formable, can be made translucent or opaque, are low in density and hardness compared with metals, and are poor conductors of temperature and electricity. Of the four classes of materials presented, polymers have the lowest stiffness, lowest long-term stability in an aqueous environment, and the lowest melting or glass transition point.

Basic Nature of Polymers

Chemical Composition

The term *polymer* denotes a molecule that is made up of many (poly) parts (mers). The *mer* ending represents the simplest repeating chemical structural unit from which the polymer is composed, a monomer. Thus poly(methyl methacrylate) is a polymer having chemical structural units derived from methyl methacrylate monomers, as indicated by the simplified reaction and structural formula I.

I

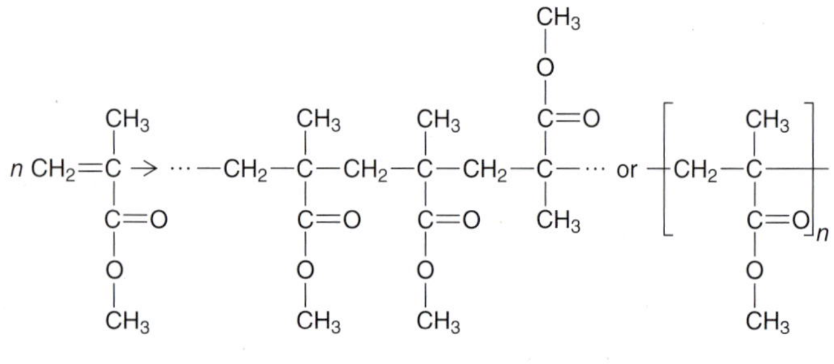

Methyl methacrylate — Poly(methyl methacrylate)

Polymer molecules may be prepared from a mixture of different types of monomers. They are called *copolymers* if they contain two or more different chemical units and *terpolymers* if they contain three different units, as indicated by the structural formulas II and III.

II

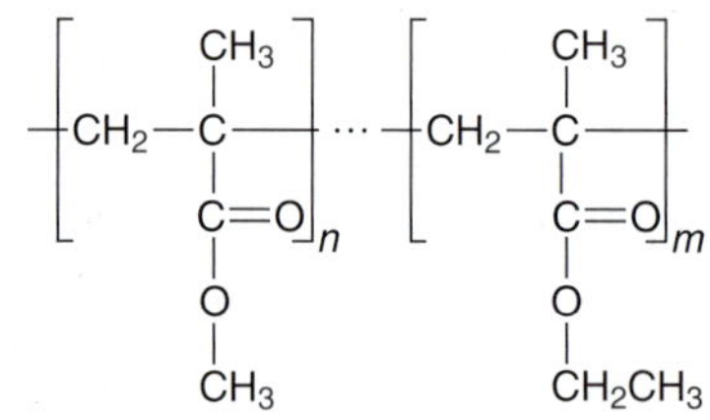

Methyl methacrylate–ethyl methacrylate copolymer

III

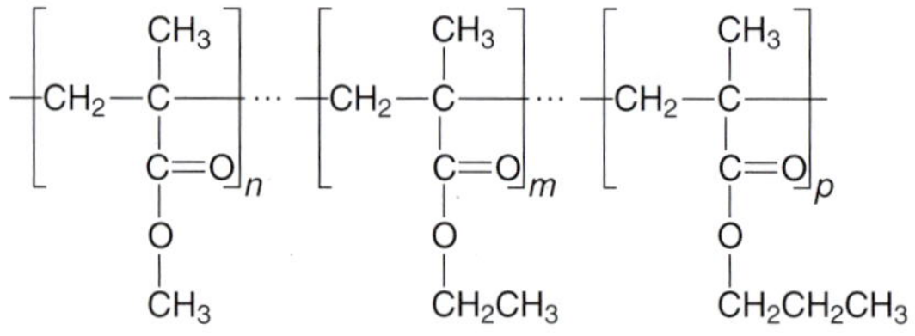

Methyl-, ethyl-, propyl methacrylate copolymer or terpolymer

As a convenience in expressing the structural formulas of polymers, the *mer* units are enclosed in brackets, and subscripts such as n, m, and p represent the average number of the various mer units that make up the polymer molecules. Notice that in normal polymers, the mer units are spaced in a random orientation along the polymer chain. It is possible, however, to produce copolymers with mer units arranged so that a large number of one mer type is connected to a large number of another mer type. This special type of polymer is called a *block polymer.* It is also possible to produce polymers having mer units with a special spatial arrangement with respect to the adjacent units; these are called *stereospecific* polymers.

The mers of the polymers are joined through covalent, C–C, bonds. Typically, during the polymerization process, C=C double bonds are converted to C–C single bonds, and a mer is attached to one of the carbon atoms that was part of the C=C double bond. The next section describes various network configurations for mers, including crosslinking, in which chains are linked in a nonlinear configuration.

Molecular Weight

The molecular weight of the polymer molecule, which equals the molecular weight of the various mers multiplied by the number of the mers, may range from thousands to millions of molecular weight units, depending on the preparation conditions. The higher the molecular weight of the polymer made from a single monomer, the higher the degree of polymerization. The term *polymerization* is often used in a qualitative sense, but the *degree of polymerization* is defined as the total number of mers in a polymer molecule. In general, the molecular weight of a polymer material is reported as the average molecular weight because the number of repeating units may vary greatly from one polymer molecule to another. As would be expected, the fraction of low-, medium-, and high-molecular-weight molecules in a material—or in other words, the molecular weight distribution—has as pronounced an effect on the physical properties as does the average molecular weight. Therefore two poly(methyl methacrylate) specimens can have the same chemical composition but greatly different physical properties because one of the specimens has a high percentage of low-molecular-weight molecules, whereas the other has a high percentage of high-molecular-weight molecules. Variation in the molecular weight distribution may be obtained by altering the

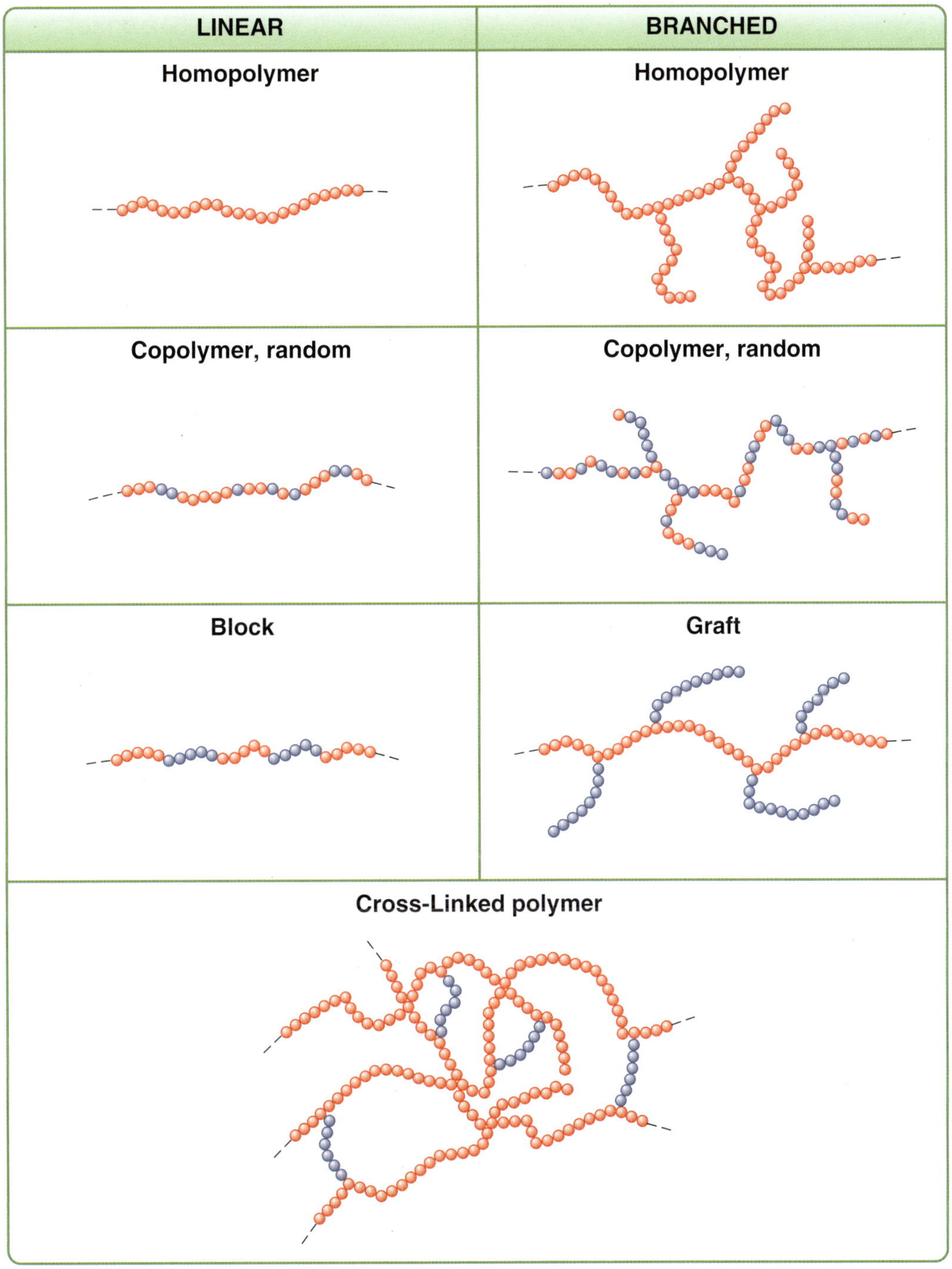

• **Fig. 5.7** Linear, branched, and crosslinked homopolymers and copolymers. *Red circles*, One type of mer unit; *blue circles*, another type of mer unit; *dashed lines*, continuation of the polymer segment.

polymerization procedure. These materials therefore do not possess any precise physical constants, such as melting point, as do ordinary small molecules. For example, the higher the molecular weight, the higher the softening and melting points, and the stiffer the polymer.

Spatial Structure

In addition to chemical composition and molecular weight, the physical or spatial structure of the polymer molecules is also important in determining the properties of the polymer. There are three basic types of structures: linear, branched, and crosslinked. They are illustrated in Fig. 5.7 as segments of linear, branched, and crosslinked polymers. The linear homopolymer has mer units of the same type, and the random copolymer of the linear type has two mer units randomly distributed along the chain. The linear block copolymer has segments, or blocks, along the chain, whereas the mer units are the same. The branched homopolymer again consists of the same mer units, whereas the graft-branched copolymer consists of one type of mer unit on the main chain and another mer for the branches. The crosslinked polymer shown in Fig. 5.7 is made up of a homopolymer crosslinked with a single crosslinking agent.

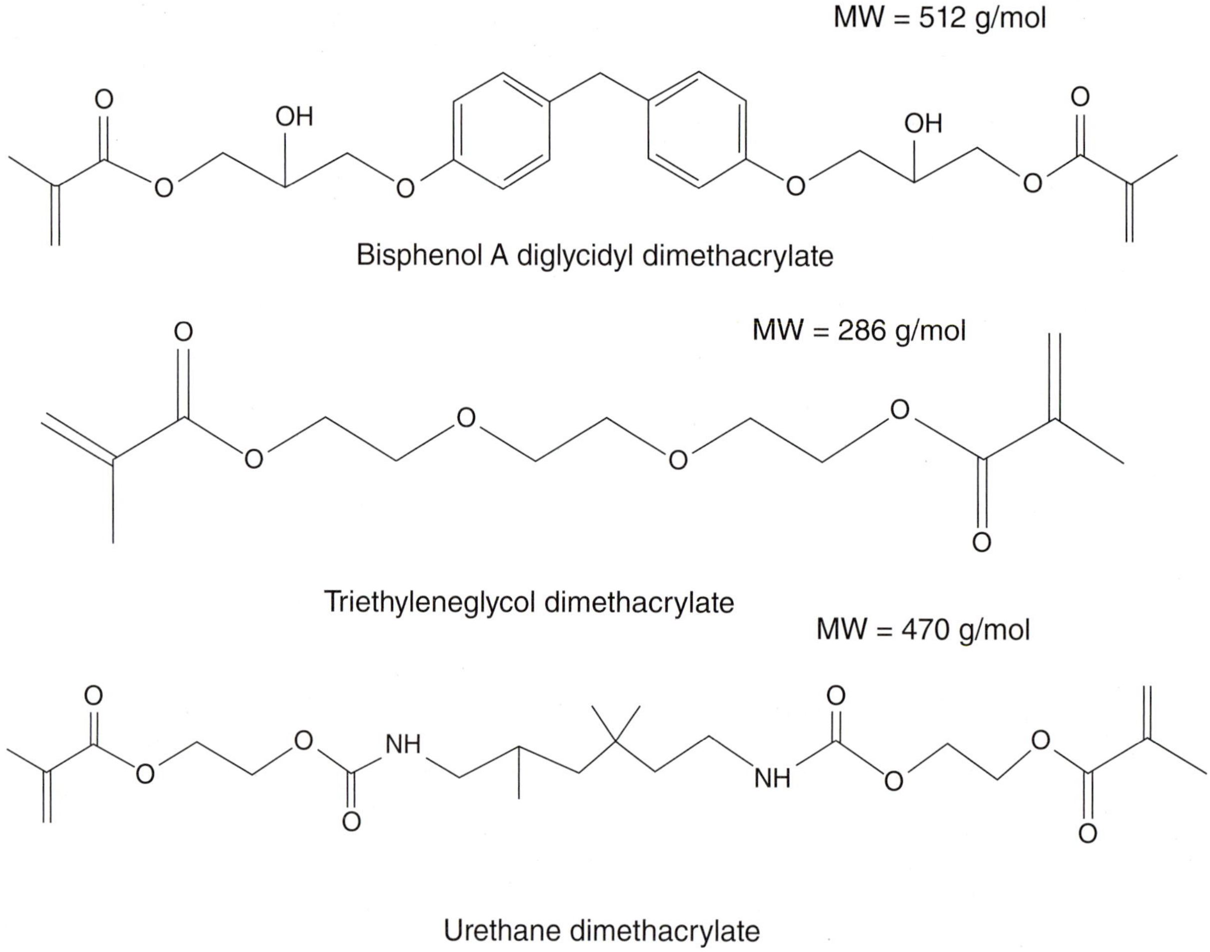

• **Fig. 5.8** Molecular structure of some of the most common monomers used in dental materials.

The linear and branched molecules are separate and discrete, whereas the crosslinked molecules are a network structure that may result in the creation of one giant polymeric molecule. The spatial structure of polymers affects their flow properties, but generalizations are difficult to make because either the interaction between linear polymer molecules or the length of the branches on the branched molecules may be more important in a particular example. In general, however, the crosslinked polymers flow at higher temperatures than linear or branched polymers. Another distinguishing feature of some crosslinked polymers is that they do not absorb liquids as readily as either linear or branched materials.

Thermoplastics and Thermosets

An additional method of classifying polymers other than by their spatial structure is according to whether they are thermoplastic or thermosetting. The term *thermoplastic* refers to polymers that may be softened by heating and hardened on cooling, the process being repeatable. Typical examples of polymers of this type are poly(methyl methacrylate) and polyethylene-polyvinyl acetate. The term *thermosetting or thermoset* refers to polymers that solidify during fabrication but cannot be softened by reheating. These polymers generally become nonfusible because of a crosslinking reaction and the formation of a spatial structure. Typical dental examples are crosslinked poly(methyl methacrylate), silicones, *cis*-polyisoprene, and dimethacrylates.

Polymers, as a class, have unique properties, and by varying the chemical composition, molecular weight, molecular weight distribution, or spatial arrangement of the mer units, the physical and mechanical properties of polymers may be altered.

Principles of Polymerization

Polymers are ubiquitous in our daily lives and also in dentistry. Examples include denture bases, impression materials, orthodontic appliances, bleaching trays, and a whole range of direct and indirect restorations. Dental adhesives and dental composites are also mainly organic polymers in nature. With the exception of

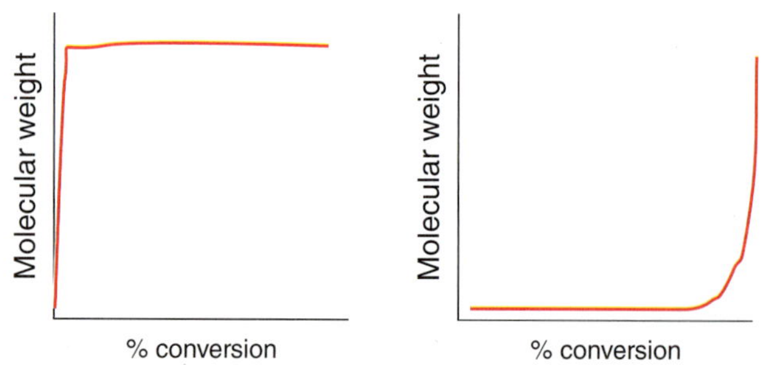

• **Fig. 5.9** Molecular weight increases as a function of conversion for chain-growth (*left*) and step-growth (*right*) polymerizations.

impression materials, which will be detailed in their specific chapter, most other polymers in dentistry are vinyl-based, more commonly composed of methacrylates. The basic structure of commonly used methacrylates is shown in Fig. 5.8.

Polymerization Mechanism

There are two mechanisms by which monomers can be joined together to form polymers: condensation (or step-growth) and addition (or chain-growth) polymerization. In condensation polymerization, monomers are usually difunctional and polymerize in a step-wise fashion (dimers link together to form tetramers, etc.) in such a way that the molecular weight increases slowly initially but presents a sharp increase toward the tail end of the polymerization. These reactions generally, but not necessarily, result in the elimination of a low-molecular-weight by-product such as water or ethanol. Some examples in dentistry include certain impression materials (condensation silicones and polysulfides). This chapter will focus on addition polymerization, the mechanism through which methacrylates polymerize. In this mechanism, individual monomers join a growing chain, so the increase in molecular weight is significant at relatively low conversions. Fig. 5.9 contrasts molecular weight development for the two different mechanisms. The implication of a fast increase in molecular weight is the rise of diffusion limitations for the growing polymer chain and for still unreacted monomers, which ultimately leads to incomplete mono mer conversion at room temperature. This is especially true for crosslinked polymers, such as resin composites and adhesives.

Phases of Addition Polymerization

There are three specific stages of polymerization in chain-growth/addition polymerization: initiation (or induction), propagation, and termination. They will be didactically described as being exclusively sequential, but it is important to note that these events overlap to some extent during polymerization.

Initiation requires the presence of compounds known as initiators, as well as a source of activation energy. Initiators can be classified into anionic (not common), cationic (a few examples in dentistry), and free radical (by far the most common in dentistry). Cationic initiators are required to polymerize epoxy-based materials and are usually composed of at least two components: one electron donor and one electron acceptor. This mechanism is very sensitive to moisture in the environment. Free-radical initiators are used to polymerize vinyl- (carbon double bond) containing monomers, such as methacrylates. The classes of free-radical initiators most commonly used in dentistry are Norrish-type II (e.g., camphorquinone, which requires a proton donor such as an amine to be effective) or alpha cleavage type I (e.g., benzoyl peroxide (BPO); bisacylphosphine oxides (BAPOs); or 1-phenyl-1,2-propanedione (PPD), the latter two known as alternative initiators for highly aesthetic materials).

In free-radical polymerization, the initiator requires energy input to overcome the activation energy barrier and move into an excited state, forming a radical that then interacts with the monomer, driving the monomer now into a reactive state. As far as sources of energy input, there are three main categories: thermal, redox (cold cure), and photopolymerization. In thermal initiation, the specific initiator has a bond that can be broken at high temperatures. For example, in benzoyl peroxide, the most common thermal initiator, also the one used in denture base materials, the oxygen-oxygen bond is thermolabile. Once the material is exposed to temperatures above 70°C for a number of hours, these bonds are broken, radicals are formed, then those radicals interact with the vinyl bond to start propagation. In redox initiation, instead of having a source of heat, an electron donor molecule (or hydrogen abstracting molecule, usually an amine) is added, which then that interacts with the benzoyl peroxide to start the radical formation, analogous to the role the temperature played in the previous example. This is also known as cold cure, self-curing, autopolymerization, or chemical cure. In those types of materials, each component (e.g., benzoyl peroxide and amine) must be kept separate until right before use, so they are usually formulated with two pastes that are mixed chair-side. Photopolymerization requires a light source to excite the photoinitiator (in the case of direct cleavage-type initiators) or the photosensitizer (in the case of Norrish-type initiators requiring co-initiators such the camphorquinone/amine systems). Specifically for camphorquinone-based materials, the sequence of events is as follows: photoenergy in the blue wavelength (around 470 nm) leads the photosensitizer into an exciplex state when it leads to proton abstraction in the amine co-initiator, which in turn becomes a free radical. This amine free radical then reacts with the first vinyl monomer, leading to the generation of a monomer radical. This monomer radical then continues the reaction in the propagation and termination phases. Finally, there are dual-cure materials that combine redox and photopolymerization mechanisms. This is useful in cases where light access is complicated, such as in the cementation of thick ceramic or metallic restorations. This will be discussed in Chapter 12.

Once the monomer radicals are formed, regardless of the initiator type and energy source, they start reacting with other monomers in the **propagation** phase. This process is exothermic, and for methacrylates, approximately 13 kcal/mol of vinyl functionalities are lost in the form of heat energy. This is an important consideration when polymerizing denture bases since the concentration of heat may cause the monomer to boil, leading to the formation of pores that weaken the structure. In the case of dental composites, the heat generated may be sufficient to cause injury to the dental pulp, especially in deep cavity preparations. During the course of propagation in multi-vinyl monomers, a tridimensional network is formed, which leads to diffusion limitations. Termination actually occurs concomitantly with propagation, and it relies either on close proximity of two growing polymer chains (bi-radical termination) and/or on the decay of the terminal radical (disproportionation). Because of the growing polymer chains and increasing diffusional limitations in the reaction medium, it becomes less likely that these long-range molecular motions take place, so propagation actually dominates this stage, since smaller molecules such as monomers and initiators have much greater degrees of freedom, so they continue adding to the ends of the polymer chains. This phenomenon is known as autoacceleration or cage effect. Eventually, the reaction medium becomes so restricted that even smaller molecules, such as monomers, which are also less abundant in this stage, lose mobility and end up being trapped in the forming network. These unreacted monomers may eventually leach out of the restoration into the oral environment and may cause cytotoxicity concerns to pulp and gingival cells. This is why it is important to pay close attention to the clinical procedures described for composites and adhesives to ensure as high monomer conversion as possible.

Initiation stage

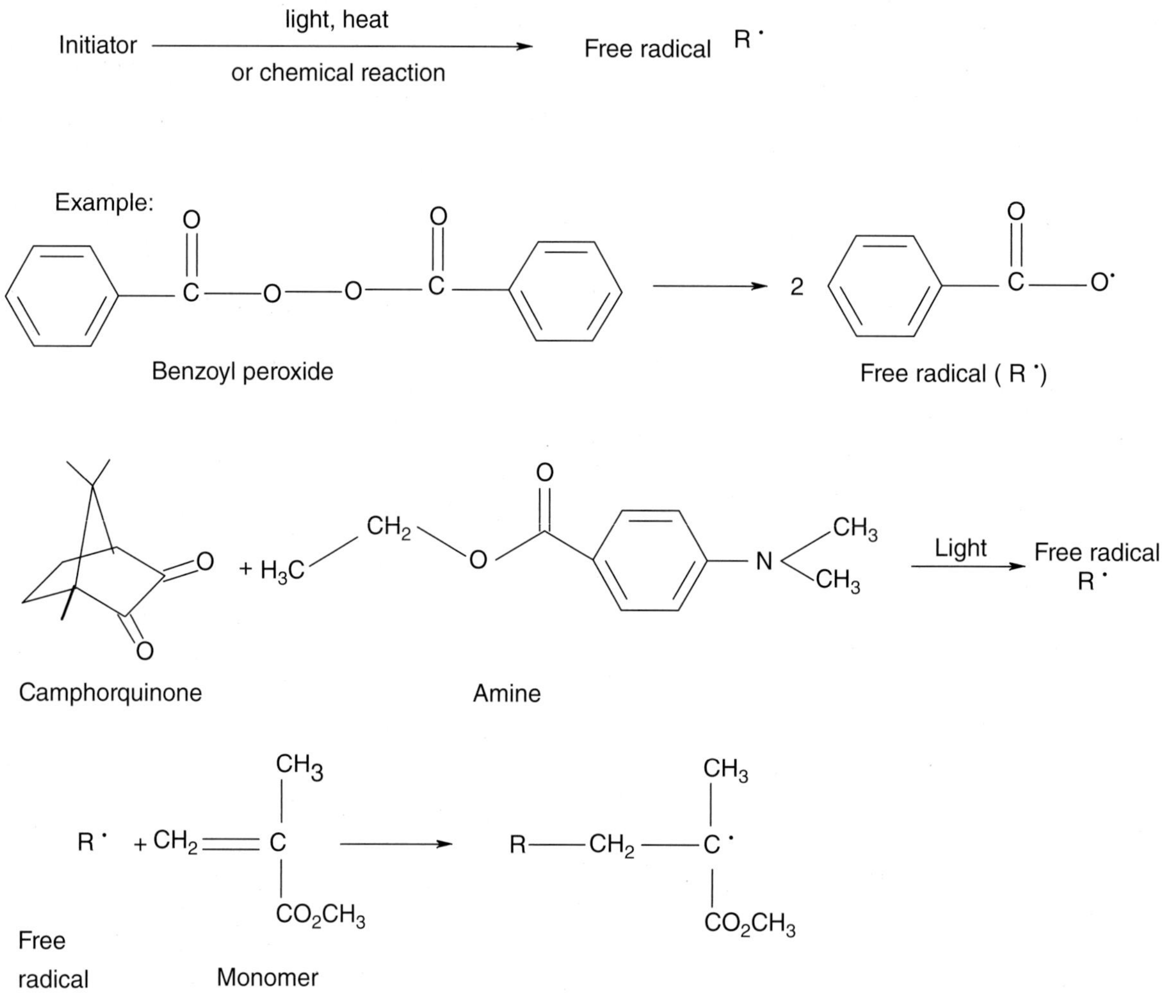

Propagation stage

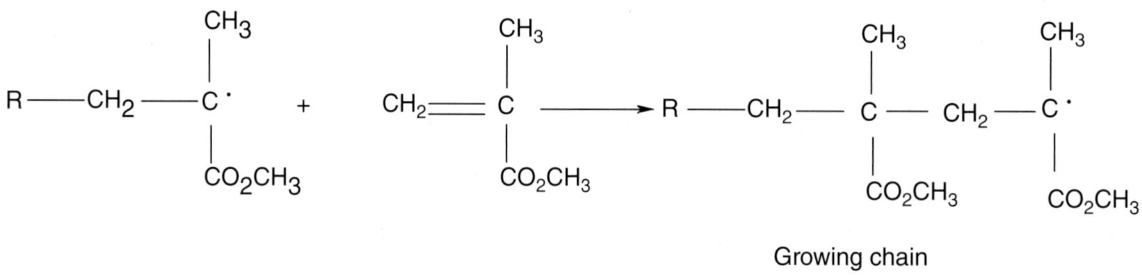

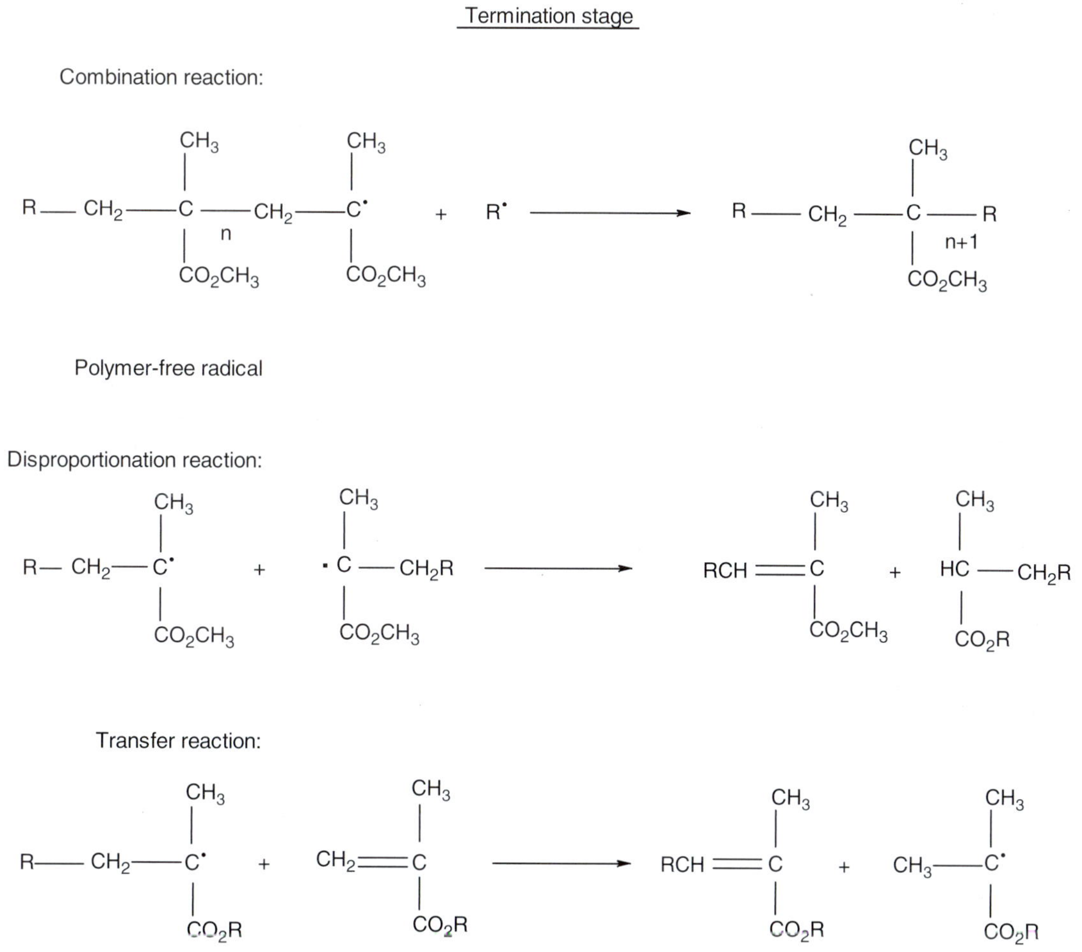

The polymerization can be controlled by several factors, such as the concentration of initiators, the light intensity (in the case of photopolymerizations), and the addition of inhibitors. Inhibitors are highly reactive molecules and work as radical scavengers, since newly formed radicals are more prone to react with the inhibitors than with the vinyl groups. These can be useful to increase the shelf life of products, and the most common examples are monomethyl ether hydroquinone (MEHQ) and butyl hydroxytoluene (BHT). Inhibitors are also responsible for a delay in the onset of polymerization, exactly because they slow down the reaction of vinyls. In addition to inhibitor compounds that are purposefully added to the materials, ambient and dissolved oxygen is also a very efficient free-radical inhibitor. It inhibits the reaction on the surface of the material, up to 10–20 microns, which helps different layers of composite to bond together. This inhibition layer is not usually a concern on the surface of the finished restoration because it gets eliminated by finishing and polishing procedures. Additional discussion of polymers is included in Chapter 8.

Ceramics

The term *ceramic* refers to any product made essentially from a nonmetallic inorganic material usually processed by firing at a high temperature to achieve desirable properties. They are oxides of metals. A comparison of the amorphous structure of a silicon dioxide glass versus a crystalline silica where the atoms are regularly arranged is shown in Fig. 5.10. Ceramics may be totally crystalline or semi-crystalline. As a class, ceramics are hard, low in toughness compared to metals, stiff, poor thermal and electrical conductors, and can be cast or machined to fabricate dental restorations. The translucency and opacity of a dental ceramic can be modified for applications where color and translucency are critical. Ceramics generally demonstrate little plastic behavior and are thus considered brittle when compared to metals or polymers. Their stress-strain curves are generally linear with no plastic strain. Ceramics are used in restorative dentistry as full- and partial-coverage crowns, fixed partial dentures, denture teeth, and as particulate fillers for resin matrix composite filling materials.

The more restrictive term *porcelain* refers to a specific compositional range of ceramic materials made by mixing kaolin, quartz, and feldspar and firing at high temperatures. Dental ceramics for *ceramic-metal* restorations belong to this compositional range and are commonly referred to as *dental porcelains.* Dental porcelain is used as veneers on metal frameworks (metal–ceramic restoration), on high-strength ceramic frameworks, as veneers on minimally prepared anterior teeth, and for denture teeth.

The properties of dental ceramics depend on their composition, microstructure, and flaw population. The nature and amount of reinforcing crystalline phase present dictate the material's strength and resistance to crack propagation as well as its optical properties.

Ceramics are brittle and contain at least two populations of flaws: fabrication defects and surface cracks. The fracture

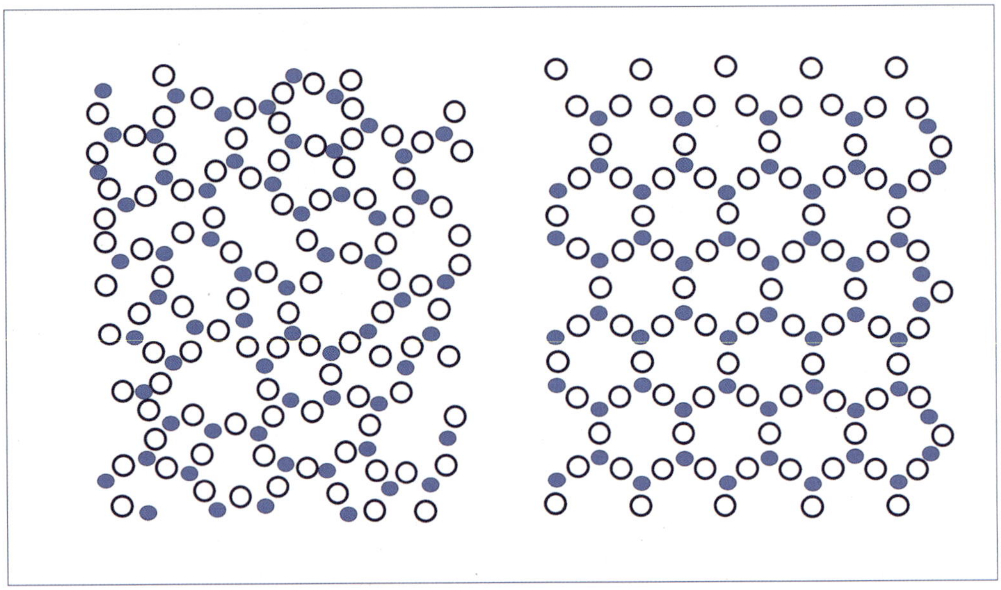

• **Fig. 5.10** Structure of amorphous glass with an irregular arrangement of atoms and crystalline ceramic. Blue circles represent silicon atoms and white circles represent oxygen atoms.

mechanisms involve crack propagation from these flaws. Fabrication defects are created during processing and consist of inclusions at the condensation stage or voids generated during sintering. Inclusions are often linked to improper cleaning of the metal framework or the use of unclean instruments. Porosity on the internal side of clinically failed glass-ceramic restorations has been identified as the fracture initiation site. Microcracks also develop upon cooling in feldspathic porcelains and can be due to thermal contraction mismatch between the leucite crystals and the glassy matrix or to thermal shock if the porcelain is cooled too rapidly.

Surface cracks are induced by machining or grinding. The average natural flaw size varies from 20 to 50 μm. Usually, failure of the ceramic originates from the most severe flaw.

Dental ceramics are subjected to repeated (cyclic) loading in a humid environment (chewing), conditions that are ideal for the extension of the preexisting defects or cracks. This phenomenon, called *slow crack growth*, can contribute to a severe reduction of the survival probability of ceramic restorations.

Composites

Composites are a combination of two or more classes of materials. In dentistry, the most common composite is a combination of a polymer and ceramic or glass, where the polymer is used to bind the inorganic particles. The polymer functions as the matrix in dental composites and the particles are reinforcing materials, commonly referred to as fillers. Polymer matrix composites, also known as *resin composites*, are used as sealants, intracoronal and extracoronal restorations, provisional restorations, veneers, denture teeth, cements, and core buildups. As a class, dental composites are formable, can be made to be machineable, opaque or translucent, moderate in stiffness and hardness, thermal and electrical insulators, and sparingly soluble. Many advances have been made in particle technology and are discussed in Chapter 8.

In a composite, the properties are intermediate between the two compositional materials. A benefit of combining two material classes is the ability to fabricate a new material that has desirable handling properties that are not achievable with one material alone. For example, individual glass particles do not adhere to each other, but the addition of a polymer to bind them enables the composite to be used as a paste. Use of a polymer alone will not achieve sufficient stiffness and stability, which are properties contributed by the filler particles. The polymer used in many dental composites, bisphenol A-glycidyl methacrylate (Bis-GMA), has shown no significant health risks when used in dental resin composites.

In industries and professions other than dentistry, other classes are combined to form composites, such as metal-ceramic composites used in aerospace. A commonly used material in the construction industry, concrete, is a composite of sand, gravel, and Portland cement. As with dental resin composites, the cement in concrete is the binder for the sand and gravel particles. Composites differ from alloys in that, at the microscopic level, the individual components of the composite are visible.

In the case of concrete, a limiting factor is the adhesion between the Portland cement and sand-gravel particles. At the surface, the cement washes away with use, leaving the particles incompletely surrounded by cement. These particles are then easily dislodged, leaving a void in the surface of the concrete. In dental resin composites, coupling agents are used to enhance the adhesion between the ceramic particles and polymer matrix, thereby increasing its wear resistance and long-term surface integrity.

During polymerization of resin composites, a volumetric contraction of the polymer matrix occurs that results in strain within the matrix. This contraction strain is coupled with the increase in elastic modulus as the composite cures. The combination of contraction strain and the development of elastic modulus produces stress within the composite because the periphery of the restoration is constrained by adhesion to the enamel and dentin cavity walls. Methods to reduce residual stress include the development of polymers with reduced shrinkage during cure and modifications to the clinical placement technique. More detail on the measurement of polymerization shrinkage can be found in the supplemental material and the mechanism for polymerization can be found in Chapter 8.

Bibliography

Anusavice KJ, Shen C, Rawls HR. *Phillips' Science of Dental Materials*. 12th ed. Saunders; 2012.

Denry I, Holloway JA. Ceramics for dental applications: a review. *Materials*. 2010;3(1):351.

Denry I, Kelly JR. State of art of zirconia for dental applications. *Dent Mater*. 2008;24(3):299.

Dieter G. *Mechanical Metallurgy*. 3rd ed. McGraw-Hill; 1986.

Flinn RA, Trojan PK. *Engineering Materials and Their Applications*. 4th ed. John Wiley & Sons; 1990.

Gettleman L. Noble alloys in dentistry. *Current Opinion Dent*. 1991;2:218.

Höland W, Beall G. *Glass-Ceramic Technology*. The American Ceramic Society; 2002.

Imazato S, Ma S, Chen J, Xu HK. Therapeutic polymers for dental adhesives: loading resins with bio-active components. *Dent Mater*. 2014;30(1):97.

Kelly JR, Nishimura I, Campbell SD. Ceramics in dentistry: historical roots and current perspectives. *J Prosthet Dent*. 1996;75:18.

Khvostenko D, Mitchell JC, Hilton TJ, Ferracane JL, Kruzic JJ. Mechanical performance of novel bioactive glass containing dental restorative composites. *Dent Mater*. 2013;29(11):1139.

Kingery WD, Bowen HK, Uhlmann DR. *Introduction to Ceramics*. 2nd ed. John Wiley & Sons; 1976.

Lawn BR, Pajares A, Zhang Y, et al. Materials design in the performance of all-ceramic crowns. *Biomaterials*. 2004;25(14):2885.

Malhotra ML. Dental gold casting alloys: a review. *Trends Tech Contemp Dent Lab*. 1991;8:73.

O'Brien WJ. Recent developments in materials and processes for ceramic crowns. *J Am Dent Assoc*. 1985;110:547.

Odian G. *Principles of Polymerization*. 4th ed. John Wiley & Sons; 2004.

Paravina RD, Powers JM, eds. *Esthetic Color Training in Dentistry*. Mosby; 2004.

Powers JM, Wataha JC. *Dental Materials: Foundations and Applications*. 11th ed. Mosby; 2017.

Rekow ED. A review of the developments in dental CAD/CAM systems. *Curr Opin Dent*. 1992;2:25.

Zhang Y, Lawn BR. Long-term strength of ceramics for biomedical applications. *J Biomed Mater Res*. 2004;69B(2):166.

6

Preventive Dental Materials: Compounds Increasing Mineral Saturation and Diffusion Barriers

JULIANA BRANCO DA COSTA, DANIELLE P. WINGROVE

CHAPTER OUTLINE

Dental caries is a multifactorial disease that results from complex interactions between host, agents, environment, and time. Cavitation resulting from this infectious disease is caused by acidogenic bacteria, whose metabolites lead to the dissolution of enamel, coronal dentin, cementum, and root dentin. According to the World Health Organization (WHO) 2022, globally, an estimated 2 billion people suffer from caries of permanent teeth and 514 million children suffer from caries of primary teeth. The prevalence of the main oral diseases continues to increase globally with growing urbanization and changes in living conditions.

Caries prevention is the cornerstone of dentistry. Currently, more emphasis is being placed on dental caries detection, diagnosis, and risk analysis than detection of cavities that require immediate invasive treatment such as a restoration. While in the past, the cavities were filled at the earliest sign of detection, now preventive measures, including remineralization, are emphasized in order to reverse the dental caries process and avoid surgical intervention.

Remineralization is a natural repair process for carious lesions. Dental remineralization is the process of bringing minerals from the surrounding environment (i.e., saliva and biofilm) into partially demineralized tooth structures. Remineralization can replace minerals in partially demineralized enamel and dentin or create amorphous mineral precipitates in the inter-crystal and inter-rod spaces. Calcium and phosphate are essential elements for remineralization, while fluoride plays a crucial role in enhancing the process. Remineralization can occur naturally or be induced by therapies. Among the therapies, fluoride-based treatments have the highest level of supporting evidence and the widespread use of fluoride is considered the main reason for dental caries reduction in most populations. However, currently available fluoride therapy has limited efficacy in some individuals and remineralization can be hampered by limited bioavailability of calcium and phosphate. Therefore new product formulations designed to ensure a constant supply of these critical ions have been developed. These materials were designed to work by increasing mineral saturation in the environment around caries lesions (in saliva and biofilm).

Fluoride uptake differs depending on the tooth surface. Pits and fissures on the occlusal surfaces of posterior teeth are more resistant to fluoride uptake because of the irregular morphology of the occlusal surface. This, combined with the retention of food and the difficulty of proper brushing in the posterior segment, can lead to the start of a carious lesion. A preventive therapy consisting of a sealant to fill in the occlusal irregularities, creating a diffusion barrier, can reduce the risk of caries by creating a smoother surface that is easier to clean and less likely to retain food and harbor bacteria. Another type of diffusion barrier that can hinder caries progression on smooth and proximal surfaces is resin infiltration.

Glass ionomers are fluoride-releasing materials that can be used as liners, bases, or temporary restorations with the aim of inhibiting further tooth demineralization.

This chapter discusses the prevention of caries by therapies that either induce tooth remineralization by increasing mineral saturation, such as fluoride varnish, silver diamine fluoride (SDF), casein phosphopeptide-amorphous calcium phosphate (CPP-ACP), and glass ionomers; or by creating diffusion barriers to prevent caries formation, such as pit and fissure sealants and resin infiltration (Table 6.1).

TABLE 6.1 Preventive Dental Materials Classification

Material	Examples
Compounds increasing mineral saturation	– Fluoride varnish – Silver diamine fluoride – Casein phosphopeptides-amorphous calcium phosphate (CCP-ACP) – Sodium trimetaphosphate (STMP) – Bioactive glass (BAG) – Calcium Hydroxide – Tricalcium silicate cements and bioceramics – Glass ionomer
Diffusion barriers	– Sealant – Resin infiltration

Fluoride-Containing Agents and Materials

Low-level fluorides in water supplies have provided tremendous benefits in reducing the incidence of dental caries in children. Fluorides can be introduced into community water supplies to ensure systemic ingestion during early life when the teeth are forming. Fluoride can also be provided as a dietary supplement to inhibit caries where drinking water is not fluoridated. Patients who are at high risk for developing caries in spite of receiving systemic fluoride can be given additional fluoride via topical application in toothpastes, mouth rinses, gels, and varnishes. A combination of systemic and topical fluoride applications has contributed to a dramatic reduction in the prevalence of smooth surface caries since the 1960s.

Elevated levels of fluoride in toothpaste have been shown to be effective in rehardening root caries lesions that are cavitated. A 5000-ppm-F toothpaste rehardened 76% of lesions compared with 35% in an 1100-ppm-F group. The concept of the caries balance proposed by Featherstone describes three pathological factors and three protective factors for dental caries. The pathological factors are (1) acid-producing bacteria, (2) frequent consumption of fermentable carbohydrates, and (3) below-normal salivary flow and function. The three protective factors are (1) a normal salivary flow and components, (2) fluoride, and (3) antibacterial agents. Two salivary components required for remineralization are calcium and phosphate, and fluoride enhances this process.

Fluoride Varnishes

Fluoride varnish was first introduced in Europe in 1964 but did not become available in the United States until 1991 when it was approved by the US Food and Drug Administration. Studies have since demonstrated that fluoride varnish is a safe and highly effective means of preventing caries. Fluoride-containing varnishes deliver fluoride topically to the surfaces of teeth in patients at risk for caries, and usually after prophylaxis.

Composition

Products contain either 5% sodium fluoride (2.26% F^- or 22,600 ppm) or 1% difluorosilane (0.1% F^- or 1000 ppm).

Properties and Application

The fluoride is dissolved in an organic solvent that evaporates when applied or sets when exposed to moisture, leaving a thin film of material covering all exposed tooth surfaces. The mechanism of action for a fluoride varnish is similar to that of a fluoride mouthwash. Calcium fluoride is deposited on the tooth surface and later the hydroxyapatite (HA) of the tooth is converted through a reaction to the more acid-resistant fluorapatite.

One advantage of fluoride varnish is the extended time of exposure to the active fluoride ingredient against the tooth surface. Instead of seconds, as with a mouthwash, it may be hours before a varnish wears off. One resin-modified glass ionomer (RMGI)-based varnish has been reported to release fluoride for up to 6 months.

Clinical Studies

Clinical trials have documented the efficacy of fluoride varnish in treating young children at risk for caries, with reductions reported as high as 70%. Another potential use for this type of material is in the prevention of root caries in an older population having exposed root surfaces. Semiannual application of 2.26% fluoride varnishes seems to provide optimum efficacy for patients at risk of developing dental caries.

Silver Diamine Fluoride

Silver has long been used in the medical arts for its known antibacterial properties. Some of the earliest uses were for water disinfection and storage. The Greeks and Romans stored water in silver vessels to keep it fresh. The first use of silver in dentistry was through silver nitrate and Howe's solution that could penetrate affected dentine, having an antibacterial effect. At the end of the 20th and beginning of the 21st century, many researchers began studying potential caries-arresting properties of silver fluoride compounds. The success of these studies led to their commercial use in Mexico, Japan, and Australia.

Composition

SDF, or silver ammonium fluoride ($Ag[NH_3]_2F$), is a colorless, alkaline solution containing silver and fluoride and combines with ammonia to form a complex solution. SDF is a solution of about 38% SDF (of which approximately 25% is silver, 5% is fluoride, and 8% is ammonia) in water with a pH of approximately 10. The ammonium ions combine with the silver ions to produce diamine-silver, which is more stable than silver fluoride. The high pH makes it a strong neutralizer of acids, but perhaps more important is its strong antibacterial effect, predominantly due to the presence of silver, a known antimicrobial. The material was preceded by silver nitrate used in a similar way, that is, the application of the colorless liquid to frank caries. There is growing evidence that caries is arrested in the presence of the material, and this has great advantages for use in children and geriatric populations especially. The problem with the material is that it stains tooth structure, as well as other objects such as skin or clothing.

Properties

Two concentrations of SDF have been studied in the literature, 12% and 38% (Fig. 6.1), with 38% being more effective in arresting caries. Each milliliter of SDF contains 380 mg of $Ag(NH_3)_2F$. Thirty-eight percent SDF contains a high concentration of fluoride ions, 44,800 ppm. SDF can treat hypersensitivity and arrest caries when applied to tooth structure by blocking dentinal tubules. SDF can also lead to bacterial death, remineralization of demineralized tooth structure, and inhibition of collagen degradation. Silver precipitates and calcium fluoride form on the external surface of dentin and reduce tubule patency.

Many mechanisms have been proposed for the bactericidal effect of SDF (Fig. 6.2). When in high concentrations, fluoride ions can inhibit biofilm formation by binding to the bacteria's cellular components, interfering with both carbohydrate metabolism and sugar uptake. Silver ions exert antibacterial effects in at least three different ways. The first is through cell wall destruction and preventing the synthesis of a new cell wall. The second is interacting with bacterial proteins and enzymes, reducing the bacteria's metabolic processes. The final method by which SDF is antibacterial is inhibiting the bacteria's DNA replication.

A systematic review showed that demineralized dentin treated with SDF had significantly lower counts of cariogenic bacteria *Streptococcus mutans, Lactobacillus acidophilus,* and *Actinomyces naeslundii.* The growth of *S. mutans, Lactobacillus casei,* and *Streptococcus oralis* was reduced after the application of SDF on contaminated dentin. The authors also stated that SDF inhibited the adherence of *S. mutans* to tooth surfaces, and SDF was more effective than silver ammonia nitrate and sodium fluoride.

SDF's ability to remineralize affected dentin is related to the fluoride ions and the interaction of SDF and HA. This interaction creates silver phosphate and calcium fluoride, which both help raise the pH of the area. Silver phosphate and calcium fluoride eventually dissolve and form insoluble fluorapatite at the tooth surface. The incorporation of fluorapatite into the tooth structure creates a surface that is less susceptible to acid dissolution. Teeth treated with SDF show higher fluoride uptake and the depth of penetration of calcium and phosphorus increases with SDF use.

SDF has been shown to have an inhibitory effect on matrix metalloproteinases (MMP) and cysteine cathepsins, contributing to a reduction in dentin collagen degradation. SDF was shown to inhibit MMP-2, MMP-8, and MMP-9, and after treatment with SDF, dentin showed less hydroxyproline liberation than water.

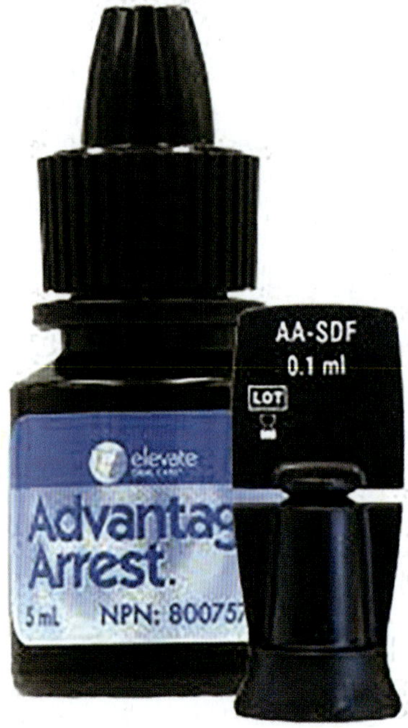

• **Fig. 6.1** Silver diamine fluoride—advantage arrest 38%. (Courtesy Elevate Oral Care, West Palm Beach, FL.)

Applications

The most common form of SDF is a colorless liquid applied as a caries-preventative and caries-arresting agent. Other uses for SDF have been proposed in the literature to include desensitizing agents, endodontic irrigants, vital pulp therapy, and endodontic intracanal medicaments. Contraindications for using SDF include a silver allergy, desquamative gingivitis or mucositis, pregnancy, caries and restorations in the aesthetic zone, and periapical pathosis.

Studies have not shown any reduction in the bond strength of resin composites to sound dentin treated with SDF. However, more research is necessary to evaluate all potential issues with bonding to dentin treated with SDF. One of SDF's most common side effects is a black discoloration of the dentin where the liquid has been applied. One approach to reducing the discoloration of SDF is to apply potassium iodide (KI) after SDF application. The KI salt reacts with the free silver ions, preventing the formation of silver phosphate and black discoloration. The combination of the salt and SDF forms silver iodide, a white or colorless precipitate, but this precipitate can turn dark when exposed to light.

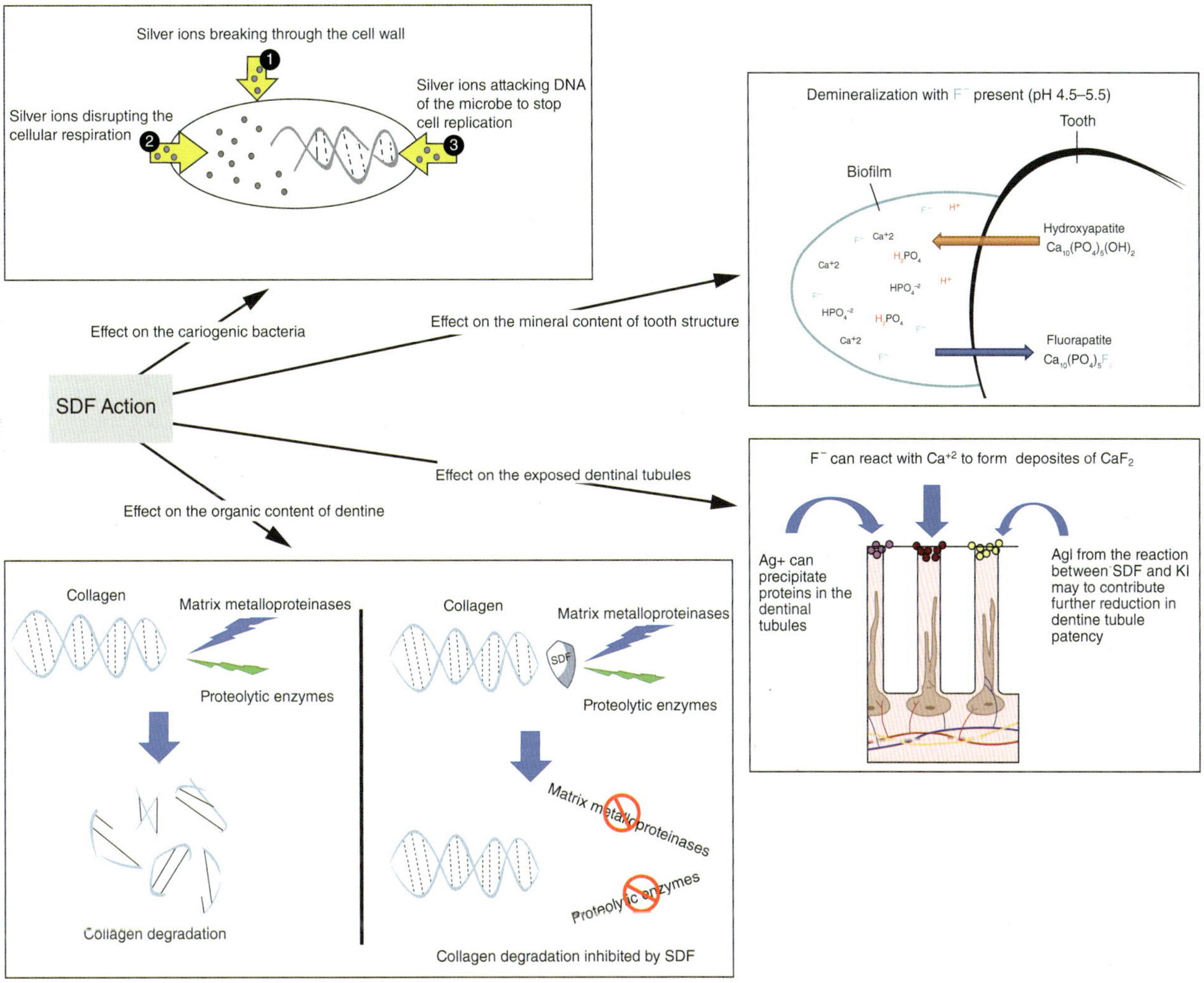

• **Fig. 6.2** Diagrammatic representation summarizing main actions of SDF on (1) biofilm bacteria, (2) tooth tissue mineral content, (3) exposed dentinal tubules, and (4) inhibition of collagen (dentin) degradation. (From Seifo N, Robertson M, MacLean J, et al. The use of silver diamine fluoride (SDF) in dental practice. *Br Dent J*. 2020;228(2):75–81.)

Clinical Studies

A systematic review indicated that SDF, at concentrations of 30% and 38%, is more effective than other preventive management strategies for arresting dentinal caries in the primary dentition. Additionally, both concentrations of SDF show potential as a caries preventive treatment in primary teeth and permanent first molars. Standardized SDF protocols must be developed to allow meaningful study comparisons and establish treatment guidelines.

Glass Ionomer to Prevent Progression of Caries

Glass Ionomers (GIs) were developed in the 1960s and are based on an acid-base cement-forming reaction between fluoroalumino-silicate (FAS) glass powder similar to those used in silicate cements and aqueous solutions of polycarboxylic acids. These were less prone to dissolution than silicates but the early materials suffered from difficulty of manipulation, technique sensitivity, and poor aesthetics. Advances in these materials have continued and modern materials have improved properties. RMGIs were invented in the late 1980s to preserve the advantages of fluoride release and clinical adhesion of the conventional GIs yet provide the ease of light curing and good aesthetics of resin-based materials. The use of nano-technology in RMGI has resulted in enhanced aesthetics of these materials. Because of their documented slow release of fluoride, glass ionomers are used in cervical restorations when the highest aesthetics are not critical. They are specifically recommended for patients with high caries risk. A video showing a provisional glass ionomer cement restoration can be found online. A description of glass ionomer for cementation/luting applications can be found in Chapter 12.

Composition and Setting

Glass ionomers are water-based, self-adhesive restorative materials in which the filler is a reactive glass called FAS glass and the matrix is polymer or copolymer of carboxylic acids. They are supplied in various shades as two-part powder-liquid systems that require mixing, and there are two main types: conventional glass ionomer cement (GIC) and resin-modified glass ionomer cement (RMGIC). The polymeric matrix of most GIs is a copolymer of acrylic acid and itaconic acid or maleic acid. In most cases, this is formulated as a concentrated aqueous liquid. Tartaric acid is added to control the working and setting characteristics of the material. The powder consists of an acid-reactive comminuted FAS glass and has ions such as calcium, strontium, and lanthanum. When heavy-metal ions are used, the set material is radiopaque to x-rays. An initial set is achieved within 3 to 4 minutes of mixing, but the ionic reaction continues for at least 24 hours or more so that maturation is achieved much later. Maturation time has been improved in newer formulations to allow finishing after 15 minutes of placement of the mix. The actual process of ion extraction and complex formation is quite elaborate; however, the essential steps are described in the scheme shown.

All carboxylic acids have a common organic functional group denoted by COOH. In the presence of water, the COOH group undergoes partial ionization to yield a carboxylate anion COO^{-1} and a hydrated proton, H_3O^+ (Reaction 1). The hydrated proton attacks the surface of the glass particles releasing calcium and aluminum ions. The carboxylate ions from the polymer react with these metallic ions to form a salt bridge, resulting in gelation and setting. During the initial setting, calcium ions are more rapidly bound to the polyacrylate chains; binding to the aluminum ions occurs at a later stage. The strength of the cement builds with time. Silicic acid is initially formed when the glass breaks down but rapidly polymerizes to form silica hydrogel (Reaction 4). A very important by-product of the setting reaction is the release of fluoride ions from the glass matrix. This fluoride release process is sustained and occurs over a long period. It is important to understand that this fluoride ion release is a result of the setting reaction and the ion-exchange process in the cement. In this process, the fluoride from the glass is being replaced by carboxylates and water. Hence, if properly formulated, there is little chance of the cement losing its strength with time. Considerable research has shown no loss of strength of the cement during years of storage in water.

Water plays several important roles in the overall setting. First, it provides for the ion transport needed for the acid-base setting reaction and fluoride release. Second, a portion of the water is also chemically bound in the set complex and provides stability to the restorative material. Water also provides plasticity during the manipulative stages.

The set cement is constituted by a hydrogel of calcium, aluminum, and fluoroaluminum polyacrylates involving the unreacted glass particles sheathed by a weakly bonded siliceous hydrogel layer. About 20% to 30% of the glass is dissolved in the reaction. Smaller glass particles may be entirely dissolved and replaced by siliceous hydrogel particles containing fluorite crystallites. The stability of the matrix is given by an association of chain entanglement, weak ionic cross-linking, and hydrogen bonding.

Significant advances have been made in formulation of conventional GIs in recent years to improve their manipulation and mechanical properties. Fast hardening has been achieved by altering the particle size and particle size distribution of the glass powder. One manufacturer coats the powder particles with a polymeric material for easy mixing.

A similar ionic interaction called "chelation" takes place between the negatively charged polymer and the calcium on the exposed tooth surface, creating an adhesive bond (more details are shown in Chapter 12, Fig. 12.1). The surfaces of new restorations should be protected from saliva during the initial set with a protective coating of varnish or light-cured resin.

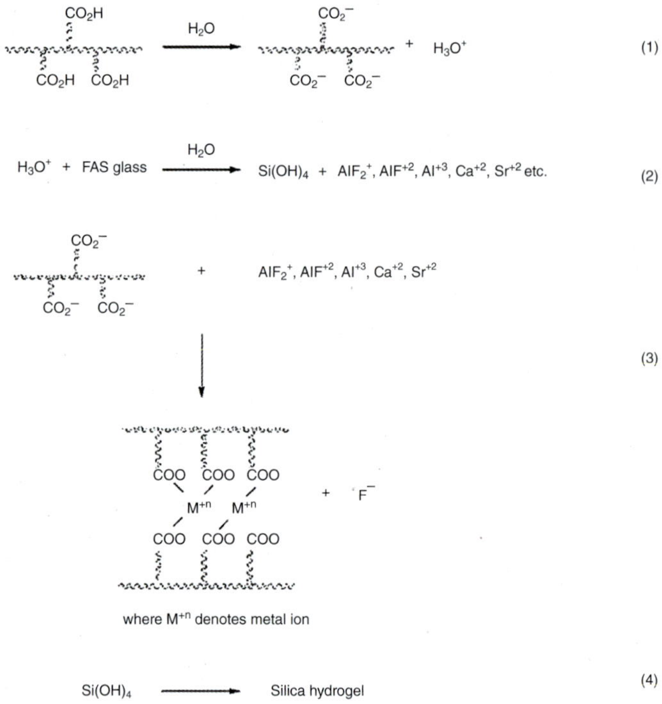

Setting mechanism of conventional glass ionomers

Resin-Modified Glass Ionomers

To create a longer working time yet quick setting time so that immediate finishing can take place, the concept of RMGIs was introduced in the late 1980s. The essential components are similar to those in conventional GIs in which an aqueous polycarboxylic acid undergoes an acid-base setting reaction with FAS glass. To this methacrylate, components are added in limited amounts so a photoinitiated and/or redox-curing reaction of the double bonds can also occur. RMGI, at one time known as *hybrid ionomers*, are used for restorations in low stress–bearing areas and are recommended for patients with high caries risk (Table 6.2). These restorations are more aesthetic than glass ionomers because of their resin content. Examples of RMGIs in cervical erosions, abfractions, and other restorations are shown in Fig. 6.3.

Composition

The powder of RMGI is similar to that used in the conventional glass ionomers. The liquid contains methacrylate monomers, polyacids, and water. RMGIs are set by a combined acid-base ionomer reaction and light-cured resin polymerization of monomers, typically 2-hydroxyethyl methacrylate. In some commercial brands, the polyacid is functionalized with methacrylates, so they can copolymerize and cross-link with the methacrylate monomers (typical 2-hydroxyethyl methacrylate, and/or glycerol dimethacrylate) and at the same time react with Ca^{2+} in the powder and the tooth structure via the COOH units. Free radical initiators are added to trigger the curing of the methacrylate groups. Visible light initiators and/or self-cure redox initiators are employed to affect this curing and covalent cross-linking reaction. RMGIs are typically light-cured like dental composites for 10 to 20 seconds, depending on the manufacturer's instructions.

TABLE 6.2 Uses of Composites, Compomers, Resin-Modified Glass Ionomers, and Glass Ionomers

Type	Uses
Hybrid/microfilled/ multipurpose composite (this needs to align with RC chapter)	Classes 1, 2, 3, 4, 5 Classes 1, 3, 4, medium caries–risk patients
Compomer (this needs to align with information in other chapters)	Primary teeth, classes 1, 2 restorations in children Cervical lesions, classes 3, 5, medium caries–risk patients
Resin-modified glass ionomer	Cervical lesions, root caries, Classes 3, 5 for primary teeth, Class 5 for adult teeth, high caries–risk patients, closed and open sandwich technique, pulp capping, intermediate restoration
Glass ionomer	Cervical lesions, root caries, Class I and Class II restorations in deciduous teeth, Class 5 restorations in adults where aesthetics are less important, pulp capping, closed sandwich technique, intermediate restoration

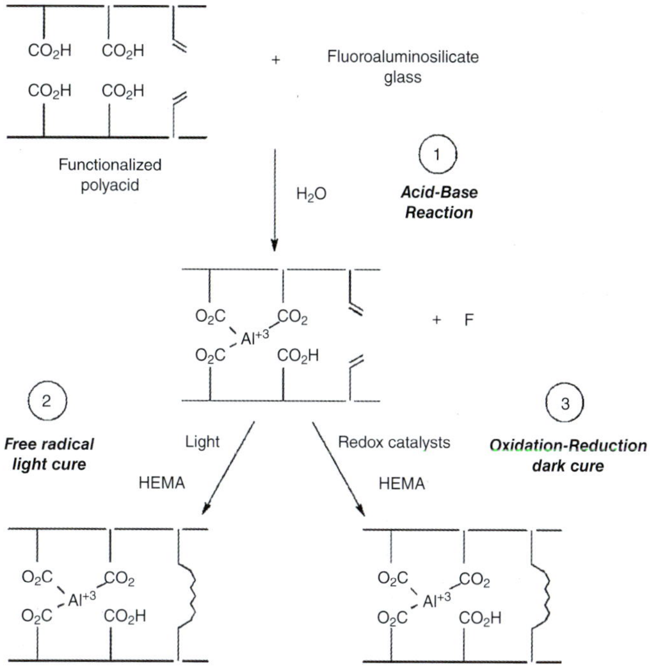

Setting reactions in tri-cure glass ionomer system

Some RMGIs have an additional curing mode. If only photoinitiators are used for cross-linking of the methacrylate groups, the RMGI has to be cured in layers because penetration of visible light can occur only to a limited depth. This is not a disadvantage in applications where thin layers of materials are to be placed; for example, for lining or basing. However, for restorative and core build-up applications, the need for incremental filling is a drawback. This problem has been overcome in the so-called tri-cure GI system. Here, in addition to the photoinitiators, self-cure redox imitators are added so that the methacrylate polymerization can proceed in the absence of light. The three curing reactions are as follows:

1. Acid-base GI reaction
2. Light-activated polymerization
3. Chemically activated polymerization

Reactions 2 and 3 are chemically similar but differ in the mode of initiation. Reactions 1 and 3 take place spontaneously when the powder and liquid are mixed. Reaction 2 occurs only when initiated by light. The introduction of tri-cure technology has allowed RMGIs to be used as bulk-cured materials, thus saving time for the practitioner. In one commercial system, the redox initiators are microencapsulated separately in polymers and added to the powder. The spatulation and mixing of the powder and liquid trigger the release of the catalysts from the microcapsules resulting in autocuring.

Although several commercial products claim to have tri-cure chemistry, it is important to become familiar with the instructions for use and realize that there are very important differences between them. In a true tri-cure, the redox cure is quite rapid to allow the material to be placed in bulk if desired.

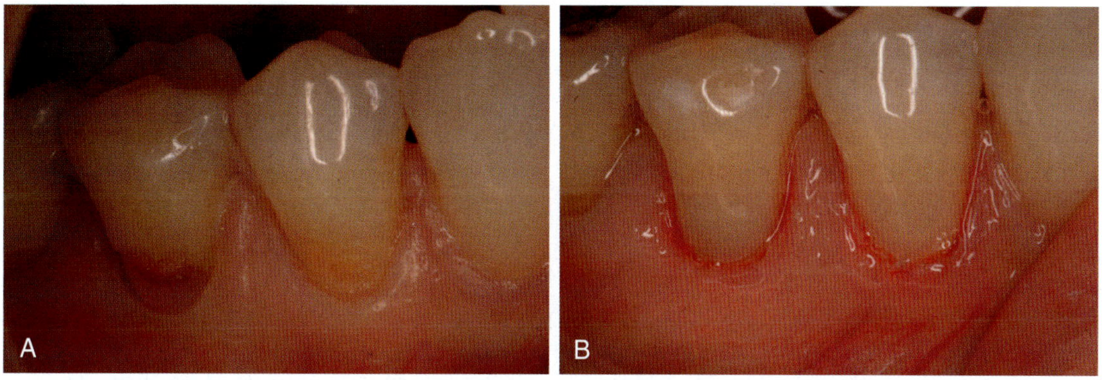

• **Fig. 6.3** Restoration of root surface lesions. (A) Abrasion/erosion lesions on the facial surface of mandibular premolars. (B) Restorations with resin-modified glass ionomer cement and composite. (Courtesy Dr. Thomas J. Hilton, Portland, OR.)

TABLE 6.3 Ranking of Selected Properties of Resin-Modified Glass Ionomers and Glass Ionomers

Property	Resin-Modified Glass Ionomer	Glass Ionomer
Compressive strength	Med	Low–Med
Flexural strength	Med	Low–Med
Flexural modulus	Med	Med–High
Wear resistance	Med	Low
Fluoride release	Med–High	High
Fluoride rechargeability	Med–High	High
Aesthetics	Good	Acceptable

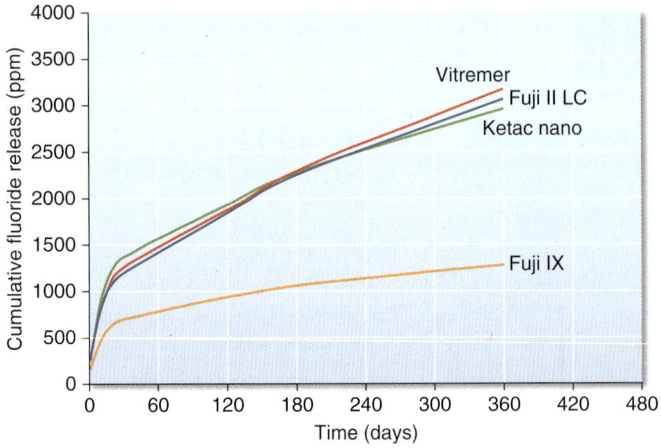

• **Fig. 6.4** Fluoride release from typical glass ionomers. (From Mitra SB, Oxman JD, Falsafi A, Ton TT. Fluoride release and recharge behavior of a nano-filled resin-modified glass ionomer compared with that of other fluoride releasing materials. *Am J Dent*. 2011;24(6):372–378.)

Properties

Physical, Mechanical, and Thermal Properties

Like many two-part systems, the properties of GIs, both conventional type and resin-modified, are quite dependent on the ratio of polycarboxylic acid and FAS glass components dispensed. Particular care has to be exercised for powder-liquid hand-mixed systems to ensure accurate proportions. The ISO standard 9917 for water-based cements provides some requirements of GIs as restorative materials, whereas the ISO standard 9917-2 covers the properties of RMGIs. The properties of conventional glass ionomers are compared qualitatively with other restorative materials in Table 8.3 (Chapter 8). Significant properties are (1) elastic modulus that is similar to dentin, (2) bond strength to dentin of 2 to 3 MPa, (3) expansion coefficient comparable to tooth structure, (4) low solubility, and (5) fairly high opacity. The physical properties of the RMGIs, including wear resistance and dimensional stability, are improved over the conventional counterparts (Table 6.3). The additional covalent cross-linking in the matrix due to the polymerization of the methacrylate groups contributes toward this improvement. The modulus of the RMGIs is low during the initial set by light activation but increases over time as the acid-base reaction completes. This unique characteristic makes the RMGI particularly attractive when used as a liner or as the base in sandwich restorations under resin composites because it can relieve the stress associated with the polymerization shrinkage of the latter.

The thermal diffusivity and coefficient of thermal expansion of several conventional and RMGIs have been shown to be closer to tooth structure (dentin) than resin composites. Therefore such materials should serve as good insulation against thermal shock particularly when used as liners and bases. However, because products from different manufacturers vary widely in their thermal expansion coefficient values, it is advisable to check the values of individual materials. In general, the products that have the smallest proportion of resin components exhibit the lowest coefficient of thermal expansion values.

Fluoride Ion Release and Uptake

A particularly beneficial characteristic of GIs, conventional or resin modified, is that these materials act as a reservoir of fluoride ions. The fluoride is released by an ion-exchange mechanism from these materials. Research has shown that the released fluoride ions are taken up by the associated enamel and dentin, rendering those tooth structures less susceptible to acid challenge by a combination of decreased solubility and disruption of the activity of cariogenic bacteria. The release of fluoride ion is sustained over prolonged periods (Fig. 6.4). These materials also have been shown to act as fluoride reservoirs in the oral environment by taking up salivary fluoride from dentifrices, mouthwashes, and topical fluoride solutions. Fluoride ion dynamics is particularly advantageous for those with high susceptibility to dental caries.

RMGIs release more fluoride than compomers and composites but almost the same as conventional glass ionomers. Fig. 6.5 illustrates the release of fluoride ions from a glass ionomer and RMGI over a 30-day period. There is an early period of high release, which tapers after about 10 days to 1 ppm. Both ionomer materials recharge when exposed to fluoride treatments or fluoride dentifrices. Fig. 6.6 illustrates this recharge capability with a similar time-dependent release curve. In evaluating the effectiveness of this release, fluoride has been measured in plaque samples immediately adjacent to glass ionomer–based restorations (Fig. 6.7). For these two materials from the same manufacturer, plaque adjacent to the RMGI had significantly higher fluoride content than plaque adjacent to compomer restorations at 2 and 21 days after insertion of the restorations.

Adhesion

GI materials have good clinical adhesion to tooth structure. Unlike the resin-based composite materials, etching of the enamel or dentin surface by phosphoric acid is not needed. Hence these materials are sometimes referred to as being "self-adhesive." The mechanism of adhesion to the tooth structure is mostly chemical in nature and proceeds through an exchange of ions arising from both the tooth and restoration. Calcium-polyacrylate bonds have been shown by some products by in vitro electron spectroscopy for chemical analysis (ESCA) studies. RMGIs bond to tooth structure without the use of a bonding agent, and because they are somewhat stronger than conventional glass ionomers, RMGIs tend to have higher bond strength. Typically, the tooth is conditioned with polyacrylic acid or another primer before placing the material. A small amount of micromechanical bonding has been exhibited by some RMGIs.

Laboratory measurements of bond strengths of conventional and RMGIs to tooth structure have generally yielded lower values than with the combination of resin adhesives and composites. The failure is usually cohesive in the GI; hence it is doubtful if these laboratory measurements reflect the actual interfacial adhesion.

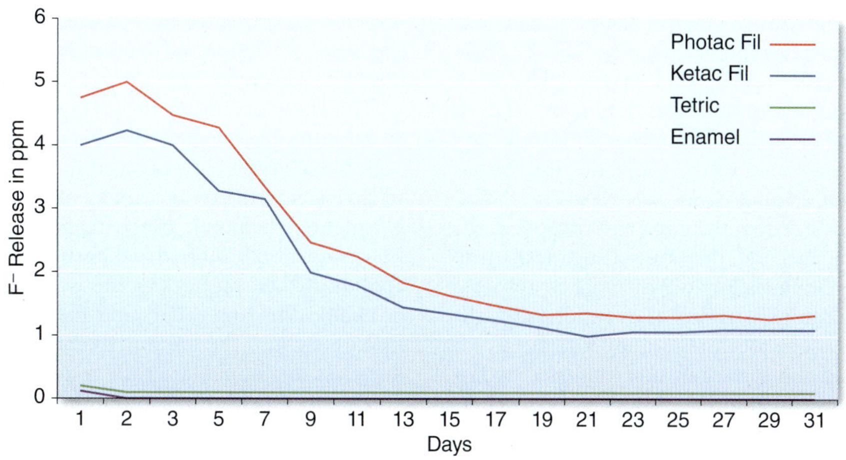

• **Fig. 6.5** Fluoride release from glass ionomer cements and composite resin in distilled water over 30 days. (From Strother JM, Kohn DH, Dennison JB, et al. Fluoride release and re-uptake in direct tooth-colored restorative materials. *Det Mater*. 1998;14:129–136.)

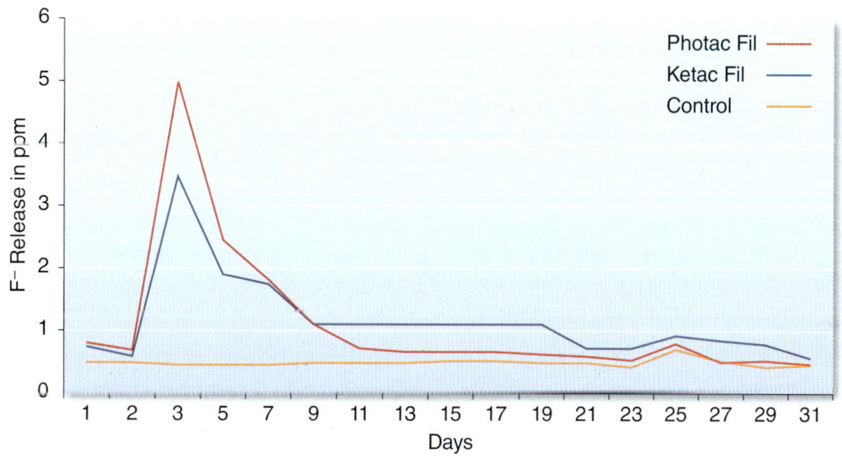

• **Fig. 6.6** Fluoride reuptake and release from glass ionomer cements after recharging the material with 1.1% neutral sodium fluoride gel. (From Strother JM, Kohn DH, Dennison JB, et al. Fluoride release and re-uptake in direct tooth-colored restorative materials. *Det Mater*. 1998;14:129–136.)

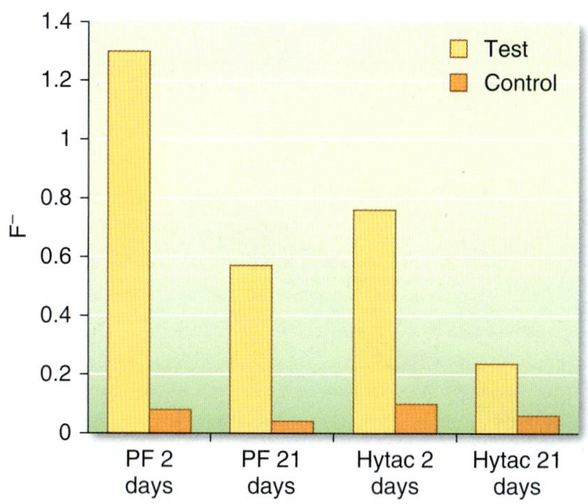

• **Fig. 6.7** Total fluoride concentration in plaque (microgram fluoride per milligram plaque) adjacent to resin-modified glass ionomer and compomer restorations over 21 days; restored test teeth versus nonrestored control teeth.

However, retrospective clinical analyses of in vivo studies have shown RMGIs to provide excellent retention and sealing of the tooth. One of the reasons for this is due to the relief of external stress provided by the dual-curing reactions of this class of materials. Although the bond strength of glass ionomers to dentin is lower than that of resin composites, clinical studies have shown that the retention of glass ionomers in areas of cervical erosion is considerably better than for composites. When the dentin is conditioned (etched) using a dilute solution (15% to 25%) of polyacrylic acid, the glass ionomer may be applied without a cavity preparation. Four-year clinical data showed a retention rate for glass ionomer cervical restorations of 75%.

Surface Characteristics and Biocompatibility

The surfaces of the restorations seen in the studies were noticeably rough, and some shade mismatches were present. Pulp reaction to glass ionomers is mild; however, if the thickness of dentin is less than 1 mm, a calcium hydroxide liner is recommended. Although the polished surface remains slightly rough, cervical restorations did not contribute to inflammation of gingival tissues. In fact, gingival response to glass ionomers is typically very good. Fewer *Streptococcus mutans* organisms exist in plaque adjacent to glass ionomer restorations than in controls without glass ionomers. RMGIs have been recognized as one of the best treatments for minimizing postoperative sensitivity in restored teeth. There are two reasons for this. First, because prior etching is not needed during placement, the collagen fibrils are not demineralized and collapse of the denuded layers cannot occur. Second, the dual-setting mechanism and gradual build-up of modulus allow the material to absorb a considerable amount of shrinkage stresses thus minimizing the effect of contraction forces at the tooth-restoration interfaces.

Color can be maintained and surface texture improved by finishing the restorations in a wet environment (water spray or water-soluble lubricant) and then recoating with a protective varnish or light-cured resin. Glass ionomer materials are an increasingly important material in operative dentistry for both an aging population with high incidence of root caries, patients with xerostomia and reduced salivary flow, and children who have high caries–risk factors.

Packaging of Glass Ionomers

Glass ionomers are packaged in bottles and in vacuum capsules for mixing in a mechanical mixer. When supplied in bulk, the powder and liquid are dispensed in proper amounts on a paper pad, and half the powder is initially incorporated to produce a homogeneous milky consistency. The remainder of the powder is then added for a total mixing time of 30 to 40 seconds. The typical initial setting time is about 4 minutes. After placing the restorative and developing the correct contour, the surface should be protected from contamination by applying a protective barrier.

Recently, the RMGIs have been formulated in paste-liquid or two-paste systems. During manufacture the FAS powder component is mixed with a small amount of resin to provide a paste-like consistency. The liquid may be left as such or alternatively formulated with a nonreactive glass and also provided as a paste. The manufacturer provides the two components in a dual-barrel syringe type of construction (Fig. 6.8). During use the two components are extruded by a lever in a predetermined ratio in the amount needed for the clinical preparation. The variability in dispensing is expected to be less in these types of dispensers. Furthermore, mixing by spatulation is more facile than with powder-liquid materials.

The latest advancement in dispensing of two-paste systems is an automixable, single-unit direct delivery device (Fig. 6.9). An example of an RMGI packaged in capsules is shown in Fig. 6.10. In this device, the two pastes are placed in two side-by-side compartments. The nozzle of the capsule contains a ministatic mixer. In use, the nozzle is lifted and positioned parallel to the barrels. An applicator then pushes out the two pastes into the nozzle where mechanical mixing occurs and the paste is extruded through the tip directly into the tooth preparation. The system is said to produce less microbubbles in the restoration, a condition that could potentially arise during trituration.

Consistent and accurate powder-to-liquid ratio is critical to the long-term maintenance of physical properties and the clinical success of restorations. Unlike conventional glass ionomer restorations, RMGIs set immediately when light-cured and can be finished 5 to 10 minutes after initial set. Optimum results are achieved if the manufacturer's instructions are followed carefully such as by maintaining adequate isolation and using adequate cavity conditioner procedures.

Manipulation of GIs can be found on the book's website at http://evolve.elsevier.com/sakaguchi/restorative.

Applications of GI and RMGI

GICs exhibit a number of advantages over other restorative materials. By bonding a restorative material to tooth structure, the cavity is theoretically sealed, protecting the pulp, eliminating secondary caries, and preventing leakage at the margins. These materials provide tooth-colored restorations with a low technique sensitivity.

Clinically, both conventional and RMGIs are used for a variety of restorative applications, particularly in situations of high caries activity or where caries is likely to recur. The main clinical indications are for small lesions (long-term non-stress–bearing restorations in permanent teeth, interim restoration in permanent teeth, and atraumatic restoration technique), especially where one or more margins are on dentin. They make an excellent liner or

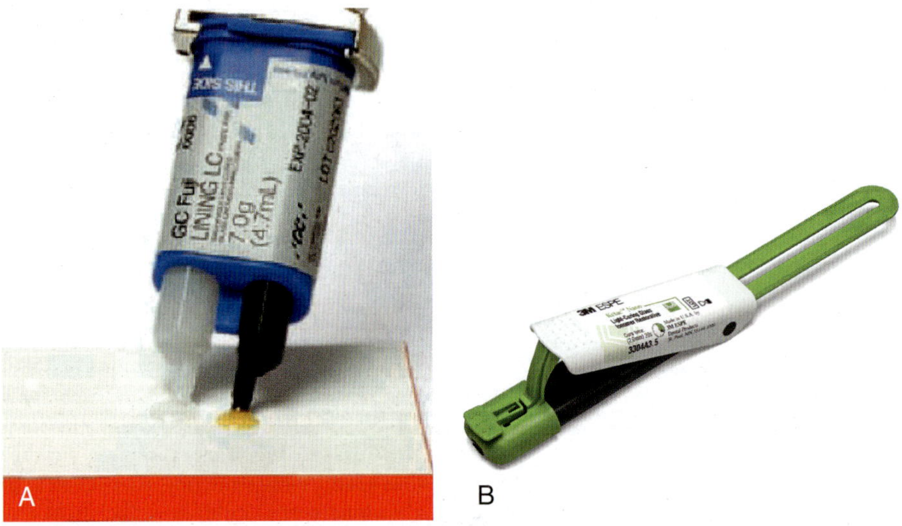

• **Fig. 6.8** Paste-liquid resin-modified glass ionomer dispensers. (A) Paste-Pak; (B) Clicker. (A, Courtesy GC America, Alsip, IL; B, Courtesy 3M Company, St. Paul, MN.)

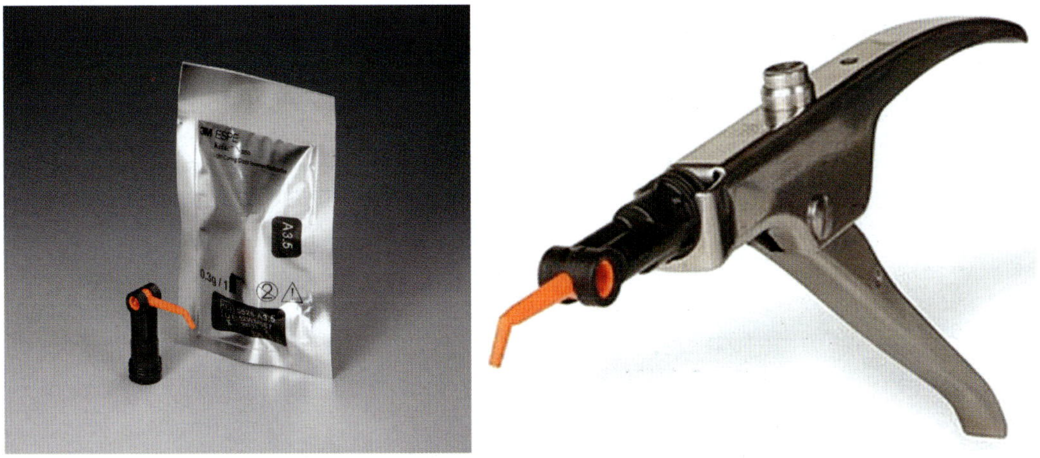

• **Fig. 6.9** Single-unit automix dispensing "Quick Mix" Capsule for a two-paste resin-modified glass ionomer. The dispensing tip contains a ministatic mixer for automixing when expressed by a delivery gun device. (Courtesy 3M Company, St. Paul, MN.)

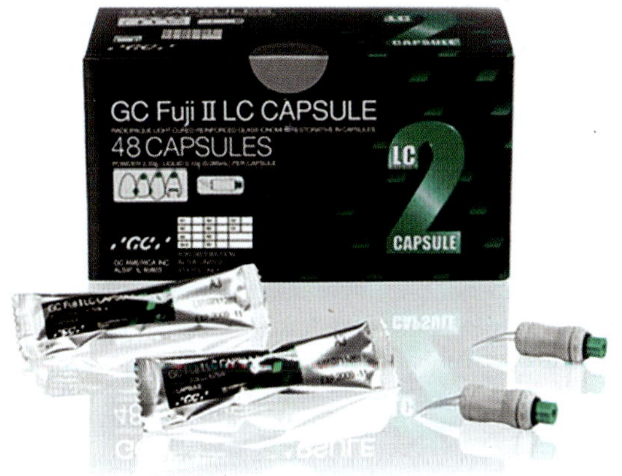

• **Fig. 6.10** RMGI materials available encapsulated for mechanical mixing. (Courtesy GC America Inc, Alsip, IL.)

base in all deep lesions where demineralized dentin remains on the cavity floor to be remineralized. When used as a cavity liner, these materials provide thermal insulation. They also advocated for a technique known as "sandwiching," "layering," or "stratification," where a resin composite is bonded over a base of the GI. A *sandwich technique* uses an RMGI as a liner to seal the dentin and provide the benefit of fluoride release, followed by a surface layer of resin composite to fill the remainder of the cavity. Some advocate the use of the glass ionomer as a liner under class I and II composite restorations to relieve stresses that result from shrinkage of the composite during cure. Glass ionomer lining materials bond to dentin with bond strengths varying from 2.0 to 4.9 MPa. These materials also adhere to composite restorative materials, by mechanical retention for conventional glass ionomer and mechanical and chemical bonding for RMGI. Glass ionomer lining materials release fluoride ions and are radiopaque. One video showing an open sandwich restoration with a dental composite can be found online.

Because of their low modulus, they are often advocated for class V restorations and abfraction lesions where tooth flexure is more pronounced. RMGI has often been recommended for use as an interim or definitive restoration in caries-active patients. Similarly, RMGIs are often the material of choice for pediatric restorations and preventive applications (direct filling as well as core build-up), because they are one-step procedures and require minimal isolation during placement. Some products are indicated for erupting permanent first and second molars with partially exposed grooves that are not yet able to be sealed with conventional resin sealant. The indications for both GI and RMGI materials are described in Table 6.2. More discussion of glass ionomers as cements can be found in Chapter 12.

Casein Phosphopeptides-Amorphous Calcium Phosphate

CPP-ACP is a stabilized system of calcium and phosphate that has been considerably studied in the last 20 years. Calcium phosphate formulations have been developed for addition to toothpastes, varnishes, and gums. CPP-ACP was designed to remineralize enamel subsurface lesions by stabilizing high levels of calcium and phosphate ions.

Composition

ACP is a glassy solid that is formed from the chemical decomposition of a mixture of dissolved phosphate and calcium salts (e.g., $[NH_4]_2HPO_4$+ $Ca[NO_3]_2$). The resulting amorphous mixture consists mostly of calcium and phosphate. It also contains varying amounts of water, hydrogen, and hydroxide ions, depending on the synthesis conditions. Such mixtures are also known as calcium phosphate cement.

ACP is generally categorized into either "amorphous tricalcium phosphate" (ATCP) or hydroxyapatite (CDHA). CDHA is sometimes termed "apatitic calcium triphosphate." The composition of ACP is CaxHy(PO4)z•nH2O, where n is between 3 and 4.5. CDHA has a general formula of $Ca_9(HPO_4)(PO_4)_5(OH)$. Precipitation from a moderately supersaturated and basic solution of a magnesium salt produces amorphous magnesium calcium phosphate (AMCP), in which magnesium is incorporated into the ACP structure.

A commercial preparation of ACP is CPP-ACP. Casein is predominant phosphoprotein in bovine milk. The concentration of CPP-ACP varies from 2% to 10% w/w. It is sold under various brand names, including GC mousse, MI paste, and MI paste plus, intended to be applied directly to teeth (Fig. 6.11).

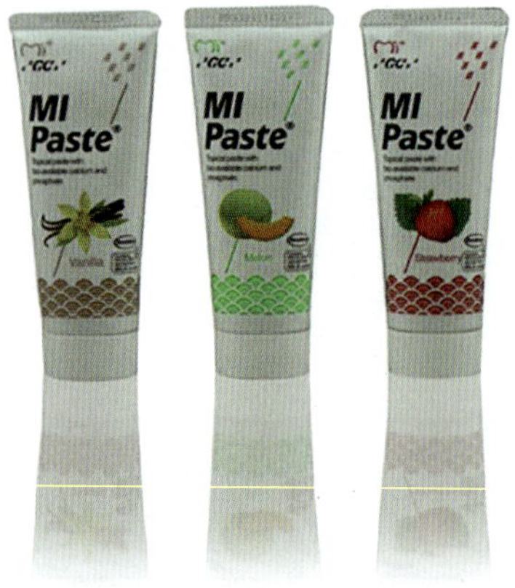

• **Fig. 6.11** Paste of CPP-ACP for enamel remineralization. (Courtesy GC America Inc, Alsip, IL.)

Properties

CPP-ACP was considered to be a calcium phosphate reservoir, buffering the activities of free calcium and phosphate ions, consequently helping maintain a state of supersaturation that inhibits demineralization and enhances remineralization. In recent years, studies have shown its potential to remineralize early caries lesions and also its anticariogenic characteristics in laboratory, animal, and human in situ experiments. Nevertheless, there remains some controversy regarding the efficacy of CPP-ACP and fluorides in the prevention of caries.

Application

Casein phosphopeptide can deliver ACP and can also help the ACP bind with the dental enamel. The action of the CPP-ACP complex ranges from buffering pH, preventing demineralization to enhancing remineralization, and reducing dentinal sensitivity.

In many recent studies that focused on the treatment of early caries lesions, CPP-ACP has shown promising outcomes as an adjunctive treatment to fluorides. Moreover, CPP-ACP is a unique protein derived from milk and therefore has a high safety level. A number of in vitro, in situ, and in vivo experiments have indicated the possible anticariogenic ability of CPP-ACP by its remineralizing effects. However, other studies demonstrate that fluorides combined with CPP-ACP achieved no clinical advantage over fluorides alone, which might question the anticariogenic ability of CPP-ACP by itself.

Clinical Studies

The clinical benefits of using CPP-ACP supplements over fluoride are still unclear. Systematic reviews on long-term remineralizing effect of CPP-ACP on early caries lesions in vivo found that CPP-ACP has a long-term remineralization effect on early caries lesions in comparison with placebo, although this effect was not significantly different from that of fluoride agents. Additionally, most remineralization studies have been conducted on orthodontics-related incipient lesions, thus limiting the generalizability of the results to other lesions.

Sodium Trimetaphosphate

To aid in the remineralization of dentin, the collagen matrix must be preserved and stabilized. By doing so, the collagen matrix can serve as a scaffold for mineral deposition. Researchers have speculated that sodium trimetaphosphate (STMP, $Na_3P_3O_9$) can phosphorylate type I collagen by integrating a phosphate ion onto the collagen surface, thereby inducing mineralization. STMP can attach to the demineralized collagen matrix by covalent bonds but also attracts ACP nano-precursors and induces apatite nucleation within the collagen matrix. The authors also speculate that the phosphate groups of STMPs immobilized on the collagen fibrils attract calcium ions by electrostatic force and direct apatite nucleation within the gap zones of collagen fibrils.

Composition

STMP is a chemical phosphorylation reagent in the food industry and has a cyclic structure that contains three phosphorus atoms in a six-membered ring. The composition of STMP is $Na_3P_3O_9$. In an alkaline environment, STMP can react with the hydroxyl groups on proteins, thereby introducing phosphate functional groups to protein molecules. Calcium ions can then be adsorbed onto the phosphorylated collagen surface by static electricity, and a calcium phosphate crystal cluster forms, gradually growing until a HA nucleus is formed.

Properties

STMP is reported to have a dual effect in that it hinders demineralization and promotes remineralization. STMP strongly binds to phosphate on enamel, blocking the release of calcium and phosphate ions. This leads to a layer on the enamel surface that limits acid ion diffusion. While limiting acid diffusion, this layer of STMP on the surface of the enamel does not seem to inhibit the diffusion of Ca^+ and F^- ions into the enamel. In addition, STMP can minimize mineral loss even in the presence of low-fluoride concentrations.

Applications

STMP can be added to many topical dental applications. These can include toothpastes, gels, and varnishes (Fig. 6.12).

Clinical Studies

In situ models have shown that supplementing a low-fluoride product with STMP produced similar remineralization effects to a 1100-ppm fluoride formulation. Similarly, the addition of STMP

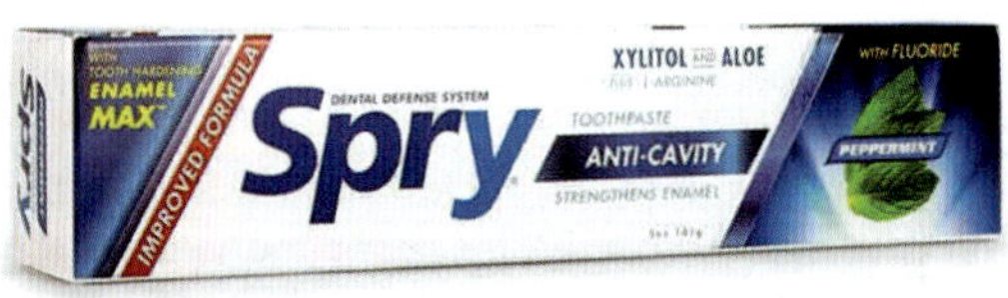

• **Fig. 6.12** Spry toothpaste with STMP. (Courtesy Xlear Inc, American Fork, UT.)

to conventional fluoride dentifrices and varnishes significantly enhanced their remineralization of artificial caries lesions.

A recent study showed that children using 500 ppm fluoride toothpaste with phosphates developed less carious lesions than toothpaste alone. In another study, an application of hydrolyzed STMP was tested in an artificial caries model with and without adhesive dentin bonding, and the demineralized dentin treated with STMP without adhesive bonding was more heavily mineralized than the group with adhesive bonding.

Bioactive Glass

Bioactive glass (BAG) has been used in the medical field to regenerate bone damaged by trauma or diseases. The first BAG was introduced in 1969 as a combination of sodium, calcium, and phosphorus silicate glass. BAG is both bioactive and biocompatible. The combination of both attributes allows it primarily to be used in the human body as a scaffold to guide bone regeneration. BAGs can raise the local pH, release beneficial ions, and facilitate apatite formation. They also have some activity against bacterial biofilm formation.

Composition

BAGs are based on a calcium sodium phosphosilicate (SiO_2–P_2O_5–CaO–Na_2O) system. Different BAGs utilize different compositions of these elements.

Properties

When the BAG is in contact with an aqueous solution, its particles will change to a mesoporous shape, followed by a pH rise. The pH rise promotes the precipitation of HA. Using BAGs in particle sizes between 5 and 45 μm ensures that there is degradation of the BAG filler, and apatite is formed within 28 days. Calcium and phosphate ions from BAG and mineralizing agents in saliva may enhance the mineralization process.

When used in a dental resin-based material, the resins and BAG particles must match their refractive index (RI) (within 0.02) to eliminate excessive light scattering at the glass-resin interface. This is important for the composite's efficient light-curing and final aesthetics to give translucency. Most commonly used dental resins have an RI ranging from 1.47 to 1.56, depending on the composition of the resin. Changing the BAG composition can alter the RI; for example, modifying oxides such as SrO or ZnO increases the RI whereas CaF_2 decreases it. Sodium in the BAG absorbs water and can weaken the composite, so most BAG fillers aim for low sodium content.

Applications

BAG can be used in multiple dental materials, from toothpastes, resin composites, GICs, and adhesives. These materials have been shown in vitro to enhance the remineralization of enamel and dentin.

Typical forms of BAGs found commercially are NovaMin and BioMinF. NovaMin is composed primarily of calcium, sodium, phosphorus, and silica). It is incorporated into toothpastes to aid in remineralization. NovaMin releases ions in the presence of saliva to shift the pH to a more alkaline state. This allows the formation of calcium-phosphate complexes, which can serve as a reservoir for calcium-potassium ions. These complexes can release these ions over several days.

BioMinF is a BAG containing dentifrice that includes calcium, phosphate, and fluoride. Adding fluoride ions in this complex allows for the prolonged delivery of fluoride ions into saliva. This formulation has been shown to enhance phosphate concentration three times that of NovaMin, thereby creating an optimal environment for apatite formation. Fluorapatite formed from BioMinF is more resistant to extrinsic and intrinsic acids. BioMinF dissolves in an accelerated manner in an acidic environment, which is beneficial in the oral cavity due to repeated acid encounters.

Clinical Studies

A systematic review on BAG for dentin remineralization confirmed that BAG can stimulate apatite formation on dentin, but there is insufficient evidence for BAG to effectively remineralize dentin. The size of the BAGparticles is an important aspect influencing the rate of apatite formation with nanoparticles having the fastest formation. The authors contend that more research is necessary to evaluate the mechanical properties of mineralized dentin and new apatite development.

Calcium Hydroxide

Hermann introduced calcium hydroxide in the United States in 1920, and the first reports of using calcium hydroxide to promote pulpal healing appeared in the literature between 1934 and 1941. Since World War II, indications for using calcium hydroxide expanded, becoming the primary material for inducing hard tissue deposition and promoting the healing of vital pulpal and periapical tissues.

Composition

Calcium hydroxide is a white, odorless powder with the chemical formula of $Ca(OH)_2$. Calcium hydroxide has a low solubility in water, decreasing with a temperature rise. The pure powder of calcium hydroxide has a high pH, ranging from 12.5 to 12.8, and is insoluble in alcohol. Its main action is dissociating Ca^{2+} and OH^- ions.

Radiopacity is produced by adding calcium tungstate or barium sulfate fillers. The product contains a base and catalyst component when used as a cavity liner. The base comprises calcium tungstate, tribasic calcium phosphate, and zinc oxide suspended in a glycol salicylate liquid. The catalyst consists of calcium hydroxide, zinc oxide, and zinc stearate in ethylene toluene sulfonamide liquid. The calcium hydroxide liner is low in strength and highly soluble in water. Resin-based restorative materials do not bond to conventional calcium hydroxide bases and liners.

Properties

The mechanism of action of calcium hydroxide has been an issue of discussion since its inception. It does dissociate into calcium and hydroxide ions in an aqueous solution; however, that is not the only mechanism of action for calcium hydroxide. More recent research has shown that calcium hydroxide acts to release bioactive molecules sequestered within the dentin. Calcium hydroxide has been shown to have antibacterial effects and stimulate complex tissue deposition.

The antibacterial effects of calcium hydroxide include inducing lipid peroxidation resulting in the destruction of phospholipids in the bacterial cell membrane. It also reacts with bacterial DNA to induce the splitting of the DNA strands inhibiting replication and cellular activity. The third antibacterial mechanism is through the alkalinization of calcium hydroxide, which induces the breakage of ionic bonds of bacterial proteins. This results in the loss of biological activity of enzymes and cellular metabolism.

Applications

Calcium hydroxide has been used in many facets of dentistry, including in deep cavity lining, indirect pulp capping, direct pulp capping, pulpotomy procedures, as an intracanal medicament, apexification, apexogenesis, and root resorption repair. There are limitations with using calcium hydroxide, especially when used in direct contact with vital pulp tissue. Calcium hydroxide has been shown to leave tunnel defects in the dentin bridge formed over pulp tissue when used in either a partial pulpotomy or a direct pulp cap. These tunneling defects can allow the passage of bacteria if an adequate coronal seal is not present.

Calcium hydroxide also creates a layer of necrosis up to 1.5 mm in vital pulp tissue after placement directly on the tissue. This necrosing action can compromise the vascularity of the pulp tissue, and the formation of a blood clot can interfere with the dentin bridge formation. On the positive side, calcium hydroxide has been shown to increase the recruitment, migration, proliferation, and mineralization of dental pulp stem cells, facilitating the process of reparative dentinogenesis.

The specific calcium hydroxide material to be used depends on the dental procedure it is intended for. Using calcium hydroxide in a vital pulp therapy procedure requires using a nonsetting calcium hydroxide product that contains mainly calcium hydroxide powder and an aqueous vehicle. Using calcium hydroxide in a deep carious lesion as a liner or base requires using a setting product containing the base and catalyst.

Hard-setting calcium hydroxide has two- to three fold less hydroxy ion release than the nonsetting version. Hard-setting calcium hydroxides (Life, Dycal, and Prisma VLC Dycal) are cavity liners and bases (Fig. 6.13).

These hard-setting liners have a low compressive strength that is not compatible with the condensation forces used when placing some definitive restorations. Life and Dycal are both degraded by acid etching and rinsing before restoration. This can lead to leakage and dissolution over time. Prisma VLC Dycal has calcium hydroxide incorporated into urethane dimethacrylate with initiators and accelerators, which bind to dentin and resist acid dissolution.

Clinical Studies

Systematic reviews and meta-analyses comparing calcium hydroxide and mineral trioxide aggregate (MTA) for direct pulp-capping procedures concluded pulp capping with MTA had higher success rates than those capped with calcium hydroxide. MTA showed less pulpal inflammation and a more predictable dentin bridge formation. The authors suggest that MTA may be a suitable replacement for calcium hydroxide in treatment of the vital pulp.

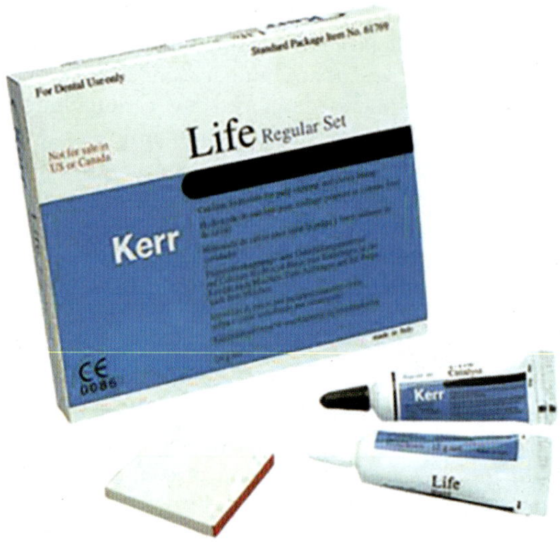

• **Fig. 6.13** Calcium Hydroxide, Life paste/paste. (Courtesy Kerr, Orange, CA.)

Tricalcium Silicate Cements

Tricalcium silicate cements and bioceramics were introduced to dentistry in the 1990s as an endodontic retrograde filling material. These materials and their uses were expanded into other areas of endodontics, such as perforation repair, root canal sealers, and coatings for gutta-percha. Torabinejad introduced a modified Portland cement product named MTA in the 1990s, and since then, multiple other formulations of tricalcium silicate cements have come to market).

Composition

MTA is a mixture of dicalcium silicate, tricalcium silicate, tricalcium aluminate, calcium sulfate, tetracalcium aluminoferrite, and bismuth oxide. This powder is mixed with water to create a thick paste-like material. MTA is becoming the gold standard against which other materials are tested. Today, newer products on the market, such as Biodentine, behave similarly to MTA while not having the staining issues seen with MTA.

Biodentine contains tricalcium silicate, calcium carbonate, zirconium oxide, and a water-based liquid containing calcium chloride as the setting accelerator. Zirconium oxide is the radiopacifier added for visualization on radiographs. Biodentine has a setting time of around 10 to 12 minutes and is marketed as a dentin substitute, which can be used as a coronal restoration material, for perforation repair, and as a pulp-capping material. The pH of Biodentine has been reported to be 11.7 after 1-day immersion in Hank's balanced salt solution and demonstrates no significant change over 28 days. Biodentine exhibited high compressive strength, push-out strength, and microhardness.

Another popular tricalcium silicate cement material is Endosequence Root Repair Material (ERRM). ERRM was created to overcome some of the adverse effects of MTA, specifically the less-than-ideal handling properties and staining of tooth structure. According to the manufacturer, ERRM comprises calcium silicates, monobasic calcium phosphate, zirconium oxide, tantalum oxide, proprietary fillers, and thickening agents.

Properties

The mechanism of action of each of these materials is similar. Bioceramic cements or tricalcium cements are materials that enable the release of other bioactive materials sequestered in the dentin matrix, similar to calcium hydroxide. These released bioactive molecules have been found to include growth factors, chemokines, cytokines, extracellular matrix molecules, and bioactive peptides (transforming growth factor, bone morphogenetic proteins, insulin growth factor, and platelet-derived growth factor). Calcium silicate cements induce odontoblastic differentiation and can promote dental pulp cell migration and pulp repair.

These cements can set in a wet environment, whether blood, water, saliva, or dentinal fluid, though one must be cautious that the environment is not flooded with fluid. The initial setting time for tricalcium silicate cements is around 40 to 50 minutes, with the final setting around 120 to 170 minutes. All tricalcium silicate cements have an alkaline pH ranging from 10.2 after the initial setting time to 12.5 after the final setting time. Each of these cement has high compressive strength, does not shrink over time, and is antibacterial. The compressive strength of MTA was reported to be lower than amalgam and Super EBA at 24 hours. Still, after 3 weeks, the compression strength of MTA increased and was similar to that of Super EBA, although still less than amalgam. Tricalcium silicate cements demonstrate minimal cellular cytotoxicity.

Applications

Tricalcium silicate cements are used in many dental procedures, including direct pulp caps, pulpotomies, root perforation repair, internal and external resorption repair, root end fillings, apexification, apexogenesis, regenerative endodontics, root canal sealers, and indirect pulp caps.

Clinical Studies

A systematic review of different types of bioceramics used as direct pulp-capping materials showed that MTA and Biodentin were the most studied and also the most successful. Bioceramic materials used for direct pulp capping showed high biocompatibility and bioactivity, and possessed antimicrobial properties. Calcium silicate-based materials are currently the most effective bioceramic materials used for direct pulp capping.

Systematic reviews and meta-analyses have concluded that MTA produced better clinical effects than calcium hydroxide regarding dental pulp protection in capping of mechanical exposures. The authors also found that MTA showed a higher rate of hard tissue barrier formation than calcium hydroxide.

Pit and Fissure Sealants

Dental sealants were introduced in the 1960s to help prevent dental caries, mainly in the pits and fissures of occlusal tooth surfaces. Sealants act to prevent bacteria growth that can lead to dental decay. Evidence suggests that fissure sealants are effective in preventing caries in children and adolescents compared to no sealants. Effectiveness may, however, be related to caries incidence level of the population.

Clinicians have used resin-based materials (conventional fissure sealants or flowable composites), polyacid-modified resin sealants (compomers), and GICs (low viscosity, high viscosity, or resin modified) for this purpose.

Resin-Based Pit and Fissure Sealants

Composition

Resin-based pit and fissure sealants contain different methacrylate monomers, including bisphenol A-glycidyl methacrylate (Bis-GMA), and are light-cured, although some self-cured products are also available. The chemistry of Bis-GMA sealants is the same as that described for resin composites in Chapter 8. The principal difference is that sealants are much more fluid to enable them to penetrate the pits, fissures, and etched areas on the enamel, which promotes retention of the sealant. The viscous Bis-GMA resin is mixed with a diluent, such as triethylene glycol dimethacrylate, to produce a reasonably low-viscosity, flowable resin. An alternative but similar oligomer base is urethane dimethacrylate; some materials are formulated from a combination of the two base resins. To provide stiffness to the material and improve wear resistance, filler particles of fumed silica or silanated inorganic glasses can be added to form low-viscosity composites.

The polymerization of light-cured sealants is initiated by a photosensitive diketone in conjunction with a tertiary amine. The complete reactions for similar resin composites are given in Chapter 8. Light-cured sealants are supplied in light-proof containers and should have a shelf life of more than 12 months.

Properties

Because sealants are completely circumscribed by enamel and should not be subjected to heavy occlusal stresses without support of the underlying enamel, the mechanical properties of sealants are less important than those of resin composite restoratives that must support occlusal loads in bulk. By adding ceramic or glass filler particles up to 40% by weight, most properties show improvement as compared to unfilled resins. The modulus of elasticity shows the most dramatic improvement, and the increased rigidity makes the filled material less subject to deflection under occlusal stress. Filler is also added with the goal of improving wear resistance and making the material more visible on clinical inspection (Fig. 6.14).

Optimal adhesion of the sealant to enamel occurs when the sealant has a low surface tension, good wetting, and a low viscosity. These properties permit the sealant to flow and spread easily along the enamel surface. The surface wettability is demonstrated by the contact angle of a drop of liquid on the enamel surface. A drop that spreads readily produces a low contact angle. This highly wetted surface is conducive to a strong adhesive bond because it increases the amount of surface area in contact. Polymer tags form when the resin flows into the surface irregularities created by acid etching and are responsible for the mechanical bond that retains the sealant to enamel. Functional durability of the sealant bond is related to stresses induced by shrinkage of the resin during curing, thermal cycling, deflection from occlusal forces, water sorption, and abrasion, with total failure manifested by the clinical loss of material.

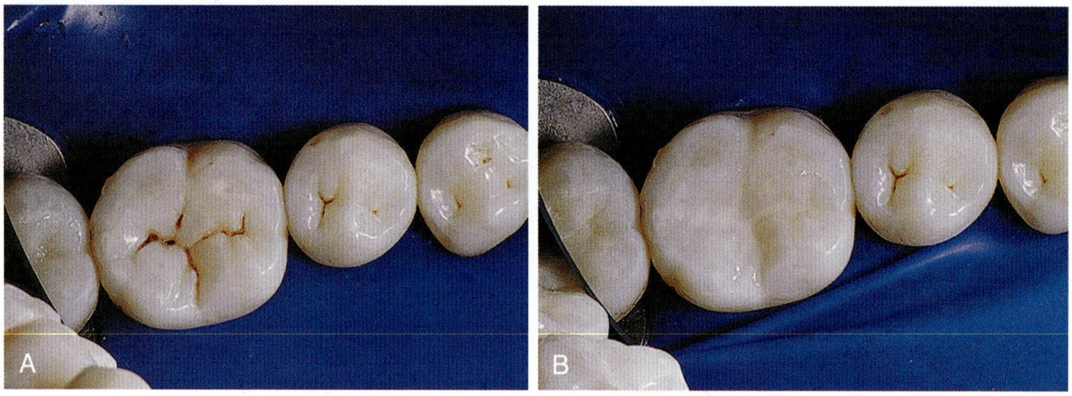

• **Fig. 6.14** Typical molar with stained fissures and no diagnosable caries. (A) Before sealing and (B) after sealing with a natural-colored sealant material. (From Hatrick CD, Eakle WS, Bird WF. *Dental Materials: Clinical Applications for Dental Assistants and Dental Hygienists*. 2nd ed. Saunders; 2011.)

Sealant materials have a variety of features that must be selected carefully by the health care provider. Most current materials are light-cured rather than self-cured because of the ease of use and controlled rate of cure. Tooth-colored or clear resins are available that are natural looking on the tooth surface, but they are also available in opaque or tinted materials to make the recall examination process easier (Fig. 6.15). Color-reversible, photosensitive sealants include photosensitive pigments that are normally colorless but change to green or pink when exposed to the dental curing light to help determine whether the sealant adequately covers the pit and fissures. The color change lasts for about 5 to 10 minutes after exposure but can be repeated at recall visits with another exposure to a dental curing light.

An increasing number of resin sealants are marketed with the claim that they release fluoride. The release is highest in the first 24 hours after placement and then tapers to a low maintenance level, which to date has not been proven to provide any significant improvement in clinical protection against caries.

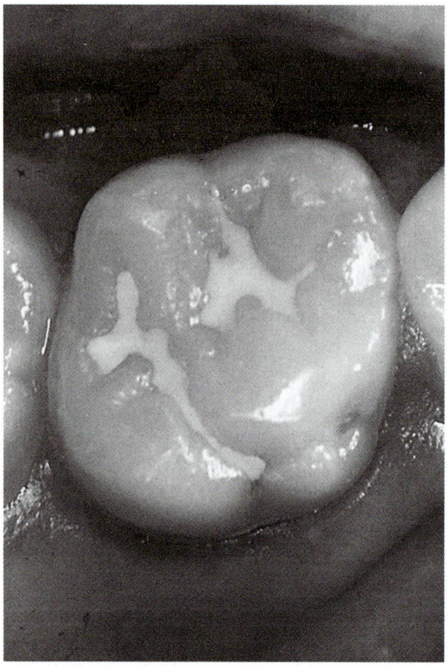

• **Fig. 6.15** Maxillary molar tooth wit opaque sealant that has been in place for 5 years.

Application of Resin-Based Pit and Fissure Sealant

The handling characteristics of a sealant depend on the composition of the material and the surface to which it is applied. Optimal preparation of the surface will lead to close adaptation of the sealant to the tooth enamel, a strong seal against the ingress of oral fluids and debris, and long-term material retention.

The penetration of any of the sealants to the bottom of the pits and fissures and filling them without voids is important. Air or debris can be trapped in the bottom of the fissure that prevents it from being completely filled, as shown in Fig. 6.16. Control of the viscosity of the sealant is important to obtain optimum results, and sealants that are too thick and viscous will not penetrate the pits and fissures, or the etched enamel itself as well. Penetration of sealant into etched enamel, forming tags to a depth of 25 to 50 μm, is shown in Fig. 6.17.

One technique that maximizes the benefits of conservative, adhesive dentistry is preventive resin restoration (PRR). PRR is indicated when some areas of the fissure system of the tooth are associated with carious dentin and others are not. Once the lesion is removed, no further preparation is performed. If the resultant preparation is restricted to narrow and shallow opening of the fissure, a resin sealant or flowable composite is placed. If additional tooth structure of the tooth is removed, a posterior dentin composite is placed in that area, and the remaining fissures and the surface of the composite restoration are sealed with resin sealant or flowable composite.

Glass Ionomers Sealants

Because of their demonstrated ability to release fluoride and provide some caries protection on tooth surfaces at risk, glass ionomers have been suggested and tested for their ability to function as a fissure sealant. Glass ionomers are generally more viscous than their resin-based counterparts, which somewhat reduces their penetration to the depth of a fissure and mechanical retention to the enamel surface compared with resins. They are also more

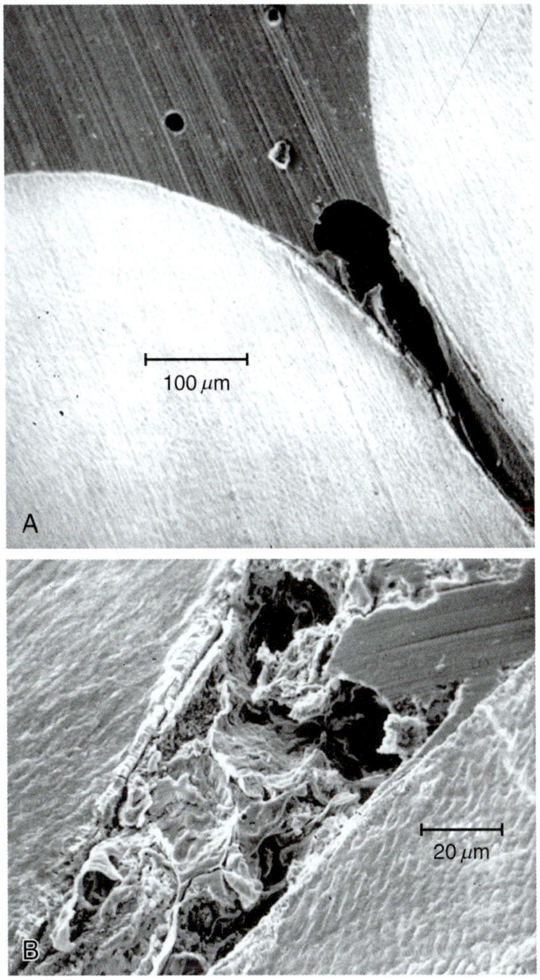

• **Fig. 6.16** Section showing a fissure incompletely filled with sealant as a result of (A) air and (B) debris. (From Gwinnett AJ. The bonding of sealants to enamel. *J Am Soc Prevent Dent*. 1973;3:21–29.)

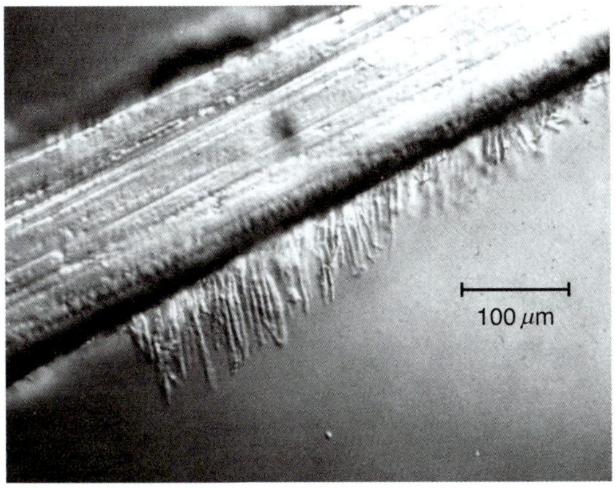

• **Fig. 6.17** Penetration of sealant into etched enamel. These tags are responsible for the bonding to enamel. (From Gwinnett AJ. The bonding of sealants to enamel. *J Am Soc Prevent Dent*. 1973;3:21–29.)

brittle and less resistant to occlusal wear. However, clinical studies using various formulations of glass ionomers have shown that, in spite of the significantly lower retention rates than resin sealants, glass ionomer–based sealants have a much greater fluoride deposition in the enamel surfaces. Thus there is a greater potential for latent caries protection after sealant loss. In summary, although glass ionomer retention appears to be poorer than for resins, clinical outcomes in terms of caries recurrence are similar if not better than with resins.

In areas where high-risk children do not have access to definitive treatment, a conservative caries management technique can seal remaining caries in a fluoride-rich environment and establish some degree of remineralization. Atraumatic restorative treatments (ARTs) involve opening a lesion, removing soft surface decay with hand instruments, and filling or sealing the surface with highly filled glass ionomer with a fast setting time. Two-year survival rates of single- and multiple-surface ART restorations in primary teeth have been reported as 93% and 62%, respectively. Five-year survival rate of single-surface ART restorations in permanent teeth was reported as 80%.

Flowable Composites as Sealants

Low-viscosity composites referred to as *flowable composites* are marketed for a wide variety of applications, such as PRR, cavity liners, restoration repairs, and cervical restorations. The properties of flowable composites are described in Chapter 8.

Flowable composites are usually packaged in syringes or in capsules (Fig. 6.18) for direct application to the pit or fissure. As with lower-viscosity resin sealants, trapping of air in the sealant must be avoided. Because they have higher filler content than most resin sealants, flowable composites should have better wear resistance. Flowable composites appear to provide good retention and caries resistance after 24 months.

When flowable composites are used as preventive restorations, their low viscosity is a benefit in extending the restoration into adjacent fissures as a sealant. A 24-month study showed the retention and caries incidence of a flowable composite to be equivalent to that of a fluoride-containing fissure sealant.

Clinical Outcomes Using Different Types of Sealants

Many clinical studies using Bis-GMA–based resins have been documented. In earlier studies on effectiveness of treatment with

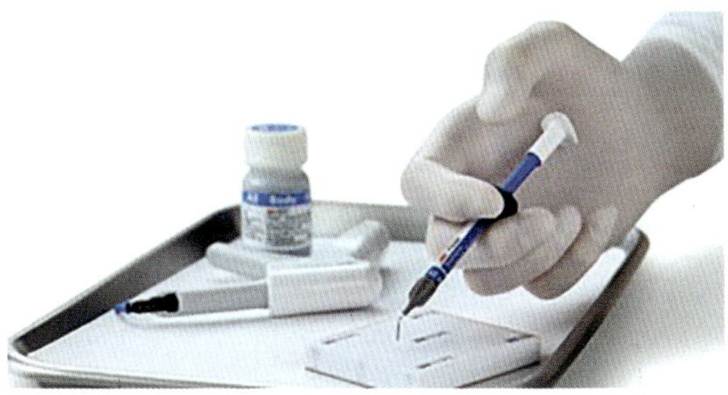

• **Fig. 6.18** Flowable composite resin in syringe delivery system and capsule. (Courtesy of Solventum, San Diego, California, United States.)

sealant in newly erupting teeth, a light-cured sealant demonstrated a retention rate of 42% and an effectiveness of 35% in caries reduction after 5 years. In a similar study, a filled resin sealant showed a retention rate of 53% and a clinical effectiveness of 54% after 4 years. Results involving a quicker-setting unfilled resin sealant with very good penetration showed a retention rate of 80% and an effectiveness of 69% after 3 years. The longest published study on sealant effectiveness is a 15-year evaluation of a self-cured unfilled material, which showed 27.6% complete retention and 35.4% partial retention.

In pairwise comparisons, the treated first molars had 31.3 decayed and filled primary tooth surfaces, compared to 82.8 for the untreated controls. In a more current 4-year study comparing a fluoride-releasing sealant with one that did not have fluoride, retention rates were 91% for the fluoride material (77% complete and 14% partial) and 95% for the nonfluoride sealant (89% complete and 6% partial). Although the retention was somewhat lower in the fluoride-containing sealant, the caries incidence for both groups was identical (10%). In a study conducted in private practice, the 2-year retention rates for two newer fluoride-containing resins were greater than 90%, and no caries was detected on the test teeth. In a continuing study with retreatment of all defective sealant surfaces at 6-month recalls, the teeth were maintained caries free for a 5-year period. The retreatment rate was highest (18%) at 6 months, and then diminished as time progressed, but at each recall period, at least two teeth (about 4%) required reapplication.

Resin-based sealants (RBSs) applied on occlusal surfaces of permanent molars are effective in preventing caries in children and adolescents. A Cochrane review (2017) found moderate-quality evidence that RBSs reduced caries by between 11% and 51% compared to no sealant when measured at 24 months. Similar benefit was seen at timepoints up to 48 months; after longer follow-up, the quantity and quality of evidence were reduced. There was insufficient evidence to judge the effectiveness of glass ionomer sealant or the relative effectiveness of different types of sealants. Information on adverse effects was limited, but none occurred where this was reported.

There was no difference between the percentage of caries development with use of GICs as fissure-sealing material compared with that for the conventional RBSs, but the retention rate of conventional RBSs was much higher than that of the GICs.

Almost all studies show a direct correlation between sealant retention and caries protection. Therefore it is important to use materials that are retentive to enamel, resistant against occlusal wear, and easily applied with minimal opportunities for surface contamination. Current evidence indicates that sealants are most effective on occlusal surfaces where pits and fissures are well defined and retentive to food and in patients with elevated risk for pit and fissure caries.

Resin Infiltration

Resin infiltration is a minimally invasive technique that aims to halt the progression of incipient carious lesions and restore the appearance of affected teeth without the need for removal of healthy tooth structure. The concept of arresting caries by infiltration of resins was introduced in the mid-1970s and was more extensively studied in the early 1990s. Researchers at the University of Göttingen developed a resin material with low viscosity that could penetrate and stabilize the demineralized enamel. The first commercial product, Icon (initially known as DMG Penetrating Sealant) was introduced in 2009 specifically to treat smooth surface and noncavitated interproximal lesions.

Composition

The resin infiltration system is a two-step process involving an etchant followed by the infiltrant. The etchant is composed of hydrochloric acid, pyrogenic silicic acid, and surface-active substances. The resin infiltrant is composed of methacrylate-based resin matrix, initiators, and additives, and ethanol as the solvent (99% solvent).

Properties

The resin infiltration technique is based on a low-viscosity resin with a high penetration coefficient filling the enamel intercrystalline spaces and blocking diffusion pathways for cariogenic acids. In contrast to conventional sealants, with this technique, the diffusion barrier is created inside the lesion and not on the surface. Additionally, the Icon resin is unfilled and has optical properties similar to those of natural enamel, effectively transmitting the natural shade of the tooth and masking white spot lesions (WSLs).

Applications

Dental resin infiltration is indicated for treating early noncavitated proximal carious lesions up to one-third of outer dental (D1 lesion) and smooth surface lesions. Resin infiltration can serve as a preventive treatment option for patients at high risk of developing caries. By treating early demineralized enamel, the progression of carious lesions can be halted, potentially avoiding the need for more invasive restorative procedures in the future. Resin infiltration can also help blend the color of WSLs, areas of demineralized enamel that appear as chalky white spots on the tooth surface. WSLs can result from the early stages of caries, enamel demineralization due to acid exposure, fluorosis, or as a consequence of orthodontic treatment. Resin infiltration is particularly useful for addressing aesthetic concerns associated with WSLs, especially on the visible front teeth. By reducing the appearance of white spots and discolorations, the treatment can enhance aesthetics without compromising healthy tooth structure. After orthodontic treatment, some patients may develop WSLs around orthodontic brackets or bands due to plaque accumulation and enamel demineralization. Resin infiltration can be used to treat these WSLs, restoring a more even and uniform tooth appearance.

It is important to note that dental resin infiltration is most effective when applied to early and superficial lesions that have not extended into the dentin or deeper layers of the tooth. In cases of cavitated lesions, other restorative treatments, such as direct and indirect restorations, are more appropriate.

Clinical Studies

A systematic review of clinical trials concluded that resin infiltration appears to be an effective method to arrest the progression of noncavitated proximal caries lesions, but longer-term studies are required. In two studies, infiltration of proximal noncavitated lesions was shown to reduce caries lesion progression compared to a placebo over 3 years. One study reported that only 4% of caries lesions treated with resin infiltration progressed and 42% of lesions without treatment progressed.

Another systematic review of clinical trials concluded that the resin infiltration technique seems to be a feasible option for color masking of white-colored enamel discolorations resulting from both WSLs and enamel development defects.

Bibliography

Introduction (caries prevention and remineralization)

Cochrane NJ, Cai F, Huq NL, Burrow MF, Reynolds EC. New approaches to enhanced remineralization of tooth enamel. *J Dent Res.* 2010;89(11):1187–1197.

Featherstone JD. The caries balance: the basis for caries management by risk assessment. *Oral Health Prev Dent.* 2004;2(suppl 1):259–264.

Featherstone JDB. Remineralization, the natural caries repair process: the need for new approaches. *Adv Dent Res.* 2009;21(1):4.

Gonzalez-Cabezas C, Fernandez CE. Recent advances in remineralization therapies for caries lesions. *Adv Dent Res.* 2018;29(1):55–59.

Philip N. State of the art enamel remineralization systems: the next frontier in caries management. *Caries Res.* 2018;53(3):284–295. https://doi.org/10.1159/000493031.

Fluorides (fluoride varnish)

Banting DW, Papas A, Clark DC, et al. The effectiveness of 10% chlorhexidine varnish treatment on dental caries incidence in adults with dry mouth. *Gerodontology.* 2000;17:67.

Beltran-Aguilar ED, Goldstein JW. Fluoride varnishes: a review of their clinical use, cariostatic mechanism, efficacy and safety. *J Am Dent Assoc.* 2000;131:589.

Marinho VC, Worthington HV, Walsh T, Clarkson JE. Fluoride varnishes for preventing dental caries in children and adolescents. *Cochrane Database Syst Rev.* 2013;7:CD002279.

Petersson LG, Twetman S, Pakhomov GN. The efficiency of semiannual silane fluoride varnish applications: a two-year clinical study in preschool children. *J Public Health Dent.* 1998;58:57.

Weyant R, Tracy S, Anselmo T, et al. Topical fluoride for caries prevention. *JADA.* 2013;144(11):1279–1291.

Silver Diamine Fluoride

Contreras V, Toro MJ, Elias-Boneta AR, Encarnacion-Burgos A. Effectiveness of silver diamine fluoride in caries presention prevention and arrest: a systematic literature review. *Gen Dent.* 2017;65(3):22–29.

Crystal YO, Niederman R. Evidence-based dentistry update on silver diamine fluoride. *Dent Clin N Am.* 2019;63(1):45–68. https://doi.org/10.1016/j.cden.2018.08.011.

Greenwall-Cohen J, Greenwall L, Barry S. Silver diamine fluoride—an overview of the literature and current clinical techniques. *Br Dent J.* 2020;228(11):831–838. https://doi.org/10.1038/s41415-020-1641-4.

Horst JA, Ellenikiotis H, Milgrom PL. UCSF protocol for caries arrest using silver diamine fluoride: rationale, indications and consent. *J Calif Dent Assoc.* 2016;44(1):16.

Peng JJ, Botelho MG, Matinlinna JP. Silver compounds used in dentistry for caries management: a review. *J Dent.* 2012;40(7):531.

Seifo N, Robertson M, MacLean J, et al. The use of silver diamine fluoride (SDF) in dental practice. *Br Dent J.* 2020;228(2):75–81. https://doi.org/10.1038/s41415-020-1203-9.

Zhao I, Gao S, Hiraishi N, et al. Mechanisms of silver diamine fluoride on arresting caries: a literature review. *Int Dent J.* 2018;68(2):67–76. https://doi.org/10.1111/idj.12320.

Glass Ionomers and Resin-Modified Glass Ionomers to Prevent Caries Progression

Cattani-Lorente MA, Dupuis V, Moya F, et al. Comparative study of the physical properties of a polyacid-modified composite resin and a resin-modified glass ionomer. *Dent Mater.* 1999;15:21.

Farah JW, Powers JM. Fluoride-releasing restorative materials. *Dent Advis.* 1998;15:2.

Fleming GJ, Faroog AA, Barralet JE. Influence of powder/liquid mixing ratio on the performance of a restorative glass-ionomer dental cement. *Biomaterials.* 2003;24:4173.

Forss H. Release of fluoride and other elements from light-cured glass ionomer in neutral and acidic conditions. *J Dent Res.* 1993;72:1257.

Holmgren CJ, Roux D, Domejean S. Minimal intervention dentistry: part 5. Atraumatic restorative treatment (ART)—a minimum intervention and minimally invasive approach for the management of dental caries. *Br Dent J.* 2013;214:1.

Müller J, Brucker G, Kraft E, et al. Reaction of cultured pulp cells to eight different cements based on glass ionomers. *Dent Mater.* 1990;6:172.

Quackenbush BM, Donly KJ, Croll TP. Solubility of a resin-modified glass ionomer cement. *J Dent Child.* 1998;65:310.

Ribeiro AP, Serra MC, Paulillo LA, et al. Effectiveness of surface protection for resin-modified glass-ionomer materials. *Quint Int.* 1999;30:427.

Strother JM, Kohn DH, Dennison JB, et al. Fluoride release and reuptake in direct tooth colored restorative materials. *Dent Mater.* 1998;14:129.

Weidlich P, Miranda LA, Maltz M, et al. Fluoride release and uptake from glass ionomer cements and composite resins. *Braz Dent J.* 2000;11:89.

Wellbury RR, Shaw AJ, Murray JJ, et al. Clinical evaluation of paired compomer and glass ionomer restorations in primary teeth. *Br Dent J.* 2000;189:93.

Ylp HK, Smales RJ. Fluoride release and uptake by aged resin-modified glass ionomers and a polyacid-modified resin composite. *Int Dent J.* 1999;49:217.

Glass Ionomers and Resin-Modified Glass Ionomers

Billington RW, Williams JA, Pearson GJ. Ion processes in glass ionomer cements. *J Dent.* 2006;34:544–555.

Burke FJT, Wilson NH. Glass-ionomer restorations in stress bearing and difficult to access cavities. In: Davidson CL, Mjor IA, eds. *Advances in Glass Ionomer Cements.* Quintessence; 1999:253–268.

Croll TP, Berg JH. Resin-modified glass-ionomer restoration of primary molars with proximating class II caries lesions. *Compend Contin Educ Dent.* 2007;28:372 376.

Croll TP, Nicholson JW. Glass-ionomer cements: history and current status. *Inside Dentistry.* 2008;4:76–84.

Donly KJ, Segura A, Kanellis M, Erickson RC. Clinical performance and caries inhibition of resin-modified glass ionomer cement and amalgam restorations. *J Am Dent Assoc.* 1999;13:1459–1466.

Falsafi A, Mitra SB, Oxman JD, Bui HT, Ton TT. Mechanisms of setting reactions and interfacial behavior of a nano-filled resin-modified glass ionomer. *Dent Mater.* 2014;30(6):632–642.

Forsten L. Fluoride release and uptake by glass ionomers and related materials and its effect. *Biomaterials.* 1998;19:503–508.

Haveman CW, Summit JB, Burgess JO, Carlson K. Three restorative materials and topical fluoride gel used in xerostomic patients: a clinical comparison. *J Am Dent Assoc.* 2003;134:177–184.

Hunt PR. Glass ionomers: the next generation. A summary of the current situation. *J Esthet Dent.* 1994;6(5):192-194. doi: 10.1111/j.1708-8240.1994.tb00859.x.

McComb D, Erickson RL, Maxymiw WG, Wood RE. A clinical comparison of glass ionomer, resin-modified glass ionomer and resin composite restorations in the treatment of cervical caries in xerostomic head and neck cancer patients. *Oper Dent.* 2002;27:430–437.

Mitra S. Glass ionomers and related filling materials. In: Dhuru VB, ed. *Contemporary Dental Materials.* Oxford University Press; 2004:66–80.

Mitra SB, Kedrowski BL. Long-term mechanical properties of glass ionomers. *Dent Mater.* 1994;10:78–82.

Mitra SB, Lee C-Y, Bui HT, Tantbirojn D, Rusin RP. Long-term adhesion and mechanism of bonding of a paste-liquid resin-modified glass-ionomer. *Dent Mater.* 2009;25:459–466.

Mitra SB, Oxman JD, Falsafi A, Ton T. Fluoride release and recharge behavior of a nano-filled resin-modified glass ionomer compared with that of other fluoride releasing materials. *Am J Dent.* 2011;24(6):372–378.

Mount GJ, Tyas MJ, Ferracane JI, Berg JH, Ngo HC. A revised classification for direct tooth-colored restorative materials. *Quintessence Int.* 2009;40:691–697.

Mount GJ. Description of glass ionomers. In: *An Atlas of Glass Ionomer Cements: A Clinician's Guide*. 3rd ed. Martin Dunitz Ltd; 2002:1–42.
Peumans M, Kanumilli P, De Munck J, van Landuyt K, Lambrechts P, Van Meerbeek B. Clinical effectiveness of contemporary adhesives: a systematic review of current clinical trials. *Dent Mater*. 2005;21:864–881.
Ruiz JL, Mitra S. Using cavity liners with direct posterior composite restorations. *Compend Contin Educ Dent*. 2006;27:347–351.
Tantbirojn D, Rusin RP, Mitra SB. Inhibition of dentin demineralization adjacent to a glass ionomer/composite sandwich restoration. *Quintessence Int*. 2009;40:287–294.
Van Meerbeek B, Peumans M, Poitevin A, et al. Relationship between bond-strength test and clinical outcomes. *Dent Mater*. 2010;26:100–121.
Wilson AD, McLean JW. *Glass-Ionomer Cements*. Quintessence; 1988.

Casein Phosphopeptides-amorphous Calcium Phosphate

Destainville A, Champion E, Bernache-Assollant D, Laborde E. Synthesis, characterization and thermal behavior of apatitic tricalcium phosphate. *Mater Chem Phys*. 2003;80(1):269–277. https://doi.org/10.1016/S0254-0584(02)00466-2.
Dorozhkin SV. Amorphous calcium (ortho)phosphates. *Acta Biomater*. 2010;6(12):4457–4475. https://doi.org/10.1016/j.actbio.2010.06.031.
Gonzalez-Cabezas C, Fernandez CE. Recent advances in remineralization therapies for caries lesions. *Adv Dent Res*. 2018;29(1):55–59.
Indraprivadharshini K, Kumar PD, Sharma K, Iyer K. Reminerizing potential of CPP-ACP in the white spot lesions—a systematic review. *Indian J Dent Res*. 2018;29(4):487–496.
Li J, Xie X, Wang Y, et al. Long-term remineralization effect of casein phosphopeptide-amorphous calcium phosphate (CPP-ACP) on early caries lesions in vivo: a systemic review. *J Dent*. 2014;42:769–777.
Reynolds EC. Casein phosphopeptide-amorphous calcium phosphate: the scientific evidence. *Adv Dent Res*. 2009;21(1):25.
Tao S, Zhu Y, Yuan H, et al. Efficacy of fluorides and CPP-ACP vs fluorides monotherapy on early caries lesions: a systematic review and meta-analysis. *PLoS One*. 2018;13(4):e0196660.

Sodium Trimetaphosphate

Gonçalves RS, Candia Scaffa PM, Giacomini MC, Rabelo Buzalaf MA, Honório HM, Wang L. Use of sodium trimetaphosphate in the inhibition of dentin matrix metalloproteinases and as a remineralizing agent. *J Dent*. 2018;68:34–40. https://doi.org/10.1016/j.jdent.2017.10.009.
Grohe B, Mittler S. Advanced non-fluoride approaches to dental enamel remineralization: the next level in enamel repair management. *Biomater Biosyst*. 2021;4:100029. https://doi.org/10.1016/j.bbiosy.2021.100029.
Liu Y, Li N, Qi Y, et al. The use of sodium trimetaphosphate as a biomimetic analog of matrix phosphoproteins for remineralization of artificial caries-like dentin. *Dent Mater*. 2011;27(5):465–477. https://doi.org/10.1016/j.dental.2011.01.008.
Zhong B, Peng C, Wang G, Tian L, Cai Q, Cui F. Contemporary research findings on dentine remineralization. *J Tissue Eng Regen Med*. 2013;9(9):1004–1016. https://doi.org/10.1002/term.1814.

Bioactive Glass

Dai L, Mei M, Chu C, Lo E. Mechanisms of bioactive glass on caries management: a review. *Materials*. 2019;12(24):4183. https://doi.org/10.3390/ma12244183.
Fernando D, Attik N, Pradelle-Plasse N, Jackson P, Grosgogeat B, Colon P. Bioactive glass for dentin remineralization: a systematic review. *Mater Sci Eng C Mater Biol Appl*. 2017;76:1369–1377. https://doi.org/10.1016/j.msec.2017.03.083.
Ramadoss R, Padmanaban R, Subramanian B. Role of bioglass in enamel remineralization: existing strategies and future prospects—a narrative review. *J Biomed Mater Res B Appl Biomater*. 2021;110(1):45–66. https://doi.org/10.1002/jbm.b.34904.
Tiskaya M, Shahid S, Gillam D, Hill R. The use of bioactive glass (BAG) in dental composites: a critical review. *Dent Mater*. 2021;37(2):296–310.

Calcium Hydroxide

Fava LG, Saunders WP. Calcium hydroxide pastes: classification and clinical indications. *Int Endod J*. 1999;32(4):257–282. https://doi.org/10.1046/j.1365-2591.1999.00232.x.
Freire IR, Pessan JP, Amaral JG, Martinhon CC, Cunha RF, Delbem AC. Anticaries effect of low-fluoride dentifrices with phosphates in children: a randomized, controlled trial. *J Dent*. 2016;50:37–42. https://doi.org/10.1016/j.jdent.2016.04.013.
Philip N. State of the art enamel remineralization systems: the next frontier in caries management. *Caries Res*. 2018;53(3):284–295. https://doi.org/10.1159/000493031.
Sangwan P, Sangwan A, Duhan J, Rohilla A. Tertiary dentinogenesis with calcium hydroxide: a review of proposed mechanisms. *Int Endod J*. 2013;46(1):3–19. doi: 10.1111/j.1365-2591.2012.02101.x.
Siqueira JF, Lopes HP. Mechanisms of antimicrobial activity of calcium hydroxide: a critical review. *Int Endod J*. 1999;32(5):361–369. https://doi.org/10.1046/j.1365-2591.1999.00275.x.
Weiner R. Liners and bases in general dentistry. *Aust Dent J*. 2011;56:11–22. https://doi.org/10.1111/j.1834-7819.2010.01292.x.

Tricalcium Silicate Cements

da Rosa WO, Cocco AR, da Silva TM, et al. Current trends and future perspectives of dental pulp capping materials: a systematic review. *J Biomed Mater Res B Appl Biomater*. 2017;106(3):1358–1368. https://doi.org/10.1002/jbm.b.33934.
Davaie S, Hooshmand T, Ansarifard S. Different types of bioceramics as dental pulp capping materials: a systematic review. *Ceram Int*. 2021;47(15):20781–20792. https://doi.org/10.1016/j.ceramint.2021.04.193.
Didilescu AC, Cristache CM, Andrei M, Voicu G, Perlea P. The effect of dental pulp-capping materials on hard-tissue barrier formation. *J Am Dent Assoc*. 2018;149(10):903–917.e4. https://doi.org/10.1016/j.adaj.2018.06.003.
Wang Z. Bioceramic materials in endodontics. *Endod Topics*. 2015;32(1):3–30. https://doi.org/10.1111/etp.12075.

Pit and Fissure Sealants

Ahovuo-Saloranta A, Forss H, Walsh T, Nordblad A, Mäkelä M, Worthington, HV. Pit and fissure sealants for preventing dental decay in permanent teeth. Cochrane Oral Health Group. *Cochrane Database Syst Rev*. 2017;7(7):CD001830. https://doi.org/10.1002/14651858.CD001830.pub5.
Alirezaei M, Bagherian A, Shirazi AS. Glass ionomer cements as fissure sealing materials: yes or no? A systematic review and meta-analysis. *JADA*. 2018;149(7):640–649.
Arenholt-Bindslev D, Breinholt V, Preiss A, et al. Time-related bisphenol-A content and estrogenic activity in saliva samples collected in relation to placement of fissure sealants. *Clin Oral Investig*. 1999;3:120–125.
Boksman L, Carson B. Two-year retention and caries rates of UltraSeal XT and FluoroShield light-cured pit and fissure sealants. *Gen Dent*. 1998;46:184.
De Amorim RG, Leal SC, Frencken JE. Survival of atraumatic restorative treatment (ART) sealants and restorations: a meta-analysis. *Clin Oral Investig*. 2012;16:429.
Erdemir U, Sancakli HS, Yaman BC, Ozel S, Yucel T, Yildiz E. Clinical comparison of a flowable composite and fissure sealant: a 24-month split-mouth, randomized, and controlled study. *J Dent*. 2014;42(2):149.
Feigal RJ, Quelhas I. Clinical trial of a self-etching adhesive for sealant application: success at 24 months with Prompt-L-Pop. *Am J Dent*. 2003;16:249.
Folke BD, Walton JL, Feigal RJ. Occlusal sealant success over ten years in a private practice: comparing longevity of sealants placed by dentists, hygienists and assistants. *Pediatr Dent*. 2004;26:426.
Fortin D, Vargas MA. The spectrum of composites: new techniques and materials. *J Am Dent Assoc*. 2000;131:26S.
Frencken JE, Leal SC, Navarro MF. Twenty-five year atraumatic restorative treatment (ART) approach: a comprehensive overview. *Clin Oral Investig*. 2012;16:1337.

Gungor HC, Altay N, Alpar R. Clinical evaluation of a polyacid-modified resin composite-based fissure sealant: two year results. *Oper Dent.* 2004;29:254.

Gwinnett AJ. The bonding of sealants to enamel. *J Am Soc Prevent Dent.* 1973;3:21.

Hannig M, Grafe A, Atalay S, et al. Microleakage and SEM evaluation of fissure sealants placed by use of self-etching priming agents. *J Dent.* 2004;32:75.

Hatrick CD, Eakle WS, Bird WF. *Dental Materials: Clinical Applications for Dental Assistants and Dental Hygienists.* 2nd ed. Saunders; 2011.

Hori M, Yoshida E, Hashimoto M, et al. In vitro testing of all-in-one adhesives as sealants. *Am J Dent.* 2004;17:177.

Manabe A, Kaneko S, Numazawa S, et al. Detection of Bisphenol-A in dental materials by gas chromatography-mass spectrometry. *Dent Mater.* 2000;19:75.

Myers CL, Rossi F, Cartz F. Adhesive taglike extensions into acid-etched tooth enamel. *J Dent Res.* 1974;53:435.

O'Brien WJ, Fan PL, Apostolidis A. Penetrativity of sealants and glazes. *Oper Dent.* 1978;3:51.

Pahlavan A, Dennison JB, Charbeneau GT. Penetration of restorative resins into acid-etched human enamel. *J Am Dent Assoc.* 1976;93:1170.

Pardi V, Pereira AC, Mialhe FL, et al. Six-year clinical evaluation of polyacid-modified composite resin used as fissure sealant. *J Clin Pediatr Dent.* 2004;28:257.

Pereira AC, Pardi V, Mialhe FL, et al. A 3-year clinical evaluation of glass ionomer cements used as fissure sealants. *Am J Dent.* 2003;16:23.

Tarumi H, Imazato S, Narimatsu M, et al. Estrogenicity of fissure sealants and adhesive resins determined by reporter gene assay. *J Dent Res.* 1838;79:2000.

Taylor CL, Gwinnett AJ. A study of the penetration of sealants into pits and fissures. *J Am Dent Assoc.* 1973;87:1181.

Unterbrink GL, Liebenberg WH. Flowable resin composites as "filled adhesives": literature review and clinical recommendations. *Quint Int.* 1999;30:249.

Resin Infiltration

Domejean S, Ducamp R, Leger S, Homgren C. Resin infiltration of non-cavitated caries lesions: a systematic review. *Med Princ Pract.* 2015;24(3):216–221.

Kentovitz KR, Pascon FM, Nobre-dos-Santos M, Puppin-Rontani RM. Review the effects of infiltrants and sealers on non-cavitated enamel lesions. *Oral Health Prev Dent.* 2010;8:295–305.

Martignon S, Ekstrand KR, Gomez J, et al. Infiltrating/sealing proximal caries lesions: a 3-year randomized clinical trial. *J dent Res.* 2012;91(3):288–292.

Meyer-Lueckel H, Bitter K, Paris S. Randomized controlled clinical trial on proximal caries infiltration: three-year follow up. *Caries Res.* 2012;46(6):544–548.

Meyer-Lueckel H, Paris S. Improved resin infiltration of natural caries lesions. *J Dent Der.* 2008;87:1112–1116.

Paris S, Hopfenmuller W, Meyer-Lueckel H. Resin infiltration of caries lesions: an efficacy randomized trial. *J Dent Res.* 2010;89:823–826.

Paris S, Meyer-Lueckel H. Masking labial enamel white spot lesions by resin infiltration: aclinical report. *Quintessence Int.* 2009;40(9):713–718.

Soveral M, Machado V, Botelho J, et al. Effect of resin infiltration on enamel: a systematic review and meta-analysis. *J Funct Biomater.* 2021;12(3):1–16.

7

Principles of Adhesion and Adhesive Systems

CARMEM PFEIFER

CHAPTER OUTLINE

It can be argued that the ability to bond to enamel and dentin has revolutionized the field of aesthetic dentistry. Tooth-colored resin-based direct and indirect composites, metal-ceramic and all-ceramic dental prostheses (e.g., inlays, onlays, veneers, crowns, and bridges), endodontic posts, and resin cores must all be bonded to the remaining tooth structure to function adequately. Advancements in dental adhesive materials have facilitated the growth of conservative dentistry, strengthening and supporting the remaining tooth structure without the need to remove healthy tooth tissue. The creation of a strong, durable, and bonded interface with enamel or dentin provides important benefits. It significantly protects the restoration's interface against the penetration of bacteria that may cause secondary caries. It reduces the need for retentive areas in the preparation that would require the removal of sound tooth structure. In some cases, bonding may help strengthen the remaining tooth structure. The development of adhesive luting techniques also broadened the application of materials such as low-strength ceramics and indirect composites for crowns, inlays, and onlays as they reduce the risk of crack propagation within the bulk of the restoration, which ultimately may lead to its catastrophic failure.

This chapter presents the basic aspects of the application of adhesion science to dentistry and describes the composition, properties, and indications for use of various types of adhesives. Their fundamental technologies and chemistries will be detailed and related to the requirements for different clinical situations. Finally, the most current evidence on clinical outcomes will be presented to help guide the selection of the most appropriate materials for each situation.

Principles of Adhesion

The term *adhesion* refers to the establishment of molecular interactions between a substrate (*adherend*) and an adhesive brought into close contact, creating an adhesive joint (Fig. 7.1). In contrast, *cohesion* is used to describe the interaction of similar atoms and molecules within a material, involving primary (i.e., covalent or ionic) or strong secondary forces (i.e., hydrogen bonding).

There are certain aspects and characteristics of the adherend and adhesive that need to be considered, as they significantly affect outcomes. The wetting of the substrate by the adhesive depends on the contact angle formed when the two interact, which in turn depends on their hydrophobic/hydrophilic characteristics, as well as surface energies. In other words, how well an adhesive spreads on the substrate depends on its composition and physical state. The most basic aspect to be observed in creating any adhesive joint is the cleanliness of the substrate. Saliva, biofilm, and other organic debris are always present on the tooth surface, and the walls of a cavity preparation are covered with a smear layer. All of these contaminants reduce the surface energy of the bonding substrate and, consequently, its wettability. Therefore it is very important for the surface that will contact the adhesive to be thoroughly clean and, in some cases, for the smear layer to be removed by acid etching. Indirect restorations also need to have their internal surface cleaned and free from films that may impede the penetration of the adhesive.

Wettability is the result of molecular interactions between the adhesive and the substrate, as well as the cohesion forces of the adhesive, particularly its surface tension. Liquids tend to form spheres when placed on a surface because that is the shape with the lowest surface area and therefore the minimum surface energy (Fig. 7.2). Wetting is usually evaluated by the contact angle (θ), that is, the internal angle between the liquid and the substrate. Generally, small contact angles are achieved when a low surface tension liquid is placed on a high-energy surface substrate. Contact angles less than 90 degrees indicate a favorable wetting of the surface. Ideal wetting occurs when the liquid spreads over the surface with $\theta \approx 0$ degrees. Surface roughness increases the wettability of the surface by liquids.

Viscosity influences the contact of the adhesive with the substrate. It should be low enough to allow the adhesive to flow readily and penetrate into the details of the substrate surface without leaving porosities at the interface. Finally, the adhesive must harden sufficiently to create strong interlocks with the substrate microstructure to achieve micromechanical retention. The ideal conditions for bonding are summarized below:

- High-energy surface—clean
- Adherend with high surface energy—wetting
- Adhesive with low surface tension—flows
- Adhesive with low viscosity—flows
- Adhesive with low dimensional change

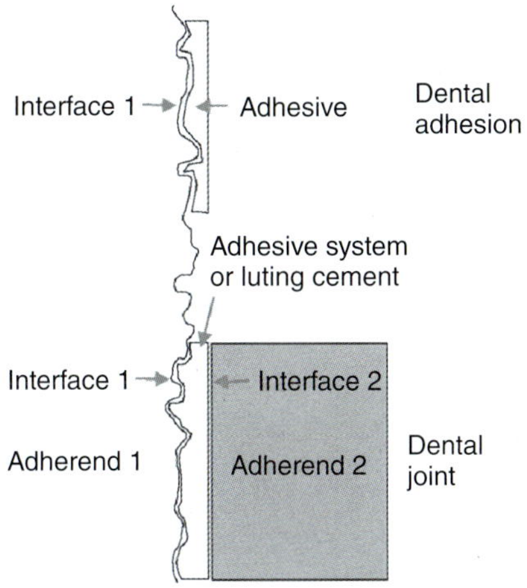

• **Fig. 7.1** Definitions of the terminology associated with adhesive systems (adhesives, adherents, or substrates, and interfaces). Most dental joints involve at least one adhesive, two substrates, and two interfaces.

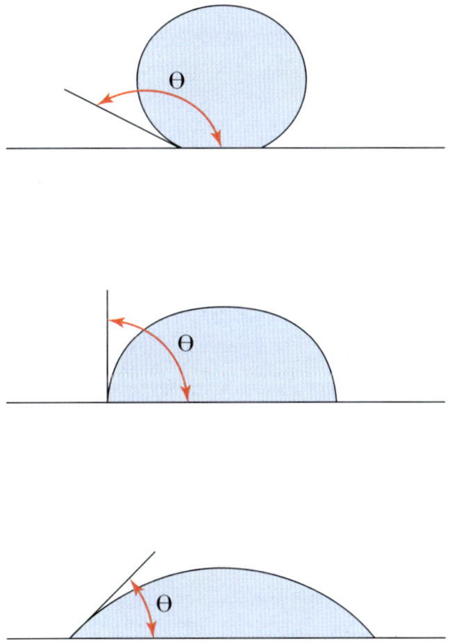

• **Fig. 7.2** Relation of contact angle to the spreading or wetting of a liquid on a solid.

Types of Adhesion

There are basically two types of adhesion in dentistry: true chemical adhesion and micromechanical interlocking. Chemical adhesion entails the formation of true ionic or covalent bonds between the adhesive and the tooth substrate, and these are very difficult to achieve because of the complex composition of substrates such as dentin, the presence of contaminants, and the presence of water. Zinc polycarboxylate, glass ionomer, resin-modified glass ionomer, calcium aluminate/glass ionomer, and self-adhesive resin cements are examples of dental materials capable of establishing chemical interaction with hydroxyapatite. However, in daily practice, adhesion is most often accomplished by micromechanical interlocking between the adhesive and the substrate. This interlocking is created through roughening the surface of the substrate by acid etching and/or by use of abrasion (with burs or specialized compressed air jets loaded with particles). It is important to point out that when two materials are in close contact, physical bonding is always present (e.g., van der Waals dipoles); however, it is weak, especially in a wet environment, and does not really contribute significantly to the integrity of the adhesive joint.

A dental sealant attached to enamel is an example of a simple adhesive joint with one interface. Often, however, adhesive joints involve more than one interface (e.g., tooth/adhesive and adhesive/restorative or luting material), which presents an extra challenge because an adhesive does not necessarily bond equally well to different substrates.

Adhesive Systems

Classification and Basic Components

Adhesive systems rely on different approaches to obtain a strong and durable bond to dentin and enamel. There are basically three main components in adhesive systems: one etching system, one priming system, and one bonding system. Adhesives are then classified according to the etching strategy as *etch-and-rinse* or *self-etch*. Additionally, *universal systems* (or *multimode systems*) can be applied following either etching approach. Etch-and-rinse (also referred to as *total-etch*) systems can be presented as three-step systems (fourth generation), that is, etching, priming, and bonding in separate application steps. Alternatively, two-step systems present primer and bonding resin mixed in a single component (fifth generation). Self-etch adhesives are also available as two- (sixth generation) or single-step systems. The latter can be subclassified into conventional seventh-generation adhesives and universal adhesives, as will be explained later. A summary of the different generations of adhesives is shown in Fig. 7.3. As for the basic composition of each component:

A. Etching uses 30% to 40% phosphoric acid gels to demineralize the tooth structure. Originally, etching solutions were free-flowing liquids and were difficult to control during placement. Gel etchants were developed by adding small amounts of microfillers or cellulose-thickening agents. These gels flow under slight pressure but not under their own weight.
B. Primers are hydrophilic monomers, oligomers, or polymers, usually carried in a solvent. The solvents used in primers are acetone, ethanol-water, or primarily water. In some primers, the solvent levels can be as high as 90%. Therefore primers have different evaporation rates, drying patterns, and penetration characteristics, all of which can influence the resulting bond strength. Dimethacrylate oligomers and lower-molecular-weight monomers can be added to the primer in two-step etch-and-rinse systems or presented as a separate step in three-step systems or in self-etch two-step systems.
Self-etch systems contain ester monomers with grafted carboxylic or phosphate acid groups dissolved in water. According to their aggressiveness, these systems can be characterized as *strong* (pH of 1 or less), *moderate* (pH between 1 and 2), or *mild* (pH of 2 or greater). They can be presented as two-step systems, with a hydrophobic bonding resin in a separate bottle (also known as *self-etching primers*) or single-component systems (*all-in-one* systems). Several different monomers can be used, but the most commonly used self-etching monomer used in commercial formulations is 10-methacryloyloxydecyl dihydrogen phosphate (MDP) (10-MDP, Fig. 7.4). As with any phosphate-bearing molecule, these monomers can chelate the mineral content in enamel and dentin and, analogous to what is observed with glass ionomers, form a true covalent bond with the tooth substrate (Fig. 7.4).

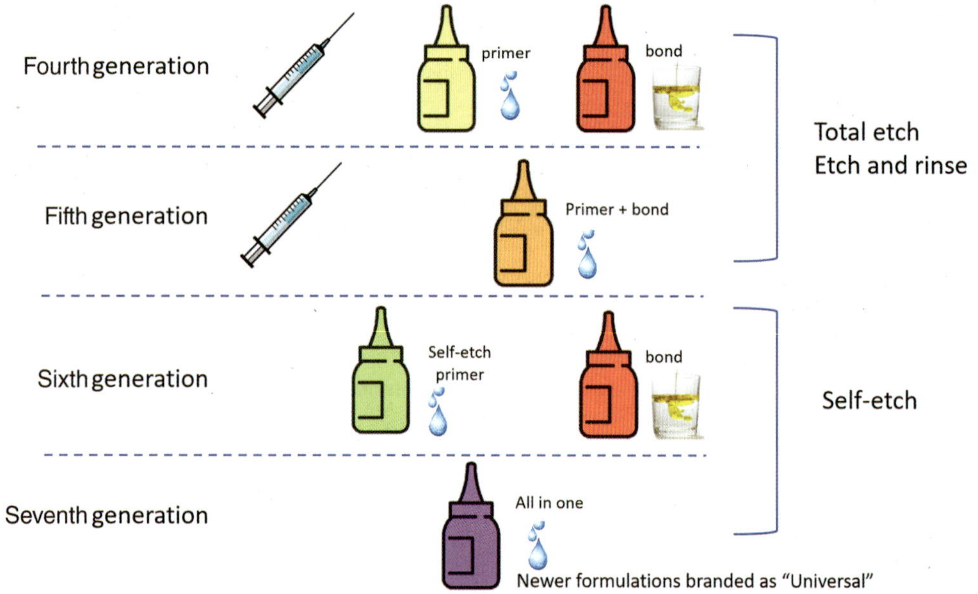

• **Fig. 7.3** Different types of adhesives currently available on the market. Each adhesive type requires a different number and/or type of application steps. Fourth- and fifth-generation adhesives are classified as total-etch (or etch and rinse), and sixth- and seventh-generation adhesives are classified as self-etch. The water or oil droplets represent the hydrophilic and hydrophobic nature of each component, respectively.

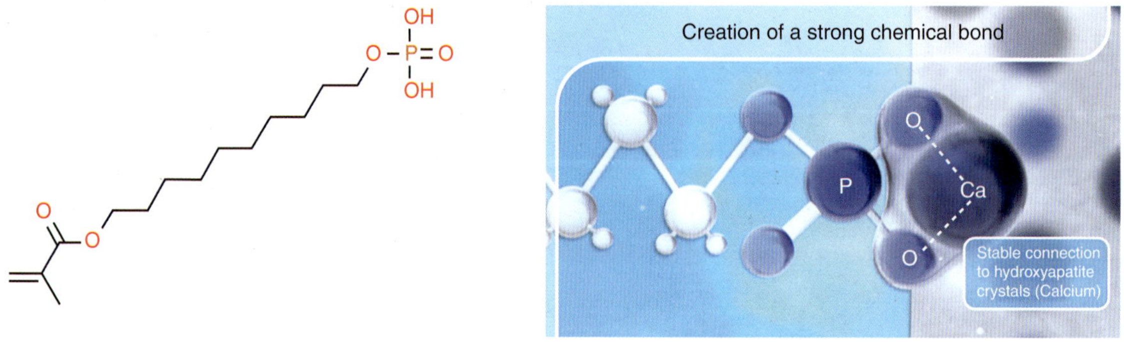

• **Fig. 7.4** Molecular structure of 10-MDP and schematic representation of its chemical interaction with the mineral content (hydroxyapatite) on the tooth substrate.

Universal systems are so called because they can be used following either an etch-and-rinse, two-step technique, or a self-etch (one-step) approach, depending on the practitioner's preference (Fig. 7.5). When used as self-etch systems, universal adhesives can be classified as mild based on the micromorphology of the bonded interface. These versatile systems were developed to be used with other bonding substrates and contain components such as silanes and acidic monomers to also mediate bonding to ceramics and metals.

C. Most bonding agents are light-cured and contain an activator such as camphorquinone and an organic amine. Dual-cured bonding agents include a catalyst to promote self-curing. Although most bonding agents are unfilled, some products contain nanofillers and submicron glasses ranging from 0.5% to 40% by weight. Fillers are described in more detail in Chapter 8. Filled bonding agents may be easier to place on the tooth and may produce higher in vitro bond strengths. Bonding agents may contain fluoride, antimicrobial ingredients, or desensitizers, such as glutaraldehyde. The true clinical effectiveness of fluoride and antimicrobial release from a bonding agent has not been demonstrated.

The sheer number of available commercial products can make adhesive selection in clinical practice a daunting experience. As the systems evolved, especially in the past two decades, a trend can be identified for "simplified," faster-to-apply adhesive systems with fewer than two application steps. Table 7.1 summarizes the application steps and times for each of those classes of adhesives. The advantages and disadvantages of each generation of adhesive will be discussed later in the chapter.

It can be argued that the greater the number of application steps, the greater the risk for operator error to be introduced. The bonding procedure is intrinsically technique-sensitive, and the risks being referred to include under- or overetching enamel and/or dentin, under- or overdrying dentin, insufficient removal of solvent from primer/adhesive, residual acidity in the hybrid layer (and consequent incompatibility with self- or dual-cured resin cements), hybrid layer permeability (overly hydrophilic adhesives), and inadequate light curing. Each of these aspects will be discussed below as they pertain to enamel and dentin bonding substrates—a summary is provided in Table 7.2.

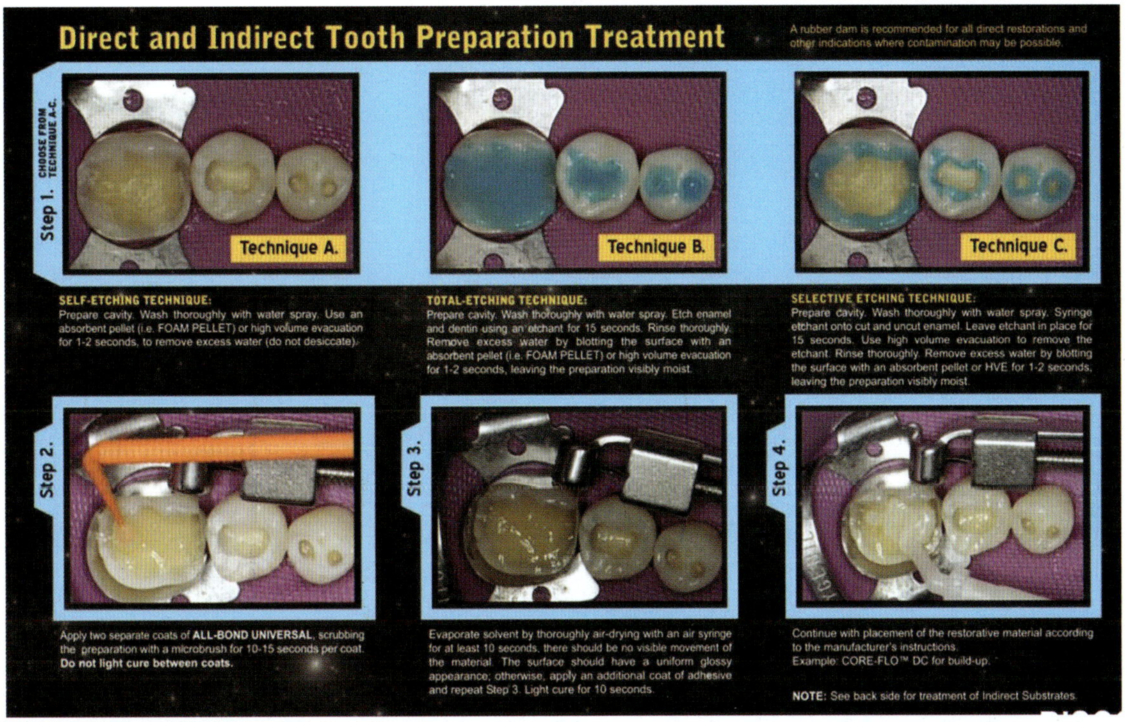

• **Fig. 7.5** Different possible etching techniques for use with universal adhesives. In technique A, no prior etching is done, and the universal adhesive is applied to the cavity preparation in one step. In technique B, etching is performed in both dentin and enamel—this may be used in cases where sclerotic dentin is present. In technique C, selective etching of enamel is performed to ensure adequate bonding to that substrate.

TABLE 7.1 Different Steps for Each Type of Adhesive System Currently Available. The Last Row Provides an Estimate Time of Length of Application for Each of Them

Step	Fourth-generation, etch-and-rinse, three steps	Fifth-generation, etch-and-rinse, two steps	Sixth-generation, self-etch, two steps	Seventh-generation and universal, self-etch, one step
1	PA etch	PA etch	–	–
2	Rinse and dry (dentin left moist)	Rinse and dry (dentin left moist)	–	–
3	Apply hydrophilic primer	Apply hydrophilic primer/adhesive	Apply acidic primer	Apply acidic primer/adhesive
4	Dry gentle air	Dry gentle air	Dry gentle air	Dry gentle air
5	Apply adhesive and brush thin	–	Apply adhesive and brush thin	
6	Light-cure	Light-cure	Light-cure	Light-cure
time	75–80 s	70–75 s	70–75 s	40–45 s

Bonding Substrates

Enamel Bonding

Bonding to enamel occurs by micromechanical retention after acid etching is used to preferentially dissolve hydroxyapatite crystals in the enamel outer surface (Fig. 7.6). Fluid adhesive constituents penetrate into the newly produced surface irregularities and become locked into place after polymerization.

Gel etchants (typically phosphoric acid) are dispensed from a syringe onto tooth surfaces. Etching times for enamel vary depending on the type and quality of enamel. Generally, a 15-second etch with 30% to 40% phosphoric acid is sufficient to reach the characteristic clinical endpoint of a frosty enamel appearance. Deciduous unground enamel generally contains some aprismatic enamel that has not yet worn away and requires longer etching times (20 to 30 seconds) to create a retentive pattern. Enamel may have been rendered more insoluble as a result of fluorosis, and in such cases, extended etching times (15 to 30 seconds) are required to ensure that sufficient micromechanical bonding can occur. The only caution is that dentin should not be etched for the same extended time because fluorotic dentin is more susceptible to acid than regular dentin, and extensive dentin demineralization should be avoided. There really is no risk of overetching enamel, as the peaks and valleys created during dissolution would still form with longer etching times (Table 7.2). The etching procedure can be seen in the companion video online.

After the intended etching time, the acid gel is rinsed away, and the tooth structure is dried to receive the bonding resin. If a hydrophilic primer or a two-step etch-and-rinse system is used, the surface can be left moist for the next stage of bonding. Then, primer can be flowed onto the surface to penetrate into the available surface irregularities. After curing, primer and adhesive

TABLE 7.2 **Potential Pitfalls That May Arise During the Application of Modern Adhesive Systems. Generations Fourth to Seventh Are Divided in Etch and Rinse (E&R) or Self-etching (SE). The X Marks the Type of Adhesive for Which Each of the Pitfalls Is More Likely to Be Observed**

Potential Pitfalls With Modern Adhesives X = More Critical	Gen 4 E&R - 3	Gen 5 E&R - 2	Gen 6 SE - 2	Gen 7 SE - 1
Under Etch Enamel			X	X
Over Etch Enamel				
Under Etch Dentin			X	X
Over Etch Dentin	X	X		
Dentin Wetness/Dryness	X	X		
Solvent Removal		X		X
Overthinning Adhesive	X	X	X	X
Residual Acidity in Hybrid Layer		X		X
Semipermeable Hybrid Layer		X		X
Inadequate Light Curing	X	X	X	X

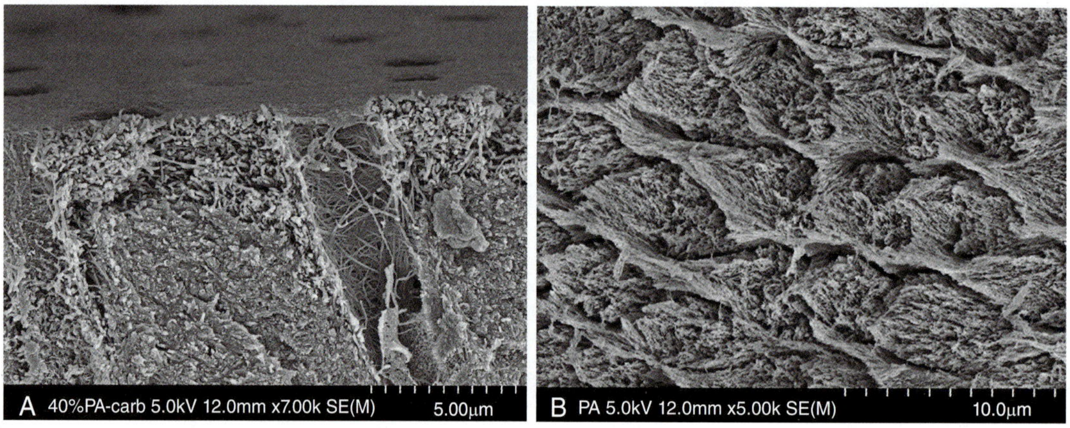

• **Fig. 7.6** Scanning electron micrograph (SEM) of etched enamel and dentin. (A) Field emission SEM of dentin etched with 40% phosphoric acid for 15 seconds. Note the collagen fibers deprived of hydroxyapatite crystals as a result of acid demineralization. The more intense decalcification around the peritubular area may be a result of both the high mineral content of the peritubular region and the easier penetration of the acid through the tubular lumen. (B) Enamel etched with 38% phosphoric acid for 15 seconds. (From Perdigão J. New developments in dental adhesion. *Dent Clin N Am*. 2007;51(2):333–357, viii).

produce resin *macrotags* by penetrating the space surrounding the enamel prisms. Microtags form where adhesive flows into the etched prisms involving individual hydroxyapatite crystals. Microtags are much more numerous and contribute to most of the micromechanical retention.

Strong self-etch adhesives produce a similar pattern on enamel as that obtained with phosphoric acid. Mild self-etch systems present lower bond strength to enamel compared to etch-and-rinse systems, probably because of a shallower etching pattern. In those cases, selective etching of the enamel can be performed using 30% to 40% phosphoric acid gel. This should be carefully applied to enamel only, after which the application of the self-etch adhesive can follow the usual manufacturer-recommended steps (Fig. 7.5, Technique C).

Dentin Bonding

The high water content in dentin represents an extra challenge for the establishment of an interdiffusion zone. To manage this problem, primers have hydrophilic components, such as 2-hydroxyethyl methacrylate (HEMA), that wet dentin and penetrate its structure. In etch-and-rinse systems, etching with phosphoric acid removes the mineral content, unclogging and widening the dentin tubules, as well as exposing the collagen network. Once the hydroxyapatite component of the outer layer of dentin is removed, the remaining dentin contains about 50% unfilled space and about 20% water. After the acid is rinsed off, drying of dentin must be done cautiously. Even a short air blast from an air-water spray can inadvertently dehydrate the outer surface and cause the remaining collagen scaffold to collapse onto itself. Once this happens, the collagen mesh readily excludes the penetration of primer, and bonding will fail. In other words, the risk of overdrying dentin cannot be understated. However, excess moisture tends to dilute the primer and interfere with resin interpenetration, so the operator also must be careful to avoid "pooling" of excess water on the line angles of the cavity preparation. The ideal dentin moisture level varies according to the solvent present in the adhesive, but in general, the appearance of properly moist dentin is of a "glistening surface." One advantage of self-etch systems is the elimination of this rather subjective step of the bonding procedure (Table 7.2).

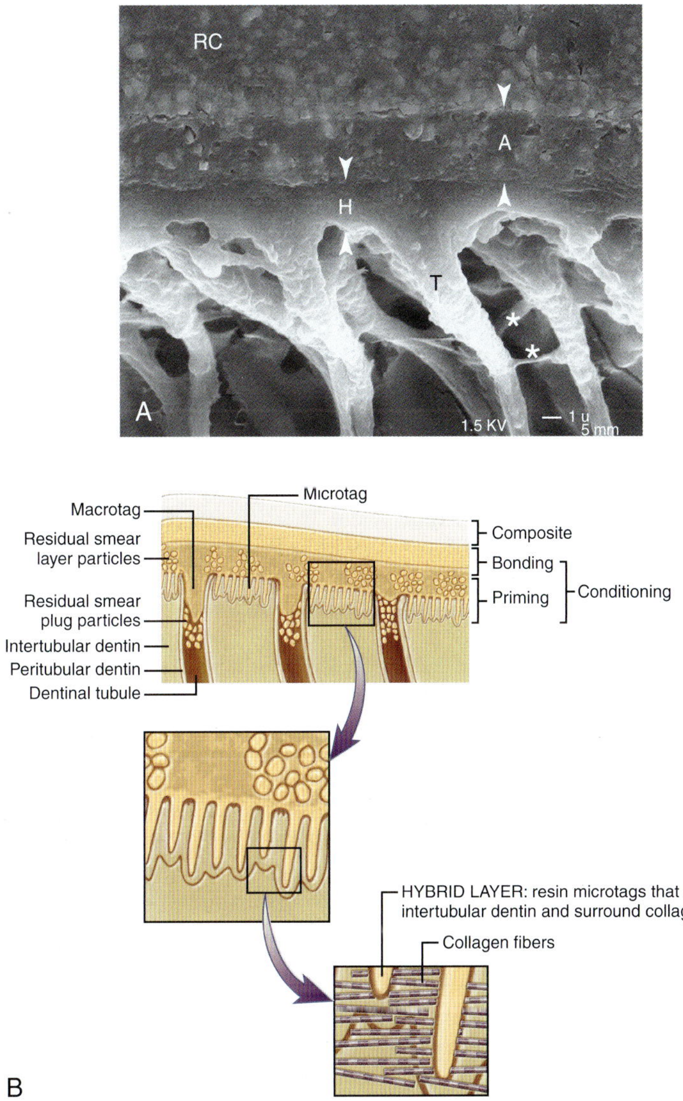

• **Fig. 7.7** Adhesion to dentin. (A) Scanning electron micrograph (SEM) of interface bonded with a dental adhesive (final magnification: × 4000). Note the visible thickness of the adhesive layer *(A, arrowheads)* beneath the resin composite (RC). The hybrid layer *(H, arrowheads)* is 2 μm thick. The tubular resin tags *(T)* show lateral branches *(asterisks).* (B) Schematic showing that etching removes hydroxyapatite crystals within intertubular dentin and along peritubular dentin. Primer penetrates intertubular spaces and fluid-filled tubular spaces. Cured primer forms microtags within intertubular dentin and macrotags within tubules. A, (From Frankenberger R, Perdigão J, Rosa BT, et al. "No-bottle" vs "multi-bottle" dentin adhesives—a microtensile bond strength and morphological study. *Dent Mater*. 2001;17(5):373–380).

The infiltration of resin within the collagen scaffold is termed *hybridization* (Fig. 7.7). The result of this diffusion process is called the *resin-interpenetration zone* or *resin-interdiffusion zone*, or simply *hybrid layer.* Concurrent with hybrid layer formation is the penetration of primer into the fluid-filled dentinal tubules. This may generate long resin tags, though these appear to be of little value to overall bonding because this resin is generally undercured and behaves as soft, flexible tags. During application of the primer, most of the solvent evaporates quickly. Thus several layers usually must be applied to ensure a complete impregnation. The rule of thumb is that one should apply as many layers as are necessary to produce a persistent glistening appearance on dentin. If dentin becomes dehydrated before priming and bonding, the collagen fibers collapse and hinder penetration of the primer into the collagen network layer. If the dentin is overly wet, the solvents contained in the primers are not able to displace the water and carry the monomers into the microporosities within the collagen network. In addition, if the dentin is etched for too long (this only applies to etch-and-rinse systems), there is a chance that the thickness of the demineralized band is too great for the adhesive to completely penetrate—this is particularly concerning for fifth-generation adhesives, which combine primer and bond in the same step and tend to be more viscous. If this happens, underneath the hybridized layer, there will be a band of demineralized dentin that is weakened by the absence of polymerized primer/adhesive. The thickness of a hybrid layer itself is not a critical requirement for success. Dentin bond strength is probably proportional to the interlocking between resin and collagen, as well as to the "quality" of the hybrid layer, but not to its thickness. Effective etching of dentin does not require long times to produce acceptable dentin bond strengths, and usually 15 seconds is employed.

After priming the surface, an adhesive is applied and light-cured. Surfaces of the cured bonding agents are initially air-inhibited and do not immediately react. However, as the composite is placed against the surface, much of the air is displaced, and copolymerization occurs.

Self-etch systems have the great advantages of eliminating the risk of incomplete primer/adhesive penetration into the collagen scaffold and also eliminating the subjectivity when determining the ideal amount of moisture on the dentin surface for primer diffusion. With these systems, the smear layer is dissolved and incorporated into the hybrid layer. The bonding mechanism for strong self-etch adhesives is very similar to that of etch-and-rinse systems. Their bond strength, particularly for all-in-one systems, is relatively low, probably because of their high initial acidity and high water content. Mild self-etch systems demineralize dentin only superficially (a few micrometers) and leave residual hydroxyapatite attached to collagen fibrils. Although the main bonding mechanism is the interlocking between collagen fibrils and the polymerized resin, monomers such as 4-methacryloxyethyl trimellitic anhydride (4-META) and 10-MDP may bond chemically to this residual hydroxyapatite, as already mentioned. In addition, the presence of hydroxyapatite may, in the future, help protect the collagen against degradation that weakens the bonded interface. Mild self-etch systems may present relatively low bond strength values when applied to sclerotic dentin or enamel, hence the recommendation for selective etching of the enamel with phosphoric acid in certain cases, as already pointed out.

Another draw back associated with all-in-one systems is that, due to their high water content, the polymers formed from these adhesives behave as semipermeable membranes, which increases degradation by hydrolysis. This is also true for fifth-generation adhesives, whose application does not include a standalone adhesive component. This may lead to accelerated degradation of the hybrid layer by water seepage, in a phenomenon sometimes referred to as "water-tree formation." Conversely, in fourth- and sixth-generation adhesives, where the bond step is separate from the primer, the last layer of the adhesive system is always highly hydrophobic and provides a barrier that prevents/reduces the contact of dentinal fluid with the overlaying composite restoration. It also must be noted that the acidity of some fifth- and seventh-generation adhesives may interfere with the redox polymerization of self-cure and dual-cure resin cements, making it prudent to use adhesive systems and cements from the same manufacturer during luting procedures.

Universal Bonding

Universal adhesives have been more recently designed by manufacturers as an evolution in relation to the first few formulations of all-in-one adhesives. As the name implies, these are meant to be a single-component adhesive system, which can be used for bonding to all surfaces relevant to restorative dentistry. The main difference between the early iterations and the more recent universal adhesives is the incorporation of silanes, other copolymers (in some brands), and the addition of 10-MDP as the phosphate-containing monomer. Silanes are added to provide bonding to silica-based ceramic restorations; however, the use of zirconia primers (see "Bonding to other substrates") is advisable for zirconia-based restorations. One commonly used commercial product uses a proprietary methacrylate-functionalized polycarboxylic acid copolymer (also used in some popular resin-modified glass ionomers, see Chapter 6) in the formulation to provide consistent adhesive strength under the varying humidity conditions often encountered in clinical situations. Like the other types of adhesives, these materials also contain common monomers such as bisphenol A-glycidyl methacrylate (Bis-GMA), urethane dimethacrylate (UDMA), and HEMA to control the hydrophilic-hydrophobic balance. Photoinitiators and stabilizers are used as with other materials. Water and alcohol are used as carrier solvents.

Ideally a universal adhesive should be a single-bottle, no-mix adhesive that can be used reliably in total-etch, self-etch, and selective-etch (i.e., phosphoric etch of enamel only) modes according to the clinicians' needs for all direct and indirect restorations. Thus it should bond to tooth surfaces (enamel and dentin), direct restoratives (methacrylate resin-based and glass ionomer or resin-modified glass ionomer), and indirect restoratives (e.g., metals, glass-ceramics, and high-strength zirconia without the need for an extra primer step). Furthermore, it should be compatible with self-cure, light-cure, and dual-cure resin-based cements. Care should be taken in the choice and use of such adhesives because, in actuality, many commercial universal adhesives still require an additional component or step. Thus certain products require a separate "activator" to be used for self-cure or dual-cure resin cements. Others may need two components to be mixed prior to use, whereas for some sequential application of two separate components is essential.

The key to the successful performance of a universal adhesive is to have the right hydrophilic-hydrophobic balance in the formulation. Hydrophilicity is needed to properly wet the dentin while hydrophobicity is essential after polymerization of the adhesive to minimize hydrolysis and water absorption with time. The adhesive should have adequate acidity to be effective in etching all substrates yet not be so acidic that it deactivates the initiators needed for the polymerization of self-cured and dual-cured cements. The best performance is seen for such adhesives when they are in the pH range of 2.2 to 3.2. Optimal cohesive strength is also necessary to withstand the stresses due to polymerization shrinkage of resin restoratives.

Biocompatibility

Solvents and monomers in bonding agents are typically skin irritants. For example, HEMA may produce local and systemic reactions in dentists and dental assistants sufficient to preclude their further use in the dental office. It is critical that dental personnel protect themselves from recurring exposure. Protective techniques include wearing gloves, immediately replacing contaminated gloves, using high-speed suction, keeping all bottles tightly closed or using unit-dose systems, and disposing of materials in such a way that the monomers cannot evaporate into the office air. Even with double gloves, contact with aggressive solvents and monomers will produce actual skin contact in a few minutes. All reasonable precautions should be followed, and if unwanted contact occurs, affected areas should be flushed immediately with copious amounts of water and soap. Once the materials are polymerized, there is very little risk of side effects. Although patients should be protected during bonding operations, properly polymerized materials have not been shown to be hazardous to the patient.

Clinical Performance

American Dental Association guidelines require adhesives to be tested in restorations for nonretentive class 5 lesions. The lesions, which may be saucer or notch shaped, have enamel along the

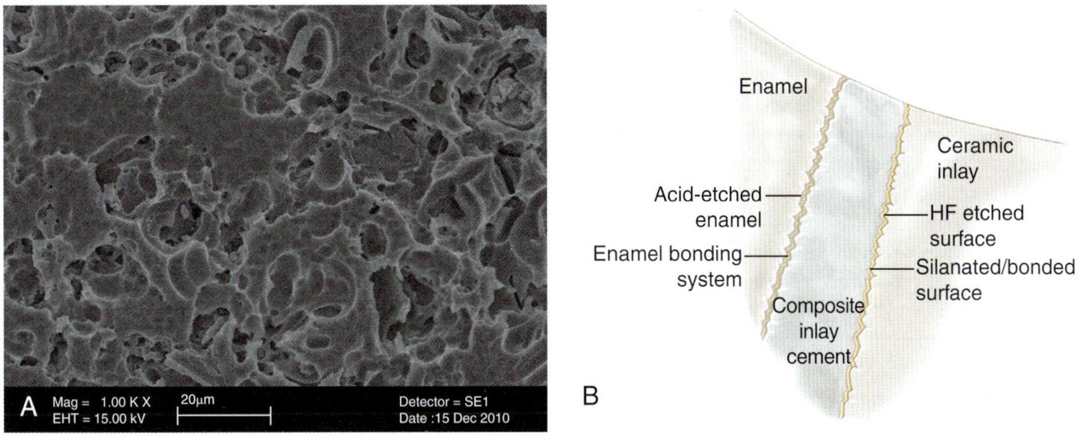

• **Fig. 7.8** Etched porcelain. (A) Scanning electron micrograph (SEM) of etched porcelain. (B) Schematic of materials and interfaces involved in bonding all-ceramic restorations to tooth structure. *HF*, Hydrofluoric acid. A, (From Cesar PF, Yoshimura HN, Miranda Júnior WG, et al. Correlation between fracture toughness and leucite content in dental porcelains. *J Dent*. 2005;33:721–729).

coronal margin and dentin along the apical margin. The success of a bonding agent is evaluated indirectly by examining the performance of the restorations for (1) postoperative sensitivity, (2) interfacial staining, (3) secondary caries, and (4) retention or fracture followed for 18 months. These clinical trials test short-term retention and initial sealing.

Most commercial adhesive systems are successful in clinical trials. However, these clinical trials generally combine enamel and dentin bonding. There is no acceptable clinical regimen for critically testing only dentin bonding in nonretentive preparations. Because clinical trials are usually highly controlled, they are often not predictive of routine clinical use in general practice. Longevity of the bond in general practice may be only 40% of that achieved in clinical trials. While long-term clinical performance is not known for all bonding systems, there are reports of studies of longer than 10 years duration showing excellent results for some two-step self-etch and three-step etch-and-rinse materials.

Sites of failure for most bonded restorations occur along cervical margins where the bonding is primarily to dentin. Studies of bonded composites in class 2 restorations have shown that 95% of all secondary caries associated with the composite restoration are in the interproximal area. These margins are the most difficult to seal during placement of the restoration because they are typically bonded to dentin and cementum rather than enamel and are hard to access with a light guide for adequate polymerization.

Based on the most extensive clinical evidence, the three-step etch-and-rinse systems as a group remain the "gold standard" for adhesive systems in both laboratory and clinical evaluations.

Bonding to Other Substrates

Cast Alloys

Sandblasting with aluminum oxide is the most commonly used method to prepare metal substrates for receiving bonding resins or resin cements. It creates a microretentive, high-energy surface.

Electrolytic etching can be used with base-metal alloys but is not as effective with noble alloys because of its more homogeneous microstructure. Tin plating can be used to improve the retention of noble alloys in resin cements. Commercial systems using silica coating at high temperatures or tribochemical application of a silica layer using aluminum oxide modified by silicic acid have also been available for many years. In both cases, a silane solution is applied to the treated metal to create a surface capable of bonding to dimethacrylate-based resins.

Monomers such as 10-MDP and 4-META are used in formulations of resin cements to improve retention of cast alloy restorations. They seem to be more effective with base-metal alloys compared to noble alloys. Metal primers developed for improving the bond strength between alloy and resin cements are also available. However, research results are inconsistent.

Silica-Based Ceramics

Silica-based ceramics have been successfully bonded to resin cements by etching the restoration's inner surface with a hydrofluoric acid solution, followed by the application of a silane primer (Fig. 7.8). Different acid concentrations are commercially available, from 2.5% to 10%, in liquid or gel forms, and recommended etching times vary from 1 to 4 minutes. Hydrofluoric acid attacks the glass phase of ceramics to the point where crystals are removed, leaving a microretentive honeycomb-like, high-energy surface. Silane application improves the wettability of the resin cement on the ceramic surface and establishes covalent bonds with both the ceramic surface (via siloxane bonds, –Si–O–Si–) and the resin cement (by carbon double bond polymerization). Hydrolysis of the silane molecule is necessary to convert the methoxy groups ($–OCH_3$) to silanol (–Si–OH). Silanes are presented in a nonhydrolyzed form (two bottles) or prehydrolyzed (one bottle).

Zirconia Ceramics

The clinical success of indirect ceramic restorations is highly dependent on the cementation procedure employed. In recent years, there has been an increase in the popularity of zirconia-based prosthetics such as crowns and bridges due to the material's superior mechanical strength, aesthetic properties, versatility of clinical indications, and ability to be used in digital procedures involving computer-aided design/computer-aided manufacturing milling. However, conventional adhesive cementation procedures involving hydrofluoric acid treatment and the application of silane primers do not work for zirconia restorations. This is because zirconia is a polycrystalline material with no amorphous silica glass component, thus making it resistant to acid etching by hydrofluoric acid and also unreactive toward silane primers.

Several strategies have been employed for formulating commercial zirconia primers. The primary approach has been to roughen the bonding surface of the zirconia by sandblasting and then use a specially formulated zirconia primer containing phosphate or phosphonate monomers as the key reactive ingredient. These acidic groups are believed to form a stable Zr–O–P bond with the surface of the zirconia. In addition to the phosphate or phosphonate functionality, these monomers contain a hydrophobic backbone and a methacrylate group that can copolymerize with the adhesive resin cement upon initiation to build up cohesive strength. The most widely used monomer in zirconia primers is 10-MDP. It has also been reported that combining phosphate/dithione and phosphate/carboxyl monomers produces a synergistic effect in bonding. Some manufacturers also incorporate a silane component in addition to the organophosphate monomer in the primer in order to expand their use to both zirconia and porcelain surfaces. However, the shelf stability of the silanes in the acidic environment of these primers has been questioned and refrigerated storage of the primers is indicated. In another approach, laboratory or chair-side air abrasion with 110- and 30-μm silica-coated aluminum particles have been used on the interior surface of the zirconia device to create a siliceous surface followed by the treatment with conventional silane-based primer (tribochemical bonding). This technique has given mixed results.

Bonding glass-infiltrated or densely sintered alumina, as well as yttria-stabilized tetragonal zirconia polycrystalline (Y-TZP) ceramics, remains a subject of debate among clinicians and researchers. Hydrofluoric acid etching is not efficient in highly crystalline ceramics. Therefore other methods, such as airborne particle abrasion with 35 to 110 μm alumina, are indicated to increase surface roughness. Tribochemical coating of Y-TZP surfaces using silica-modified alumina particles followed by silanization is also efficient. Organophosphate monomers such as 10-MDP, present in *primers* developed specifically for zirconia bonding, universal adhesive systems, and self-adhesive resin cements were shown to form stable Zr–O–P bonds on the zirconia surface and improve its bond strength to other substrates, particularly when the surfaces were previously modified by air abrasion with alumina.

Indirect (Laboratory) Composites

A microretentive bonding surface is obtained with alumina sandblasting. Etching with 37% phosphoric acid is used to clean debris from the surface prior to the application of the resin cement. Etching with hydrofluoric acid is not recommended because it causes degradation of the composite surface by etching away the silica glass and leaving a weak and porous polymer matrix.

Amalgam

Adhesive systems, filled adhesives, and resin cements can be used in association with amalgam in the so-called *bonded amalgam* restoration. The purpose of this technique is to reduce the need for macromechanical retention, which would save tooth structure, and reinforce the remaining structure by creating a bonded interface between the restorative material and the cavity walls. The bonding between the adhesive and the amalgam is achieved by the establishment of an interpenetration zone. Although laboratory studies show better results for bonded amalgams compared to conventional, nonbonded amalgam in terms of bond strength, microleakage, and retention, these findings are not supported by clinical data, which show no difference between bonded restorations and those retained by mechanical undercuts.

Fiber Posts

Bonding fiber-reinforced resin posts to dentin is one of the most challenging situations faced by the clinician. Adhesive application is critical because it is virtually impossible to control moisture inside the root canal. The use of self-etching adhesive systems is not indicated because their acidity would impede the chemical activation of the resin cement. The use of self-adhesive resin cements (see later) has shown promising results in laboratory evaluations. The surface treatment of the post has also been debated. Silanization, sandblasting, or the association of both treatments are often quoted as being effective procedures to improve the bonding between the resin cement and the fiber post.

Repair of Composite, Ceramic, and Ceramic-Metal Restorations

Repair of fractured restorations is indicated when the extent of the fracture is not severe enough to warrant the replacement of the restoration or when there are other factors taken into consideration, such as conservation of the tooth structure, cost, time, or in case of fixed prostheses, the replacement of multiple units. For example, when completely replacing a composite restoration, the cavity volume tends to increase by the removal of sound tooth structure, given the difficulty in visualizing the remains of the old material.

Aging of composite restorations in the oral environment severely decreases the composite-to-composite bond strength. Therefore the use of adhesive systems to mediate the bond between the aged and the fresh composite is recommended. The surface can be roughened with the use of an intraoral sandblaster or a diamond bur, followed by phosphoric acid application for cleaning prior to adhesive application. Some clinical studies have also demonstrated the advantages of applying a layer of silane to the surface to be repaired for extra adhesion with the exposed surface of filler particles. The repaired composite only reaches 50% to 80% of the cohesive strength of the original restoration; however, so these patients need to be monitored closely. The great advantage of repair is it increases the longevity of a restoration that would otherwise need to be replaced by about 10% over 10 years, according to a practice-based study.

The repair of chipped ceramic restorations includes conditioning with hydrofluoric acid, silanization, application of a bonding resin, and restoration with a resin composite. Intraoral use of hydrofluoric acid gel must be performed with rubber dam isolation because of its caustic effect on soft tissues.

Repair of metal-ceramic restorations includes bonding to different substrates. When there is a large area of the metal infrastructure exposed, sandblasting with alumina or alumina modified with silicic acid is recommended, followed by the application of silane and adhesive resin, prior to composite application. Fractured porcelain surfaces can be sandblasted and etched with hydrofluoric acid gel prior to silanization, adhesive application, and restoration with composite.

Amalgam restorations can also be repaired with composites. The clinical steps involve removing the affected portion of the amalgam restoration, air-abrading the amalgam surface to be repaired, etching the exposed enamel/dentin, followed by application of adhesive and flowable composite.

Bibliography

Abo-Hamar SE, et al. Effect of temporary cements on the bond strength of ceramic luted to dentin. *Dent Mater*. 2005;21(9):794–803.

Alex G. Universal adhesives: the next evolution in adhesive dentistry? *Compend Cont Educ Dent*. 2015;36(1):15–26.

Amaral M, et al. The potential of novel primers and universal adhesives to bond to zirconia. *J Dent*. 2014;42:90–98.

Berry 3rd EA, Powers JM. Bond strength of glass ionomers to coronal and radicular dentin. *Oper Dent*. 1994;19(4):122–126.

Bertolotti RL. Adhesion to porcelain and metal. *Dent Clin North Am*. 2007;51(2):433–451 , ix–x.

Boeckh C, et al. Antibacterial activity of restorative dental biomaterials in vitro. *Caries Res*. 2002;36(2):101–107.

Braga RR, et al. Adhesion to tooth structure: a critical review of "macro" test methods. Dent Mater. 26(2):e38–e49.

Braga RR, Ferracane JL, Condon JR. Polymerization contraction stress in dual-cure cements and its effect on interfacial integrity of bonded inlays. *J Dent*. 2002;30(7–8):333–340.

Brauer GM. New developments in zinc oxide-eugenol cement. *Ann Dent*. 1967;26(2):44–50.

Bunek SS. Looking back over 30 years—composites and bonding agents. *Dent Advis*. 2014;31(3):2–9.

Bunek SS. Update on adhesion—universal bonding agents and resin cements. *Dent Advis*. 2014;31(7):1.

Cardoso PE, Braga RR, Carrilho MR. Evaluation of micro-tensile, shear and tensile tests determining the bond strength of three adhesive systems. *Dent Mater*. 1998;14(6):394–398.

Casagrande L, Laske M, Bronkhorst EM, Huysmans MCDNJM, Opdam NJM. Repair may increase survival of direct posterior restorations – A practice based study. *J Dent*. 2017;64:30–36. https://doi.org/10.1016/j.jdent.2017.06.002.

Chen C, et al. Bonding of universal adhesives to dentine—old wine in new bottles? *J Dent*. 2015;43:525–536.

Chin MY, et al. Fluoride release and cariostatic potential of orthodontic adhesives with and without daily fluoride rinsing. *Am J Orthod Dentofacial Orthop*. 2009;136(4):547–553.

Christensen G. Ask Dr. Christensen. *Dent Econ*. 2008;98(5). https://www.dentaleconomics.com/practice/practice-management-software/article/16387374/ask-dr-christensen.

Civjan S, Brauer GM. Physical properties of cements, based on zinc oxide, hydrogenated rosin, O-Ethoxybenzoic acid, and eugenol. *J Dent Res*. 1964;43:281–299.

Davidson CL, Mjör IA. Advances in Glass-Ionomer Cements. *Quintessence*;. 1999.

de Melo M, et al. *Braz Oral Res*. 2011;25:485–491.

de Oyague RC, Monticelli F, Toledano M, Osorio E, Ferrari M, Osorio R. Influence of surface treatments and resin cement selection on bonding to densely-sintered zirconium- oxide ceramic. *Dent Mater*. 2009;25(2):172–179.

Di Hipólito V, Figueiredo Rei A, Mitra SB, de Goes MF. Interaction morphology and bond strength of nanofilled simplified-step adhesives to acid etched dentin. *European J Dent*. 2012;6:349–360.

Dias A, et al. *Gen Dent*. 2011;59:e82–e86.

dos Santos JG, et al. Shear bond strength of metal-ceramic repair systems. *J Prosthet Dent*. 2006;96(3):165–173.

Eisenburger M, Addy M, Rossbach A. Acidic solubility of luting cements. *J Dent*. 2003;31(2):137–142.

Farah JW, Powers JM. Self-etching bonding agents. *Dent Advis*. 2010;27(9):1.

Farah JW, Powers JM. Traditional crown and bridge cements. *Dent Advis*. 2006;23(2):1.

Ferracane JL, Stansbury JW. Self-adhesive resin cements—chemistry, properties and clinical considerations. *J Oral Rehabilitation*. 2011;8(4):295–314.

Fonseca RG, et al. Effect of metal primers on bond strength of resin cements to base metals. *J Prosthet Dent*. 2009;101(4):262–268.

Frankenberger R, Perdigão J, Rosa BT, Lopes M. "No-bottle" vs "multi-bottle" dentin adhesives–a microten- sile bond strength and morphological study. *Dent Mater*. 2001;17(5):373–380.

Fujisawa S, Kadoma Y. Effect of phenolic compounds on the polymerization of methyl methacrylate. *Dent Mater*. 1992;8(5):324–326.

Furuchi M, et al. Effect of metal priming agents on bond strength of resin-modified glass ionomers joined to gold alloy. *Dent Mater J*. 2007;26(5):728–732.

Garcia-Godoy F, Donly KJ. Dentin/enamel adhesives in pediatric dentistry. *Pediatr Dent*. 2002;24(5):462–464.

Goracci C, Sadek FT, Monticelli F, Cardoso PE, Ferrari M. Influence of substrate, shape, and thickness on microtensile specimens' structural integrity and their measured bond strengths. *Dent Mater*. 2004;20(7):643–654.

He LH, Purton DG, Swain MV. A suitable base material for composite resin restorations: zinc oxide eugenol. J Dent. 38(4):290–295.

Hembree Jr JH, George TA. Hembree ME. Film thickness of cements beneath complete crowns. *J Prosthet Dent*. 1978;39(5):533–535.

Hibino Y, et al. Correlation between the strength of glass ionomer cements and their bond strength to bovine teeth. *Dent Mater J*. 2004;23(4):656–660.

Hibino Y, et al. Relationship between the strength of glass ionomers and their adhesive strength to metals. *Dent Mater*. 2002;18(7):552–557.

Hitz T, Stawarczyk B, Fisher J, Hämmerle CH, Sailer I. Are self-adhesive resin cements a valid alternative to conventional resin cements? A laboratory study of the long-term bond strength. *Dent Mater*. 2012;28(11):1183–1190.

Hunter A, et al. *Oper Dent*. 1995;20:2–6.

Ilie N, Hickel R. Can CQ be completely replaced by alternative initiators in dental adhesives? *Dent Mater J*. 2008;27(2):221–228.

Ilie N, Oberthür M-T. Effect of sonic-activated resin composites on the repair of aged substrates: an in vitro investigation. *Clin Oral Invest*. 2013;18:1605–1612. doi:10.1007/s00784-013-1136-7.

Inokoshi M, Kameyama A, de Munck J, Minakuchi S, van Meerbeek B. Durable bonding to mechanically and/or chemically pre-treated dental zirconia. *J Dent*. 2013;41(2):170–179.

Irie M, Suzuki K, Watts DC. Marginal and flexural integrity of three classes of luting cement, with early finishing and water storage. *Dent Mater*. 2004;20(1):3–11.

Jemt T, Stalblad PA, Oilo G. Adhesion of polycarboxylate- based dental cements to enamel: an in vivo study. *J Dent Res*. 1986;65(6):885–887.

Jivraj SA, Kim TH, Donovan TE. Selection of luting agents, part 1. *J Calif Dent Assoc*. 2006;34(2):149–160.

Johnson GH, et al. Retention of metal-ceramic crowns with contemporary dental cements. *J Am Dent Assoc*. 2009;140(9):1125–1136.

Jongsma LA, Kleverlaan CJ, Feilzer AJ. Influence of surface pretreatment of fiber posts on cement delamination. *Dent Mater*. 2010;26(9):901–907.

Kim TH, Jivraj SA, Donovan TE. Selection of luting agents: part 2. *J Calif Dent Assoc*. 2006;34(2):161–166.

Kious AR, Roberts HW, Brackett WW. Film thicknesses of recently introduced luting cements. *J Prosthet Dent*. 2009;101(3):189–192.

Knobloch LA, et al. Solubility and sorption of resin-based luting cements. *Oper Dent*. 2000;25(5):434–440.

Li Z, White S. Mechanical properties of dental luting cements. *J Prosthet Dent*. 1999;81(5):597–609.

Lööf Jet, et al. A comparative study of the bioactivity of three materials for dental applications. *Dent Mater*. 2008;24:653–659.

Lööf Jet, et al. Mechanical property aspects of a biomineral based dental restorative system. *Key Eng Mater*. 2005;284–286:741–744.

Machado C, et al. *Oper Dent*. 2007;32:341–346.

Magne P, Paranhos MPG, Burnett Jr LH. New zirconia primer improves bond strength of resin-based cements. *Dent Mater*. 2010;26(4):345–352.

Magni E, et al. Evaluation of the mechanical properties of dental adhesives and glass-ionomer cements. *Clin Oral Investig*. 2010;14(1):79–87.

Mair L, Padipatvuthikul P. Variables related to materials and preparing for bond strength testing irrespective of the test protocol. Dent Mater. 26(2):e17–e23.

Marcusson A, Norevall LI, Persson M. White spot reduction when using glass ionomer cement for bonding in orthodontics: a longitudinal and comparative study. *Eur J Orthod.* 1997;19(3):233–242.

Marshall SJ, et al. A review of adhesion science. *Dent Mater.* 2010;26(2):e11–e16.

Mausner IK, Goldstein GR, Georgescu M. Effect of two dentinal desensitizing agents on retention of complete cast coping using four cements. *J Prosthet Dent.* 1996;75(2):129–134.

Mesu FP. Mechanical mixing of zinc oxide-eugenol cements. *J Prosthet Dent.* 1982;47(5):522–527.

Mitra SB. Dental cements: formulation and handling techniques. In: Curtis RV, Watson T, eds. *Dental Biomaterials: Imaging, Testing and Modelling.* Elsevier; 2014.

Mojon P, et al. Early bond strength of luting cements to a precious alloy. *J Dent Res.* 1992;71(9):1633–1639.

Moura JS, et al. Effect of luting cement on dental biofilm composition and secondary caries around metallic restorations in situ. *Oper Dent.* 2004;29(5):509–514.

Nakamura T, et al. Mechanical properties of new self-adhesive resin-based cement. J Prosthodont Res. 54(2):59–64.

Negm MM, Beech DR, Grant AA. An evaluation of mechanical and adhesive properties of polycarboxylate and glass ionomer cements. *J Oral Rehabil.* 1982;9(2):161–167.

Nicholson JW, Czarnecka B. Review paper: role of aluminum in glass-ionomer dental cements and its biological effects. *J Biomater Appl.* 2009;24(4):293–308.

Nicholson JW, Czarnecka B. The biocompatibility of resin-modified glass-ionomer cements for dentistry. *Dent Mater.* 2008;24(12):1702–1708.

Oilo G, Espevik S. Stress/strain behavior of some dental luting cements. *Acta Odontol Scand.* 1978;36(1):45–49.

Osborne JW, et al. A method for assessing the clinical solubility and disintegration of luting cements. *J Prosthet Dent.* 1978;40(4):413–417.

Ozcan M, et al. Bond strength durability of a resin composite on a reinforced ceramic using various repair systems. *Dent Mater.* 2009;25(12):1477–1483.

Perdigao J. New developments in dental adhesion. *Dent Clin North Am.* 2007;51(2):333–357 , viii.

Peutzfeldt A, Asmussen E. Influence of eugenol-containing temporary cement on bonding of self-etching adhesives to dentin. *J Adhes Dent.* 2006;8(1):31–34.

Peutzfeldt A. Dual-cure resin cements: in vitro wear and effect of quantity of remaining double bonds, filler volume, and light curing. *Acta Odontol Scand.* 1995;53(1):29–34.

Pilo R, Kaitsas V, Zinelis S, Eliades G. Interaction of zirconia primers with yttria-stabilized zirconia surfaces. *Dent Mater.* 2016;32(3):353–362.

Piwowarczyk A, Lauer HC, Sorensen JA. In vitro shear bond strength of cementing agents to fixed prosthodontic restorative materials. *J Prosthet Dent.* 2004;92(3):265–273.

Piwowarczyk A, Lauer HC, Sorensen JA. The shear bond strength between luting cements and zirconia ceramics after two pre-treatments. *Oper Dent.* 2005;30(3):382–388.

Piwowarczyk A, Lauer HC. Mechanical properties of luting cements after water storage. *Oper Dent.* 2003;28(5):535–542.

Powis DR, Prosser HJ, Wilson AD. Long-term monitoring of microleakage of dental cements by radiochemical diffusion. *J Prosthet Dent.* 1988;59(6):651–657.

Radovic I, Monticelli F, Goracci C, Vulicevic ZR, Ferrari M. Self-adhesive resin cements: a literature review. *J Adhes Dent.* 2008;10(4):251–258.

Rinastiti M, Ozcan M, Siswomihardjo W, Busscher HJ. Effects of surface conditioning on repair bond strengths of non-aged and aged microhybrid, nanohybrid, and nanofilled composite resins. *Clin Oral Investig.* 2011;15(5):625–633.

Robertello FJ, et al. Fluoride release of glass ionomer-based luting cements in vitro. *J Prosthet Dent.* 1999;82(2):172–176.

Rosa WL, Piva E, Silva AF. Bond strength of universal adhesives: a systematic review and meta-analysis. *J Dent.* 2015;43(7):765–776.

Schmid-Schwap M, et al. Cytotoxicity of four categories of dental cements. *Dent Mater.* 2009;25(3):360–368.

Schulman A, Vaidyanathan TK. Dental cements for luting and lining. *N Y J Dent.* 1977;47(5):142–146.

Setcos JC, Staninec M, Wilson NH. Bonding of amalgam restorations: existing knowledge and future prospects. *Oper Dent.* 2000;25(2):121–129.

Shaw AJ, Carrick T, McCabe JF. Fluoride release from glass-ionomer and compomer restorative materials: 6-month data. *J Dent.* 1998;26(4):355–359.

Sidhu SK, Schmalz G. The biocompatibility of glass-ionomer cement materials: a status report for the American journal of dentistry. *Am J Dent.* 2001;14(6):387–396.

Smith D. A new dental cement. *Br Dent J.* 1968;5:381–384.

Smith D. The setting of zinc oxide/eugenol mixtures. *Br Dent J.* 1958;105(9):313–321.

Sousa A, et al. *J Adhes Dent.* 2012;15:137–144.

Spinell T, Schedle A, Watts DC. Polymerization shrinkage kinetics of dimethacrylate resin-cements. *Dent Mater.* 2009;25(8):1058–1066.

Summers A, et al. Comparison of bond strength between a conventional resin adhesive and a resin-modified glass ionomer adhesive: an in vitro and in vivo study. *Am J Orthod Dentofacial Orthop.* 2004;126(2):200–206; quiz 254–255.

Swartz ML, Phillips RW, Clark HE. Long-term F release from glass ionomer cements. *J Dent Res.* 1984;63(2):158–160.

Van Meerbeek B, et al. Buonocore memorial lecture. Adhesion to enamel and dentin: current status and future challenges. *Oper Dent.* 2003;28(3):215–235.

Areti D Vrochari 1, George Eliades, Elmar Hellwig, Karl T Wrbas. Water sorption and solubility of four self-etching, self-adhesive resin luting agents. *J Adhes Dent.* 2010;12(1):39–43. doi: 10.3290/j.jad.a17539.

White SN, Kipnis V. Effect of adhesive luting agents on the marginal seating of cast restorations. *J Prosthet Dent.* 1993;69(1):28–31.

White SN, Yu Z. Compressive and diametral tensile strengths of current adhesive luting agents. *J Prosthet Dent.* 1993;69(6):568–572.

Wiegand A, Buchalla W, Attin T. Review on fluoride-releasing restorative materials–fluoride release and uptake characteristics, antibacterial activity and influence on caries formation. *Dent Mater.* 2007;23(3):343–362.

Wilson AD, McLean JW. *Glass-Ionomer Cement.* Quintessence Books; 1988.

Wilson AD, Nicholson J. *Acid-Base Cements: Their Biomedical and Industrial Applications.* Cambridge University Press; 1993:398.

Wilson AD, Prosser HJ, Powis DM. Mechanism of adhesion of polyelectrolyte cements to hydroxyapatite. *J Dent Res.* 1983;62(5):590–592.

8 Polymeric Restorative Materials

CARMEM PFEIFER

CHAPTER OUTLINE

Resin Composites

The concept of a composite biomaterial, introduced in Chapter 5, can be described as a solid that contains two or more distinct constituent materials or phases when considered at greater than an atomic scale. In these materials, mechanical properties such as elastic modulus are significantly altered in comparison with a homogenous material consisting of either of the phases alone. Enamel, dentin, bone, and reinforced polymers are considered composites, but alloys such as brass are not. The ability to change properties of the macroscale object based on control of the individual constituents is a significant advantage for the use of composite materials. In dentistry, the term "resin composite" generally refers to a reinforced polymer system used for restoring hard tissues, such as enamel and dentin. The proper materials science term is "polymer matrix composite," or for those composites with filler particles often used as direct-placed restorative composites, "particulate-reinforced polymer matrix composite." In this chapter, the term "resin composite" will refer to the reinforced polymer matrix materials used as restorative materials. The class of materials called conventional glass ionomers (GIs) and resin-modified glass ionomers (RMGIs) also fall in the scientific class of composite materials, but because these are water-based materials and have a distinct acid-base setting reaction, they have been traditionally categorized as a class of their own (see Chapter 6). It is important to remember, however, that most biological materials, including enamel, dentin, bone, connective tissue, muscle, and even cells, are classified as composites within the broad range of biological engineering materials.

Resin composites are used to replace missing tooth structures and modify tooth color and contour, thus enhancing aesthetics. A number of commercial resin composites are available for various applications. Traditionally, some have been optimized for aesthetics, and others were designed for higher stress-bearing areas. More recently, nanocomposites have become available, which are optimized for both excellent aesthetics and high mechanical properties for stress-bearing areas. GIs and RMGIs are used selectively as filling materials, usually for small lesions, or can be used in conjunction with composites, especially where one or more margins are in dentin and in areas of caries activity.

Resin-based composites were first developed in the early 1960s and provided materials with higher mechanical properties than acrylics and silicates, lower thermal coefficient of expansion, lower dimensional change on setting, and higher resistance to wear, thereby improving clinical performance. Early composites were chemically activated, followed by photoactivated composites initiated with ultraviolet (UV) wavelengths. These were later replaced by composites activated in the visible wavelengths. Continued improvements in composite technology have resulted in modern materials with excellent durability, wear resistance, and aesthetics mimicking natural teeth. In particular, the incorporation of nanotechnology in controlling the filler architecture has made dramatic improvements in these materials. Moreover, the development of bonding agents for bonding composites to tooth structure (see Chapter 7) has also improved the longevity and performance of composite restorations. However, the overall lifetime of a composite restoration is still, on average, 10–12 years, with the most common reasons for replacement being fracture and recurrent decay.

TABLE 8.1 Types of Restorations and Recommended Resin Composites

Type of Restoration	Recommended Resin Composite
Class 1	Multipurpose, nanocomposite, bulk filled, microfilled (posterior),[a] compomer (posterior)[a]
Class 2	Multipurpose, nanocomposite, bulk filled, laboratory, microfilled (posterior),[a] compomer (posterior)[a]
Class 3	Multipurpose, nanocomposite, microfilled, compomer
Class 4	Multipurpose, nanocomposite
Class 5	Multipurpose, nanocomposite, microfilled, resin-modified glass ionomer, compomer
Class 6 (MOD)	Bulk-filled, nanocomposite
Cervical lesions	Flowable, resin-modified glass ionomer, compomer
Pediatric restorations	Flowable, resin-modified glass ionomer, compomer
3-unit bridge or crown	Laboratory (with fiber reinforcement)
Alloy substructure	Laboratory (bonded)
Core build-up	Core
Temporary restoration	Provisional
High caries-risk patients	GIs, resin-modified glass ionomer

GIs, Glass ionomers; *MOD*, mesial-occlusal-distal.
[a]Special microfilled composites and compomers are available for posterior use.

TABLE 8.2 Characteristics of Various Types of Resin Composites

			HANDLING CHARACTERISTICS AND PROPERTIES	
Type of Composite	Size of Filler Particles (mm)	Volume of Inorganic Filler (%)	Advantages	Disadvantages
Multipurpose	0.04, 0.2–3.0	60–70	High strength, high modulus	
Nanocomposite	0.002–0.075	72–79	High polish, high strength, high modulus, polish retention	
Microfilled	0.04	32–50	Best polish, best aesthetics	Higher shrinkage, lower strength
Bulk filled	0.04, 0.2–20	59–80	Deep cure, reduced step	Questionable marginal adaptation
Flowable	0.04, 0.2–3.0	42–62	Syringeable, lower modulus	Higher wear
Laboratory	0.04, 0.2–3.0	60–70	Best anatomy and contacts, lower wear	Laboratory cost, special equipment, requires resin cement

Therefore, there is still an opportunity for improvement in these materials, particularly in terms of bioactivity, as well as resistance to degradation and bacterial attachment in the oral environment. Rather than being simply "inert placeholders," ideally those materials would be able to reinforce the tooth structure, along with adhesives to provide a long-lasting seal to the tooth and discourage the formation of cariogenic biofilm. One example of resin composite restoration placement is shown in the video available online.

A classification of preparation type and recommended composite category is listed in Table 8.1. Characteristics of these composite categories are summarized in Table 8.2.

Multipurpose Resin Composites

Composition

A resin composite is composed of four major components: organic polymer matrix, inorganic filler particles, coupling agent, and the initiator-accelerator system. The organic polymer matrix in most commercial resin composites today is a cross-linked matrix of dimethacrylate monomers. The double bonds at each end of these molecules undergo addition polymerization by free-radical initiation. While some of these monomers can provide an optimum of optical, mechanical, and clinical properties, they are rather viscous and have to be blended with low-molecular-weight diluent monomers so that a clinically workable consistency may be obtained upon incorporation of the fillers. More recently, other higher-molecular-weight, low-viscosity diluents have been introduced, as have low-shrink composites, which contain, for example, monomers with epoxy (also known as oxirane) functional groups at the ends and whose polymerization is initiated by cations. Other commercial resin composites utilize various monomers and filler technology to reduce polymerization shrinkage or stress.

The dispersed inorganic filler particles may consist of one or more inorganic materials such as finely ground quartz or glass, sol-gel-derived ceramics, microfine silica, or, more recently, nanoparticles. Two-dimensional diagrams of fine and microfine particles surrounded by a polymer matrix are shown in Fig. 8.1.

The coupling agent, an organosilane (often referred to as "silane"), is applied to the inorganic particles by the manufacturer to surface treat the fillers before being mixed with the unreacted

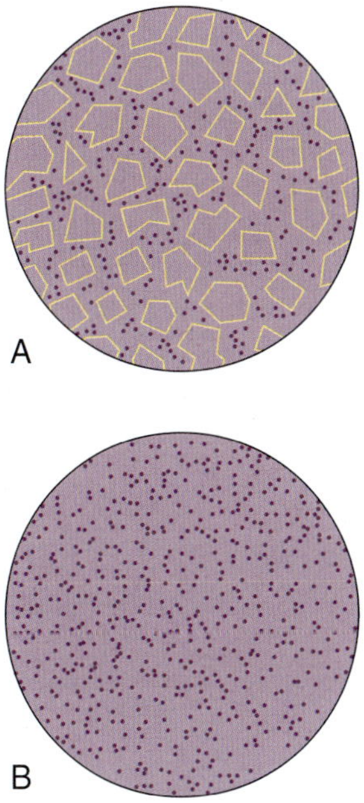

• **Fig. 8.1** Two-dimensional diagrams of composites with (A) fine and (B) microfine particles. (From Powers JM, Wataha JC. *Dental Materials: Foundations and Applications*. 11th ed. Elsevier; 2017).

monomer mixture. Silanes are called *coupling agents* because they form a bond between the inorganic and organic phases of the composite. One end of the molecule contains functional groups (such as methoxy), which hydrolyze and react with the inorganic filler, whereas the other end has a methacrylate double bond that copolymerizes with the monomers.

The role of the initiator-accelerator system is to polymerize and cross-link the system into a hardened mass. The polymerization reaction can be triggered by light activation, self-curing (chemical activation), and dual curing (chemical and light curing).

Resin Matrix

Methacrylate Monomers

The vast majority of monomers used for the resin matrix are dimethacrylate compounds. Two monomers that have been commonly used are 2,2-bis(4[2-hydroxy-3-methacryloxypropyloxy]-phenyl) propane (bisphenol A-glycidyl methacrylate [Bis-GMA]), and urethane dimethacrylate (UDMA). Both contain reactive carbon double bonds at each end that can undergo addition polymerization initiated by free-radical initiators. The use of aromatic groups affords a good match of refractive index with the radiopaque glasses and thus provides better overall optical properties of the composites. A few products use both Bis-GMA and UDMA monomers.

The viscosity of the monomers, especially Bis-GMA (Mw = 512 g/mol), is rather high, and diluents must be added so a clinical consistency can be reached when the resin mixture is compounded with the filler. Low-viscosity compounds with difunctional carbon double bonds, for example, triethylene glycol dimethacrylate (TEGDMA, MW = 286 g/mol) or bisphenol A ethoxylate dimethacrylate (Bis-EMA6, MW = 540 g/mol), are added by the manufacturer to reduce and control the viscosity of the compounded composite. TEGDMA, in particular, is considered to be a low-molecular-weight monomer, and this has implications for the polymerization shrinkage and shrinkage stress, as will be discussed later in the chapter. In general, smaller monomers lead to greater polymerization shrinkage.

Low-Shrink Methacrylate Monomers

A variety of other methacrylate monomers have been used in the newer commercial products introduced since the mid-2000s for controlling the volumetric shrinkage and polymerization stress of composites (Fig. 8.2). In summary, three different approaches were taken to reducing polymerization shrinkage and/or shrinkage stress: (1) develop higher molecular weight monomers, such as dimer acids (MW > 800 g/mol) and monomers incorporating cycloaliphatic units (MW > 700 g/mol), which essentially reduce the amount of free volume available prior to polymerization; (2) develop monomers with photocleavable units to relieve stress

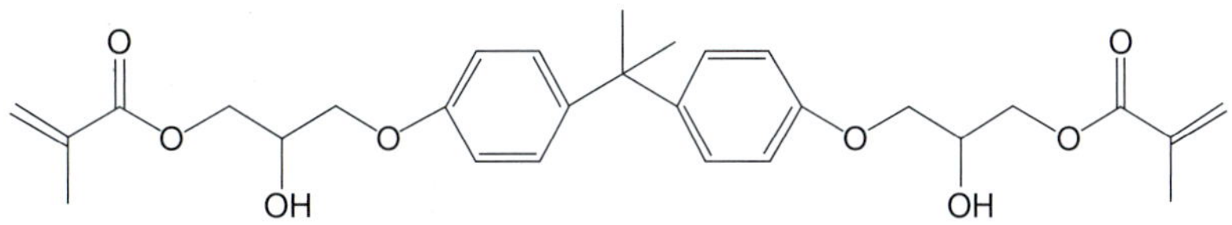

Structure of Bis-GMA

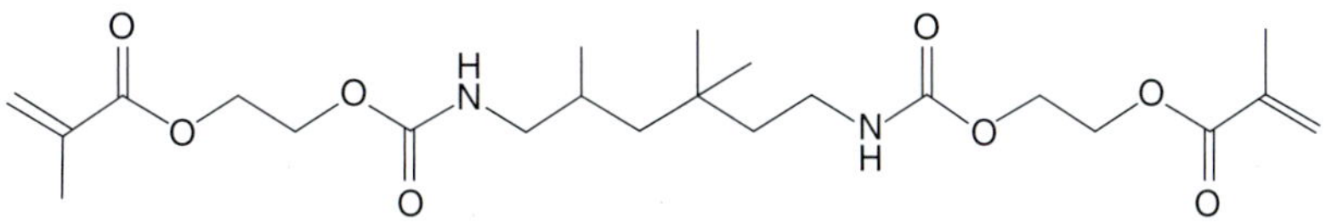

Structure of UDMA

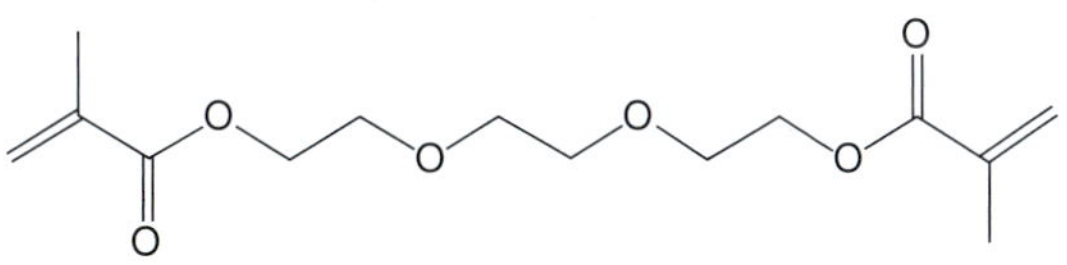

Structure of TEGDMA

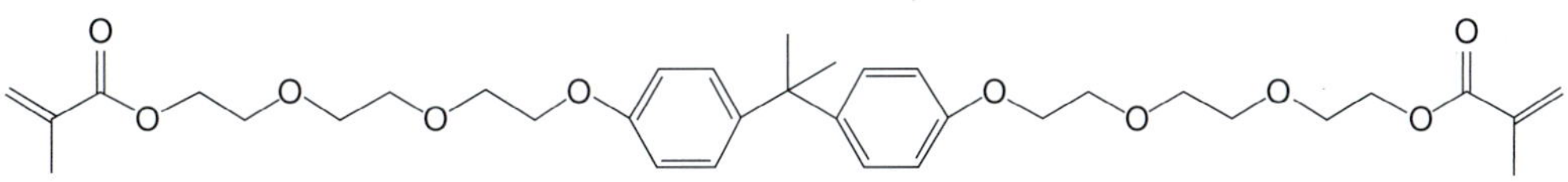

Structure of Bis-EMA6

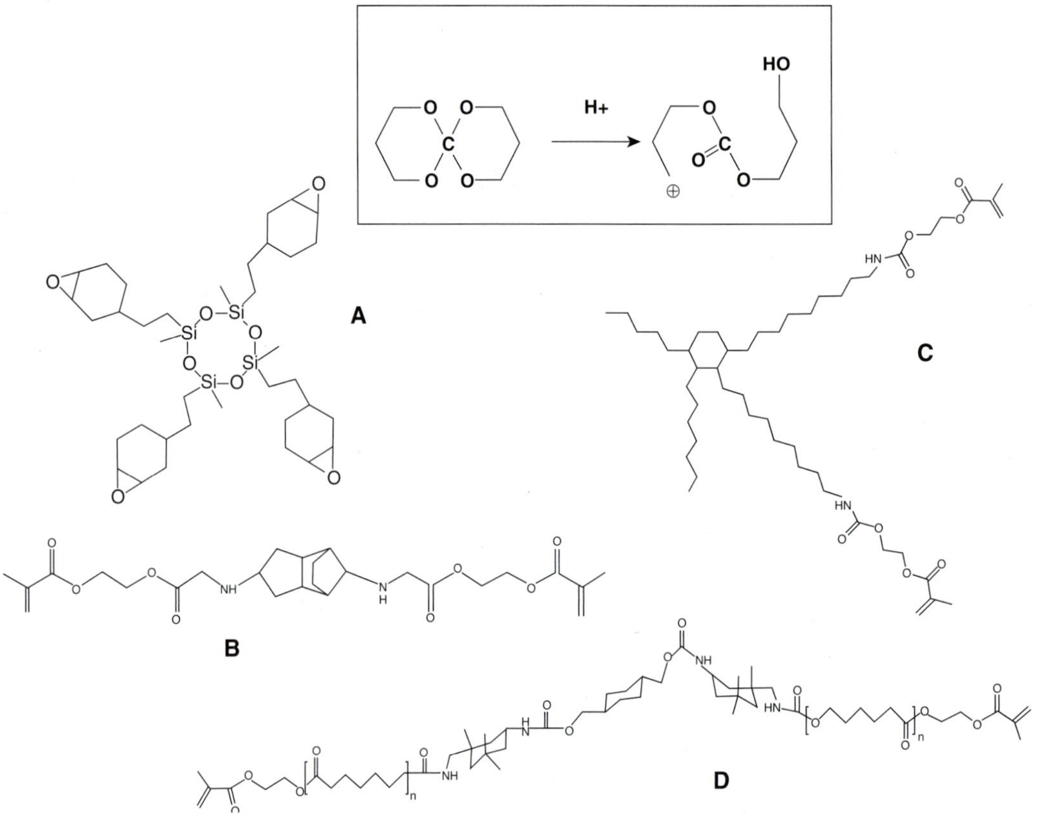

• **Fig. 8.2** Molecular structure of alternative monomers currently used in commercial products. (A) Oxirane (Filtek LS, 3M-ESPE); (B) TCD-urethane (Venus Diamond, Heraeus Kulzer); (C) Dimeracid dimethacrylate (N'Durance, ConfiDental-Septodont); (D) DuPont DX-511 (Kalore, GC America). The insert shows a spiro-orthocarbonate molecule, which expands upon polymerization but has not been used in any commercial materials.

during and after polymerization, such as allyl disulfides, which produce covalently adaptable networks; and (3) develop a monomer with intrinsically lower molar shrinkage coefficient, such as spiro-orthocarbonates, or the silorane. The oxirane functionalities on the silorane undergo ring-opening cross-linking via cationic polymerization, and that at least partially compensates the loss in free volume among the polymerizing molecules. The name silorane was coined from its chemical building blocks, *silo*xane and oxi*rane* (also known as epoxy). The siloxane functionality provides hydrophobicity to the composite. There was one commercial material using this technology, but it is no longer available on the market.

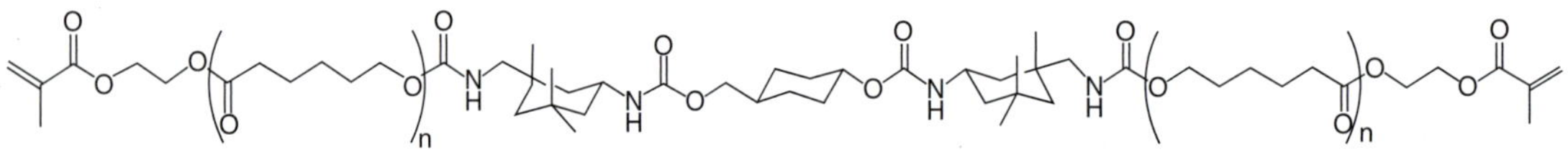

Structure of a monomer with cycloaliphatic units

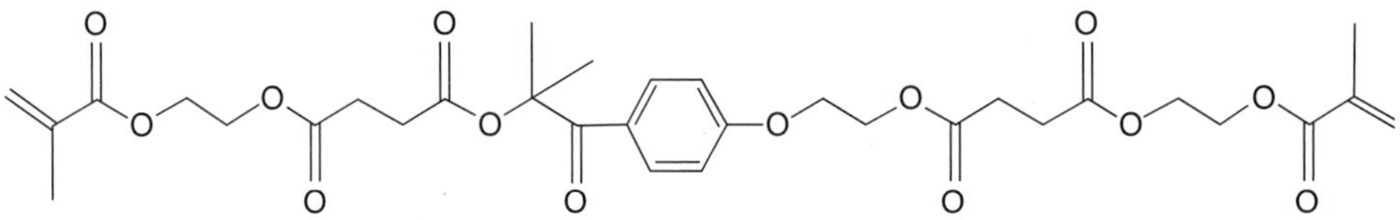

Structure of monomer with photocleavable units

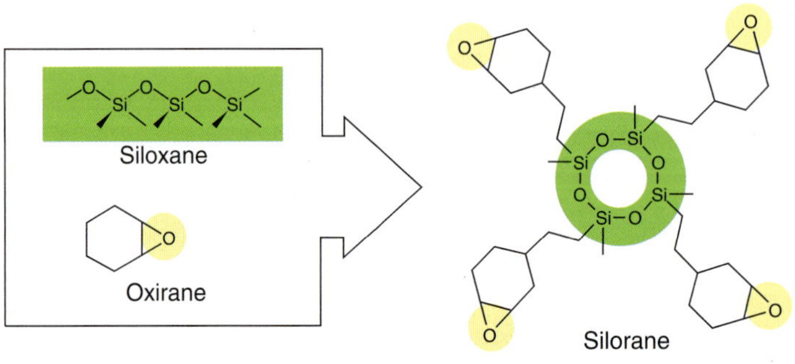

Structure of silorane

Fillers and Classification of Composites

Fillers make up a major portion by volume or weight of the composite. The function of the filler is to reinforce the resin matrix, provide the appropriate degree of translucency, and control the volume shrinkage of the composite during polymerization. Fillers have been traditionally obtained by grinding minerals such as quartz, glasses, or sol-gel-derived ceramics. Most glasses contain heavy-metal oxides such as barium or zinc so that they provide radiopacity for visualization when exposed to X-rays. It is advantageous to have a distribution of filler diameters so that smaller particles fit in the spaces between larger particles and provide more efficient packing. Recently nanofillers have been introduced into composites. These are described in the section Nanofillers and Nanocomposites.

A helpful method of classifying dental composites is by the particle size, shape, and particle-size distribution of the filler. This classification is presented in the following section.

Macrofills

The early composites were macrofills. These composites contained large spherical or irregular-shaped particles of average filler diameter of 20 to 30 µm. The resultant composites were rather opaque, difficult to polish to restore aesthetics, and had low resistance to wear.

Microfills

In these materials, the average particle size is 50 nm, and the main type of filler is fumed silica. Because of the small particle size, volume loading becomes challenging, so the manufacturers prepolymerize the composite at high temperatures, grind the polymerized composite, and reintroduce that powder, along with more fumed silica, into the resin matrix. This allows for about 32 to 50 vol% overall filler to be added (see Table 8.2) and also decreases polymerization shrinkage.

Typical properties of microfilled composites are listed in Table 8.3. Because they are less highly filled, microfilled composites exhibit more water sorption and thermal expansion than microhybrid composites or nanocomposites. Depending on the amount of prepolymerized resin added, the shrinkage can be more than that which occurs with microhybrids or nanocomposites. Because of the small particle size, these materials are highly polishable and aesthetic, but also have lower mechanical properties.

Hybrid and Microhybrid Composites

In hybrid composites, two types of fillers are blended together: fine particles of average particle size 2 to 4 µm and 5% to 15% of microfine particles, usually silica, of particle size 0.04 to 0.2 µm. In microhybrid composites, the fine particles of lower average particle size (0.04–1 µm) are blended with microfine silica. The fine particles may be obtained by grinding glass (e.g., borosilicate glass, lithium or barium aluminum silicate glass, strontium, or zinc glass), quartz, or ceramic materials and have irregular shapes. The distribution of filler particles provides efficient packing so that high filler loading is possible while maintaining good handling of the composite for clinical placement. Microhybrid composites may contain 60% to 70% filler by volume, which, depending on the density of the filler, translates into 77% to 84% by weight in the composite. Most manufacturers report filler concentration in weight percent (wt%). A micrograph of a typical, fine glass filler is shown in Fig. 8.3A. Hybrids and microhybrids have good clinical wear resistance and mechanical properties and are suitable for stress-bearing applications. However, they lose their surface polish with time and become rough and dull.

Nanocomposites

The latest advancement in composite technology has been the utilization of nanotechnology in development of fillers. Nanotechnology is the production of functional materials and structures in the range of 1 to 100 nm—the nanoscale—by various physical and chemical methods. Nanotechnology requires devices and systems to create structures that have novel properties and functions because of their small sizes. Thus it implies the ability to control and manipulate structures at the atomic and/or molecular scale. Although true nanocomposites should have all filler particles in the nanometer size, the term "nanotechnology" has some hype associated with it, and it is sometimes misused in describing a material. To date, oxide nanoparticles have been the most prevalent type of nanomaterials used in dental composites. At present, there are two distinct types of resin composites available that contain nanoparticles:

1. Nanofills: These contain nanometer-sized particles (1–100 nm) throughout the resin matrix. Larger primary particles are not present.
2. Nanohybrids: These consist of large particles (0.4–5 µm) with added nanometer-sized particles. Thus they are hybrid materials, not true nanofilled composites.

It is important to highlight the difference between the fumed silica particles used in microfill composites and the nanoparticles used in the nanocomposites. Fumed silica is produced via flame hydrolysis synthesis. The carbon-based raw material is vaporized at high temperatures (1100°C) in the presence of oxygen, followed by cooling and condensation, which results in precipitated fumed silica particles. There is not a lot of control of the surface properties of the resulting particles. Nanoparticles are produced using much more controlled methods, some of which are proprietary, which allow for strict tunability of size, surface area, and surface treatment—these are the characteristics that allow for the incorporation of adequate amounts of filler particles in composites in spite of the small particle size. Different types of nanoparticles are described in the following section.

Nanofill Composites

All filler particles of true nanofilled composites are in the nanometer range. There are several purposes for incorporating nanofillers in dental composites. First, the size of nanomeric particles is below that of visible light (400–800 nm), which provides the opportunity of creating highly translucent materials. In addition, the surface area-to-volume ratio of the nanoparticles is quite large. The sizes of the smallest nanoparticles approach those of polymer molecules so they can form a molecular-scale interaction with the host resin matrix.

Two types of nanoparticles have been synthesized and utilized for preparing this class of composite. The first type consists of nanomeric particles that are essentially monodispersed nonaggregates and nonagglomerated particles of silica or zirconia. The surface of the nanoparticles is treated with silane coupling agents that allow them to be bonded to the resin matrix when the composite is cured after placement. Nanomers are synthesized from sols, creating particles of the same size. Because of this, if nanomeric particles alone are used to make highly filled composites, the rheological properties are rather poor. To overcome this disadvantage, one manufacturer has designed a second type of nanofiller, which is called nanocluster. The nanoclusters are made by lightly sintering nanomeric oxides to form clusters of a controlled particle size distribution. Nanoclusters have been synthesized from silica sols alone as well as from mixed oxides of silica and zirconia. The

TABLE 8.3 Properties of Various Types of Resin Composites, Compomers, Conventional Glass Ionomers, and Resin-Modified Glass Ionomers

Property	Nanocomposite[a]	Multipurpose Composite	Microfill Composite	Packable Composite	Flowable Composite	Laboratory Composite	Core Composite	Conventional Glass Ionomer	Resin-Modified Glass Ionomer
Flexural strength (MPa)	180	80–160	60–120	85–110	70–120	90–150[b]	—	7–15	50–60
Flexural modulus (GPa)	—	8.8–13	4.0–6.9	9.0–12	2.6–5.6	4.7–15[b]	—	—	—
Flexural fatigue limit (MPa)	—	60–110	—	—	—	—	—	—	—
Compressive strength (MPa)	460	240–290	240–300	220–300	210–300	210–280	210–250	10–15	200–250
Compressive modulus (GPa)	—	5.5–8.3	2.6–4.8	5.8–9.0	2.6–5.9	—	7.5–22	7.2–10.3	3.2–6.9
Diametral tensile strength (MPa)	81	30–55	25–40	—	33–48	—	40–50	7–15	30–40
Linear polymerization shrinkage (%)	—	0.7–1.4	2–3	0.6–0.9	—	—	—	—	—
Color stability, accelerated aging: 450 kJ/m^2 (ΔE^*)[c]	—	1.5	—	—	15	1.1–2.3	—	—	—
Color stability, stained by juice/tea (ΔE^*)[c]	—	4.3	—	—	—	1.7–3.9	—	—	—

[a]From Mitra SB, Wu D, Holmes BN. An application of nanotechnology in advanced dental materials. *J Am Dent Assoc.* 2003;134(10):1382–1390.

[b]Without fiber reinforcement.

[c]$\Delta E < 3.3$ is considered not clinically perceptible.

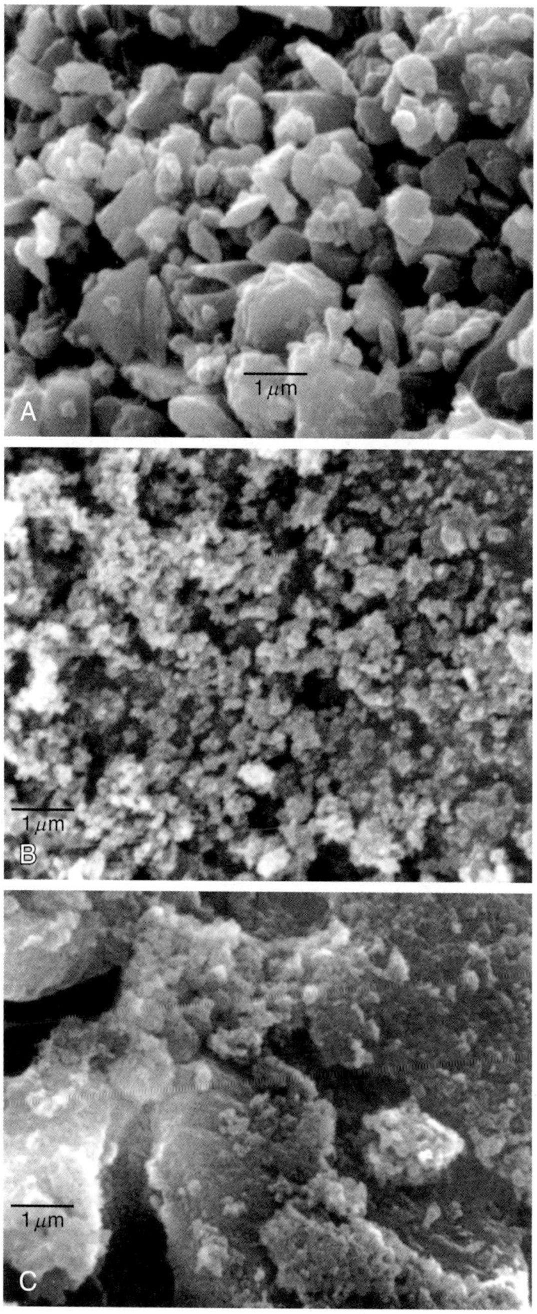

• **Fig. 8.3** Scanning electron micrographs of types of filler. (A) Fine inorganic filler; (B) microfine silica filler; (C) microfine silica in organic polymer filler.

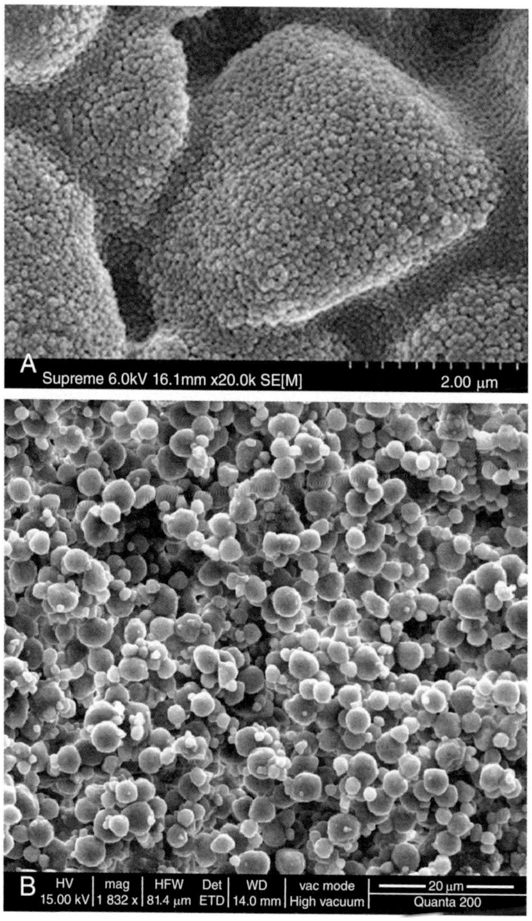

• **Fig. 8.4** (A) Scanning electron micrograph image of a nanocluster of silica in a commercial composite 3M ESPE Filtek Supreme. (B) Image of a nanocluster of zirconia-silica in Filtek Supreme Ultra. (A, Courtesy Dr. Jorge Perdigao, University of Minnesota. B, From Rodrigues SA Jr, Scherrer SS, Ferracane JL, Della Bona A. Microstructural characterization and fracture behavior of a microhybrid and a nanofill composite. *Dent Mater.* 2008;24(9):1281–1288).

primary particle size of the nanomers used to prepare the clusters ranges from 5 to 75 nm.

It is important to remember that in a nanocluster, the nanoparticles still maintain their individual form, much as in a cluster of grapes. The clusters can be made to have a wide size distribution ranging from 100 nm to submicron level and have an average size of 0.6 μm. Fig. 8.4A shows a scanning electron micrograph (SEM) image of a nanocluster of silica in the composite in a commercial composite after the resin matrix was removed by washing with acetone. In this material, the surface of the nanoclusters is treated with a silane coupling agent to provide compatibility and chemical bonding with the resin system. Fig. 8.4B shows the micrograph image of a nanocluster composed of silica and zirconia. The differences in particle architecture of nanomers, nanoclusters, and conventional microhybrid fillers are readily apparent from transmission electron micrographs (TEMs) of composites prepared from these fillers. Fig. 8.5A shows the TEM image of a nanocomposite filled with 75-nm diameter nanoparticles only; Fig. 8.5B is that of a nanocomposite filled with a mixture of nanoclusters alone; and Fig. 8.5C is of a conventional microhybrid composite. To date, there is only one true nanofilled dental composite available. In this manufactured composite, a combination of nanomeric particles and nanoclusters is used in optimum combinations. Fig. 8.6A shows a schematic diagram of this nanocomposite containing a blend of nanocluster and nanomeric fillers, whereas Fig. 8.6B shows a TEM of the nanocomposite showing the presence of the two types of nanofillers.

The uniqueness of the nanofilled composite is that it has the mechanical strength of a microhybrid but, at the same time, retains smoothness during service like a microfill. The initial gloss of many restoratives is quite good, but in hybrid composites (microhybrids and nanohybrids), plucking the larger fillers causes loss of gloss. By contrast, in the nanofilled composite, the nanoclusters shear at a rate similar to the surrounding matrix during abrasion. This allows the restoration to maintain a smoother

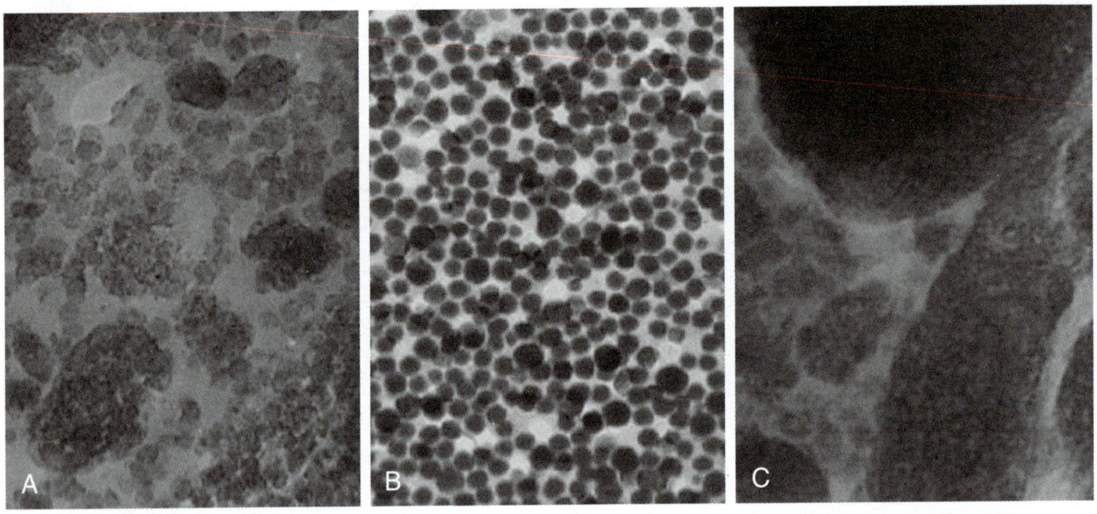

• **Fig. 8.5** (A) Transmission electron micrograph (TEM) image of composite with nanomeric particles (×60,000 magnification). (B) TEM image of composite with nanocluster particles (×300,000 magnification). (C) TEM image of composite with hybrid fillers (×300,000 magnification). (A, B, and C From Mitra SB, Wu D, Holmes BN. An application of nanotechnology in advanced dental materials. *J Am Dent Assoc*. 2003;134(10):1382–1390).

surface for long-term polish retention. Optical analysis of the polish retention can be done using atomic force microscopy after extended toothbrush abrasion.

Nanofillers also offer advantages in optical properties. In general, it is desirable to provide low visual opacity in unpigmented dental composites. This allows for the creation of a wide range of shades and opacities so the clinician can design a highly aesthetic restoration. In hybrid types of composites, the filler particles are 0.4 to 3.0 µm in size. When particles and resin are mismatched in the refractive index, which measures the ability of the material to transmit light, the particles will scatter light and produce opaque materials. Nanomeric filler particles are far smaller than the wavelength of light, making them unmeasurable by refractive index. When light enters, long-wavelength light passes directly through, and materials show high translucency. As shown by Fig. 8.7, the disks made with hybrid and microfill fillers are rather opaque. The nanofill composite sample made predominantly with the nanomeric filler is quite clear, as the background can be easily seen through the composite. In addition, when placed on a black background, the nanomeric and nanocluster particles preferentially scatter blue light, giving the composite an opalescent effect. This gives a more lifelike appearance because natural enamel also exhibits the same effect.

The ability to create a nanocomposite with very low opacity provides the ability to formulate a vast range of shade and opacity options, from the very translucent shades needed for the incisal edge and for the final layer in multilayered restorations to the more opaque shades desired in the enamel, body, and dentin shades. This allows the clinician the flexibility of choosing a single shade or a multishade layering technique depending on the aesthetic needs. The wear resistance of this material after

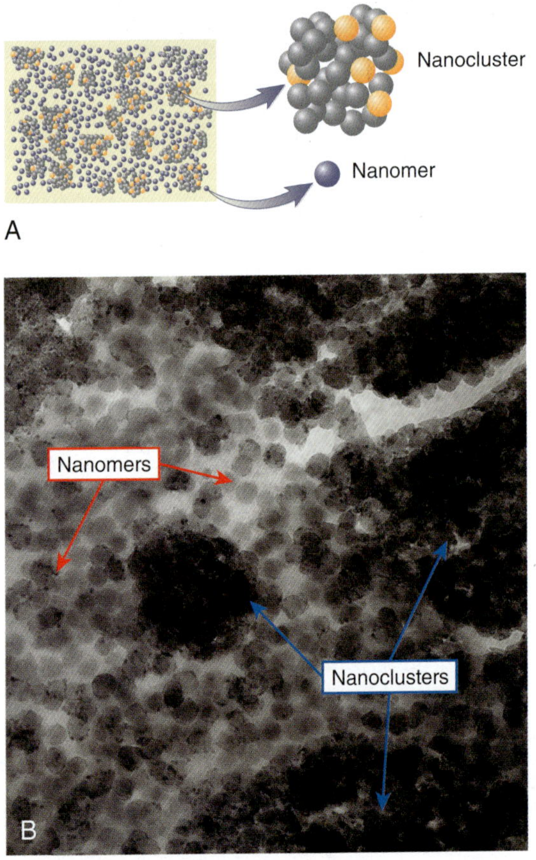

• **Fig. 8.6** (A) Schematic diagram of a nanofilled composite containing nanoclusters and nanomers. (B) Transmission electron micrograph image of a nanocomposite with nanocluster and nanomeric fillers in Filtek Supreme Plus. (Courtesy 3M Company, St. Paul, MN.)

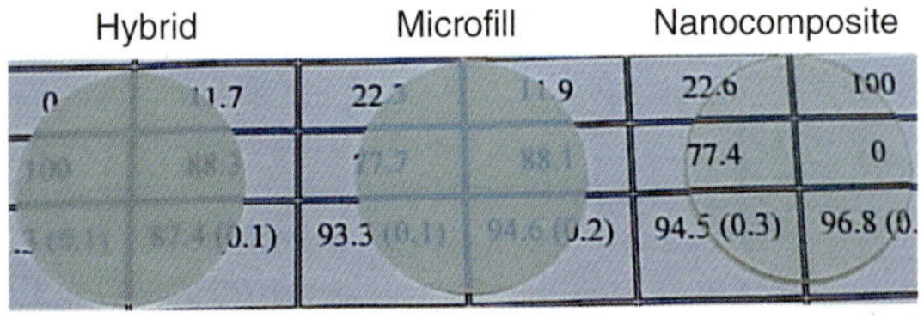

• **Fig. 8.7** Translucency of a hybrid composite, microfill composite, and a nanocomposite. (From Mitra SB, Wu D, Holmes BN. An application of nanotechnology in advanced dental materials. *J Am Dent Assoc*. 2003;134(10):1382–1390).

3 and 5 years of clinical use was found to be similar to human enamel.

Nanohybrid Composite

Several manufacturers have placed nano-sized particles in their microhybrids. These composites have been described as nanohybrids. Because the smoothness and wear of any composite are often determined by the size of its largest filler particles, as with microhybrids, the surface of nanohybrids becomes gradually dull after a few years of clinical service.

Interfacial Phase and Coupling Agents

For a composite to have successful clinical performance, a good bond must form between the inorganic filler particles and the organic resin matrix during setting. This is achieved through the use of compounds called coupling agents, the most common of which are organic silicon compounds called silane coupling agents. The surface of the filler is treated with a coupling agent during the manufacture of the composite. A typical silane coupling agent is 3-methacryloxypropyltrimethoxysilane, the chemical structure of which is shown below.

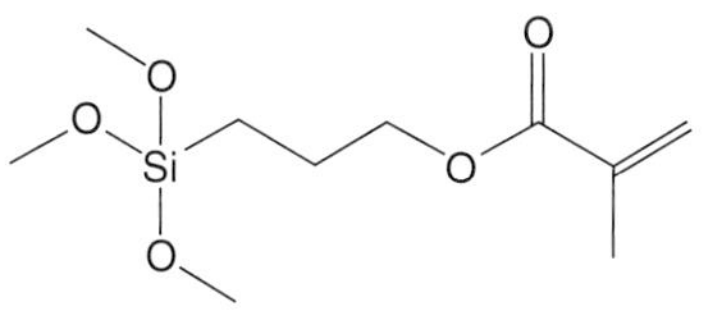

Structure of 3-Methacryloxypropyltrimethoxysilane

During the filler treatment process, the methoxy groups hydrolyze to generate hydroxyl groups through an acid- or base-catalyzed reaction. These hydroxyl groups then undergo condensation with the hydroxyl groups on the surface of the filler and become attached by covalent bonds (see the following schematic sketch). Condensation is also possible with the adjacent –OH groups of the hydrolyzed silanes or with water absorbed on the surface of the filler. This results in the formation of a very thin monolayer or multilayer polymeric film on the surface of the filler with unreacted double bonds. During the curing of the composite, the double bonds of the methacryloxy groups of the treated surface coreact with the monomer resins. The coupling agent plays a critical role in the composite. Its functions are as follows:

- It forms an interfacial bridge that strongly binds the filler to the resin matrix.
- It enhances the mechanical properties of the composite and minimizes the plucking of the fillers from the matrix during clinical wear.
- The resulting interfacial phase provides a medium for stress distribution between adjacent particles and the polymer matrix.
- It provides a hydrophobic environment that minimizes water absorption of the composite.

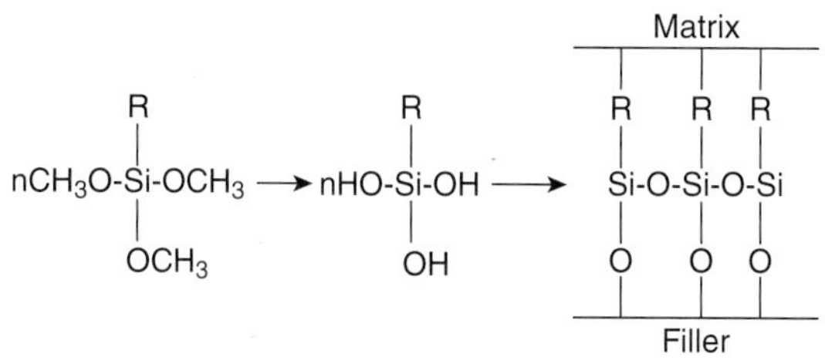

Initiators and Accelerators

The curing of composites is triggered by light or a chemical reaction, with the former being more common. Light activation is typically accomplished with blue light at a peak wavelength of about 465 nm, which is absorbed usually by a photosensitizer, such as camphorquinone, added to the monomer mixture during the manufacturing process in amounts varying from 0.1% to 1.0%. As briefly mentioned earlier, the increase in popularity of tooth whitening treatments has brought forth the need for restorative materials with lighter shades, which is difficult to be achieved if high concentrations of camphorquinone, a bright yellow compound, are used. For that reason, alternative, colorless initiators have been introduced, which absorb light in the near-UV range (390–420 nm). It is important to ensure matching of the absorption spectra of the initiators and the emission spectra of the light-curing unit, as will be detailed later in the chapter.

Once the photoinitiator is exposed to light, the polymerization reaction initiates. In methacrylate composites, free radicals are generated upon activation. If camphorquinone is the photoinitiator being used, there is a need for a coinitiator to be added, the most efficient of which are usually aromatic compounds. The amine and the camphorquinone are stable in the presence of the oligomer at room temperature as long as the composite is not exposed to light.

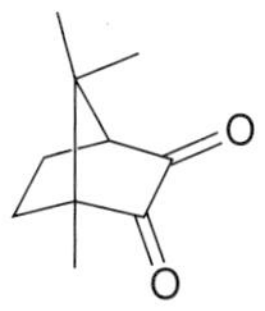

Camphorquinone

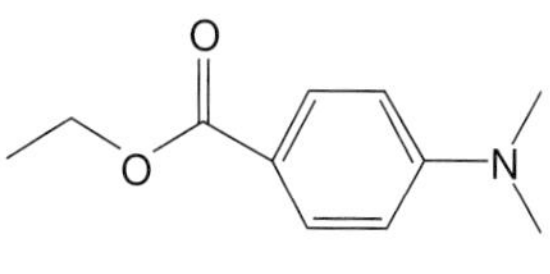

A typical amine

The alternative initiators, such as 1-phenyl-1,2 propanedione (PPD) and Bisacylphosphine oxides (BAPO), are α-cleavage-type initiators, which are directly cleaved by energy of light of the appropriate wavelength, typically in the near-UV range. They do not require the addition of an amine coinitiator, which is also advantageous from the aesthetics standpoint. Amines are typically added in excess and, over time, can oxidize and contribute to shade-matching deterioration. Some materials use a three-component initiator system, containing an electron acceptor such as an iodonium salt.

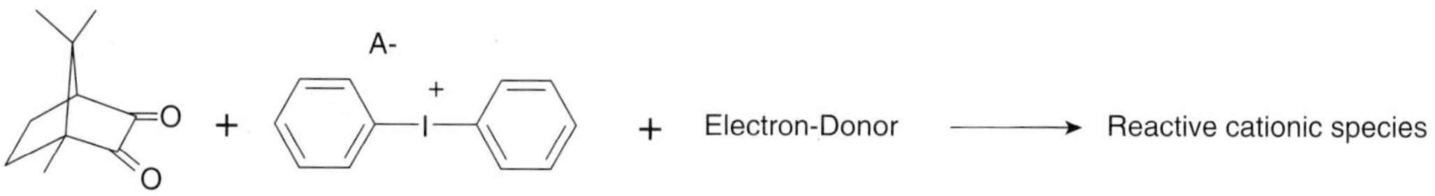

Chemical or dual activation products require that the organic amine (catalyst paste) and the organic peroxide (universal paste) are kept separate, each in a different container, just until before mixing. Once the two pastes are mixed, the polymerization reaction proceeds rapidly, as discussed in Chapter 5.

Some composites, such as core and provisional products, are dual-cured. These formulations contain initiators and accelerators that allow light activation followed by self-curing, or self-curing alone.

Pigments and Other Components

Inorganic oxides are usually added in small amounts to provide shades that match the majority of tooth shades. The most common pigments are oxides of iron. Numerous shades are supplied, ranging from very light shades to yellow to gray. Various color scales are used to characterize the shades of the composites. A UV absorber may be added to minimize color changes caused by oxidation. Darker and more opaque shades of composites cannot be cured to the same depth as the lighter translucent shades.

Fluorescent agents are sometimes added to enhance the optical vitality of the composite and mimic the appearance of natural teeth. These are dyes or pigments that absorb light in the UV and violet region (usually 340 to 370 nm) of the electromagnetic spectrum and reemit light in the blue region (typically 420–470 nm). These additives are often used to enhance the appearance of color, causing a perceived "whitening" effect, making materials look less yellow by increasing the overall amount of blue light reflected.

Polymerization Reactions

Polymerization of Methacrylate Composites

Methacrylate composites form the workhorse of direct restorative materials. The polymer network of these composites is formed by a process called free-radical addition polymerization of the corresponding methacrylate monomers, as already discussed in Chapter 5. This is shown in the following scheme:

Composites can actually be classified according to their polymerization reaction in self-cured, photo-cured, or dual-cured. The polymerization reaction of self-cured composites is chemically initiated at room temperature with a peroxide initiator and an amine accelerator. Polymerization of light-cured composites is triggered by visible blue light. The photoinitiators used are described in the section Initiators and Accelerators. Dual-cured products use a combination of chemical and light activation to carry out the polymerization reaction.

The polymerized resin is highly cross-linked because of the presence of difunctional carbon double bonds. The degree of polymerization varies, depending on whether it is in the bulk or in the air-inhibited layer of the restoration. Polymerization of light-cured composites varies by the distance of the light from the restoration and the duration of light exposure. The percentage of double bonds that react may vary from 35% to 80%. The degree of polymerization is higher for laboratory composites that are postcured at elevated temperatures and light intensities.

During polymerization, molecules have to approach their "neighbors" to form chemical bonds with them. Reduction of volume, or shrinkage, is generally observed during polymerization because two factors are reduced: the van der Waals volume and the free volume. The van der Waals volume is the volume of the molecule itself derived from the atoms and bond lengths. Reduction in the van der Waals volume takes place during polymerization because of a change in the bond lengths (conversion of double bonds to single bonds). The free volume of a molecular species, whether a monomer or a polymer, is the volume occupied by it due to its random rotational and thermal movement. When monomers are converted to polymers, reduction in the free volume occurs because the rotation of the polymer chain is more restricted than in unpolymerized monomer molecules. Shrinkage can be of concern because it may lead to the formation of gaps at the interface between the tooth and the restoration, which may lead to recurrent caries formation.

Manufacturers have taken several steps to minimize the polymerization contraction in composites by adopting one or more of the following methods:

- Filling the monomer resins with prepolymerized resins
- Maximizing the amount of inorganic filler
- Using high-molecular-weight methacrylate monomers
- Using monomers with a lower molar shrinkage coefficient, such as in epoxide-based materials.

Packaging of Composites

Composites, as supplied by the manufacturer, are in their uncured state and hence have to be packaged with adequate protection against inadvertent settings. The primary package is made from a plastic material that allows the diffusion of oxygen (which works as an inhibitor for methacrylate polymerization) and also prevents moisture absorption in humid environments.

Light-Cured Composites

Because the setting of light-cured composite is triggered by visible light, these materials have to be protected from premature curing when supplied by the manufacturer and stored in the dental office. Hence, they are packaged in opaque, most often black, plastic syringes or unit-dose capsules, sometimes referred to as compules. In the latter case, a delivery gun for direct intraoral placement is provided. An advantage of the capsule delivery is the lower risk of cross-infection. Composite packaging and delivery systems are shown in Fig. 8.8. The composites are supplied in a variety of shades and opacities. Some manufacturers color code their capsule caps or syringe plungers for ease of identification of the shades and/or opacities.

Self-Cured and Dual-Cured Composites

These materials are supplied in two syringes. Two pastes are mixed to initiate the chemical cure. An example of a two-paste core build-up composite is shown in Fig. 8.9. It is advisable to store these materials at a cool temperature to prolong their shelf-life.

Properties of Composites

To have good clinical service life, composites have to meet certain performance criteria. Important physical, mechanical, and clinical properties are described in this section. Selected properties of various types of composites are listed in Table 8.3. Values of properties for polymer-based filling and restorative materials based on ISO 4049 (ANSI/ADA No. 27) are summarized in Table 8.4.

Physical Properties

Working and Setting Times

For light-cured composites, curing is considered to be "on demand." Polymerization is initiated when the composite is first exposed to the curing light. Stiffening takes place within seconds after light exposure by a high-intensity curing light source.

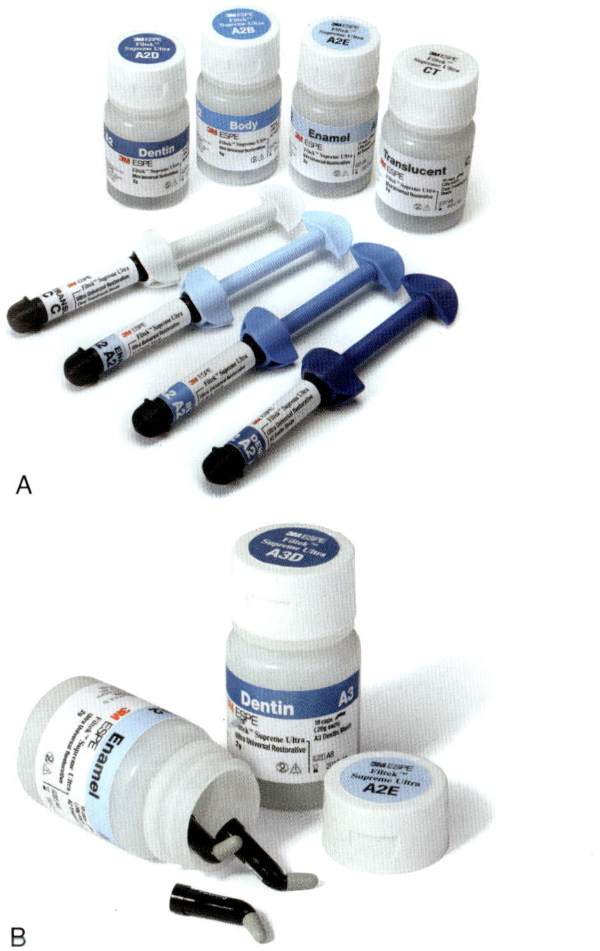

• **Fig. 8.8** Single-paste, visible light-initiated composite in syringe (A) and capsules (B) (Courtesy 3M Company, St. Paul, MN.)

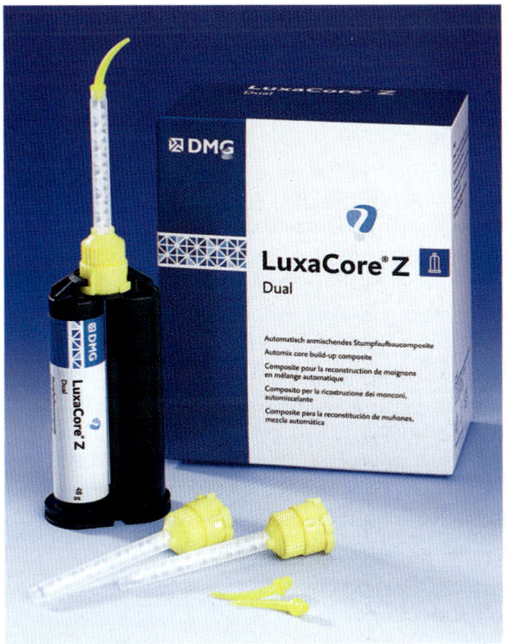

• **Fig. 8.9** Dual-curing composite for core build-ups. (Courtesy DMG Chemisch-Pharmazeutische Fabrik GmbH, Hamburg, Germany.)

TABLE 8.4 Requirements for Polymer-Based Filling and Restorative Materials Based on ISO 4049

Property	Class 1	Class 2	Class 3
Working time (min, seconds)	90	—	90
Setting time (max, min)	5	—	10
Depth of cure (min, mm)			
Opaque shades	—	1.0	—
Other shades	—	1.5	—
Water sorption (max, μg/mm³)	40	40	40
Solubility (max, μg/mm³)	7.5	7.5	7.5
Flexural strength (MPa)			
Type 1	80	80[a] 100[b]	80
Type 2	50	50[a]	50

[a]Group 1: cured intraorally.
[b]Group 2: cured extraorally.

Although the composite restoration appears hard and fully cured after exposure to the curing light source, the setting reaction continues for a period of 24 hours. All of the available unsaturated carbon double bonds of methacrylate-based composites do not react; studies report that about 25% remain unreacted in the bulk of the restoration. A thin layer of air-inhibited, unpolymerized material remains on the surface of the polymerized layer, which is advantageous for subsequent incremental placement during layering. It is useful to protect the surface of the contoured restoration with a transparent matrix, to minimize the amount of unpolymerized resin in the final restoration. Although for some composites, the final physical properties may not be reached until about 24 hours after the reaction is initiated, enough of the mechanical strength is attained immediately after curing, so the restoration can be finished and polished with abrasives and is functional.

For most composites that are initiated by visible light, bright operatory lights can initiate cure prematurely if the composite is left unprotected on a mixing pad. Within 60 to 90 seconds after exposure to ambient light, the surface of the composite may lose its capability to flow readily against the tooth, and further work with the material becomes difficult. The dispensed paste can be covered with an opaque or orange cover to present premature exposure to light.

The setting times for chemically activated composites range from 3 to 5 minutes. These short setting times have been accomplished by controlling the concentration of initiator and accelerator.

Polymerization Shrinkage and Stress

As explained in the section Polymerization Reactions, all composites undergo volumetric shrinkage upon setting. Typical shrinkage values are listed in Table 8.3. The issue with polymerization shrinkage is that it takes place under confinement within the cavity preparation. The composite is bonded to the cavity walls by the adhesive system, and as it shrinks, tensile contraction stresses as high as 13 MPa can be generated between the composite and the tooth structure. These stresses severely strain the interfacial bond between the composite and the tooth and, if the stresses are higher than the bond strength, this can lead to the formation of a very small gap that can allow marginal leakage of saliva and microorganisms. Recurrent caries and marginal staining may result. This stress can actually exceed the tensile strength of enamel and result in stress cracking and enamel fractures along the interfaces. Other than volumetric shrinkage, the overall degree of conversion and the stiffness of the composite also modulates the level of stress generated at the interface. In general, the greater the conversion, the greater the volumetric shrinkage (and therefore the higher the stress) and the greater the stiffness (or elastic modulus). Therefore, it is conceivable that low-shrinkage composites might exhibit high stress if it has a high elastic modulus. Adding the composite in 2-mm increments and polymerizing each increment independently can reduce the net effect of polymerization shrinkage. Net shrinkage stress is less because a smaller volume of composite is allowed to shrink before successive additions. A recent paper has reviewed the clinical and laboratory properties of several low-shrink/low-stress composites. Most of these products are universal composites but two products are described as flowable composites. The shrinkage values are dependent on the method used. Volumetric polymerization shrinkage for low-shrink universal composites using pycnometer varies from 0.9% to 1.8%, whereas that of low-shrink flowables is 2.4% to 2.5%. When the ACTA* linometer was used, the values were 1.0% to 1.4% and 2.6% to 2.9%, respectively. The polymerization stress was measured from 1.2 to 1.6 MPa. In comparison, traditional universal composites have been reported to have polymerization stress of 0.8 to 2.4 MPa, whereas flowables were reported to have stress values ranging from 1.3% to 3.2%. In any event, it is important to highlight that any measures taken in an attempt to modulate stress should not be at the expense of the conversion or the stiffness. Lower conversion increases cytotoxicity concerns due to the augmented potential for unreacted monomer leaching, and lower stiffness might lead to excessive deformation and fracture of the restoration.

Thermal Properties

The linear coefficient of thermal expansion (α) of composites ranges from 25 to 38 × 10^{-6}/°C for composites with fine particles to 55 to 68 × 10^{-6}/°C for composites with microfine particles. The α values for composites are less than the mean of the constituents added together; however, the values are higher than those for dentin (8.3 × 10^{-6}/°C) and enamel (11.4 × 10^{-6}/°C). The higher values for the microfilled composites are related mostly to the greater amount of polymer present. Certain glasses may be more effective in reducing the effect of thermal change than others, and some resins have more than one type of filler to compensate for differential rates.

Thermal stresses place an additional strain on the bond to tooth structure, which adds to the detrimental effect of the polymerization shrinkage. Thermal changes are also cyclic in nature, and although the entire restoration may never reach thermal equilibrium during the application of either hot or cold stimuli, the cyclic effect can lead to material fatigue and early bond failure. If a gap forms, the difference between the thermal coefficient of expansion of composites and teeth could permit *percolation* of oral fluids.

The thermal conductivity of composites with fine particles (25–30 × 10^{-4} cal/s/cm² [°C/cm]) is greater than that of composites with microfine particles (12–15 × 10^{-4} cal/s/cm² [°C/cm]) because of the higher conductivity of the inorganic fillers compared with the polymer matrix. However, for highly transient temperatures, the composites do not change temperature as fast as tooth structure, and this difference does not present a clinical problem.

Water Sorption

The water sorption of composites with hybrid particles (5–17 μg/mm³) is lower than that of composites with microfine particles (26–30 μg/mm³) because of the lower volume fraction of polymer in the composites with fine particles. The quality and stability of the silane coupling agent are important in minimizing the deterioration of the bond between the filler and polymer and the amount of water sorption. Expansion associated with the uptake of water from oral fluids could relieve some polymerization stress, but water sorption is a slow process when compared to polymerization shrinkage and stress development. In the measurement of hygroscopic expansion starting 15 minutes after the initial polymerization, most resins required 7 days to reach equilibrium and about 4 days to show the majority of expansion. Because composites with fine particles have lower values of water sorption than composites with microfine particles, they exhibit less expansion when exposed to water.

Solubility

The water solubility of composites varies from 0.25 to 2.5 mg/mm³. Inadequate light intensity and duration can result in insufficient polymerization, particularly at greater depths from the surface. Inadequately polymerized composites have greater water sorption and solubility, possibly manifested clinically with early color instability.

During the storage of microhybrid composites in water, the leaching of inorganic ions can be detected; such ions are associated with a breakdown in interfacial bonding. Silicon leaches in the greatest quantity (15–17 μg/mL) during the first 30 days of storage in water and decreases with time of exposure. Microfilled composites leach silicon more slowly and show a 100% increase in amount during the second 30-day period (14.2 μg/mL). Boron, barium, and strontium, which are present in glass fillers, are leached to various degrees (6–19 μg/mL) from the various resin-filler systems. Breakdown and leakage can be a contributing factor to the reduced resistance to wear and abrasion of composites.

Color and Color Stability

The color and blending of shades for the clinical match of aesthetic restorations are important. The characteristics of color are discussed in Chapter 4, and these principles can be applied specifically to composites for determining appropriate shades for clinical use. Universal shades vary in color among currently marketed products. Modern-day composites are often supplied by the manufacturer in multiple opacities. This allows for better aesthetic outcomes using multiple shades of different opacities to construct the restoration.

Change of color and loss of shade match with surrounding tooth structure are reasons for replacing restorations. Stress cracks within the polymer matrix and partial debonding of the filler to the resin as a result of hydrolysis tend to increase opacity and alter appearance. Discoloration can also occur by oxidation and result from water exchange within the polymer matrix and its interaction with unreacted polymer sites and unused initiator or accelerator.

Color stability of current composites has been studied by artificial aging in a weathering chamber (exposure to UV light and elevated temperatures of 70°C) and by immersion in various stains (coffee/tea, cranberry/grape juice, red wine, and sesame oil). As shown in Table 8.3, composites are resistant to color changes caused by oxidation but are susceptible to staining.

Mechanical Properties

Although composites take advantage of selected properties of each constituent material, the physical and mechanical properties of the composites are different from those of the separate phases.

*Academisch Centrum Tandheelkunde Amsterdan [Academic Center for Dentistry Amsterdan].

Factors that affect the properties of composites include (1) the state of matter of the second (dispersed) phase, including its degree of conversion; (2) the geometry of the second phase; (3) the orientation of the second phase; (4) the composition of the dispersed and continuous phases; (5) the ratio of the phases; and (6) bonding of the phases. Examples of properties that can be changed (improved if the composites are judiciously developed) are (1) modulus, (2) strength, (3) fracture toughness, (4) wear resistance, (5) thermal expansion, and (6) chemical and corrosion resistance.

Strength and Modulus

Values of compressive, tensile (tested by the diametral method), and flexural strengths and modulus for dental composites are listed in Table 8.3. Compressive strength is of importance because of the chewing forces. The flexural and compressive moduli of microfilled and flowable composites are about 50% lower than values for multipurpose hybrids and packable composites, which reflects the lower volume percent filler present in the microfilled and flowable composites (see Table 8.2). For comparison, the modulus of elasticity in compression is about 62 GPa for amalgam, 19 GPa for dentin, and 83 GPa for enamel.

Knoop Hardness

Knoop hardness for composites (22–80 kg/mm^2) is lower than enamel (343 kg/mm^2) or dental amalgam (110 kg/mm^2). The Knoop hardness of composites with fine particles is somewhat greater than values for composites with microfine particles because of the hardness and volume fraction of the filler particles. These values indicate a moderate resistance to indentation under functional stresses for more highly filled composites, but this difference does not appear to be a major factor in resisting functional wear.

A microhardness measurement such as Knoop can be misleading on composites with large filler particles (>10 μm in diameter), in which the small indentation could be made solely on the organic or the inorganic phase. However, with most current products, filler particle sizes are much smaller (<1 μm), and the microhardness values appear more reliable.

Bond Strength to Substrates Other Than the Tooth

Composite can be bonded to existing composite restorations, ceramics, and alloys when the substrate is roughened and appropriately primed (see Chapter 7). In general, the surface to be bonded is sandblasted (microetched) with 50-μm alumina and then treated with a resin-silane primer for composite, a silane primer for silica-based ceramics, an acidic phosphate monomer for zirconia, or a special alloy primer. Bond strengths to treated surfaces are typically greater than 20 MPa.

Clinical Properties

Clinical requirements for composites accepted for unrestricted use, including cuspal replacement in posterior teeth, as defined by the American Dental Association (Proposed) Guidelines for Resin-based Composites for Posterior Restorations, are listed in Table 8.5.

TABLE 8.5 Clinical Requirements for Resin Composites Accepted for Unrestricted Use, Including Cuspal Replacement, in Posterior Teeth

Property	Criteria
Maintenance of color (18 months)	No more than 10%
Marginal discoloration (18 months)	No more than 10%
Marginal integrity (18 months)	No more than 5%
Caries: recurrent or marginal (18 months)	No more than 5%
Maintenance of interproximal contact (18 months)	95% showing no observable broadening of contacts
Postoperative sensitivity	Thorough history of adverse sensitivity to hot, cold, and biting stimuli
Failure (18 months)	No more than 5%
Wear between 6 and 18 months	No more than 50 μm

Proposed American Dental Association guidelines for resin-based composites for posterior restorations.

Marginal Integrity

Marginal integrity refers to the non-disrupted sealing of the tooth-restoration interface. A composite restoration might lose its marginal integrity if: (1) the adhesive layer fails through hydrolysis of the adhesive materials and/or the collagen substrate network (Chapter 7); (2) the polymerization stress exceeds the bond strength of the adhesive to the tooth substrate; (3) the composite undergoes wear/fracture; or (4) the tooth itself cracks or chips. A breakdown in marginal integrity may lead to aesthetic concerns, such as staining and/or recurrent caries, which in turn can compromise the pulpal and, subsequently, periodontal tissues. It goes without saying that ensuring marginal integrity through proper technique and material selection is paramount to the longevity of the restoration. In some instances, the use of resin-modified glass ionomers (RMGI) in an open sandwich technique is recommended to preserve interfacial integrity when margins are in dentin (see video online for an example). More information on RMGIs can be found in Chapter 6.

Depth of Cure (Light-Cured Composites)

Light intensity decreases as the light source is moved away from the surface of an object. Furthermore, as the light travels through a scattering medium like a composite with filler particles, the light intensity is reduced. The depth of light penetration into a composite restoration depends on the wavelength of light, its irradiance, and the scattering that takes place within the restoration. A number of factors influence the degree of polymerization at given depths from the surface after light curing. The concentration of photoinitiator or light absorber in the composite must be such that it will react at the proper wavelength and be present in sufficient concentration. Both filler content and particle size are critical to dispersion of the light beam. For this reason, microfilled composites with smaller and more numerous particles scatter more light than microhybrid composites with larger and fewer glass particles. Longer exposure times are needed to obtain adequate polymerization of microfilled composites.

Another important consideration is the particular shade and opacity of the composite used. Many shades are intentionally opacified and have more pigments to mask discolored teeth after the removal of carious tissue. These materials have higher concentrations of opacifying agents and pigments that scatter more light and hence have lower depth of cure. In such cases, longer exposure times and smaller increments are essential for clinical success.

Light intensity at the surface is a critical factor in completeness of cure at the surface and within the material. The tip of the light source should be held within 1 mm of the surface to provide optimum exposure. More opaque shades reduce light transmission and cure only to minimal depths (1 mm). A standard exposure time using most dental curing lights is 20 seconds. In general, this is sufficient to cure a light shade of resin to a depth of 2 or 2.5 mm, assuming that the light guide is immediately adjacent to the restoration surface. The anatomy of the tooth often precludes the positioning of the light guide close to the restoration surface. A 40-second exposure improves the degree of cure at all depths and is required to obtain sufficient cure with the darker shades. Because the light beam is partially collimated and does not spread sufficiently beyond the diameter of the tip at the emitting surface, it is necessary to "step" the light across the surface of large restorations so the entire surface receives a complete exposure. Larger tips have been manufactured for placement on most light-curing units. However, as the light beam is distributed over a larger surface area, the intensity at a given point is reduced. A longer exposure time of up to 60 seconds should be used when larger emitting tips are used.

Bulk-fill composites, which theoretically allow for curing of up to 4 mm thick increments, have been introduced in recent years. Those will be discussed separately.

Radiopacity

It is rather difficult to locate enamel-composite margins radiographically because of the relatively low radiopacity of composites. Modern composites include glasses having atoms with high atomic numbers, such as barium, strontium, and zirconium. Some fillers, such as quartz, lithium–aluminum glasses, and silica, are not radiopaque and must be blended with other fillers to produce a radiopaque composite. Even at the highest volume fraction of filler, the amount of radiopacity is noticeably less than that exhibited by a metallic restorative like amalgam. Some microhybrid composites achieve some radiopacity by incorporating finely divided heavy-metal glass particles. Others use ceramic particles containing heavy-metal oxides. In the nanofilled composite, radiopacity is achieved by using nanomeric zirconia (5–7 nm) or by incorporating the zirconia in the nanoclusters along with silica.

Wear Rates

Under clinical conditions, a composite restoration comes in contact with other surfaces, such as the opposing tooth, food particles, and oral fluids, which can result in surface wear and degradation. The extent of wear is a complex phenomenon and depends on several intrinsic and extrinsic factors that are elaborated in Chapter 4 and in the online-only materials. Many in vitro wear studies have been reported but because there are many different methodologies used, standardization and direct comparison of these results with actual clinical performance are not available. It is advisable to look at controlled clinical studies when choosing a composite, particularly for posterior restorations.

Clinical studies have shown that composites are ideal for anterior restorations in which aesthetics are essential and occlusal forces are low. Wear rates are a larger concern in the posterior segments, where occlusal forces and lateral excursive contacts are higher than in the anterior segment. Although earlier generations of composites exhibited attrition and abrasion wear, newer formulations minimize the problem. Marginal degradation is still evident and is attributed to improper preparation design, inadequate adhesion, polymerization contraction of the composite, and marginal microcracks. Marginal degradation and stain are sometimes interpreted as recurrent caries, although this is not always the case. Currently, accepted composites for posterior applications require clinical studies that demonstrate, over an 18-month period, a loss of surface contour less than 50 μm. Several clinical studies have been published showing that the newest generation of filled composite (nanocomposite) has excellent wear resistance. The nanofilled composite has been shown to exhibit wear resistance similar to that of natural human enamel in a 3-year and 5-year clinical study.

Biocompatibility

Details about the biocompatibility of composites are discussed in the online-only materials, but some of the central issues are discussed here. Nearly all of the major components of composites (Bis-GMA, TEGDMA, and UDMA, among others) are cytotoxic in vitro if tested as the bulk monomer, but the biological liability of a cured composite depends on the extent of release of these components from the composite. Although composites may release some low levels of components for weeks after curing, there is considerable controversy about the biological effects of these components. The amount of release depends on the type of composite and the method and efficiency of the cure of the composite. A dentin barrier markedly reduces the ability of components to reach pulpal tissues, but these components can traverse dentin barriers, albeit at reduced concentrations. The effects of low-dose, long-term exposures of cells to resin components are not generally known. By contrast, the use of composite materials as direct pulp-capping agents poses a higher risk for adverse biological responses because no dentin barrier exists to limit exposure of the pulp to the released components.

The effects of released components from composites on oral or other tissues are not known with certainty, although no studies have documented any adverse biological effects. The ISO standard for testing of toxicity of dental materials requires the testing of composites after immersion in various aqueous and organic elution media followed by the testing of the eluants for adverse biological response. The tissue at highest risk from this type of release would appear to be the mucosa in close, long-term contact with composites. Components of composites are known allergens, and there has been some documentation of contact allergy to composites. Most of these reactions occur with dentists or dental personnel who regularly handle uncured composite and, therefore, have the greatest exposure. There are no good studies documenting the frequency of allergy to composites in the general population.

Finally, there has been some controversy about the ability of components of composites to act as xenoestrogens. Studies have proved that bisphenol A is estrogenic in in vitro tests that measure this effect using breast cancer cell growth. Trace levels of these components have been identified in some commercial uncured composites; however, estrogenicity from cured commercial composites has not been demonstrated. Furthermore, there is considerable controversy about the accuracy and utility of in vitro tests using breast cancer cells to measure a true estrogenic effect. An early study in this area, which claimed that dental sealants and composites were estrogenic in children, has since been discredited.

Manipulation of composites can be found on the book's website at http://evolve.elsevier.com/sakaguchi/restorative

Composites for Special Applications

Bulk-Fill Composites

Bulk-fill composites (Fig. 8.10) have been developed to enable the restoration to be built up in thick layers of up to 4 mm and are recommended by manufacturers to simplify clinical technique and save time compared to traditional incremental placement.

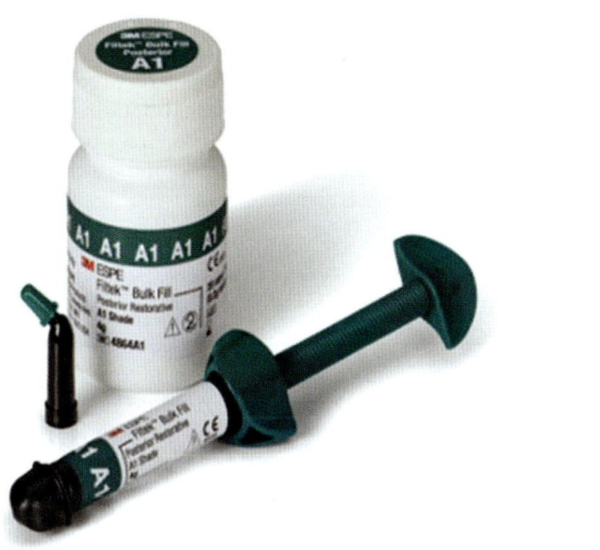

• **Fig. 8.10** A bulk-fill composite. (Filtek, Courtesy 3M Company, St. Paul, MN.)

Although the idea of bulk fill is not new, and several materials have been available over the years, recently, there has been a surge of interest in these materials. A host of new products, including both flowable and high-viscosity pastes, have become available from various manufacturers. There are several approaches that the manufacturers use in an attempt to achieve greater depth of cure through the bulk of the material. The first one is to use either lower filler concentration or fillers with a refractive index that more closely matches that of the organic matrix, both aiming to facilitate light penetration. Because of the translucency limitation, these materials are available only in a limited range of shades. Another strategy is to use initiators that are capable of more efficiently reacting even as light intensity decreases with depth, one such example being a product incorporating a new germanium initiator to enable greater cure depths. These composites are recommended for use primarily in class 1 and 2 cavity preparations, although their use is not contraindicated for other classes as long as there is adequate shade match with the surrounding tooth (see Table 8.1).

A number of approaches have been taken to control polymerization shrinkage stress as well as provide good marginal adaptation to the axial walls and floor of the cavity due to bulk filling. In one approach, a rheology modifier that responds to sonic energy has been incorporated into the composite paste. This allows for a decrease in viscosity of the initially thick paste to provide good adaptation to the cavity surfaces. In other approaches, materials have been formulated to include modulators of the polymerization reaction and thus relieve shrinkage stress. These include the incorporation of a light-sensitive monomer that cleaves when exposed to light, the addition of an addition-fragmentation monomer that provides network rearrangement during polymerization and leads to stress relaxation, and the addition of special fillers with low elastic modulus to absorb stresses during polymerization.

The flowable bulk-fill composites appear to have better curing efficiency than the high-viscosity ones. Typical physical properties are listed in Table 8.3. In general, mechanical and physical properties cured in larger depths appear to be within normal range of incrementally placed traditional composites. In addition, important properties include greater depth of cure compared to traditional composites. In several cases, the measured volumetric shrinkage may be similar to traditional composites, but the shrinkage stress is lower. There is increasing clinical performance data on the recent bulk-fill composites and those corroborate the results reported from in vitro studies. The quality of marginal adaptation seems to be comparable to incrementally placed composites, although a few studies have shown equivocal results for bulk-fill materials. A few long-term clinical studies have become available, and several systematic reviews and meta-analysis studies seem to indicate that these materials have similar performance to their conventional counterparts. However, the ultimate clinical effectiveness of these newer bulk-fill composite materials will become apparent as more high-quality evidence clinical studies are published.

Flowable Composites

These light-activated, low-viscosity composites are recommended for cervical lesions, restorations in deciduous teeth, and other small, low- or nonstress-bearing restorations (see Table 8.1). In much of the older dental literature, these are also referred to as flowable composites. Typically, they are delivered through a needle tip attached to the head of the syringe. In some instances, they are also used as pit and fissure sealants. These composites contain dimethacrylate resin and inorganic fillers with a particle size of 0.4 to 3.0 μm and filler loading of 42% to 53% by volume (see Table 8.2). These low-viscosity composite materials typically show shear thinning (pseudoplasticity). When expressed through a syringe tip, there is a reversible structural breakdown due to disruption of the hydrogen bonds between the polymer and filler. After the material has been placed, the hydrogen bonds reform very quickly so that the material does not slump.

The newest generation of flowable composites contains nanofiller particles at a volume loading somewhat lower than universal or multipurpose composites. Recently, self-adhesive flowable composites (commonly referred to as self-adhesive flowable) have become available. Dual-cured flowable composites, in conjunction with bonding agents, have been used in the treatment of internal resorption. This technique seals the dentinal tubules and strengthens the remaining tooth structure.

Typical properties of these composites are listed in Table 8.3. Flowable composites have a low modulus of elasticity, which may make them useful in cervical abfraction areas. Because of their lower filler content, they exhibit higher polymerization shrinkage and lower wear resistance than universal composites. The viscosity of these composites allows them to be dispensed by a syringe with a needle tip for easy handling. Gentle heating of higher-viscosity composites can improve their flow and enable them to be placed as flowable composites.

Laboratory Composites

Laboratory composites are used to fabricate dental prosthetic devices extraorally and then affixed to the tooth preparation with the aid of adhesives. Although the newest generations of direct composites have excellent properties, their use can still be a challenge for large cavities with high C-factors due to concerns of polymerization stress leading to microleakage, postoperative sensitivity, poor interproximal margins, and recurrent caries. In such cases, a prefabricated and indirectly placed laboratory composite is clinically preferred. The basic composition of the laboratory composites is similar to the new generation of direct composites prior

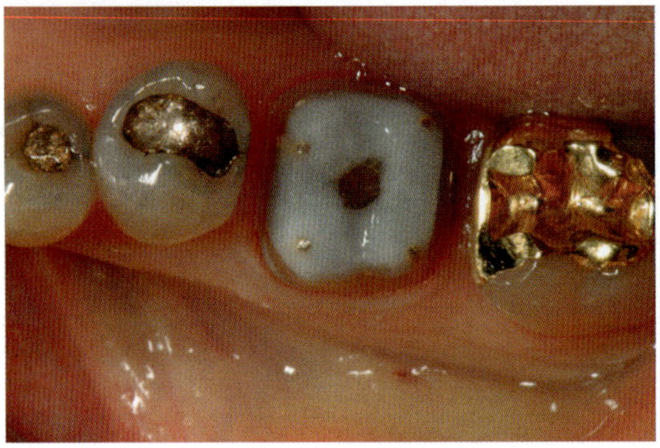

• **Fig. 8.11** A reconstructed composite resin core prepared for a cast metal crown. (Courtesy Dr. Charles Mark Malloy, Portland, OR.)

to the polymerization step. Crowns, inlays, and veneers bonded to metal copings can be prepared with composites processed in the laboratory (see Table 8.1) using various combinations of light, heat, pressure, and vacuum to increase the degree of polymerization, density, mechanical properties, and wear resistance.

Typical properties of laboratory composites are listed in Table 8.3. Although their ultimate mechanical properties are not as high as ceramic restorations, due to their lower modulus and stress absorption capacity, these polymeric composites are often the materials of choice for certain clinical situations where a considerable amount of masticatory force is transmitted to the restoration (e.g., coronal restoration on a dental implant). For increased strength and rigidity, laboratory composites can be combined with fiber reinforcement. Restorations are usually bonded with resin cements.

Core Build-Up Composites

If sufficient tooth structure remains to retain and support a full-coverage restoration, but extensive regions of dentin have been lost to disease, the core of the tooth can be restored before final preparation and impression. Composites are commonly used in this application. Core composites are available as self-cured, light-cured, and dual-cured products. Core composites are usually tinted (blue, white, or opaque) to provide a contrasting color with the tooth structure. Some products release fluoride. An example of a composite core build-up is shown in Fig. 8.11. Typical properties of core composites are listed in Table 8.3.

Composite cores have the following advantages as compared with amalgam: they can be bonded to dentin, can be finished immediately, are easy to contour, and can have a more natural color under ceramic restorations. Composite cores are bonded to remaining enamel and dentin using bonding agents. A bonding agent recommended by the manufacturer of the core material should be used because some self-cured composite core materials are incompatible with some light-cured bonding agents. Retention of the final restoration should not rely on the composite structure alone because adhesion of the composite core to remaining dentin alone is insufficient to resist rotation and dislodgement of the crown.

Provisional Composites

Provisional restorations maintain the position of the prepared tooth, seal and insulate the preparation and protect the margins, establish proper vertical dimension, aid in diagnosis and treatment planning, and help evaluate candidates for aesthetic replacements. Provisional inlays, crowns, and fixed partial dentures are usually fabricated from acrylic resins or composites. Provisional restorations fabricated from composites are generally harder, stiffer, and more color stable than those made from acrylics.

Light-Curing Units

The most common light sources used in dentistry to photoactivate composites are quartz-tungsten-halogen (QTH) and blue light-emitting diode (LED). Definitions of terms that describe light sources used to activate dental resins are listed in Table 8.6.

Quartz-Tungsten-Halogen Light-Curing Units

Quartz-tungsten-halogen light-curing units have a broad emission spectrum and can be used to activate polymerization of composites. The wavelength ranges covered are usually between 400 and 500 nm, with peak wavelength emission at 450 to 490 nm (there are some variations among the different commercial units). Typically, the irradiance ranges from 600 to 1000 mW/cm^2, but higher-intensity QTH units are available. Some units can be controlled to provide two or three different intensities (step cure) or at a continuously increasing (ramp cure) intensity. A typical 2-mm-thick resin composite restoration requires a radiant exposure of 16 J/cm^2 (800 mW/cm^2 × 20 seconds = 16 J/cm^2) for proper polymerization.

A QTH light source consists of a broad-spectrum light bulb (typically 75 W), several filters, a reflector, a fan, a power supply, and a light guide. The broad-spectrum output of the QTH bulb is clipped by a blue bandpass filter that only allows a narrow band of wavelengths centered around 470 to 480 nm (blue wavelengths) to be transferred to the light guide. A UV filter blocks the passage of UV wavelengths. A dichroic reflector focuses the light on the end of the light guide. The reflector also enables infrared wavelengths

TABLE 8.6 Definitions of Terms Used to Describe Light Sources for Polymerization of Dental Resins

Term	Unit	Definition
Spectral emission	nm	Effective bandwidth of wavelengths emitted by light source
Spectral requirement	nm	Bandwidth of wavelengths required to activate photoinitiator(s) of dental resin
Flux	mW	Number of photons per second emitted by light source
Irradiance or radiant exitance	mW/cm^2	Number of photons per second emitted by light source per unit area of curing tip
Energy	J[a]	Flux × time
Energy density	J/cm^2	Radiant exitance × time

[a]Joule (J) = 1000 mW × s

TABLE 8.7 Factors Causing Decrease in Intensity of Light from Quartz-Tungsten-Halogen Light-Curing Units and Maintenance Hints

Factors	Maintenance Hints
Dust or deterioration of reflector	Clean or replace reflector
Burn-out of bulb filament	Replace bulb
Darkening/frosting of bulb	Replace bulb
Age of components	Monitor intensity, replace unit
Chipping of light tip	Replace light tip
Resin deposit on light tip	Clean or replace light tip
Change in line voltage	Get built-in voltage regulator
Lack of uniformity across light tip	Overlap curing on larger surface
Increased distance of tip from material to be cured	Keep light tip close to material

to dissipate as heat through the back of the housing. Because substantial heat is generated by the 75 W bulb, a fan is necessary to cool the bulb and assembly. Bulb life ranges from 50 to 75 hours. Some lamps produce considerable heat at the curing tip, which may produce pulpal irritation. Maintenance of QTH lights must be provided on a regular basis, as summarized in Table 8.7.

Blue Light-Emitting Diodes

Solid-state LEDs use junctions of doped semiconductors (p-n junctions) based on gallium nitride to emit blue light. The spectral output of blue LEDs is much narrower, and there are several types on the market. All commercially available LED curing units (Fig. 8.12) have at least one chip with spectral output between 450 and 490 nm, so these units are effective for curing materials with camphorquinone photoinitiators. The first few models on the market only had this range of output and are known now as "mono-wave LEDs." More modern LED units have multiple chips ("poly-wave LEDs"), some of which cover the 450–490 nm wavelength range and some of which cover the 390–420 nm wavelength range. The need for poly-wave LED units arose from the introduction of highly aesthetic materials. Some composite shades are very light to match teeth that have undergone bleaching, so

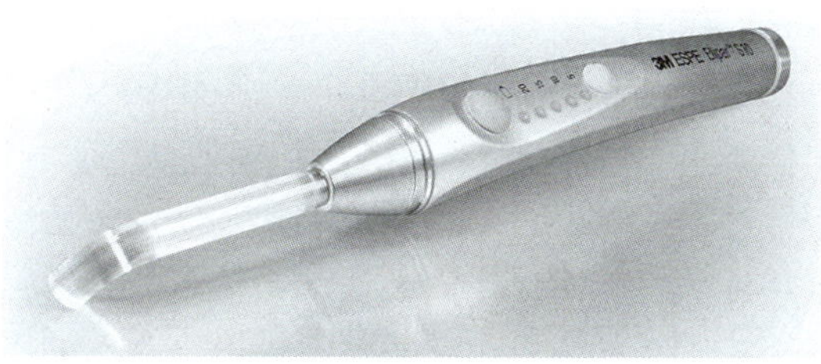

• **Fig. 8.12** LED source for photoinitiation. (Espe Elipar S10, Courtesy 3M Company, St. Paul, MN.)

there is a need to replace part of the deep yellow camphorquinone with colorless alternative photoinitiators, such as PPD or BAPO. It is then paramount to match the spectral output of the light-curing unit and the absorbance spectrum of the photoinitiator (Fig. 8.13) to ensure proper cure of the composite. LED units do not require a filter, have a long life span, and do not produce as much heat as QTH devices. However, heat becomes a concern even with LED sources when very high irradiances are produced by the light.

It is also important to note that for poly-wave LED light-curing units, as the light penetrates through the composite, the loss of intensity is not equal for each of the different wavelengths (Fig. 8.14). The intensity of the near-UV wavelength is lower, to begin with, and it decreases more rapidly. This is especially important if thicker increments were to be used, as is the case in bulk-fill composites.

Unlike the halogen lights, the heat generated from LED curing lights is much less, which means it does not require a fan to cool it; however, the heat at the tip of the light can be high. Thus these are lighter in weight and smaller than the halogen units. Because LEDs inherently have low consumption of power, they can use rechargeable batteries, making them portable. The newer generation of LED lights has dramatically decreased in size and is lighter, more ergonomic, and easier to use. They are also high powered and emit light intensity of 1000 to 1400 mW/cm^2. This feature allows more efficient and deeper curing depths. Some models are available with a "turbo" function, and can reach up to 3400 mW/cm^2, which theoretically would allow for very short exposure times. However, these should be used with extreme caution because the potential for heat generation is amplified, and damage to pulpal and gingival tissues might occur. There is also

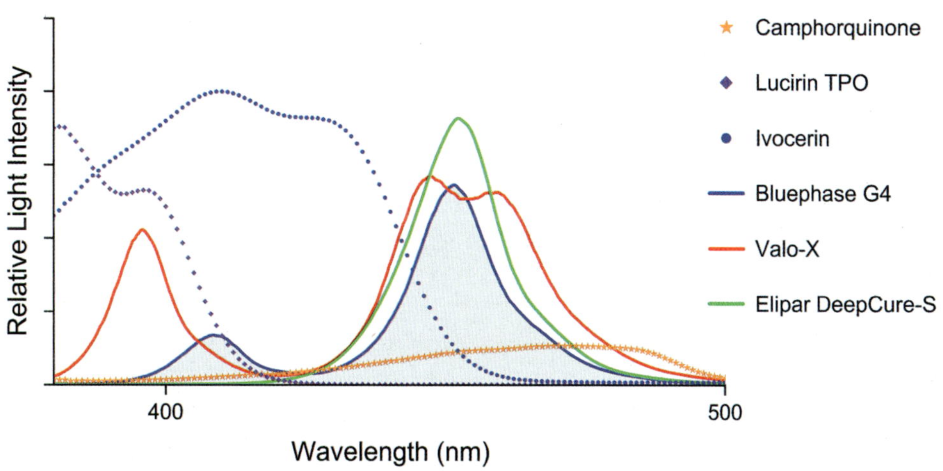

• **Fig. 8.13** Overlaying spectral output and absorbance spectra for common commercial light-curing units and initiators, respectively. Note that the single-wave LED curing units do not provide adequate spectral output for a near-UV initiator (Lucirin TPO). (Used with permission of Dr. Richard Price.)

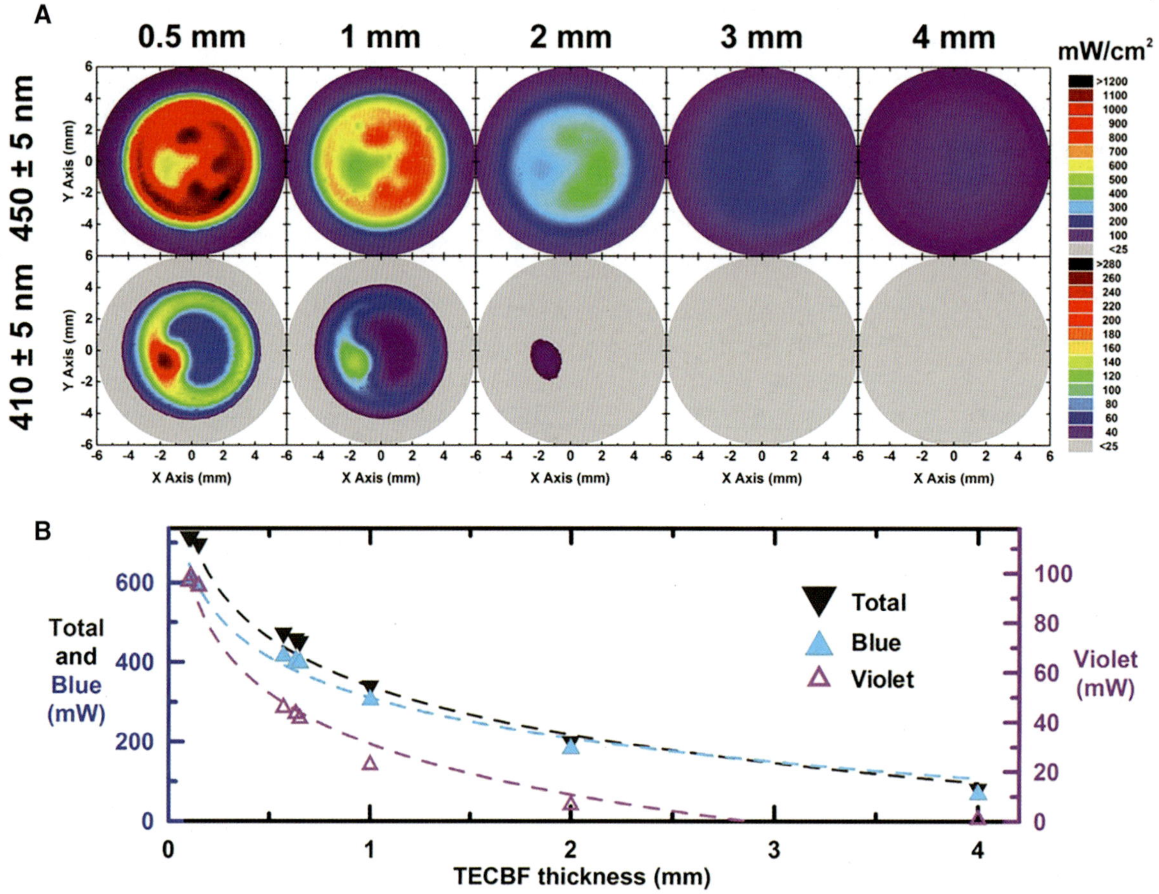

• **Fig. 8.14** Light intensity decreases through the bulk of a composite material for a poly-wave LED curing unit. Loss of energy is much more noticeable for the near-UV wavelength, which starts out lower to begin with. (From Harlow JE, Rueggeberg FA, Labrie D, Sullivan B, Price RB. Transmission of violet and blue light through conventional (layered) and bulk cured resin-based composites. *J Dent*. 2016;53:44–50. https://doi.org/10.1016/j.jdent.2016.06.007.)

the concern with the extremely short exposure times because reciprocity does not always hold true. For example, the properties of a material cured at 800 mW/cm^2 for 20 s might be different than those of a material cured at 3200 mW/cm^2 for 5 s, even if both of those regimens deliver a total energy of 16 J/cm^2. In general, extremely short exposure times at high intensity, other than the heat generation concern already mentioned, may also lead to inferior mechanical properties.

Blue Light Hazards

Irrespective of the type of light-curing unit, because of the high intensity, the operator should not look directly at the tip or the reflected light from the teeth. A number of devices are marketed, including special goggles and shields, to filter the visible-light beam so the operator can directly observe the curing procedure and protect the patient and staff. The hazard from blue light exposure has been well-documented in the past several years, and there is risk of serious damage to the retina of dental care personnel.

Prosthetic Applications of Polymers

Acrylic polymers have a wide variety of applications in restorative dentistry as denture bases, artificial teeth, denture repair materials, impression trays, provisional restorations, and maxillofacial appliances for skeletal defects.

The vast majority of dentures made today are fabricated from heat-cured poly(methyl methacrylate) and rubber-reinforced poly(methyl methacrylate). Fractures of dentures still occur but are usually associated with carelessness or unreasonable use by the patient. Considering functional stresses, the oral environment, and expected service life, denture base materials perform remarkably well.

Physical Form and Composition

Denture base plastics are commonly supplied in a powder-liquid or a gel form. The powder-liquid type may contain the materials listed in Box 8.1.

Powder

Most commercial materials contain poly(methyl methacrylate), modified with small amounts of ethyl, butyl, or other alkyl methacrylates to produce a polymer somewhat more resistant to fracture by impact. The powder also contains an initiator such as benzoyl peroxide or diisobutylazonitrile to initiate the polymerization of the monomer liquid after being added to the powder.

The peroxide initiator may be added to the polymer or be present as a residual from the polymerization reaction and is present in amounts from 0.5% to 1.5%.

• BOX 8.1 Principal Ingredients of Acrylic Denture Base: Powder and Liquid

Powder

Acrylic polymer (or copolymer) beads
Initiator
Pigments
Dyes
Opacifier
Plasticizer
Dyed organic fibers
Inorganic particles

Liquid

Monomer
Inhibitor
Accelerator
Plasticizer
Cross-linking agent

Pure polymers, such as poly(methyl methacrylate), are clear and adaptable to a wide range of pigmentation. Colorants are added to obtain the various tissue-like shades, and zinc or titanium oxides are used as opacifiers. Dyed synthetic fibers made from nylon or acrylic are usually added to simulate the small capillaries of the oral mucosa.

Plasticizers such as dibutyl phthalate may be incorporated into the powder or the monomer. Adding glass fibers and alumina (sapphire) whiskers increases the stiffness, decreases the thermal coefficient of expansion, and increases thermal diffusivity. Polyethylene-woven yarn and polyaramid fabric have also been used to reinforce acrylic polymers.

Liquid

The liquid component of the powder-liquid type acrylic resin is methyl methacrylate, but it may be modified by the addition of other monomers. Because these monomers may be polymerized by heat, light, or traces of oxygen, inhibitors are added to give the liquid adequate shelf-life. The inhibitor most commonly used to prevent premature polymerization is hydroquinone, which may be present in concentrations of 0.003% to 0.1%.

When a chemical accelerator rather than heat is used to speed up the peroxide decomposition and enable the polymerization of the monomer at room temperature, an accelerator is included in the liquid. Common accelerators are amines, such as *N,N*-dimethyl-para-toluidine, and *N,N*-dihydroxyethyl-para-toluidine. These systems are referred to as *self-curing, cold-curing*, or *autopolymerizing resins*. The pour type of denture resin is included in this category.

Plasticizers are sometimes added to produce a softer, more resilient polymer. They are generally relatively low-molecular-weight esters, such as dibutyl phthalate. Plasticizer molecules do not enter the polymerization reaction but do interfere with the interaction between polymer molecules, making the plasticized polymer softer than the pure polymer. One disadvantage of using plasticizers is that they gradually leach out of the plastic into oral fluids, resulting in hardening of the denture base. A polymer also may be plasticized by the addition of some higher ester, such as butyl or octyl methacrylate, to methyl methacrylate. The esters polymerize and form a more flexible plastic. This type of internal plasticizing does not leach out in the oral fluids, and the material remains flexible.

If a cross-linked polymer is desired, organic compounds such as glycol dimethacrylate are added to the monomer. Cross-linking compounds are characterized by reactive –CR=CH– groups at opposite ends of the molecules and serve to link long polymer molecules together. Using cross-linking agents provides greater resistance to minute surface cracking, termed "crazing", and may decrease solubility and water sorption. Cross-linking materials may be present in amounts of 2% to 14% but have little effect on the tensile strength, flexural properties, or hardness of acrylic plastics.

A discussion of the properties of denture plastics for dental bases, other properties of dental polymers, and denture teeth can be found on the book's website at http://evolve.elsevier.com/sakaguchi/restorative.

Non-restorative Uses for Polymers: Athletic Mouth Protectors

Polymers are used in fabricating mouth protectors because they can be formed to fit the occlusal surfaces, they are lightweight, and they are resilient. Mouth protectors are routinely used in football, soccer, ice hockey, basketball, wrestling, field hockey, softball, and other sports. As a result of the possibility of orofacial injury, high school athletes are required to wear internal mouth protectors, and the National Collegiate Athletic Association (NCAA) has adopted a mouth protector rule. As a result of these actions, more professional athletes are wearing mouth protectors. Because of the increased use of mouth protectors, it is estimated that 50,000 orofacial injuries are prevented each year.

The rationale for the use of mouth protectors is that the mouth protector acts like a shock absorber when the athlete receives a blow to the mouth or chin. The mouth protector absorbs 80% to 90% of the energy of the blow and distributes the remaining energy uniformly to the entire arch, resulting in less trauma to the oral structures.

Stock, mouth-formed (boil-and-bite), and custom mouth protectors are the three types available and all provide some protection to the athlete. Custom-made mouth protectors are usually vacuum formed from sheets of flexible, thermoplastic polymers about 14 cm^2 in area and 1.6 to 3 mm in thickness; they may be clear or colored. In most instances, the sheets are of a single material, but they may be laminates of two or more thermoplastic polymers. Laminated mouth protectors are fabricated so that the softer of the two layers contact the teeth and soft tissue.

Most sheets for custom mouth protectors are vinyl acetate-ethylene copolymers. Manufacturers use several different hardnesses of the material, with copolymers containing more polyethylene being harder.

The advantages of custom-made mouth protectors are (1) excellent fit, (2) comfort, (3) ease of speaking, and (4) durability; these qualities are poor for stock protectors and poor to good for mouth-formed protectors. In spite of the advantages of custom-made protectors, they are not as common as stock or mouth-formed protectors because of their higher cost.

Bibliography

History

Wilson AD, Batchelor RF. Dental silicate cements. I. The chemistry of erosion. *J Dent Res*. 1967;46:1075.

Composites

Asmussen E. Clinical relevance of physical, chemical, and bonding properties of composite resins. *Oper Dent*. 1985;10:61.

Bayne SC, Thompson JY, Swift EJ Jr, et al. A characterization of first-generation flowable composites. *J Am Dent Assoc.* 1998;129:567.

Braem M, Davidson CL, Lambrechts P, et al. In vitro flexural fatigue limits of dental composites. *J Biomed Mater Res.* 1994;28:1397.

Braem M, Finger W, Van Doren VE, et al. Mechanical properties and filler fraction of dental composites. *Dent Mater.* 1989;5:346.

Braga RR, Ferracane JL. Alternatives in polymerization contraction stress management. *Crit Rev Oral Biol Med.* 2004;15:176.

Bunek SS. Bioactive materials: where are we now? *Dent Advis.* 2015;32(8):1.

Bunek SS. Update on composites. *Dent Advis.*. 2015;32(3):1.

Choi KK, Condon JR, Ferracane JL. The effects of adhesive thickness on polymerization contraction stress of composite. *J Dent Res.* 2000;79:812.

Condon JR, Ferracane JL. Factors affecting dental composite wear in vitro. *J Biomed Mater Res.* 1997;38:303.

Condon JR, Ferracane JL. In vitro wear of composite with varied cure, filler level, and filler treatment. *J Dent Res.* 1997;76:1405.

Council on Scientific Affairs. Posterior resin-based composites. *J Am Dent Assoc.* 1998;129:1627.

Cross M, Douglas WH, Fields RP. The relationship between filler loading and particle-size distribution in composite resin technology. *J Dent Res.* 1983;62:850.

Dauvillier BS, Feilzer AJ, de Gee AJ, et al. Visco-elastic parameters of dental restorative materials during setting. *J Dent Res.* 2000;79:818.

Doray PG, Wang X, Powers JM, et al. Accelerated aging affects color stability of provisional restorative materials. *J Prosthodont.* 1997;6:183.

El Hejazi AA, Watts DC. Creep and visco-elastic recovery of cured and secondary-cured composites and resin-modified glass-ionomers. *Dent Mater.* 1999;15:138.

Eldiwany M, Powers JM, George LA. Mechanical properties of direct and post-cured composites. *Am J Dent.* 1993;6:222.

Feilzer AJ, de Gee AJ, Davidson CL. Quantitative determination of stress reduction by flow in composite restorations. *Dent Mater.* 1990;6:167.

Feilzer AJ, de Gee AJ, Davidson CL. Setting stress in composite resin in relation to configuration of the restoratives. *J Dent Res.* 1987;66:1636.

Ferracane JL, Mitchem JC, Condon JR, et al. Wear and marginal breakdown of composites with various degrees of cure. *J Dent Res.* 1997;76:1508.

Ferracane JL, Moser JB. Greener EH. Rheology of composite restoratives. *J Dent Res.* 1981;60:1678.

Ferracane JL. Current trends in dental composites. *Crit Rev Oral Biol Med.* 1995;6:302.

Ferracane JL. Developing a more complete understanding of stresses produced in dental composites during polymerization. *Dent Mater.* 2005;21:36.

Filho HN, D'Azevedo MTFS, Nagem HD, Marsola FP. Surface roughness of composite resins after finishing and polishing. *Braz Dent J.* 2003;14:37.

Geurtsen W. Biocompatibility of resin-modified filling materials. *Crit Rev Oral Biol Med.* 2000;11:333.

Hanks CT, Strawn SE, Wataha JC, et al. Cytotoxic effects of composite resin components on cultured mammalian fibroblasts. *J Dent Res.* 1991;70:1450.

Hanks CT, Wataha JC, Parsell RR, et al. Permeability of biological and synthetic molecules through dentine. *J Oral Rehabil.* 1994;21:475.

Hu X, Harrington E, Marquis PM, et al. The influence of cyclic loading on the wear of a dental composite. *Biomaterials.* 1999;20:907.

Hu X, Marquis PM. Shortall AC. Two-body in vitro wear study of some current dental composites and amalgams. *J Prosthet Dent.* 1999;82:214.

Labella R, Lambrechts P, Van Meerbeek B, et al. Polymerization shrinkage and elasticity of flowable composites and filled adhesives. *Dent Mater.* 1999;15:128.

Lee Y-K, El Zawahry M, Noaman KM, et al. Effect of mouthwash and accelerated aging on the color stability of esthetic restorative materials. *Am J Dent.* 2000;13:159.

Lu H, Roeder LB, Powers JM. Effect of polishing systems on the surface roughness of microhybrid composites. *J Esthet Restor Dent.* 2003;15:297.

Manhart J, Kunzelmann K-H, Chen HY, et al. Mechanical properties and wear behavior of light-cured packable composite resins. *Dent Mater.* 2000;16:33.

Mitra SB, Wu D, Holmes BN. An application of nanotechnology in advanced dental materials. *J Am Dent Assoc.* 2003;134:1382.

Ortengren U, Wellendorf H, Karlsson S, et al. Water sorption and solubility of dental composites and identification of monomers released in an aqueous environment. *J Oral Rehabil.* 2001;28:1106.

Paravina RD, Ontiveros JC, Powers JM. Accelerated aging effects on color and translucency of bleaching-shade composites. *J Esthet Restor Dent.* 2004;16:117.

Perry R, Kugel G, Kunzelmann K-H, et al. Composite restoration wear analysis: conventional methods vs. three-dimensional laser digitizer. *J Am Dent Assoc.* 2000;131:1472.

Powers JM, Burgess JO. Performance standards for competitive dental restorative materials. *Trans Acad Dent Mater.* 1996;9:68.

Powers JM, Hostetler RW, Dennison JB. Thermal expansion of composite resins and sealants. *J Dent Res.* 1979;58:584.

Powers JM. Lifetime prediction of dental materials: an engineering approach. *J Oral Rehabil.* 1995;22:491.

Pratten DH, Johnson GH. An evaluation of finishing instruments for an anterior and a posterior composite. *J Prosthet Dent.* 1988;60:154.

Price RB, Derand T, Loney RW, et al. Effect of light source and specimen thickness on the surface hardness of resin composite. *Am J Dent.* 2002;15:47.

Price RB, Felix CA, Andreou P. Knoop hardness of ten resin composites irradiated with high-power LED and quartz-tungsten-halogen lights. *Biomaterials.* 2005;26:2631.

Rathbun MA, Craig RG, Hanks CT, et al. Cytotoxicity of a BIS-GMA dental composite before and after leaching in organic solvents. *J Biomed Mater Res.* 1991;25:443.

Roeder LB, Powers JM. Surface roughness of resin composite prepared by single-use and multi-use diamonds. *Am J Dent.* 2004;17:109.

Sakaguchi RL, Berge HX. Reduced light energy density decreases post-gel contraction while maintaining degree of conversion in composites. *J Dent.* 1998;26:695.

Sakaguchi RL, Peters MCRB, Nelson SR, et al. Effects of polymerization contraction in composite restorations. *J Dent.* 1992;20:178.

Sakaguchi RL, Wiltbank BD, Murchison CF. Cure induced stresses and damage in particulate reinforced polymer matrix composites: a review of the scientific literature. *Dent Mater.* 2005;21:43.

Sakaguchi RL, Wiltbank BD, Murchison CF. Prediction of composite elastic modulus and polymerization shrinkage by computational micromechanics. *Dent Mater.* 2004;20:397.

Sakaguchi RL, Wiltbank BD, Shah NC. Critical configuration analysis of four methods for measuring polymerization shrinkage strain of composites. *Dent Mater.* 2004;20:388.

Sarrett DC. Clinical challenges and the relevance of materials testing for posterior composite restorations. *Dent Mater.* 2005;21:9.

Stansbury JW, Trujillo-Lemon M, Lu H, et al. Conversion-dependent shrinkage stress and strain in dental resins and composites. *Dent Mater.* 2005;21:56.

Tate WH, Friedl K-H, Powers JM. Bond strength of composites to hybrid ionomers. *Oper Dent.* 1996;21:147.

Tate WH, Powers JM. Surface roughness of composites and hybrid ionomers. *Oper Dent.* 1996;21:53.

Tirtha R, Fan PL, Dennison JB, et al. In vitro depth of cure of photo-activated composites. *J Dent Res.* 1982;61:1184.

Trajtenberg CP, Powers JM. Bond strengths of repaired laboratory composites using three surface treatments and three primers. *Am J Dent.* 2004;17:123.

Van Dijken JWV. A clinical evaluation of anterior conventional, microfiller, and hybrid composite resin fillings: a 6-year follow-up study. *Acta Odontol Scand.* 1986;44:357.

Vandewalle KS, Ferracane JL, Hilton TJ, et al. Effect of energy density on properties and marginal integrity of posterior resin composite restorations. *Dent Mater.* 2004;20:96.

Weinmann W, Thalacker C, Guggenberger R. Siloranes in dental composites. *Dent Mater.* 2005;21:68.

Nanocomposites

Curtis AR, Palin WM, Fleming GJ, Shortall AC, Marquis PM. The mechanical properties of nanofilled resin-based composites: the impact of dry and wet cyclic pre-loading on bi-axial flexural strength. *Dent Mater.* 2009;25:188–197.

Endo T, Finger WJ, Kanehira M, Utterodt A, Komatsu M. Surface texture and roughness of polished nanofill and nanohybrid resin composites. *Dent Mater J.* 2010;29:213–223.

Ernst CP, Brandenbusch M, Meyer G, Canbek K, Gottschalk F, Willershauesen B. Two-year clinical performance of a nanofiller vs a fine-particle hybrid resin composite. *Clin Oral Investig.* 2006;10:119–125.

Farah JW, Powers JM. Composite update. *Dent Advis.* 2009;26(8):1.

Mahmoud SH, El-Embaby AE, Abdallah AM, Hamama HH. Two-year clinical evaluation of ormocer, nanohybrid and nanofilled composite restorative systems in posterior teeth. *J Adhes Dentist.* 2008;19(4):315–322.

Mitra SB, Wu D, Holmes BN. An application of nanotechnology in advanced dental materials. *J Am Dent Assoc.* 2003;134:1382–1390.

Palaniappan S, Bharadwaj D, Mattar DL, Peumans M, Van Meerbeek B, Lambrechts P. Three-year randomized clinical trial to evaluate the clinical performance and wear of a nanocomposite versus a hybrid composite. *Dent Mater.* 2009;25:1302–1314.

Ure D, Harris J. Nanotechnology in dentistry: reduction to practice. *Dent Update.* 2003;30:10–15.

Yap SH, Yap AU, Teo CK, Ng JJ. Polish retention of new aesthetic restorative materials over time. *Singapore Dent J.* 2004;26:39–43.

Low-Shrink Composites

Ilie N, Jelen E, Clementino Ludeemann T, Hickel R. Low-shrinkage composite for dental application. *Dent Mater J.* 2007;26:149–155.

Lien W, Vandewalle KS. Physical properties of a new silorane-based restorative system. *Dent Mater.* 2010;26:337–344.

Mozner N, Salz U. Recent developments of new components for dental adhesives and composites. *Macromol Mater Eng.* 2007;292:245–271.

Schmidt M, Kirkevang LL, Horsted-Bindslev P, Poulsen S. Marginal adaptation of a low-shrink silorane-based composite: 1-year randomized clinical trial. *Clin Oral Investig.* 2011;15:291–295.

Weinmann W, Thalacker C, Guggenberger R. Siloranes in dental composites. *Dent Mater.* 2005;21:68–74.

Yamazaki PC, Bedran-Russo AK, Periera PN, Swift EJ Jr. Microleakage evaluation of a new low-shrinkage composite restorative material. *Oper Dent.* 2006;31:670–676.

Light-Curing Units

Antonson SA, Antonson DE, Hardigan PC. Should my new curing light be an LED? *Oper Dent.* 2008;33(4):400.

Bunek SS. Light-curing units. *Dent Advis.* 2015;21:21.

Ferracane JL, Ferracane LL, Musanje L. Effect of light activation method on flexural properties of dental composites. *Am J Dent.* 2003;16:318.

Fluent MT, Ferracane JL, Mace JG, Shah AR, Price RB. Shedding light on a potential hazard: dental light curing units. *J Am Dent Assoc.* 2019;150(12):1051–1058.

Kirkpatrick SJ. A primer on radiometry. *Dent Mater.* 2005;21:21.

Price RB, Ehrnford L, Andreou P, et al. Comparison of quartz-tungsten-halogen, light-emitting diode, and plasma arc curing lights. *J Adhes Dent.* 2003;5:193.

Sakaguchi RL, Berge HX. Reduced light energy density decreases postgel contraction while maintaining degree of conversion in composites. *J Dent.* 1998;26:695.

Sakaguchi RL, Wiltbank BD, Murchison CF. Contraction force rate of polymer composites is linearly correlated with irradiance. *Dent Mater.* 2004;20:402.

Stahl F, Ashworth SH, Jandt KD, et al. Light emitting diodes (LED) polymerization of dental composites: flexural properties and polymerisation potential. *Biomaterials.* 2000;21:1379.

Wataha JC, Lockwood PE, Lewis JB, et al. Biological effects of blue light from dental curing units. *Dent Mater.* 2004;20:150.

Wiggins KM, Hartung M, Althoff O, Wastian C, Mitra SB. Curing performance of a new-generation light-emitting diode dental curing unit. *J Am Dent Assoc.* 2004;135(10):1471–1479.

Provisional Materials

Chung K, Lin T, Wang F. Flexural strength of a provisional resin material with fibre addition. *J Oral Rehabil.* 1998;25:214.

Doray PG, Eldiwany MS, Powers JM. Effect of resin surface sealers on improvement of stain resistance for a composite provisional material. *J Esthet Restor Dent.* 2003;15:244.

Doray PG, Li D, Powers JM. Color stability of provisional restorative materials after accelerated aging. *J Prosthodont.* 2001;10:212.

Farah JW, Powers JM. Provisional composites and liquid polishes. *Dent Advis.* 2010;27(4):1.

Grajower R, Shaharbani S, Kaufman E. Temperature rise in pulp chamber during fabrication of temporary self-curing resin crowns. *J Prosthet Dent.* 1979;41:535.

Ireland MF, Dixon DL, Breeding LC, et al. In vitro mechanical property comparison of four resins used for fabrication of provisional fixed restorations. *J Prosthet Dent.* 1998;80:158.

Lepe X, Bales DJ, Johnson GH. Retention of provisional crowns fabricated from two materials with the use of four temporary cements. *J Prosthet Dent.* 1999;81:469.

Lui JL. Hypersensitivity to a temporary crown and bridge material. *J Dent.* 1979;7:22.

Robinson FB, Hovijitra S. Marginal fit of direct temporary crowns. *J Prosthet Dent.* 1982;47:390.

9 Restorative Materials: Metals

JACK FERRACANE

CHAPTER OUTLINE

Various metallic materials are used in dentistry to restore or repair individual teeth and to replace single or multiple missing teeth, as well as entire dental arches. The metals used for direct restoration of tooth structure lost due to caries or fracture include dental amalgam and direct gold, though the latter is used on a very limited basis in contemporary restorative dentistry. Many metals are used for the indirect replacement of lost or damaged teeth or parts of teeth, including high-noble metals, noble metals, and predominantly base metals. The designation of these types of dental metals is based on their composition. A variety of base metals are used in dental prosthetics, such as partial dentures, and as implants to restore lost tooth roots. These materials vary widely in terms of their composition, structures, and properties, and thus are indicated for specific applications based on the requirements of the given clinical situation.

Metals for Direct Placement: Amalgam

An amalgam is an alloy (mixture of metallic elements) of mercury and one or more other metals. Dental amalgam is produced by mixing liquid mercury with solid particles of an alloy containing predominantly silver, tin, and copper. Zinc and palladium may also be present in small amounts. It is important to differentiate between dental amalgam and amalgam alloy, the latter being the commercially produced and marketed small filings, spheroid particles, or a combination of these, which are suitable for mixing with liquid mercury to produce the dental amalgam through a chemical reaction.

Once amalgam alloy is freshly mixed with liquid mercury, it has the plasticity that permits it to be conveniently packed or condensed into a prepared tooth cavity. After condensing, the dental amalgam is carved to generate the required anatomical features and then further hardens with time. Amalgam can be used for direct, permanent, and posterior restorations and for large foundation restorations, or cores, which restore large areas of lost tooth structure prior to placing crowns. Dental amalgam restorations are reasonably easy to insert, are not overly technique sensitive, maintain anatomical form, have reasonably adequate resistance to fracture, prevent marginal leakage after a period in the mouth, can be used in stress-bearing areas, and have a relatively long service life.

The principal disadvantage of dental amalgam is that its silver color does not match tooth structure. In addition, amalgam restorations are somewhat brittle, are subject to corrosion and galvanic action, may demonstrate a degree of breakdown at the margins of tooth and amalgam, and do not help retain weakened tooth structure. Finally, there are regulatory concerns about amalgam being disposed of in the wastewater. Despite these shortcomings, dental amalgam has a long history as a cost-effective and successful restorative material.

In this chapter, the composition and morphology of the different dental amalgams are presented, followed by a discussion of low- and high-copper amalgams, the chemical reactions that occur during amalgamation, and the resultant microstructures. Various physical and mechanical properties are covered in the next section, as well as factors related to the manipulation of amalgam.

Composition and Morphology

American National Standards Institute/American Dental Association (ANSI/ADA) specification No. 1 (International Organization for Standardization [ISO] standard 24234) for amalgam alloy includes a requirement for composition, stating that it shall consist primarily of silver, tin, and copper, and that indium, palladium, platinum, zinc, or mercury may also be included in lesser amounts. This specification does prescribe a specific composition for the alloys.

The ANSI/ADA specification also includes a notation about the presence of zinc in amalgam alloys, with more than 0.01% zinc classified as zinc containing and those with less than 0.01% as nonzinc alloys. Zinc has been included in amalgam alloys as

TABLE 9.1 **Approximate Composition of Low- and High-Copper Amalgam Alloys**

		ELEMENT (WT%)					
Alloy	**Particle Shape**	**Ag**	**Sn**	**Cu**	**Zn**	**In**	**Pd**
Admixed regular	Irregular	40–70	26–30	2–30	0–2	0	0
	Spherical	40–65	0–30	20–40	0–1	0	0–1
Admixed unicomposition	Irregular	52–53	17–18	29–30	0	0	0.3
	Spherical	52–53	17–18	29–30	0	0	0.3
Unicompositional	Spherical	40–60	22–30	13–30	0	0–5	0–1

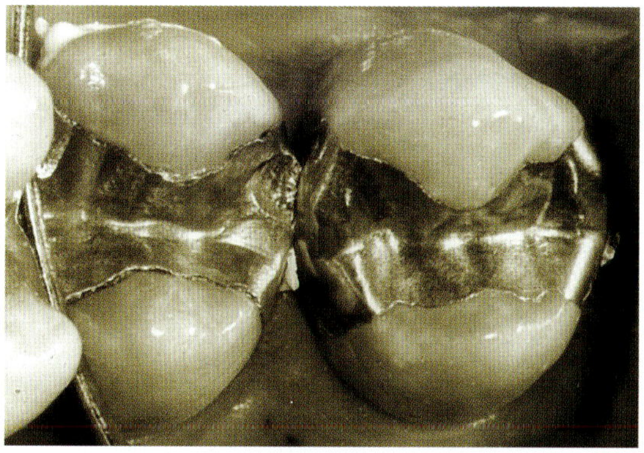

• **Fig. 9.1** Amalgam restorations from a low-copper lathe-cut alloy (*left*) and a high-copper admix alloy (*right*) after 3 years of clinical service. (Courtesy David B. Mahler, OHSU School of Dentistry, Portland, OR.)

an aid in manufacturing; it helps produce clean, sound castings of the ingots used for producing lathe-cut alloys. The presence of contamination within the amalgam must be avoided because it can degrade the integrity of the restoration. The approximate composition of commercial amalgam alloys is shown in Table 9.1.

The alloys are broadly classified as low-copper (5% or less copper) and high-copper alloys (13% to 30% copper). In modern dentistry, the low-copper formulations have been essentially totally replaced by the high-copper formulations due to the improved strength, corrosion resistance, marginal integrity, and overall clinically proven better performance, as exemplified in Fig. 9.1, where a low-copper amalgam demonstrates dramatically more marginal breakdown at 3 years than a high-copper amalgam in adjacent teeth. The remainder of the discussion in this chapter will therefore focus on the high-copper amalgam.

The powdered amalgam alloy is composed of irregularly shaped particles produced by grinding an alloy ingot on a lathe, microspheres of various sizes produced by special hot spraying techniques, or a combination of the two (so-called admix, where the composition of the two types of particles may or may not be similar). Scanning electron micrographs of the particles are shown in Fig. 9.2. The irregular lathe-cut particles are made from an alloy of silver and tin where the ratio of the two elements approximates the intermetallic compound Ag_3Sn. These are typically used in the admix alloys. The spherical particles either may contain mostly silver and copper, and be used as the second component in the admix alloy, or may be more similar to the lathe-cut particles in composition and contain silver, tin, and copper (unicompositional).

The compositional ranges of the different types of particles are shown in Table 9.1. The admixed regular alloy contains 33% to 60% spherical particles that have a composition close to the eutectic composition of Ag_3Cu_2 (see Fig. 9.2); the balance is irregular particles. The silver content of the unicompositional spherical alloys varies from 40% to 60%, copper content varies from 13% to 30%, and tin content varies from 22% to 30%. A high-copper admixed alloy is also available, in which both spherical and irregular particles have the same composition and the copper content is between 29% and 30%.

In general, alloy composition—particle size, shape, and distribution—and heat treatment control the characteristic properties of the amalgam. The following sections describing the amalgamation reaction and properties of amalgam will be devoted to the high-copper amalgams currently in use in dentistry. For an example of an amalgam restoration being placed, see video online.

Amalgamation Processes: Admixed Alloys

All dental amalgam alloys have Ag_3Sn as their primary component, which reacts with mercury to form Ag_2Hg_3, the major matrix phase of the set amalgam. The amalgam alloy is intimately mixed with liquid mercury in a process called *trituration* to wet the surface of the particles and facilitate their reaction with mercury. During this process, mercury diffuses into the alloy particles and reacts with the silver and tin portions of the particles to form predominantly a silver-mercury compound, Ag_2Hg_3, known as the *gamma one* (γ_1) phase. This phase acts as a matrix to hold the unreacted amalgam alloy together. While crystals of the γ_1 phase are being formed, the amalgam is relatively soft, easily condensable, and carvable. As time progresses, more crystals of γ_1 are formed; the amalgam becomes harder and stronger and is no longer condensable or carvable. The lapse of time between the end of the trituration and when the amalgam hardens and is no longer workable is called *working time*. Completion of the reaction may take several days to several weeks, which is reflected by the change in mechanical properties over this time. Patients are typically advised to avoid chewing directly on amalgam restorations for the first 24 hours after placement to be safe, though considerable strength has been achieved within the first few hours.

The amount of liquid mercury used to amalgamate the alloy particles is not sufficient to react with the particles completely. Therefore the set mass of amalgam contains about 27% unreacted particles, which actually enhance the strength of the final material.

In high-copper admix alloys, additional copper has typically been supplied by adding spherical particles of the silver-copper eutectic alloy to the silver-tin alloy. The solubility of silver, tin, and copper in mercury differs considerably. Approximately 1 mg of copper, 10 mg of silver, and 170 mg of tin can dissolve in mercury, all at the same temperature. Therefore while mercury is dissolving mainly the silver and tin in Ag_3Sn, as described earlier,

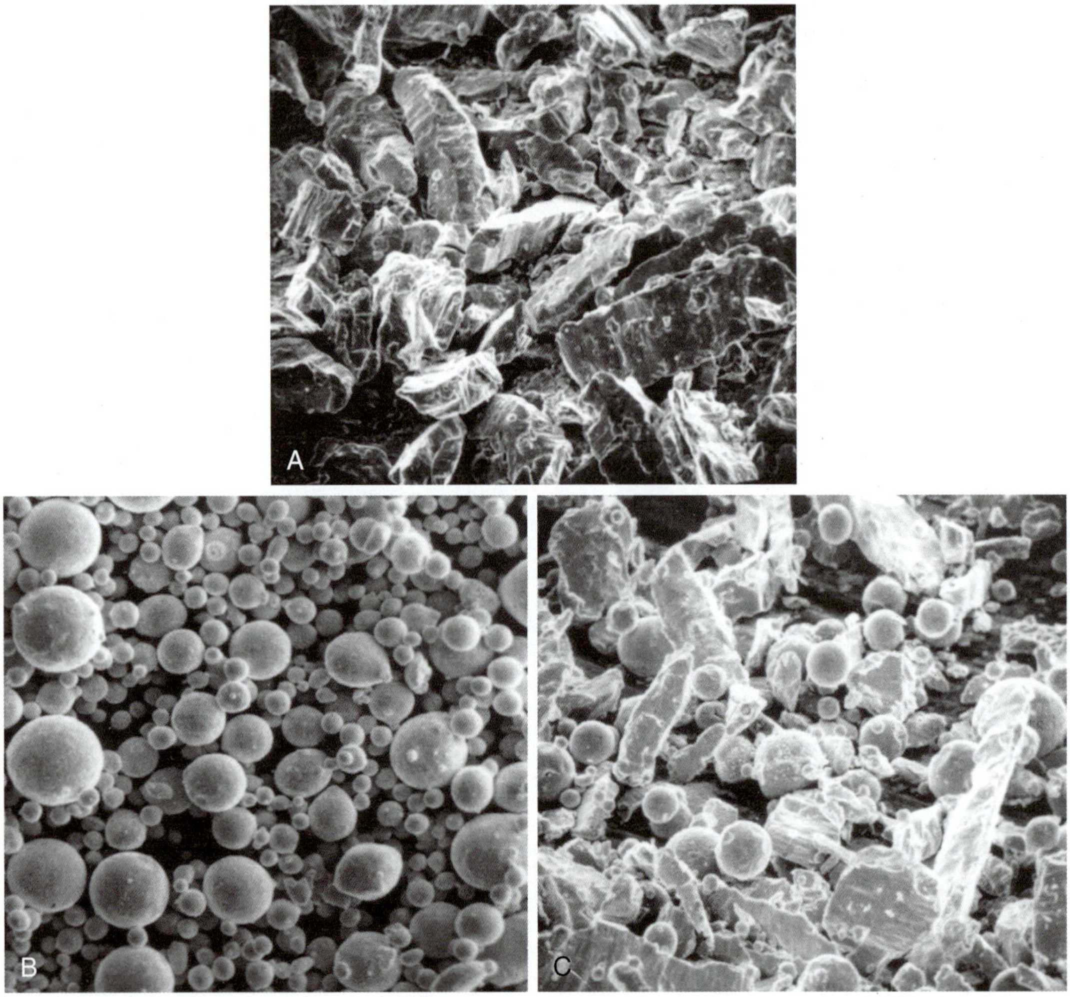

• **Fig. 9.2** Scanning electron micrographs. (A) Lathe-cut; (B) spherical; and (C) admixed amalgam alloys. The largest particles in each image are about 50 to 75 μm in size.

very little of the silver-copper eutectic particles are dissolved. However, some of the tin and copper that are dissolved by the mercury react to form a copper-tin compound, Cu_6Sn_5, referred to as the eta prime (η′) phase. It is the presence of this tin-copper compound, rather than the formation of a weak, corrosion-prone tin-mercury compound, that gives the high-copper amalgams their superior performance as compared with the older low-copper amalgams.

The amalgamation reaction may be simplified as follows:

$$\gamma(Ag_3Sn) + Ag\text{-}Cu(\text{eutectic}) + Hg \rightarrow$$
$$\gamma_1(Ag_2Hg_3) + \eta(Cu_6Sn_5) + \text{unreacted}$$
$$\gamma(Ag_3Sn) + \text{unreacted } Ag\text{-}Cu(\text{eutectic})$$

Reaction of Mercury in a Unicompositional Alloy

In high-copper unicompositional alloys, the alloy particles, typically spherical, contain both Ag_3Sn (γ) and Cu_3Sn (ε). When liquid mercury is mixed with these alloys, it diffuses into the surface of these particles and Ag_2Hg_3 and Cu_6Sn_5 are formed, as in the admixed alloy. The difference is that because all of the copper is present within the single particles, the reaction of copper and tin occurs in a ring around the spherical particles, which become surrounded by the silver-mercury matrix.

Microstructure of Amalgam

Color-coded images of the microstructures of the set amalgams of the high-copper admix and the high-copper unicompositional types are shown in Fig. 9.3. The blue/black matrix phase is A_2Hg_3 (γ_1). The tangerine color is for the Cu_6Sn_5 (η′) phase, which is very evident around spherical particles.

Physical and Mechanical Properties

ANSI/ADA Specification for Amalgam Alloy

ANSI/ADA specification No. 1 (ISO 24234) for amalgam alloy contains requirements that help control the qualities of commercially available dental amalgam. The specification lists three physical properties as a measure of amalgam quality: compressive strength, creep, and dimensional change. The minimum allowable compressive strength is 80 MPa for 1 hour after setting and 300 MPa for 24 hours after setting, the maximum allowable creep is 1%, and the dimensional change between 5 minutes and 24 hours must fall within the range of −15 to +20 μm/cm. The physical properties of several amalgams are shown in Table 9.2.

Mercury in Mix

In general, irregular particles have higher surface areas than spherical particles and therefore require more mercury to wet their

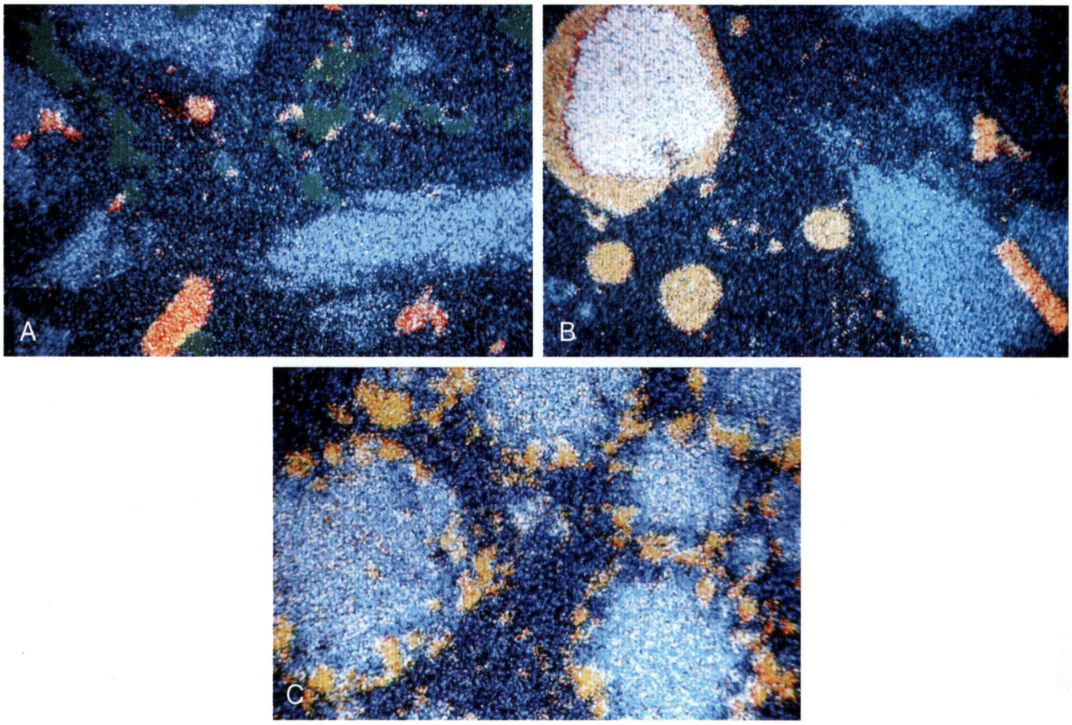

• **Fig. 9.3** Microstructures of the set amalgams of the (A) low-copper, lathe-cut; (B) the high-copper, admix; and (C) the high-copper, unicompositional types. These photographs were made by superimposing microprobe x-ray scans of the elements through colored filters: blue for silver, red for copper, and green for tin. The blue/black matrix phase is A_2Hg_3 (γ_1) for all amalgams. The green-colored $Sn_{7}–_{8}Hg$ (γ_2) phase is only present in the low-copper alloy (A). The tangerine-colored Cu_6Sn_5 (η') phase is minimal in alloy (A) but substantial in alloys (B) and (C). In alloy (B), the source of the increased copper is in the spherical silver-copper eutectic phase where the η' surrounds this spherical particle. In alloy (C), the source of the increased copper is in the additional Cu_3Sn added to the spherical Ag_3Sn particle and Cu_6Sn_5 (η') phases are present around this spherical particle. (Courtesy David B. Mahler, OHSU School of Dentistry, Portland, OR.)

TABLE 9.2 Mercury in Mix, Compressive Strength, Tensile Strength, Creep, and Dimensional Change

		COMPRESSIVE STRENGTH (MPa)		TENSILE STRENGTH (MPa)			
	Mercury in Mix (%)	**1 h**	**7 days**	**15 min**	**7 days**	**Creep (%)**	**Dimensional Change (mm/cm)**
Low Copper							
Alloys							
Lathe-cut	53.7	45	302	3.2	51	6.3	−19.7
Spherical	46.2	141	366	4.7	55	1.5	−10.6
High Copper							
Alloys							
Admixed	50.0	118	387	3.8	43	0.45	−1.9
Unicompositional	43.0	292	516	8.1	56	0.09	−8.1

(From Malhotra ML, Asgar K. Physical properties of dental silver-tin amalgams with high and low copper contents. *J Am Dent Assoc.* 1978;96:444–450.)

surfaces. In turn, higher percentages of mercury in the mix will result in higher mercury contents and lower strengths of the hardened amalgams. This effect is clearly shown in Table 9.2.

Compressive Strength

Resistance to compression forces is an important strength characteristic of amalgam. Because amalgam is strongest in compression and much weaker in tension and shear, the prepared cavity design should maximize compressive stresses in service and minimize tensile or shear stresses. When subjected to a rapid application of force either in tension or in compression, a dental amalgam does not exhibit significant deformation or elongation and, as a result, functions as a brittle material. Therefore a sudden application of excessive force to amalgam may lead to fracture of the amalgam restoration.

The early compressive strengths after 1 hour of setting for several low- and high-copper alloys are listed in Table 9.2. The high-copper unicompositional materials have the highest early compressive strengths of more than 250 MPa. High values for early compressive strength are an advantage for an amalgam because they reduce the possibility of fracture by the application of prematurely high occlusal forces by the patient before the final strength is reached. The compressive strengths at 7 days are again highest for the high-copper unicompositional alloys, with only modest differences in the other alloys.

Tensile Strength

The tensile strengths of various amalgams after 15 minutes and 7 days are also listed in Table 9.2. The tensile strengths at 7 days for low- and high-copper amalgams are about the same. The tensile strengths are only a fraction of their compressive strengths; therefore cavity designs should be constructed to reduce tensile stresses resulting from biting forces, such as eliminating bevels at margins. The tensile strengths at 15 minutes for the high-copper unicompositional alloys are significantly higher than for the other alloys.

Elastic Modulus

The elastic modulus, or the stiffness, for dental amalgam is in the range of 40 to 60 GPa. As a comparison, the elastic modulus of resin composites is only 5 to 15 GPa, which can be of significance when considering amalgam versus composites in certain clinical applications.

Creep

Creep is the time-dependent inelastic deformation of materials that are used at temperatures that are close to their melting points. Expressed in absolute temperatures, the melting point of the major matrix phase (γ_1) in dental amalgam is 400 K, whereas it is used at the mouth temperature of 310 K for a ratio of 0.8. In metals, ratios that exceed 0.5 are considered to be a forerunner for examining creep behavior. Therefore dental amalgam is an appropriate candidate for this examination.

The creep test in the specifications is conducted by applying a compressive stress of 36 MPa on a 7-day-old cylindrical specimen in a 37°C environment. Creep is measured by the shortening of the test specimen between 1 and 4 hours of testing, and the specification sets the acceptable limit for creep of 1.0%.

However, amalgams whose creep values vary within the range of less than 1.0% do not show differences in clinical performance. For example, referring to Table 9.2, unicompositional alloys with creep values of 0.05 and 0.09 do not show superior clinical performance compared to the admix alloy with a creep value of 0.45. Therefore physical properties are helpful in predicting clinical performance, but care should be exercised in the limits of their interpretation.

The ability of creep to demonstrate the permanent deformation of dental amalgam in the clinical environment is shown to be of significance in Fig. 9.1.

Dimensional Change

The dimensional change during the setting of amalgam is one of its most significant properties. Modern amalgams mixed with mechanical amalgamators usually have negative dimensional changes. The initial contraction after a short time (the first 20 minutes) is believed to be associated with the solution of the alloy particles in mercury. After this period, an expansion occurs that is believed to be a result of the reaction of mercury with silver mainly and the formation of the matrix phase. The dimensions become nearly constant after 6 to 8 hours, and thus the values after 24 hours are final values. The only exception to this statement is the excessive delayed dimensional change seen clinically when some older zinc-containing alloys were contaminated with water-based fluids during trituration or condensation.

Dimensional change is measured by the change in length of an 8-mm cylindrical specimen between 5 minutes and 24 hours after trituration. The change in length can be determined continuously, although ANSI/ADA specification No. 1 requires only the value at 24 hours.

The dimensional changes in micrometers per centimeter for various alloys are listed in Table 9.2. The lowest dimensional change of −1.9 μm/cm was for the high-copper admixed alloy. All the amalgams meet the requirements of ANSI/ADA specification No. 1 of −15 to +20 μm/cm but are susceptible to influence from various manipulative factors.

An additional clinical significance of dimensional change is related to the occasional occurrence of postoperative sensitivity associated with newly placed amalgam restorations. Amalgam does not adhere to tooth structure; therefore, a negative dimensional change would result in the presence of an interfacial gap between the amalgam restoration and tooth structure. When a cavity is prepared that cuts through dentin in a tooth requiring restoration, pulpal fluid in the tubules can flow outward into the interfacial gap. Changes in pressure of this fluid are considered to be one of the major causes of postoperative sensitivity. Apparently, the size of the interfacial gap is a key factor in determining whether sensitivity will occur, with teeth with restorations having larger gaps being more prone to being sensitive.

Although most alloys that pass ANSI/ADA specification No. 1 for negative dimensional changes of −15 μm/cm or less have not been shown to have an uncommon amount of postoperative sensitivity, some high-copper amalgams consisting of only spherical particles have been reported to show a propensity for this sensitivity. The reason for this anomaly was found by in vitro microleakage studies that showed that spherical particle alloys leaked more than lathe-cut particle alloys, even though their respective dimensional changes were not significantly different. Examination showed that the surfaces of these amalgams next to the cavity walls exhibited a relatively uneven texture for the spherical particle alloys compared to a smoother texture for the lathe-cut alloys. Thus the interfacial space filled by pulpal fluid was greater for the spherical particle alloys. In Fig. 9.4, the microleakage of a number of dental amalgams is shown where spherical particle alloys are marked with a capital *S*. It is clear that the presence of higher microleakage values is associated with the spherical alloys. Bars that are shaded refer to alloys in which data were available to indicate an unusual propensity for postoperative sensitivity.

The use of film-forming agents such as dentin bonding agents to seal the dentinal tubules before placement of an amalgam restoration has proven to be an effective solution to the problem of postoperative sensitivity of spherical particle amalgams. However, this practice has not been widely adopted by the profession.

Corrosion

In general, corrosion is the progressive destruction of a metal by chemical or electrochemical reactions with its environment. Excessive corrosion can lead to increased porosity, reduced marginal integrity, loss of strength, and the release of metallic products into the oral environment.

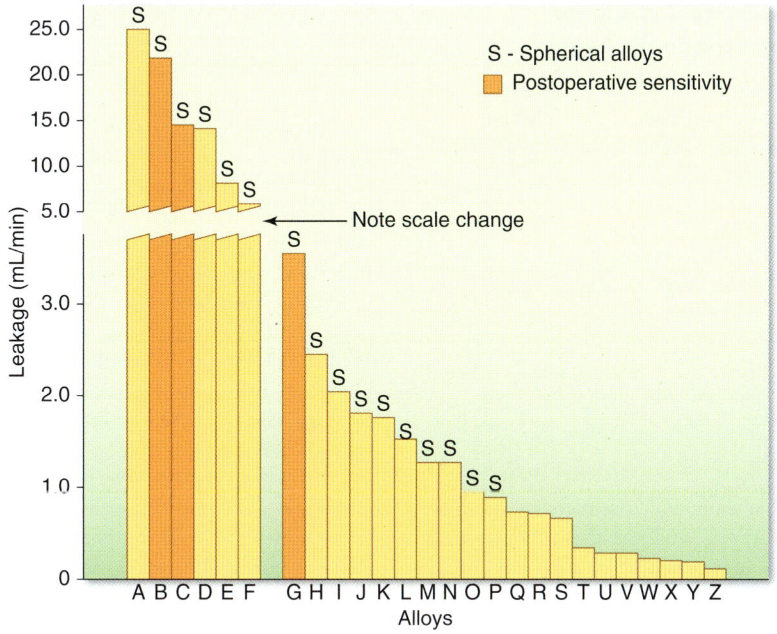

• **Fig. 9.4** In vitro microleakage of various commercial amalgams. (From Mahler DB, Nelson LW. Sensitivity answers sought in amalgam alloy microleakage study. *J Am Dent Assoc*. 1994;125:282–288.)

Corrosion products identified in dental amalgams include tin oxides, tin hydroxychlorides, copper oxides, copper chlorides, and other more complex compounds. The formation of oxides and chlorides is not surprising considering that the amalgams operate in an aerated environment containing salt solutions. Because of their different chemical compositions, the different phases of an amalgam have different corrosion potentials. Electrochemical measurements on pure phases have shown that the Ag_2Hg_3 (γ_1) phase has the highest corrosion resistance, followed by Ag_3Sn (γ), Ag_3Cu_2, Cu_3Sn (ε), Cu_6Sn_5 (η'), and $Sn_{7-8}Hg$ (γ_2). However, the presence of small amounts of tin, silver, and copper that may dissolve in various amalgam phases has a great influence on their corrosion resistance. For example, in the γ_1 phase, the silver-mercury phase always has some tin dissolved within it, and the higher the tin concentration, the lower is the corrosion resistance. The average depth of corrosion for most amalgam alloys is 100 to 500 µm, measured from the amalgam/tooth margin.

Phosphate buffer solutions inhibit the corrosion process, as does the formation of protein pellicles on the amalgam surface; thus saliva may provide some protection for dental amalgams from corrosion.

A study of amalgams that had been in service for 2 to 25 years revealed that the bulk elemental compositions were similar to newly prepared amalgams, except for the presence of a small amount of chloride and other contaminants. The compositions of the phases were also similar to new amalgams, except for internal amalgamation of the γ particles. The distribution of phases in the clinically aged amalgams, however, differed from that of new amalgams, verifying that dental amalgam is a dynamic material that changes with time.

Surface tarnish in high-copper amalgams is related to the copper-rich phases.

Bonding of Amalgam

Although amalgam has been a highly successful restorative material when used as an intercoronal restoration, it does not bond to tooth structure and therefore does not restore the original strength of the clinical crown. Features such as pins, slots, holes, and grooves must be supplied to provide retention for large restorations, but they do not reinforce the amalgam or increase its strength.

With the development of adhesive systems for dental composites came the opportunity to attempt to bond amalgams to tooth structure. Bonding agents containing 4-META, an acronym for 4-methacryloxyethyl trimellitic anhydride (see Chapter 7), have been the most successful products. Shear bond strengths of amalgam to dentin as high as 10 MPa have been reported using these adhesives, whereas comparable values for the shear bond strength of microfilled composites to dentin using these same adhesives have been 20 to 22 MPa.

There is no true adhesion between amalgam and tooth structure. Bonding that has been shown by shear bond tests is strictly produced by the commingling of the bonding agent and the amalgam at their common interface. The technique for placing a bonded amalgam consists of initially placing the bonding agent into the cavity and before the bonding agent has completely polymerized, the amalgam is condensed into the cavity. This represents the technical challenge of filling the retentive features of the preparation with amalgam mixed together with the bonding agent.

The fracture resistance of teeth restored with amalgam-bonded mesio-occlusal-distal (MOD) restorations was more than twice that of restorations containing unbonded amalgams. In addition, in spite of the lower shear-bond strength of amalgam bonded to dentin as compared to that for composites, the fracture strength of MODs in teeth restored with bonded amalgams was as high as that for composites, although neither was as high (45% to 80%) as values for the intact tooth. As expected, amalgam-bonded MODs with narrow preparations had higher strengths than those with wide preparations. Other studies showed that the retention of amalgam-bonded MODs with proximal boxes was as great as pin-retained amalgams. In addition, amalgam-bonded restorations decreased marginal leakage in class 5 restorations compared with unbonded amalgams. Finally, the bonding agents for amalgam have not been successful in increasing the amalgam-to-amalgam bond strength for the repair of amalgam restorations.

The history of dental amalgam and its manipulation can be found on the website http://evolve.elsevier.com/sakaguchi/restorative.

TABLE 9.3 Revised American Dental Association Classification of Prosthodontic Alloys

Class	Required Noble Content (%)	Required Gold Content (%)	Required Titanium Content (%)
High-noble alloys	≥60	≥40	
Noble alloys	≥25		
Predominantly base materials	<25		
Titanium and titanium alloys			≥85

Dental Casting Alloys

This section is divided into noble alloys and base-metal alloys. Fluctuations in the price of gold, platinum, and palladium influence the selection of alloys for cast dental restorations. Each alloy has specific physical and mechanical properties that affect its manipulation and application. Tooth preparation and restoration design will determine the required physical and mechanical properties of the alloy, so all factors should be kept in mind during the process of treatment planning.

Types and Composition

The ADA specification for dental casting alloys classifies alloys by composition, dividing alloys into three groups: (1) *high noble*, with a noble-metal content of at least 60 wt% and gold content of at least 40%; (2) *noble*, with a noble-metal content at least 25% (no stipulation for gold); and (3) *predominately base metal*, with a noble-metal content less than 25% (Table 9.3). It is important to keep in mind that the percentages used as boundaries in the specification are somewhat arbitrary.

ANSI/ADA specification No. 5 (ISO 1562) uses a type I through IV classification system with each alloy type recommended for specific applications, in addition to the compositional classification previously described (Table 9.4). Thus, a high-noble alloy might be type I or type IV, depending on its mechanical properties. This situation is somewhat confusing because in the old specification the alloy type was related to its composition and virtually all alloys were gold based. In the current system, each type of alloy is recommended for intraoral use based on the amount of force the restoration is likely to receive. Alloy types I and II have high elongation and are therefore easily burnished, but are appropriate only in low-stress environments, such as inlays that experience low occlusal forces. Type IV alloys are to be used in clinical situations where very high stresses are involved, such as long-span and fixed dental prostheses. Type III alloys are the most commonly used in dental practices for crowns and shorter fixed-partial dentures.

Although the number of casting alloys is immense, it is possible to subdivide each ADA compositional group into several classes (Table 9.5). These classes are simply a convenient way of organizing the diverse strategies that have been used to formulate casting alloys. For each class of alloy shown in Table 9.5, there are many variations; the compositions shown are meant only to be representative. Note that both the weight percent (wt%) and atomic percent (at%) compositions of the alloys are shown in Table 9.5. Weight percentages of the alloys are most commonly used by manufacturers in the production and sales of the alloys. However, the physical, chemical, and biological properties are best understood in terms of atomic percentages. For the sake of simplicity, the following discussion will be in terms of wt% composition. Most of the alloys contain some zinc as a deoxidizer and either iridium (Ir) or ruthenium (Ru) as grain refiners. Some of these compositions are used for both full metal castings and ceramic-metal restorations.

There are three classes of high-noble alloys: the Au-Ag-Pt alloys; the Au-Cu-Ag-Pd alloys with a gold content greater than 70 wt% (Au-Cu-Ag-Pd-*I* in Table 9.5); and the Au-Cu-Ag-Pd alloys with a gold content of about 50% to 65% (Au-Cu-Ag-Pd-*II*). The Au-Ag-Pt alloys typically consist of 78 wt% gold with roughly equal amounts of silver and platinum. These alloys have been used as casting alloys and porcelain-metal alloys. The Au-Cu-Ag-Pd-*I* alloys are typically 75 wt% gold with approximately 10 wt% each of silver and copper and 2 to 3 wt% palladium. The Au-Cu-Ag-Pd-*II* alloys typically have less than 60 wt% gold, with the silver content increased to accommodate the reduced gold content. Occasionally, these alloys will have slightly higher palladium and lower silver percentages.

There are four classes of noble alloys: the Au-Cu-Ag-Pd alloys (Au-Cu-Ag-Pd-*III* in Table 9.5); Au-Ag-Pd-In alloys; Pd-Cu-Ga alloys; and Ag-Pd alloys. The Au-Cu-Ag-Pd-*III* alloys typically have a gold content of 40 wt%. The reduced gold is compensated primarily with silver, so the copper and palladium contents are not changed much from the Au-Cu-Ag-Pd-*II* alloys. The Au-Ag-Pd-In alloys have a gold content of only 20 wt% and have about 40 wt% silver, 20 wt% palladium, and 15 wt% indium. The Pd-Cu-Ga alloys have little or no gold, with about 75 wt% palladium and roughly equal amounts of copper and gallium. Finally, the Ag-Pd alloys have no gold but have 70 wt% silver and 25 wt% palladium. By the ADA specification, these alloys are considered noble because of their palladium content.

The compositions of casting alloys determine their color. In general, if the palladium content is over 10 wt%, the alloy will be white. Thus

TABLE 9.4 ANSI/ADA Specification No. 5, Mechanical Properties of Dental Casting Alloys

Alloy Type	Description	Use	Yield Strength (annealed, MPa)	Elongated (annealed, %)
I	Soft	Restorations subjected to low stress: some inlays	<140	18
II	Medium	Restorations subjected to moderate stress: inlays and onlays	140–200	18
III	Hard	Restorations subjected to high stress: crowns, thick-veneer crowns, short-span fixed dental prostheses	201–340	12
IV	Extra-hard	Restorations subjected to very high stress: thin-veneer crowns, long-span fixed dental prostheses, removable dental prostheses	>340	10

ANSI/ADA, American National Standards Institute/American Dental Association.

TABLE 9.5 **Typical Compositions (wt%/at%) of Noble Dental Casting Alloys**

Alloy Type	Ag	Au	Cu	Pd	Pt	Zn	Other
High Noble							
Au-Ag-Pt	11.5/19.3	78.1/71.4	—	—	9.9/9.2	—	Ir (trace)
Au-Cu-Ag-Pd-*I*	10.0/13.6	76.0/56.5	10.5/24.2	2.4/3.4	0.1/0.1	1.0/2.0	Ru (trace)
Au-Cu-Ag-Pd-*II*	25.0/30.0	56.0/36.6	11.8/23.9	5.0/6.1	0.4/0.3	1.7/3.4	Ir (trace)
Noble							
Au-Cu-Ag-Pd-*III*	47.0/53.3	40.0/24.8	7.5/14.4	4.0/4.7	—	1.5/2.8	Ir (trace)
Au-Ag-Pd-In	38.7/36.1	20.0/10.3	—	21.0/33.3	—	3.8/5.8	In 16.5
Pd-Cu-Ga	—	2.0/1.0	10.0/15.8	77.0/73.1	—	—	Ga 7.0/10.1
Ag-Pd	70.0/69.0	—	—	25.0/25.0	—	2.0/3.3	In 3/2.3

TABLE 9.6 **Properties of Elements in Dental Casting Alloys**

Element	Symbol	Atomic Number	Atomic Mass	Density (g/cm^3)	Melting Temperature (°C)	Color	Comments
Noble							
Ruthenium	Ru	44	101.07	12.48	2310.0	White	Grain refiner, hard
Rhodium	Rh	45	102.91	12.41	1966.0	Silver-white	Grain refiner, soft, ductile
Palladium	Pd	46	106.42	12.02	1554.0	White	Hard, malleable, ductile
Osmium	Os	76	190.20	22.61	3045.0	Bluish-white	Not used in dentistry
Iridium	Ir	77	192.22	22.65	2410.0	Silver-white	Grain refiner, very hard
Platinum	Pt	78	195.08	21.45	1772.0	Bluish-white	Tough, ductile, malleable
Gold	Au	79	196.97	19.32	1064.4	Yellow	Ductile, malleable, soft, conductive
Base							
Nickel	Ni	28	58.69	8.91	1453.0	White	Hard
Copper	Cu	29	63.55	8.92	1083.4	Reddish	Malleable, ductile, conductive
Zinc	Zn	30	65.39	7.14	419.6	Bluish-white	Soft, brittle, oxidizes
Gallium	Ga	31	69.72	5.91	29.8	Grayish-white	Low melting
Silver	Ag	47	107.87	10.49	961.9		Soft, malleable, ductile, conductive
Tin	Sn	50	118.71	7.29	232.0	White	Soft
Indium	In	49	114.82	7.31	156.6	Gray-white	Soft

the Pd-Cu-Ga and Ag-Pd alloys in Table 9.5 are white, whereas the other alloys are yellow (gold). The Au-Ag-Pd-In alloys are an exception because they have palladium content over 20% and retain a light yellow color. The color of this alloy results from interactions of the indium with the palladium in the alloy. Among the yellow alloys, the composition will modify the shade of yellow. In general, copper adds a reddish color and silver lightens either the red or yellow color of the alloys.

Metallic Elements Used in Dental Alloys

For dental restorations, various elements are combined to produce alloys with adequate properties for dental applications because none of the elements by themselves have properties that are suitable. These alloys may be used for dental restorations as cast alloys or may be manipulated into wire or other wrought forms. The metallic elements that make up dental alloys can be divided into two major groups: the noble metals and the base metals.

Noble Metals

Noble metals are elements with a good metallic surface that retain their surface in dry air. They react easily with sulfur to form sulfides, but their resistance to oxidation, tarnish, and corrosion during heating, casting, soldering, and use in the mouth is very good. The noble metals are gold, platinum, palladium, iridium, rhodium, osmium, and ruthenium (Table 9.6). These metals can be subdivided into two groups. The metals of the first group, consisting of ruthenium, rhodium, and palladium, have atomic weights of approximately 100 and densities of 12 to 13 g/cm^3. The metals of the second group, consisting of osmium, iridium, platinum, and gold, have atomic weights of about 190 and densities of 19 to 23 g/cm^3. The melting points of members of each group decrease with increasing atomic weight. Thus ruthenium melts at 2310°C, rhodium at 1966°C, and palladium at 1554°C. In the second group, the melting points range from 3045°C for osmium to 1064°C for gold. The melting point and density are important properties when composing alloys because they affect the casting process, which affects the overall accuracy and quality of the final product. The noble metals, together with silver, are sometimes called *precious metals*. The term *precious* comes from the relatively high cost of these metals and their trading on the commodities market. Some metallurgists consider silver a noble metal, but it is not considered a noble metal in dentistry because it

TABLE 9.7 Physical and Mechanical Properties of Cast Pure Gold and Gold Alloys

Material	Density (g/cm^3)	Hardness (VHN/BHN) (kg/mm^2)	Tensile Strength (MPa)	Elongation (%)
Cast 24k gold	19.3	28 (VHN)	105	30
Cast 22k gold	—	60 (VHN)	240	22
Coin gold	—	85 (BHN)	395	30
Typical Au-based casting alloy (70 wt% Au)[a]	15.6	135/195 (VHN)	425/525	30/12

[a]Values are for softened/hardened condition.

BHN, Brinell hardness number; *VHN*, Vickers hardness number.

(From Rule RW. A further report on physical properties and clinical values of platinum-centered gold foil as compared to pure gold filling materials. *J Am Dent Assoc.* 1937;24:583–595.)

corrodes considerably in the oral cavity. Thus the terms *noble* and *precious* are not synonymous in dentistry.

Gold (Au)

Pure gold is a soft, malleable, and ductile metal that has a rich yellow color with a strong metallic luster. Although pure gold is the most ductile and malleable of all metals, it is relatively low in strength. The density of gold depends somewhat on the condition of the metal, whether it is cast, rolled, or drawn into wire. Small amounts of impurities have a pronounced effect on the mechanical properties of gold and its alloys. The presence of less than 0.2% lead causes gold to be extremely brittle. Mercury in small quantities also has a harmful effect. Therefore scrap of other dental alloys should not be mixed with gold used for dental restorations.

Air or water at any temperature does not affect or tarnish gold. Gold is not soluble in sulfuric, nitric, or hydrochloric acids. However, it readily dissolves in combinations of nitric and hydrochloric acids (aqua regia, 18 vol% nitric, and 82 vol% hydrochloric acids) to form the trichloride of gold ($AuCl_3$). It is also dissolved by a few other chemicals, such as potassium cyanide and solutions of bromine or chlorine.

Because gold is nearly as soft as lead, it must be alloyed with copper, silver, platinum, and other metals to develop the hardness, durability, and elasticity necessary in dental alloys, coins, and jewelry (Table 9.7). Through appropriate refining and purification, gold with an extremely high degree of purity may be produced. Gold can be work hardened to improve its physical properties. Without the improvement, cast gold would lack sufficient strength and hardness.

Carat and Fineness of Gold-Based Alloys. For many years the gold content of gold-containing alloys has been described on the basis of the carat, or in terms of fineness, rather than by weight percentage. The term *carat* refers only to the gold content of the alloy; a carat represents a one-twenty-fourth part of the whole. Thus 24 carat indicates pure gold. The carat of an alloy is designated by a small letter *k*, for example, 18k or 22k gold.

The use of the term *carat* to designate the gold content of dental alloy is less common now. It is not unusual to find the weight percentage of gold listed or to have the alloy described in terms of fineness. *Fineness* also refers only to the gold content and represents the number of parts of gold in each 1000 parts of alloy. Thus 24k gold is the same as 100% gold or 1000 fineness (i.e., 1000 fine). An 18k gold would be designated as 750 fine, or, when the decimal system is used, it would be 0.750 fine; this indicates that 750/1000 of the total is gold. A comparison of the carat, fineness, and weight percentage of gold is given in Table 9.8. Both the whole number and the decimal system are in common use, especially for noble dental solders. The fineness system is somewhat less relevant today because of the introduction of alloys that are not gold based. It is important to emphasize that the terms *carat* and *fineness* refer only to gold content, not noble-metal content.

TABLE 9.8 Comparison of Carat, Fineness, and Weight Percentage of Gold in Gold Alloys

Carat	Amount of Gold by Carats	Weight (%) of Gold	FINENESS	
			Parts/1000	Decimal
24	$\frac{24}{24}$	100.0	1000.00	1.000
22	$\frac{22}{24}$	91.7	916.66	0.916
20	$\frac{20}{24}$	83.3	833.33	0.833
18	$\frac{18}{24}$	75.0	750.00	0.750
16	$\frac{16}{24}$	66.7	666.66	0.666
14	$\frac{14}{24}$	58.3	583.33	0.583
9	$\frac{9}{24}$	37.5	374.99	0.375

Platinum (Pt)

Platinum is a bluish-white metal; that is, tough, ductile, and malleable; and can be produced as foil or fine-drawn wire. Platinum has hardness similar to that of copper. Pure platinum has numerous applications in dentistry because of its high fusing point and resistance to oral conditions and elevated temperatures.

Platinum increases the hardness and elastic qualities of gold, and some dental casting alloys and wires contain quantities of platinum up to 8% combined with other metals. Platinum tends to lighten the color of yellow-gold–based alloys.

Palladium (Pd)

Palladium is a white metal somewhat darker than platinum. Its density is a little more than half that of platinum and gold.

Palladium is not used in the pure state of dentistry but is used extensively in dental alloys. Palladium can be combined with gold, silver, copper, cobalt, tin, indium, or gallium for dental alloys. Alloys are readily formed between gold and palladium, and palladium quantities of as low as 5% by weight have a pronounced effect on whitening yellow-gold–based alloys. Palladium-gold alloys with a palladium content of 10% or more by weight are white. Alloys of palladium and the other elements previously mentioned are available as substitutes for yellow-gold alloys, and the mechanical properties of the palladium-based alloys may be as good as or better than many traditional gold-based alloys. Although many of the palladium-based alloys are white, some, such as palladium-indium-silver alloys, are yellow.

Iridium (Ir), Ruthenium (Ru), and Rhodium (Rh)

Iridium and ruthenium are used in small amounts in dental alloys as grain refiners to keep the grain size small. A small grain size is desirable because it improves the mechanical properties and uniformity of properties within an alloy. As little as 0.005% (50 ppm) of iridium is effective in reducing the grain size. Ruthenium has a similar effect. The grain-refining properties of these elements are largely due to their extremely high melting points. Iridium melts at 2410°C and ruthenium at 2310°C. Thus these elements do not melt during the casting of the alloy and serve as nucleating centers for the melt as it cools, resulting in a fine-grained alloy.

Rhodium also has a high melting point (1966°C) and has been used in alloys with platinum to form wire for thermocouples. These thermocouples help measure the temperature in porcelain furnaces used to make dental restorations.

Base Metals

Several base metals are combined with noble metals to develop alloys with properties suitable for dental restorations. Base metals used in dental alloys include silver, copper, zinc, indium, tin, gallium, and nickel (see Table 9.6).

Silver (Ag)

Silver is a malleable, ductile white metal. It is the best-known conductor of heat and electricity and is stronger and harder than gold but softer than copper. At 961.9°C, the melting point of silver is below the melting points of both copper and gold. It is unaltered in clean, dry air at any temperature, but combines with sulfur, chlorine, phosphorus, and vapors containing these elements or their compounds. Foods containing sulfur compounds cause severe tarnishes on silver, and for this reason, silver is not considered a noble metal in dentistry.

Pure silver is not used in dental restorations because of the black sulfide that forms on the metal in the mouth. Adding small amounts of palladium to silver-containing alloys prevents the rapid corrosion of such alloys in the oral environment.

Silver forms a series of compounds with palladium and gold, and is therefore common in gold- and palladium-based dental alloys. In gold-based alloys, silver is effective in neutralizing the reddish color of alloys containing appreciable quantities of copper. Silver also hardens the gold-based alloys via a solid-solution hardening mechanism. In palladium-based alloys, silver is important in developing the white color of the alloy. Although silver is soluble in palladium, the addition of other elements to these alloys, such as copper or indium, may cause the formation of multiple phases and increased corrosion.

Copper (Cu)

Copper is a malleable and ductile metal with high thermal and electrical conductivity and a characteristic red color. When added to gold-based alloys, copper imparts a reddish color to the gold and hardens the alloy via a solid-solution or ordered-solution mechanism. The presence of copper in gold-based alloys in quantities between approximately 40% and 88% by weight allows the formation of an ordered phase. Copper is also commonly used in palladium-based alloys, where it can be used to reduce the melting point and strengthen the alloy through solid-solution hardening and formation of ordered phases when Cu is between 15 and 55 wt%. The ratio of silver and copper must be carefully balanced in gold- and palladium-based alloys because silver and copper are not miscible. Copper is also a common component of most hard dental solders.

Zinc (Zn)

Zinc is a blue-white metal with a tendency to tarnish in moist air. In its pure form, it is a soft, brittle metal with low strength. When heated in air, zinc oxidizes readily to form a white oxide of relatively low density. This oxidizing property is exploited in dental alloys. Although zinc may be present in quantities of only 1% to 2% by weight, it acts as a scavenger of oxygen when the alloy is melted. Thus zinc is referred to as a *deoxidizing agent*. Because of its low density, the resulting zinc oxide lags behind the denser molten mass during casting and is therefore excluded from the casting. If too much zinc is present, it will markedly increase the brittleness of the alloy.

Indium (In)

Indium is a soft, gray-white metal with a low melting point of 156.6°C. Indium is not tarnished by air or water. It is used in some gold-based alloys as a replacement for zinc and is a common minor component of some noble ceramic dental alloys. Recently, indium has been used in greater amounts (up to 30% by weight) to impart a yellow color to palladium-silver alloys.

Tin (Sn)

Tin is a lustrous, soft, white metal that is not subject to tarnish in normal air. Some gold-based alloys contain limited quantities of tin, usually less than 5% by weight. Tin is also an ingredient in gold-based dental solders. It combines with platinum and palladium to produce a hardening effect, but also increases brittleness.

Gallium (Ga)

Gallium is a grayish metal that is stable in dry air but tarnishes in moist air. It has a very low melting point of 29.8°C and a density of only 5.91 g/cm^3. Gallium is not used in its pure form in dentistry but is used as a component of some gold- and palladium-based dental alloys, especially ceramic alloys. The oxides of gallium are important to the bonding of the ceramic to the metal.

Nickel (Ni)

Nickel has limited application in gold- and palladium-based dental alloys but is a common component in base-metal dental alloys. Nickel has a melting point of 1453°C and a density of 8.91 g/cm^3. When used in small quantities in gold-based alloys, nickel whitens the alloy and increases its strength and hardness.

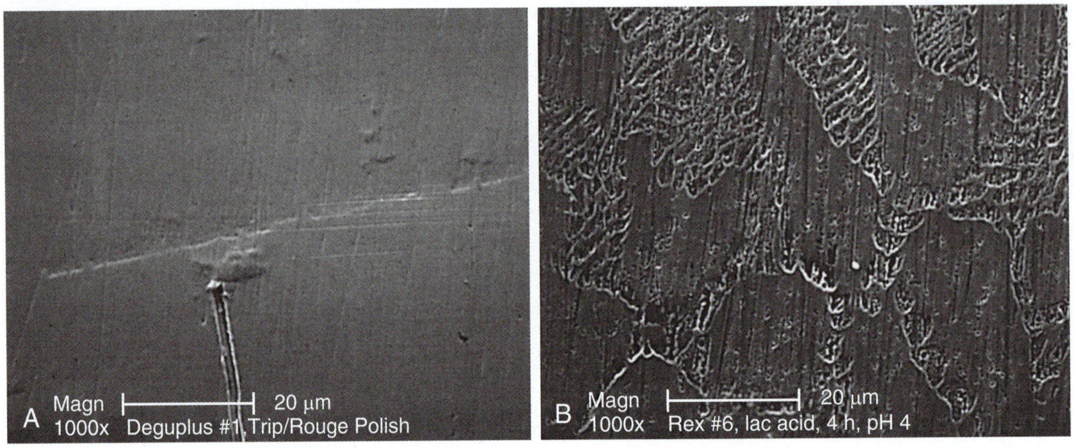

• **Fig. 9.5** Electron micrographs of single-phase (A) and multiple-phase (B) alloys. (A) Few distinguishing microstructure characteristics are seen because the alloy is nearly homogeneous. Only a few scratches from polishing and some debris on the surface are visible. (B) A rich microstructure is evident, reflecting the several phases present. Each phase has a different composition.

Noble Alloys

Phase Structure of Noble Alloys

The structure of noble alloys can consist of solid solutions, in which the elements are completely soluble in one another at all temperatures and compositions; ordered solutions, in which the elements in the alloy assume specific and regular positions in the crystal lattice of the alloy; or multiple individual phases formed because the elements are not capable of totally dissolving in one another at all compositions and temperatures.

The presence of a second phase is important because it significantly changes the corrosion properties of an alloy. Fig. 9.5 shows electron micrographs of single- and multiple-phase alloys. The single-phase alloy has little visible microstructure because its composition is more or less homogeneous. In the multiple-phase alloy, areas that have distinct compositions are clearly visible. These areas correspond to the different phases that formed during the solidification process because the elements were no longer completely able to be dissolved in one another to form a single phase as the alloy cooled. Because the different phases may interact electrochemically, the corrosion of multiple-phase alloys may be higher than for a single-phase alloy.

Hardening of Noble Alloys

The use of pure cast gold is not practical for dental restorations because cast gold lacks sufficient strength and hardness. Solid-solution and ordered-solution hardening are two common ways of strengthening noble dental alloys sufficiently for use in the mouth. By mixing two elements in the crystal lattice randomly (forming a solid solution), the force needed to distort the lattice may be significantly increased. For example, adding just 10% by weight of copper to gold, the tensile strength increases from 105 to 395 MPa and the Brinell hardness increases from 28 to 85 (see Table 9.7). If the positions of the two elements become ordered (forming an ordered solution), the properties of the alloy are improved further (see Table 9.7). For a typical gold-based casting alloy, the formation of an ordered solution may increase yield strength by 50%, tensile strength by 25%, and hardness by at least 10%. It is important to note that the elongation of an alloy is reduced by the formation of the ordered solution. For the typical gold-based alloy, the percentage elongation will decrease from 30% to about 12%.

The formation of ordered solutions has been commonly used to strengthen cast dental restorations, particularly in gold-based alloys. The process requires precise control of the cooling rate. For the correct composition capable of forming the ordered state, slow cooling will result in a harder, stronger alloy due to the formation of the ordered crystals. However, rapid cooling of the cast metal, such as by plunging it into cold water soon after the casting process, leaves the metal in the softer, disordered state because there is simply not enough time during cooling for the atoms to arrange correctly on the crystal lattice. The conversion between the ordered solution and solid solution is reversible in the solid state. Thus it is possible to heat an alloy that exists in a disordered state under appropriate conditions and temperatures to provide time for the ordered structure to form. An example of how this process can be utilized for dental castings is as follows. An alloy is cooled rapidly after casting, leaving the alloy in the softer, disordered state, and thus allowing it to be more easily ground and burnished at the margins to fit the die, and ultimately the prepared tooth. However, because it is beneficial for the alloy to be in a hardened state once placed in the mouth, the casting that has been worked in the laboratory is reheated to cause the formation of the harder, ordered structure, and this is the material that is ultimately cemented on the patient's prepared tooth.

Formulation of Noble Alloys

The desired qualities of noble dental casting alloys determine the selection of elements that will be used to formulate the alloys. The ideal noble casting alloy should have (1) a low melting range; (2) adequate strength, hardness, and elongation; (3) a low tendency to corrode in the oral environment; and (4) low cost, among other properties. Traditionally, the noble elements gold and palladium have generally been the foundation to which other elements are added to formulate dental casting alloys. Gold and palladium are preferable to other noble elements because they have relatively low melting points and low corrosion, and form solid solutions with other alloy elements, such as copper or silver. Solid-solution systems are desirable for the formulation of alloys because they are generally easier to manufacture and manipulate, have a lower tendency to corrode than multiple-phase systems, and provide increased strength through solid-solution or ordered-solution hardening. Thus it is not surprising that combinations of these

TABLE 9.9 Physical and Mechanical Properties of Several Types of Noble Dental Casting Alloys

Alloy	Melting Range (°C)	Color	Density (g/cm^3)	Yield Strength at 0.2% Offset (Soft/Hard) (MPa)	Elongation (Soft/Hard) (%)	Vickers Hardness (Soft/Hard) (kg/mm^2)
Au-Ag-Pt	1045–1140	Yellow	18.4	420/470	15/9	175/195
Au-Cu-Ag-Pd-*I*	910–965	Yellow	15.6	270/400	30/12	135/195
Au-Cu-Ag-Pd-*II*	870–921	Yellow	13.8	350/600	30/10	175/260
Au-Cu-Ag-Pd-*III*	865–925	Yellow	12.4	325/520	27.5/10	125/215
Au-Ag-Pd-In	875–1035	Light yellow	11.4	300/370	12/8	135/190
Pd-Cu-Ga	1100–1190	White	10.6	1145	8	425
Ag-Pd	1020–1100	White	10.6	260/320	10/8	140/155

elements have been extensively used in the formulation of noble dental casting alloys.

Grain Size

Studies have shown that minute quantities of various elements can influence the grain size of dental casting alloys. With the addition of small amounts (0.005% or 50 ppm) of elements such as iridium and ruthenium, fine-grained castings are produced. Adding one of these elements to the alloy is believed to develop centers for nucleating grains throughout the alloy. Most alloy manufacturers use grain refinement in present-day products. The mechanical properties of tensile strength and elongation are improved significantly (30%) by the fine grain structure in castings, which contributes to uniformity of properties from one casting to another. Other properties, however, such as hardness and yield strength, show less effect from the grain refinement.

Properties

Melting Range

Dental casting alloys do not have melting points, but rather melting ranges, because they are combinations of elements rather than pure elements. It is desirable for the dental casting alloy to have a relatively narrow melting range because if the alloy spends a long time in the partially molten state during casting, there is increased opportunity for the formation of oxides and contamination. Therefore alloys with wide melting ranges are more difficult to cast without problems.

The melting range of the alloys determines the burnout temperature, type of investment, and type of heat source that must be used during casting. In general, the burnout temperature must be about 500°C below the bottom temperature of the melting range. Therefore for the Au-Cu-Ag-Pd-*I* alloys a burnout temperature of about 450°C to 475°C should be used. If the burnout temperature approaches 700°C, a gypsum-bonded investment cannot be used because the calcium sulfate will decompose and embrittle the alloys. At temperatures near 700°C or greater, a phosphate-bonded investment is used. As shown in Table 9.9, a gypsum-bonded investment may be used with the Au-Cu-Ag-Pd-*I*, *II*, and *III* and the Au-Ag-Pd-In alloys, but a phosphate-bonded investment is advisable for the other alloys. The gas-air torch will adequately heat alloys with liquidus temperatures below 1100°C. Above this temperature, a gas-oxygen torch or electrical induction method must be used. Again, from Table 9.9, a gas-air torch would be acceptable only for the Au-Cu-Ag-Pd-*I*, *II*, and *III* and the Au-Ag-Pd-In alloys.

The maximum temperature of the melting range is important to soldering and formation of ordered phases because during both of these operations, the shape of the alloys is to be retained. Therefore during soldering or hardening-softening, the alloy may be heated only to 50°C below the maximum of the melting range to avoid local melting or distortion of the casting.

Density

Density is important during the acceleration of the molten alloy into the mold during casting. Alloys with high densities will generally accelerate faster and tend to form complete castings more easily. Among the alloys shown in Table 9.9, all have densities sufficient for convenient casting. Lower densities (7 to 8 g/cm^3) seen in the predominantly base-metal alloys are more difficult to cast. Alloys in Table 9.6 with high densities generally contain higher amounts of denser elements such as gold or platinum. Thus the Au-Ag-Pt alloys and Au-Cu-Ag-Pd-*I* alloys are among the densest of the casting alloys.

Strength

Strength of alloys can be measured by either the yield strength or tensile strength. Although tensile strength represents the maximum strength of the alloy, the yield strength is more useful in dental applications because it is the stress at which permanent deformation of the alloys occurs (see Chapter 4). Because permanent deformation of dental castings is generally undesirable, the yield strength is a reasonable, practical maximum strength for dental applications. The yield strengths for the different classes of alloys are shown in Table 9.9. Where applicable, the hard and soft conditions, resulting from the formation of ordered solutions, are shown. For several alloys, such as Au-Cu-Ag-Pd-*I*, *II*, and *III*, the formation of the ordered phase increases the yield strength significantly. For example, the yield strength of the Au-Cu-Ag-Pd-*II* alloys increases from 350 to 600 MPa with the formation of an ordered phase. For other alloys, such as the Au-Ag-Pt and Ag-Pd alloys, the increase in yield strength is more modest in the hardened condition. The Pd-Cu-Ga alloys do not support the formation of ordered phase because the ratio of palladium and copper is not in the correct range for ordered phase formation (see Table 9.9).

The yield strengths of these alloys range from 320 to 1145 MPa (hard condition). The strongest alloy is Pd-Cu-Ga, with a yield strength of 1145 MPa. The other alloys range in strength from 320 to 600 MPa. These latter yield strengths are adequate for dental applications and are generally in the same range as those for the base-metal alloys, which range from 495 to 600 MPa. The effect of solid-solution hardening by the addition of copper and silver to the gold or palladium base is significant for these alloys. Pure cast gold has a tensile strength of 105 MPa (see Table 9.7). As mentioned earlier, with the addition of 10 wt% copper (coin gold), solid-solution hardening increases the tensile strength to 395 MPa. With the further addition of 10 wt% silver and 3 wt% palladium (Au-Cu-Ag-Pd-*I*), the tensile strength increases to about 450 and 550 MPa in the hard condition.

Hardness

Hardness is a good indicator of the ability of an alloy to resist local permanent deformation under occlusal load. Although the relationships are complex, hardness is related to yield strength and gives some indication of the difficulty in polishing the alloy. Alloys with high hardness will usually have high yield strengths and are more difficult to polish. As Table 9.9 shows, the values for hardness generally parallel those for yield strength. In the hard conditions, the hardness of these alloys ranges from 155 kg/mm^2 for the Ag-Pd alloys to 425 kg/mm^2 for the Pd-Cu-Ga alloys. More typically, the hardness of the noble casting alloys is around 200 kg/mm^2. The Ag-Pd alloys are particularly soft because of the high concentration of silver, which is a soft metal. The Pd-Cu-Ga alloys are particularly hard because of the high concentration of Pd, which is a hard metal. The hardness of most noble casting alloys is less than that of enamel (343 kg/mm^2), and typically less than that of base-metal alloys. If the hardness of an alloy is greater than enamel, it may wear the enamel of the teeth opposing the restoration.

Elongation

Elongation is a measure of the ductility of the alloy. For crown and bridge applications, a low value of elongation for an alloy is generally not a big concern, because permanent deformation of the alloys is generally not desirable. However, the elongation will indicate whether the alloy can be burnished. Alloys with high elongation can be burnished without fracture. Elongation is sensitive to the presence or absence of an ordered phase, as shown in Table 9.9. In the hardened condition, the elongation will drop significantly. For example, for the Au-Cu-Ag-Pd-*II* alloys, the elongation is 30% in the soft condition versus only 10% in the hard condition. In the soft condition, the elongation of noble dental casting alloys ranges from 8% to 30%. These alloys are substantially more ductile than the base-metal alloys, which have elongation on the order of 1% to 2%.

Biocompatibility

The *biocompatibility* of noble dental alloys is equally important as other physical or chemical properties. A detailed discussion about the principles of biocompatibility can be found in Chapter 4, but a few general principles are mentioned here. The biocompatibility of noble dental alloys is primarily related to elemental release from these alloys (i.e., their corrosion). Thus any toxic, allergic, or other adverse biological response is primarily influenced by elements released from these alloys into the oral cavity. The biological response is also influenced significantly by exactly which elements are released, their concentrations, and the duration of exposure to oral tissues. For example, the short-term (more than 1 to 2 days) release of zinc may not be significant biologically, but longer-term (more than 2 to 3 years) release might have more significant effects. Similarly, equivalent amounts (in moles) of zinc, copper, or silver will have quite different biological effects because each of the elements is unique in its interactions with tissues.

Unfortunately, there is currently no way of completely assessing the biocompatibility of noble alloys (or any other material), because the effects of elemental release on tissues are not completely understood. However, in general, several principles apply to alloy biocompatibility. The elemental release from noble alloys is not proportional to alloy composition but rather is influenced by the numbers and types of phases in the alloy microstructure and the composition of the phases. In general, multiple-phase alloys release more atoms than single-phase alloys. Some elements, such as copper, zinc, silver, cadmium, and nickel, are inherently more prone to be released from dental alloys than others, such as gold, palladium, platinum, and indium. Alloys with high noble-metal content generally release less atoms than alloys with little or no noble-metal content. However, the only reliable way to assess elemental release is by direct measurement because there are exceptions to each of the generalizations just mentioned. Similarly, it is difficult to predict, even knowing the elemental release from an alloy, what the biological response to the alloy will be. Thus the only reliable way is to measure the biological response directly, either in vitro, in animals, or in humans (see online supplemental material). It is important to also remember that combinations of alloys used in the mouth may alter their corrosion and biocompatibility.

The IdentAlloy certification program was developed to make dentists and patients more aware of the composition of dental alloys. Under this program, each alloy has a certificate (Fig. 9.6) that lists the complete composition, its manufacturer, its name, and the ADA compositional classification (high noble, noble, or predominantly base metal). When the dental prosthesis is delivered by the laboratory to the dental office, a certificate is placed in the patient's chart. In this manner, all parties know the exact composition of the material used. This information can be invaluable later if there are problems with the restoration; for example, if the patient develops an allergic reaction. This information is also useful when planning additional restorations that may contact the existing restoration, or if some modification (such as occlusal adjustment or contouring) becomes necessary.

Composition and Properties of Noble-Metal Alloys for Ceramic-Metal Restorations

Ceramic-metal restorations consist of a cast metallic framework (or core) on which at least two layers of ceramic are baked. It is essential that the coefficient of thermal expansion of the alloy be slightly higher than that of the veneering ceramic to ensure that the ceramic is in slight compression after cooling. This will establish a better resistance to crack propagation of the ceramic-metal restoration. There are several requirements for the alloy in a ceramic-metal system (a complete list of requirements for both the alloy and ceramic can be found in Chapter 10):

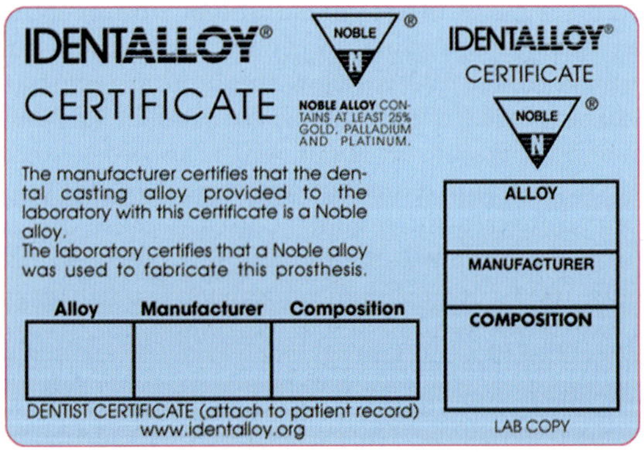

• **Fig. 9.6** An example of an IdentAlloy certificate showing the alloy name, manufacturer, composition, and American Dental Association (ADA) classification. This section of the certificate is for the dentist's records. A duplicate retained by the laboratory is not shown here. Many dentists will give this information to the patient upon delivery of the prosthesis.

1. The alloy must have a high melting temperature. The melting range must be substantially higher (greater than 100°C) than the firing temperature of the ceramic and solders used to join segments of a bridge.
2. A good bond between the ceramic and metal is essential and is achieved by the interactions of the ceramic with metal oxides on the surface of metal (Fig. 9.7) and by the roughness of the metal coping.
3. Coefficients of thermal expansion of the ceramic and metal must be compatible so that the ceramic does not crack during fabrication. The system is designed so the value for the metal is slightly higher than for the ceramic, thus putting the ceramic in compression (where it is stronger) following cooling (Fig. 9.8).

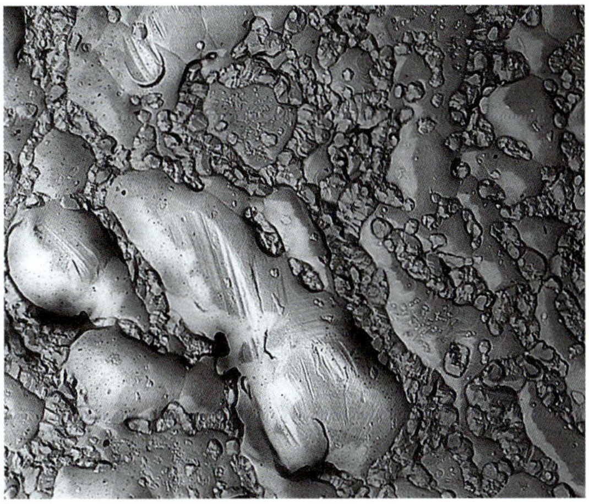

• **Fig. 9.7** Electron micrograph of replicated oxidized surface of an Au-Pt-Pd (gold-platinum-palladium) alloy (×8000). (From Kelly M, Asgar K, O'Brien WJ. Tensile strength determination of the interface between porcelain fused to gold. *J Biomed Mater Res*. 1969;3:403–408.)

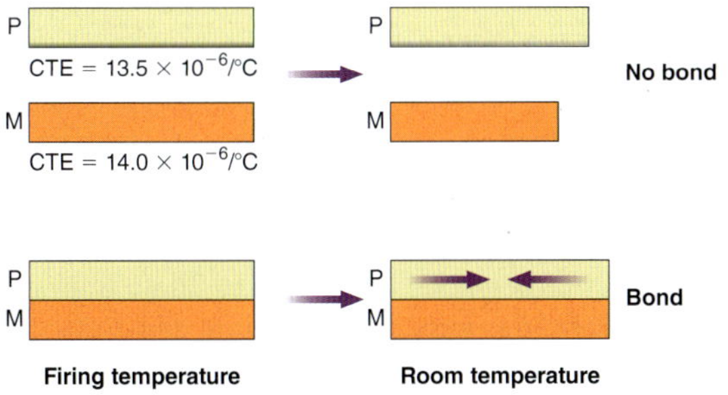

• **Fig. 9.8** Diagram of the ceramic-metal bond. Shown at the firing temperature and at room temperature, when the thermal coefficient of expansion of the metal is 0.5 × 10^{-6}/°C greater than the ceramic, thus placing the ceramic in compression at room temperature. *CTE*, Coefficient of thermal expansion; *M*, metal; *P*, porcelain. (From Powers JM, Wataha JC. *Dental Materials: Foundations and Applications*. 11th ed. Elsevier; 2017.)

4. Adequate stiffness and strength of the alloy core are especially important for fixed bridges and posterior crowns. High stiffness in the alloy reduces stresses in the ceramic by reducing deflection and strain. High strength is essential in the interproximal regions in fixed bridges.
5. High sag resistance is essential. The alloy copings are relatively thin; no distortion should occur during firing of the ceramic, or the fit of the restoration will be compromised.
6. An accurate casting of the metal coping is required even with the higher melting range of the alloy.
7. Adequate design of the restoration is critical. The preparation should provide for adequate thickness of alloy as well as enough space for an adequate thickness of ceramic to yield an aesthetic restoration.

The composition ranges and colors of five types of noble alloys for ceramic-metal restorations are listed in Table 9.10. The properties of these alloys are given in Table 9.11.

Au-Pt-Pd Alloys

The Au-Pt-Pd alloys contain very high noble-metal content, mainly gold with platinum and palladium to increase the melting range. The high noble content provides good corrosion resistance. Indium, tin, and iron (Fe) are present and form oxides to produce a ceramic-metal bond. Rhenium (Re) is added as a grain refiner. Hardening of Au-Pt-Pd alloys results from solid-solution hardening and the formation of a $FePt_3$ precipitate. Optimum heat treatment for hardening is 30 minutes at 550°C, but practically the hardening occurs during firing of the ceramic.

From Table 9.11, it is seen that these alloys have high stiffness (elastic modulus), strength, hardness, and reasonable elongation; however, they have somewhat low sag resistance. The alloys are very costly because of their high noble metal content and high density. The casting temperature is reasonably high, and although reasonably easy to solder, care must be taken because the soldering temperature is only about 50°C below the melting range of the alloys. Finally, although considerable platinum and palladium are present, these alloys are still yellow, which makes producing pleasing aesthetics with the ceramic easier than with white alloys.

Au-Pd Alloys

The Au-Pd high-noble alloys with good corrosion resistance have decreased gold but increased palladium content. These alloys contain no platinum or iron and thus are solution hardened rather than precipitation hardened. They contain indium for bonding, gallium (Ga) to decrease the fusion temperature, rhenium for grain refining, and ruthenium (Ru) for enhancing castability. Because of their high palladium content, the alloys are white (some call it gray) rather than yellow, even though they contain about 50%

TABLE 9.10 Composition Ranges and Color of Noble Alloys for Ceramic-Metal Restorations (wt%)

Type	Au (%)	Pt (%)	Pd (%)	Ag (%)	Cu (%)	Other (%)	Total Noble-Metal Content (%)	Color
Au-Pt-Pd	84–86	4–10	5–7	0–2	—	Fe, In, Re, Sn 2–5	96–98	Yellow
Au-Pd	45–52	—	38–45	0	—	Ru, Re, In 8.5, Ga 1.5	89–90	White
Au-Pd-Ag	51–52	—	26–31	14–16	—	Ru, Re, In 1.5, Sn 3–7	78–83	White
Pd-Ag	—	—	53–88	30–37	—	Ru, In 1–5, Sn 4–8	49–62	White
Pd-Cu	0–2	—	74–79	—	10–15	In, Ga 9	76–81	White

TABLE 9.11 Properties and Casting Temperatures of Noble Alloys Used in Ceramic-Metal Restorations

Type	Ultimate Tensile Strength (MPa)	Yield Strength at 0.2% Offset (MPa)	Elastic Modulus (GPa)	Elongation (%)	VHN (kg/mm^2)	Density (g/cm^3)	Casting Temperature (°C)
Au-Pt-Pd	480–500	400–420	81–96	3–10	175–180	17.4–18.6	1150
Au-Pd	700–730	550–575	100–117	8–16	210–230	13.5–13.7	1320–1330
Au-Pd-Ag	650–680	475–525	100–113	8–18	210–230	13.6–13.8	1320–1350
Pd-Ag	550–730	400–525	95–117	10–14	185–235	10.7–11.1	1310–1350
Pd-Cu	690–1300	550–1100	94–97	8–15	350–400	10.6–10.7	1170–1190

VHN, Vickers hardness number.

gold. This color causes increased difficulty in producing aesthetic restorations.

These alloys are stronger, stiffer, and harder than the Au-Pt-Pd alloys and have higher elongation (more ductile) and casting temperatures (easier to solder). They have lower densities and this means more care should be taken during casting because of the decrease in the force with which the alloy enters the casting ring. However, these alloys remain relatively easy to cast, and soldering is easy because of the higher casting temperature.

Au-Pd-Ag Alloys

The Au-Pd-Ag alloys contain less palladium and more silver than the Au-Pd alloys. However, they still have good corrosion resistance. Again, indium and tin are added for bonding with the ceramics, ruthenium for castability, and rhenium for grain refining. Hardening results from solution hardening. As seen in Table 9.11, the properties of the Au-Pd-Ag alloys are similar to those of the Au-Pd alloys.

Pd-Ag Alloys

The Pd-Ag alloys, which contain no gold and have a moderately high silver content, have the lowest noble-metal content of the five noble alloys. They contain indium and tin for bonding and ruthenium for enhanced castability. Their properties are similar to those of the Au-Pd-Ag alloys, except that they are less dense (≈11 g/cm^3 vs. 14 g/cm^3). Some ceramics used with these high-gold alloys resulted in what was called "greening" relating to a color shift toward yellow. Furnace contamination and technique were blamed to some extent for this problem.

Pd-Cu Alloys

The Pd-Cu alloys contain very high palladium content with 10% to 15% copper. They contain indium for bonding with porcelain and gallium for controlling casting temperature. These alloys have high strength and hardness, moderate stiffness and elongation, and low density. However, they have low sag resistance and form dark oxides. They are white alloys, like all the other metals except the yellow Au-Pt-Pd alloys.

Base-Metal Alloys

Base-metal alloys are used extensively in dentistry for a variety of restorations and instruments, as shown in Box 9.1. Cast cobalt-chromium alloys have been used for many years for fabricating removable dental prosthesis frameworks and have replaced type IV gold alloys almost completely for this application. Nickel-chromium and cobalt-chromium alloys are used in ceramic-metal restorations.

• BOX 9.1 Dental Applications of Cast and Wrought Base–Metal Alloys

- Cast cobalt-chromium alloys
  - Removable dental prosthesis framework
  - Ceramic-metal restorations
- Cast nickel-chromium alloys
  - Ceramic-metal restorations
- Cast titanium and titanium alloys
  - Crowns
  - Fixed-partial prosthesis
  - Removable dental prosthesis framework
  - Implants
- Wrought titanium and titanium alloys
  - Implants
  - Crowns
  - Fixed-partial prosthesis
- Wrought stainless steel alloys
  - Endodontic instruments
  - Orthodontic wires and brackets
  - Preformed crowns
- Wrought cobalt-chromium-nickel alloys: orthodontic wires and endodontic files
- Wrought nickel-titanium alloys: orthodontic wires and endodontic files

The addition of beryllium to base-metal alloys improves castability by lowering the melting temperature and surface tension and increasing the strength of the porcelain-metal bond. However, beryllium, in vapor or particulate form, is associated with several diseases, including contact dermatitis, chronic lung disease, lung carcinoma, and osteosarcoma. Laboratory personnel are at greatest risk for beryllium exposure when performing melting, grinding, polishing, and finishing procedures. Efficient local exhaust and filtration systems as well as adequate general ventilation should be used when casting, finishing, and polishing these beryllium-containing alloys. The ADA Council on Scientific Affairs recommends that, where possible, beryllium-containing alloys should not be used in the fabrication of dental restorations. If alloys containing beryllium must be used, the Occupational Safety and Health Administration (OSHA) guideline (OSHA Hazard Information Bulletin 02-04-19) must be followed. Several manufacturers have eliminated beryllium in their alloys. The ISO standard limits beryllium content to 0.02 wt%. The Food and Drug Administration (FDA) has accepted the ISO standard but has "grandfathered" beryllium-containing alloys on the market before 1976.

The presence of nickel in nickel-chromium alloys and stainless steel is of significant importance because nickel is a known allergen. The incidence of sensitivity to nickel has been reported to be from 5 to 10 times higher for females than for males, with 5% to 8% of females showing sensitivity. However, no correlation has been found between the presence of intraoral nickel-based restorations and sensitivity. A cobalt-chromium alloy without nickel or other nonnickel-containing alloy should be used on patients with a medical history indicating an allergic response to nickel. The amount of nickel in base-metal alloys used in direct soft tissue contact, such as in removable dental prosthesis frameworks, is diminishing. Nickel is mostly found in alloys for ceramic-metal restorations and for wrought applications such as wires. To minimize exposure of patients to metallic dust containing nickel or beryllium, intraoral finishing should be done with a high-speed evacuation system and preferably in a wet environment.

The use of titanium and titanium alloys is rapidly increasing for implants, orthodontic wires, and endodontic files. Stainless steel alloys are used principally for orthodontic wires, in fabricating endodontic instruments, and for preformed crowns.

General Requirements of a Dental Base-Metal Alloy

The metals and alloys used as substitutes for noble alloys in dental restorations must possess certain minimal fundamental characteristics:

1. The alloy's chemical nature should not produce toxicologic or allergic effects in the patient or the operator.
2. The chemical properties of the prosthesis should provide resistance to corrosion and physical changes when in the oral fluids.
3. The physical and mechanical properties, such as thermal conductivity, melting temperature, coefficient of thermal expansion, and strength, should all be satisfactory, meeting certain minimum values for various prosthesis designs.
4. The technical expertise needed for fabrication and use should be feasible for the average dentist and skilled technician.
5. The metals, alloys, and companion materials for fabrication should be plentiful, relatively inexpensive, and readily available, even in periods of emergency.

When base-metal alloys are used in ceramic-metal systems, the same requirements as listed for noble alloys apply.

This list of requirements for the ideal substitute for noble alloys suggests that a combination of chemical, physical, mechanical, and biological qualities is involved in the evaluation of each alloy. The properties of the alloys depend on material, compositional, and processing factors.

Cast and wrought base–metal alloys, including cobalt-chromium-nickel, nickel-chromium-iron, commercially pure titanium (CP Ti), titanium-aluminum-vanadium, stainless steel, nickel-titanium, and titanium-molybdenum (beta-titanium) alloys are discussed in this section. The discussion is based on the synergistic relationship between processing, composition, structure, and properties of the materials.

Cobalt-Chromium and Nickel-Chromium Casting Alloys for Removable Dental Prostheses

Almost all metal frameworks of removable dental prostheses are made from cobalt-chromium alloys.

ANSI/ADA Specification No. 14 (ISO 6871)

According to ANSI/ADA specification No. 14, the weight of chromium should be no less than 20%, and the total weight of chromium, cobalt, and nickel should be no less than 85%. Alloys having other compositions may also be accepted by the ADA, provided the alloys comply satisfactorily with requirements on toxicity, hypersensitivity, and corrosion. Elemental composition to the nearest 0.5% must be marked on the package, along with the presence and percentage of hazardous elements and recommendations for processing the materials. The specification also requires minimum values for elongation (1.5%), yield strength (500 MPa), and elastic modulus (170 GPa).

Composition

Principal Elements. The principal elements present in cast base metals for removable dental prostheses are chromium, cobalt, and nickel, which together account for 82 to 92 wt% of most alloys used. Representative compositions of five commercial dental casting alloys, including three that are used for ceramic-metal restorations, are listed in Table 9.12. Chromium, cobalt, and nickel compose about 85% of the total weight of these alloys, yet their effect on the physical properties is rather limited because the physical properties of these alloys are more controlled by the presence of minor alloying elements such as carbon, molybdenum, tungsten, manganese, nitrogen, tantalum, gallium, and aluminum.

Function of Various Alloying Elements. Chromium is responsible for the tarnish and corrosion resistance of these alloys. When the chromium content of an alloy is higher than 30%, the alloy is more difficult to cast and becomes more brittle. Therefore cast base–metal dental alloys should not contain more than 28% or 29% chromium. In general, cobalt and nickel, up to a certain percentage, are interchangeable elements. Cobalt increases the elastic modulus, strength, and hardness of the alloy more than nickel.

The effect of other alloying elements on the properties of these alloys is much more pronounced. One of the most effective ways of increasing the hardness of cobalt-based alloys is by increasing their carbon content. A change in the carbon content of approximately 0.2% changes the properties to such an extent that the alloy becomes too hard and brittle and should not be used for making any dental prostheses. Conversely, a reduction of 0.2% in the carbon content would reduce the alloy's yield and ultimate tensile strengths to such low values that the alloy would also not be usable in dentistry. Furthermore, almost all elements in these alloys, such as chromium, silicon, molybdenum, cobalt, and nickel, react with carbon to form carbides, which change the properties of the alloys. Note that, as shown in Table 9.12, the nickel-chromium alloys used with ceramic contain significantly less carbon than the alloys used for removable dental prostheses. The presence of 3% to 6% molybdenum contributes to the strength of the alloys.

Microstructure of Cast Base–Metal Alloys

The microstructure of a material controls its properties. In other words, a change in the physical properties of a material is a strong indication that there must have been some alteration in its microstructure. Sometimes this variation in microstructure cannot be distinguished by ordinary means. The microstructures of cobalt-chromium and nickel-chromium alloys are complex and change with slight alterations of manipulative conditions.

Many elements present in cast base-metal alloys, such as chromium, cobalt, and molybdenum, are carbide-forming elements. Depending on the composition of the alloy and its manipulative condition, it may form many types of carbide in various types of arrangements. This will affect the microstructure of the alloy, and ultimately its physical and mechanical properties.

Heat Treatment of Base-Metal Alloys

The early base-metal alloys used in removable dental prostheses were primarily cobalt-chromium and were relatively simple.

TABLE 9.12 **Composition of Major Cast Base-Metal Alloys Used in Dentistry**

	ALLOY (WT%)					
Elements	**Vitallium[a]**	**Ticonium[a]**	**Ni-Cr Alloy with Be[b]**	**Ni-Cr Alloy without Be[b]**	**Co-Cr Alloy[b]**	**Co-Cr with Some Noble Metals[c]**
Chromium (Cr)	30	17	13	22	26	20
Cobalt (Co)	Balance	—	—	—	Balance	Balance
Nickel (Ni)	—	Balance	Balance	Balance	—	—
Molybdenum (Mo)	5	5	5.5	9	6	4
Tungsten (W)	—	—	—	—	5	—
Niobium (Nb)	—	—	—	3.5	—	—
Aluminum (Al)	—	5	2.5	0.25	—	2
Iron (Fe)	1	0.5	—	1.75	0.5	—
Carbon (C)	0.5	0.1	<0.1	<0.1	<0.1	<0.1
Beryllium (Be)	—	1.0	1.9	—	—	—
Silicon (Si)	0.6	0.5	—	0.6	1	—
Manganese (Mn)	0.5	5	—	0.3	—	4
Gold (Au)	—	—	—	—	—	2
Gallium (Ga)	—	—	—	—	—	6
Rare earth	—	—	—	—	0.5	<0.25

[a](From Baran G. The metallurgy of Ni-Cr alloys for fixed prosthodontics. *J Prosthet Dent.* 1983;50:639–650.)
[b]Typical alloy compositions for ceramic-metal restorations with conventional porcelains.
[c]Alloy suitable for high-expansion porcelain.

Heat treating these alloys up to 1 hour at 1000°C did not appreciably change their mechanical properties. Base-metal alloys available today for removable dental prostheses, however, are more complex. Presently, complex cobalt-chromium alloys, nickel-chromium alloys, and iron-chromium alloys are used for this purpose.

Studies have shown that many heat treatments of cobalt-based alloys reduce both yield strength and elongation. If for any reason some soldering or welding must be performed on these removable dental prostheses, the lowest possible temperature should be used with the shortest possible heating time.

Physical Properties

Melting Temperature

Compared with cast gold alloy types I to IV, which have a melting range of 800°C to 1050°C, the melting temperature of base-metal alloys is much higher, with a range of 1150°C to 1500°C.

Density

The average density of cast base–metal alloys is between 7 and 8 g/cm^3, which is about half the density of most dental gold alloys. Density is of some importance in bulky maxillary prostheses, in which the force of gravity causes the relative weight of the casting to place additional forces on the supporting teeth. Therefore with certain prostheses, the reduction of weight resulting from the lower density of the cast base-metal alloys can be considered an advantage.

Mechanical Properties

Typical mechanical properties of the alloys for removable dental prostheses listed in Table 9.12 have been assembled in Table 9.13, together with a representative range of values for type IV casting gold alloys subjected to a hardening heat treatment.

Yield Strength

The yield strength gives an indication of when a permanent deformation of a device or part of a device, such as a partial denture clasp, will occur. As such, it is one of the important properties of alloys intended for removable dental prostheses. It is believed that dental alloys should have yield strengths of at least 415 MPa to withstand permanent deformation when used as removable prosthesis clasps. It may be seen from Table 9.13 that base-metal dental alloys have yield strengths greater than 600 MPa.

Tensile Strength

The ultimate tensile strength of cast base–metal alloys is less influenced by variations in specimen preparation and test conditions than are some other properties, such as elongation. Table 9.13 shows that the ultimate tensile strength of cast base–metal dental alloys is greater than 800 MPa. Table 9.13 also shows that hardened removable dental prosthesis gold alloys can have ultimate tensile strengths almost equal to those of cast base–metal alloys.

Elongation

The percent elongation of an alloy is important as an indication of the relative brittleness or ductility a restoration will exhibit. There are many occasions, therefore when elongation is an important property for comparison of alloys for removable dental prostheses. For example, as described in Chapter 4, the combined effect of

TABLE 9.13 Mechanical Properties of Alloys Used in Removable Dental Prostheses

	Yield Strength at 0.2% Offset (MPa)	Tensile Strength (MPa)	Elongation (%)	Elastic Modulus (GPa)	Vickers Hardness Number (kg/mm^2)
Cast base-Metal alloys[a]					
Vitallium	644	870	1.5	218	380
Ticonium	710	807	2.4	186	340
Hardened removable dental prosthesis gold alloys[b]	480–510	700–760	5–7	90–100	220–250

[a](From Asgar K, Techow BO, Jacobson JM. A new alloy for partial dentures. *J Prosthet Dent.* 1970;23:36–43; Morris HF, Asgar K. Physical properties and microstructure of four new commercial partial denture alloys. *J Prosthet Dent.* 1975;33:36–46; Moffa JP, Lugassy AA, Guckes AD, Gettlemen L. An evaluation of nonprecious alloys for use with porcelain veneers. Part I. Physical properties. *J Prosthet Dent.* 1973;30:424–431.)

[b](From Oilo G, Gjerdet NR. Dental casting alloys with a low content of noble metals: physical properties. *Acta Odontol Scand.* 1983;41(2):111–116.)

elongation and ultimate tensile strength is an indication of toughness of a material. Because of their toughness, removable dental prosthesis clasps cast of alloys with a high elongation and tensile strength do not fracture in service as often as do those with low elongation.

A small amount of microporosity will decrease the elongation of a cast metal prosthesis considerably, whereas its effect on yield strength, elastic modulus, and tensile strength is rather limited. One can therefore assume that practical castings may exhibit similar variations in elongation from one casting to another. To some degree, this is borne out in practice with some castings from the same product showing a greater tendency toward brittleness than others. This observation indicates that control of the melting and casting variables is of extreme importance if reproducible results are to be obtained.

Although nickel and cobalt are interchangeable in cobalt-nickel-chromium alloys, increasing the nickel content with a corresponding reduction in cobalt generally increases the ductility and elongation. High values of elongation are obtained by casting at the normal melting temperature and by not heating the alloy more than 100°C above its normal casting temperature. High elongation is achieved without sacrificing strength and is the result of the precise and proper combination of carbon, nitrogen, silicon, manganese, and molybdenum content.

Elastic Modulus

The higher the elastic modulus, the more rigid is the structure. Some dental professionals recommend the use of a well-designed, rigid prosthesis because it properly distributes forces on the supporting tissues when in service. With a greater elastic modulus, one can design the restoration with slightly reduced dimensions. From Table 9.13, it can be seen that the elastic modulus of base-metal alloys is approximately double the modulus of type IV cast dental gold alloys.

Hardness

Differences in composition of the cast base–metal alloys have some effect on their hardness, as indicated by the values given in Table 9.13. In general, cast base–metal alloys have hardness values about one-third greater than gold alloys used for the same purpose.

Hardness is an indication of the ease of finishing the structure and its resistance to scratching in service. The higher hardness of the cast base–metal alloys as compared with gold alloys requires the use of different polishing equipment and compounds, but the finishing operation can be completed without difficulty by experienced operators.

Fatigue

The importance of the fatigue resistance of alloys used for removable dental prostheses is obvious when one considers that these prostheses are placed and removed daily. At these times, the clasps are strained as they slide around the retaining tooth, and the alloy undergoes fatigue. Comparisons among cobalt-chromium, titanium, and gold alloys show that cobalt-chromium alloys possess superior fatigue resistance, as indicated by a higher number of cycles (putting on and taking off) required to fracture a clasp. Any procedures that result in increasing the porosity or carbide content of the alloy will reduce fatigue resistance. In addition, soldered joints, which often contain inclusions or pores, represent weak links in the fatigue resistance of the prosthesis.

Corrosion

In vitro corrosion tests have evaluated a number of important variables, including effects of electrolytic media and artificial saliva, alloy composition, alloy microstructure, and surface state of the metal. These variables account for 2 to 4 orders of magnitude variation in the amount of metal ions released. The surface state of the metal is an extremely important factor influencing corrosion because the surface composition is almost always different from that of the bulk alloy. Another important consideration is corrosion coupled with wear. Up to three times the mass of metal ions, such as nickel (Ni), is released during occlusal rubbing in combination with corrosion than during corrosion alone for nickel-chromium (Ni-Cr) alloys. No long-term studies have been performed to monitor the impact of the release of such large concentrations of metal ions on the overall health of patients.

Base-Metal Casting Alloys for Fixed Prosthodontics

Most of the nickel-chromium alloys contain 60% to 80% nickel, 10% to 27% chromium, and 2% to 14% molybdenum. As a comparison, cobalt-chromium alloys contain 53% to 67% cobalt, 25% to 32% chromium, and 2% to 6% molybdenum. They may also contain small amounts of aluminum, carbon, cobalt, copper, cerium, gallium, iron, manganese, niobium, silicon, tin, titanium, and zirconium. The range of compositions of base-metal alloys for ceramic-metal restorations is given in Table 9.14, and typical properties of these alloys are listed in Table 9.15.

TABLE 9.14 Composition Ranges of Base Metals for Ceramic-Metal Restorations (wt%)

Type	Ni	Cr	Co	Ti	Mo	Al	V	Fe	Be	Ga	Mn	Nb	W	B	Ru
Ni-Cr	69–77	13–16	—	—	4–14	0–4	—	0–1	0–2	0–2	0–1	—	—	—	—
Co-Cr	—	15–25	55–58	—	0–4	0–2	—	0–1	—	0–7	—	0–3	0–5	0–1	0–6
Ti	—	—	—	90–100	—	0–6	0–4	0–0.3	—	—	—	—	—	—	—

TABLE 9.15 Properties of Base-Metal Alloys for Ceramic-Metal Restorations

Type	Ultimate Tensile Strength (MPa)	Yield Strength at 0.2% Offset (MPa)	Elastic Modulus (GPa)	Elongation (%)	VHN (kg/mm^2)	Density (g/cm^3)	Casting Temperature (°C)
Ni-Cr	400–1000	255–730	150–210	8–20	210–380	7.5–7.7	1300–1450
Co-Cr	520–820	460–640	145–220	6–15	330–465	7.5–7.6	1350–1450
Ti	240–890	170–830	103–114	10–20	125–350	4.4–4.5	1760–1860

VHN, Vickers hardness number.

Base-metal casting alloys exhibit a higher hardness and elastic modulus than do noble-metal alloys, but they require a slightly different approach in casting and soldering to accommodate their higher solidification shrinkage and generally lower densities than noble alloys.

Nickel-Chromium (Ni-Cr) Alloys

Chromium provides tarnish and corrosion resistance, whereas alloys containing aluminum (Al) are strengthened by the formation of coherent precipitates of Ni_3Al. Molybdenum (Mo) is added to decrease the thermal coefficient of expansion. Note that because of the wide differences in atomic weight of nickel and chromium, 2 wt% is roughly equal to 6 at%.

These alloys are harder than noble alloys but usually have lower yield strengths. They also have higher elastic moduli, in some cases allowing for the use of thinner copings and frameworks. They have much lower densities (7 to 8 g/cm^3) and generally higher casting temperatures. Adequate casting compensation is at times a problem, as is the fit of the coping.

Cobalt-Chromium (Co-Cr) Alloys

Again, chromium provides tarnish and corrosion resistance. Unlike Co-Cr removable dental prosthesis alloys, the alloys for ceramic-metal restorations are strengthened by solution hardening rather than carbide formation. Molybdenum helps lower the coefficient of expansion, and ruthenium improves castability. Co-Cr alloys are stronger and harder than noble and Ni-Cr alloys and have roughly the same densities and casting temperature as Ni-Cr alloys. Casting and soldering of these alloys are more difficult than for noble alloys, as is obtaining a high degree of accuracy in the castings.

Titanium (Ti) and Titanium Alloys

Pure titanium (Ti) and titanium alloyed with aluminum and vanadium (Ti-6Al-4V) have been attempted for cast restorations, but they are mainly important in implant and orthodontic wire applications. They have superior biocompatibility compared with the other base-metal alloys, but Ti and Ti-6Al-4V present processing difficulties, as indicated by their high casting temperatures (1760°C to 1860°C), low densities, and ease of oxidation. Other processing methods, such as computer-assisted machining and spark erosion to fabricate copings, may increase the use of these metals. Additional discussion of titanium and titanium alloys appears in the following sections.

Other Applications of Cast Base-Metal Alloys

Cast cobalt-chromium alloys are also used in orthopedics in the surgical repair of bone fractures, specifically for bone plates, screws, various fracture appliances, and splints. Metallic obturators and implants for various purposes can be formed from cast base-metal alloys. The use of cobalt-chromium alloys for surgical purposes is well established, and these alloys have numerous oral surgical uses. They can be implanted directly into the bone structure for long periods without harmful reactions. This favorable response of the tissue is probably attributable to the low solubility and electrogalvanic action of the alloy; the metal is inert and produces no inflammatory response. The product known as surgical Vitallium has been used extensively for this purpose. However, the primary metal used in dental implants today is titanium (see Chapter 14).

Advanced rapid manufacturing technology called *direct metal laser sintering* is being used to create pure cobalt-chrome crowns and fixed dental prosthesis frameworks. This method uses a high-power laser to fuse successive 0.02-mm-thick layers of powdered metal. After all layers are built, the solid copings and frameworks are removed from the machine, sand blasted, polished, and cleaned, and ready for ceramic application. Cobalt-chrome can also be machined using computer-aided design and manufacturing processes. High-speed milling machines under numerical control reproduce geometries created in software originating from scanners or other dental computer-aided design systems. These devices process zirconium, cobalt-chromium, titanium, and plastics. Five-axis machining enables the creation of embrasures, undercuts, and other intricate geometries without the need for manual trimming and adjustment.

Titanium and Titanium Alloys

Titanium's resistance to electrochemical degradation; benign biological response elicited; relatively lightweight; and low density,

TABLE 9.16 Composition of CP Titanium and Alloy (wt%)

Titanium	N	C	H	Fe	O	Al	V	Ti
CP grade I	0.03	0.10	0.015	0.02	0.18			Balance
CP grade II	0.03	0.10	0.015	0.03	0.25			Balance
CP grade III	0.03	0.10	0.015	0.03	0.35			Balance
CP grade IV	0.03	0.10	0.015	0.05	0.40			Balance
Ti-6Al-4V alloy	0.05	0.08	0.012	0.25	0.13	5.50–6.50	3.50–4.50	Balance

CP, Commercially pure.

low modulus, and high strength make titanium-based materials attractive for use in dentistry. Titanium forms a very stable oxide layer with a thickness on the order of angstroms, and it repassivates in a time on the order of nanoseconds (10^{-9} seconds). This oxide formation is the basis for the corrosion resistance and biocompatibility of titanium. Titanium has therefore been called the material of choice in dentistry.

CP Ti is used for dental implants, surface coatings, and more recently, for crowns, partial removable dental prostheses, and orthodontic wires. Several titanium alloys are also used. Of these alloys, Ti-6Al-4V is the most widely used. Wrought alloys of titanium and nickel and titanium and molybdenum are used for orthodontic wires. The term *titanium* is often used to include all types of pure and alloyed titanium. However, it should be noted that the processing, composition, structure, and properties of the various titanium alloys are quite different, and also that differences exist between the wrought and cast forms of a given type of titanium.

Commercially Pure Titanium. CP Ti is available in four grades, which vary according to the oxygen (0.18–0.40 wt%) and iron (0.20–0.50 wt%) content (Table 9.16). These seemingly slight concentration differences have a substantial effect on the physical and mechanical properties.

At room temperature, CP Ti has a hexagonal close-packed crystal lattice, which is denoted as the alpha (α) phase. On heating, a phase transformation occurs. At 883°C, a body-centered cubic phase, which is denoted as the beta (β) phase, forms. A component with predominantly β phase is stronger but more brittle than a component with α-phase microstructure. As with other metals, the temperature and time of processing and heat treatment dictate the amount, ratio, and distribution of phases, overall composition and microstructure, and resultant properties. As a result, casting temperature and cooling procedure are critical factors in ensuring a successful casting.

The density of CP Ti (4.5 g/cm^3) and its elastic modulus (100 GPa) are about half the value of many of the other base metals. The yield and ultimate strengths vary, respectively, from 170 to 480 MPa and 240 to 550 MPa, depending on the grade of titanium. Table 9.17 lists the mechanical properties of CP grades 1 and 4 Ti for comparison with noble alloys and other base-metal alloys.

Titanium Alloys: General. Alloying elements are added to stabilize either the α or the β phase, by changing the β-transformation temperature. For example, in Ti-6Al-4V, aluminum is an α stabilizer, whereas vanadium, as well as copper and palladium, are β stabilizers.

In general, alpha-titanium is weldable but difficult to form or work with at room temperature. Beta-titanium, however, is malleable at room temperature and is thus used in orthodontics to make wires. The (α + β) alloys are strong and formable but difficult to weld. Thermal and thermochemical treatments can refine the postcast microstructures and improve properties.

TABLE 9.17 Mechanical Properties of Titanium and Other Selected Materials

Material	Elastic Modulus (GPa)	Ultimate Tensile Strength (MPa)	Yield Strength (MPa)
316L SS	200	965	690
Co-Cr-Mo	240	700	450
Type IV gold	90	770	>340
CP grade 1 Ti	102	240	170
CP grade 4 Ti	104	550	483
Ti-6Al-4V	113	930	860

CP, Commercially pure; *SS*, stainless steel.

Ti-6AL-4V. At room temperature, Ti-6Al-4V is a two-phase (α + β) alloy. At about 975°C, a phase transformation takes place, transforming the microstructure to a single-phase body-centered cubic β alloy. Thermal treatments dictate the relative amounts of the α and β phases and the phase morphologies and yield a variety of microstructures and a range of mechanical properties. Microstructural variations depend on whether working and heat treatments were performed above or below the β-transition temperature and on the cooling rate.

Following forging (i.e., mechanically deforming) at temperatures in the range of 700°C to 950°C, thermal treatments below the β-transition temperature (typically performed at approximately 700°C) produce recrystallized microstructures having fine equiaxed α grains (Fig. 9.9). Equiaxed microstructures are characterized by small (3–10 μm), rounded grains that have aspect ratios near unity. This class of microstructure is recommended for Ti-6Al-4V surgical implants.

The mechanical properties of (α + β) titanium alloys are dictated by the amount, size, shape, and morphology of the α phase and the density of α/β interfaces. The tensile and fatigue properties of Ti-6Al-4V have been studied extensively. Microstructures with a small (less than 20 μm) α-grain size, a well-dispersed β phase, and a small α/β interface area, such as in equiaxed microstructures, resist fatigue crack initiation best and have the best high-cycle fatigue strength (approximately 500–700 MPa). Lamellar microstructures, which have a greater α/β surface area and more oriented colonies, have lower fatigue strengths (approximately 300–500 MPa) than do equiaxed microstructures.

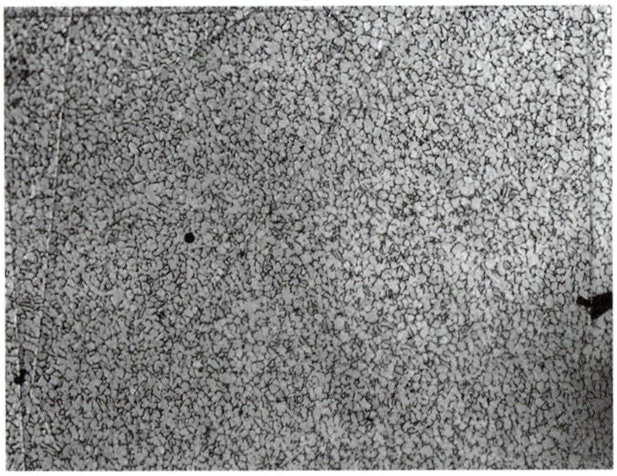

• **Fig. 9.9** Microstructure of equiaxed Ti-6Al-4V (×200). Equiaxed microstructures are characterized by small, rounded α-grains, with aspect ratios near unity.

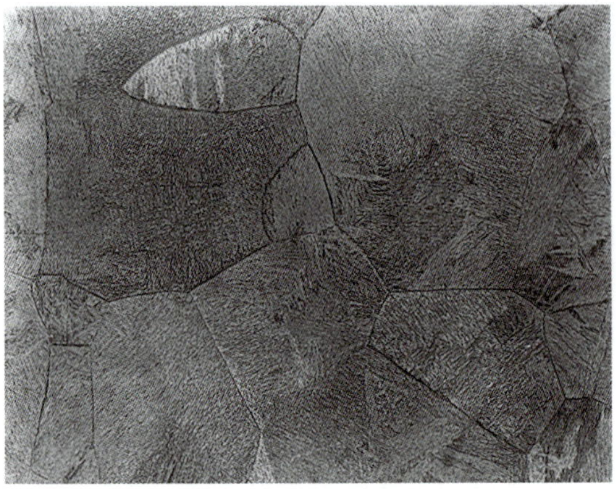

• **Fig. 9.10** Microstructure of as-cast Ti-6Al-4V.

Machined Titanium for Dental Implants. Endosseous dental implants are machined from billets of titanium. Typical materials are CP Ti or the Ti-6Al-4V alloy. Studies have been published on the potential for replacing vanadium with niobium, which might improve cell attachment. Recent research has focused on engineering specific surface textures on machined titanium to improve both the degree of osseointegration and the adaptation of soft tissue to the collar of the implant. To increase surface area for contact by bone cells, machined titanium can be grit blasted with metal oxide or hydroxyapatite particles. The surface can also be plasma sprayed with titanium or coated with hydroxyapatite. More discussion of implant surface modifications can be found in Chapter 14.

Cast Titanium. Based on the attributes, extensive knowledge, and clinical success of wrought titanium implants, interest has developed in cast titanium for dental applications. Although titanium has been cast for more than 50 years, only recently have nearly precision castings been attainable. For aerospace and medical components, hot isostatic pressing and specific finishing techniques are routinely practiced. However, these techniques are beyond the capabilities and affordability of most dental laboratories.

The two most important factors in casting titanium-based materials are their high melting point (1700°C for CP Ti) and chemical reactivity. Because of the high melting point, special melting procedures, cooling cycles, mold material, and casting equipment to prevent metal contamination are required. Titanium readily reacts with gaseous elements such as hydrogen, oxygen, and nitrogen, particularly at elevated temperatures (greater than 600°C). As a result, any manipulation of titanium at elevated temperatures must be performed in a well-controlled vacuum or inert atmosphere. Without such controls, titanium surfaces will be contaminated by an oxygen-enriched and hardened surface layer, which can be as thick as 100 μm and can reduce strength and ductility and promote cracking because of the embrittling effect of the oxygen. The technology required to overcome these factors is what makes casting titanium relatively more expensive.

Because of the high-affinity titanium has for hydrogen, oxygen, and nitrogen, standard crucibles and investment materials cannot be used. Investment materials or face coats for the wax patterns must have oxides that are more stable than the very stable titanium oxide and must also be able to withstand a temperature sufficient to melt titanium. If this is not the case, oxygen is likely to diffuse into the molten metal. Investment materials using a combination of ZrO_2-type face coat that is backed up by a phosphate-bonded silica investment or phosphate investment materials involving inert fillers (ZrO_2, Al_2O_3, MgO) achieve this goal.

Because of the low density of titanium, it is difficult to cast in conventional, centrifugal-force casting machines. In the last 20 years, advanced casting techniques, which combine centrifugal, vacuum, pressure, and gravity casting, new investment materials, and advanced melting techniques (e.g., electric arc melting) have been developed. These advances have improved the feasibility of casting titanium-based materials in the dental laboratory.

Pure titanium and Ti-alloys such as Ti-6Al-4V have been cast into crowns and removable dental prosthesis frameworks. Titanium alloys have a lower melting point than pure titanium. By alloying titanium, the melting temperature can be lowered to the same temperature as that of nickel-chromium and cobalt-chromium alloys. For example, the Ti-Pd and Ti-Cu alloys have melting points of 1350°C. Lower casting temperatures may also reduce the reactivity of titanium with oxygen and other gases.

Microstructures of cast titanium materials are similar to those described previously, namely, coarse lamellar grains, a result of slow cooling through the β to α or β to (α + β) transformation temperature (Fig. 9.10).

The mechanical properties of cast CP Ti are similar to those of types III and IV gold alloys, whereas cast Ti-6Al-4V and Ti-15V exhibit properties, except for modulus, similar to those of nickel-chromium and cobalt-chromium alloys.

Recently, cast Ti-6Al-4V microstructures have been refined by temporary alloying with hydrogen. The resulting microstructures (Fig. 9.11) can have α-grain sizes less than 1 μm, aspect ratios near unity, and discontinuous grain boundary α, microstructural attributes that increase tensile and fatigue strength. These changes in microstructural form and structure result in significant increases in yield strength (974–1119 MPa), ultimate strength (1025–1152 MPa), and fatigue strength (643–669 MPa) as compared with respective values for lamellar (902, 994, and 497 MPa) and equiaxed microstructures (914, 1000, and 590 MPa).

Pure titanium has been cast with a pressure-vacuum casting machine. Other manufacturers have developed centrifugal casting machines that use an electric arc to melt the titanium in an argon or helium atmosphere. Melting is performed in a copper crucible, followed by centrifugal casting into a mold that uses investment. Such machines provide a relatively oxygen-free environment and, with the use of a tungsten arc, can reach temperatures of 2000°C. This latter casting regime has been used to cast CP Ti crowns.

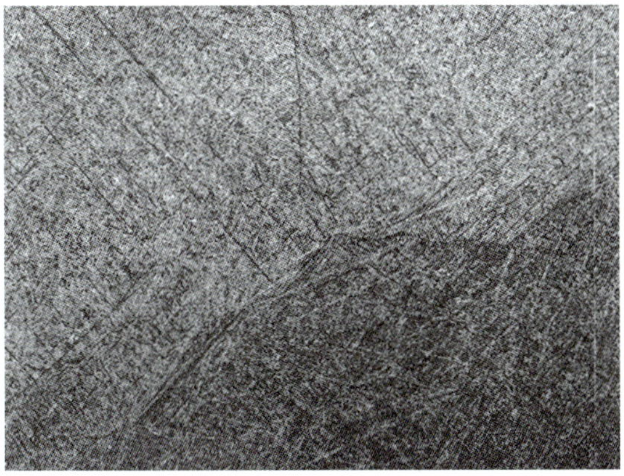

• **Fig. 9.11** Microstructure of hydrogen-alloy-treated Ti-6Al-4V (×200).

Crowns cast in this manner have been evaluated clinically, and results revealed that, although the fit was inferior to that of silver-palladium alloy, it was superior to that of nickel-chromium. Occlusal adjustment was no more difficult than with conventional crowns, and discoloration, occlusal wear, and plaque retention were similar to other metals.

Observations of randomly chosen cast crowns using old machines and silica-containing investments have revealed gross surface porosities, to a depth of 75 µm, on both the inside and outside of the surfaces. Mechanical polishing is insufficient to remove this porosity. Internal porosities, sometimes measuring up to 30% of the cross-sectional area, are also readily observed. Surfaces of castings can also be contaminated, probably due to poor atmosphere control or contamination from crucible and mold materials. For optimum functionality of the final casting, the surface layer must be removed during finishing. However, internal oxidation can remain and compromise the mechanical properties of the final prosthesis. Further examination of such castings has also revealed multiple microcracks at the edges of the margins. Some cracks are as long as 100 µm. Cracks of this length are catastrophic to a notch-sensitive material such as titanium.

As outlined, the difficulties with cast titanium for dental purposes include high melting point and high reactivity, low casting efficiency, inadequate expansion of investment, casting porosity, and difficulty in finishing this metal. From a technical standpoint, titanium is difficult to weld, solder, machine, finish, and adjust. Casting titanium requires expensive equipment.

Wrought Alloys

Alloys that are worked and adapted into prefabricated forms for use in dental restorations are described as *wrought alloys*. A wrought form is one that has been worked or shaped and fashioned into a serviceable form for a prosthesis (Fig. 9.12). The work done to the alloy is usually at a temperature far below the melting range and is therefore referred to as *cold work*. Wrought forms may include precision attachments, backings for artificial teeth, and wire in various cross-sectional shapes. Wrought alloys are used in two ways in dental prostheses. First, they can be soldered to a previously cast restoration. An example is a wrought wire clasp on a removable dental prosthesis framework. Second, they can be embedded into a cast framework by casting to the alloy, as a precision attachment is cast to the retainer of a crown, bridge, or removable prosthesis. The physical properties required of the wrought alloy will depend on the technique used and the composition of the alloy in the existing prosthesis.

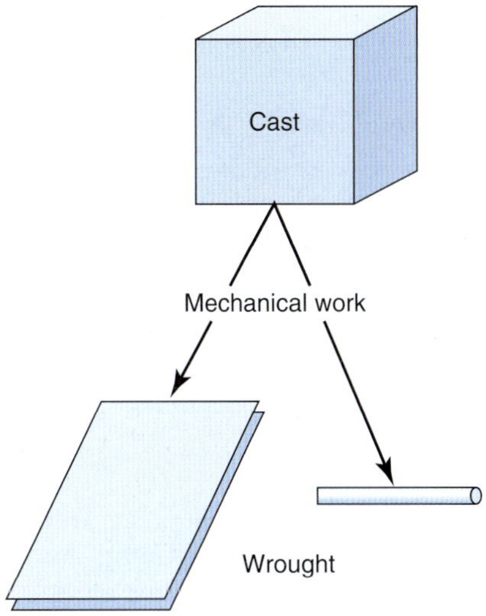

• **Fig. 9.12** Diagram of the process of mechanical work that transforms cast structures into wrought structures. The microstructure and mechanical properties of cast and wrought forms are fundamentally different.

Microstructure

The microstructure of wrought alloys is fibrous. This fibrous structure results from the cold work applied during the operations that shape the alloy into its final form. Wires or other wrought forms normally have a measurable increase in tensile strength and hardness when compared with corresponding cast structures. The increase in these properties results from the entangled, fibrous internal structure created by the cold work.

Wrought forms will recrystallize during heating operations unless caution is exercised. During recrystallization, the fibrous microstructure is converted to a grained structure similar to the structure of a cast form. In general, the amount of recrystallization increases as both the heating time and temperature become excessive. For example, in most noble dental wires, a short heating cycle during the soldering operation is not sufficient to appreciably recrystallize the wire, even though the temperature approaches the fusion temperature. However, a prolonged heating period of 30 to 60 seconds or longer may cause recrystallization, depending on the time, temperature, alloy composition, and manner in which the wire was fabricated. Recrystallization results in a reduction in mechanical properties in proportion to the amount of recrystallization. Severe recrystallization can cause wrought forms to become brittle in the area of recrystallization. Therefore, heating operations must be minimized when working with wrought forms.

Composition

By the current ADA definitions, all alloys used for wrought forms are high-noble alloys except one, which is a noble alloy (Table 9.18). As with casting alloys, several strategies have been used to formulate alloys with appropriate properties. The compositions in Table 9.18 are not inclusive of all available wrought alloys but are intended to demonstrate typical alloys. These compositions are designed to provide a range of melting ranges and mechanical properties that are appropriate for wrought alloy applications. The Pt-Au-Pd alloys contain primarily platinum with equal amounts (27 wt%) of palladium and gold. These platinum-gold-palladium alloys have been commonly used as clasping wires on removable

TABLE 9.18 Composition of Typical Wrought Dental Alloys (wt%)

Alloy	Ag	Au	Cu	Pd	Pt	Other
Pt-Au-Pd	—	27	—	27	45	
Au-Pt-Pd	—	60	—	15	24	Ir 1.0
Au-Pt-Cu-Ag	8.5	60	10	5.5	16	
Au-Pt-Ag-Cu	14	63	9	—	14	
Au-Ag-Cu-Pd	18.5	63	12	5	—	Zn 1.5
Pd-Ag-Cu	39	—	16	43	1	

dental prostheses. The Au-Pt-Pd alloys are primarily gold with platinum and palladium. The Au-Pt-Cu-Ag, Au-Pt-Ag-Cu, and Au-Ag-Cu-Pd alloys contain approximately 60 wt% gold but have adopted different strategies for the remaining 40% of the mass. The first two of these alloys contain about 15 wt% platinum with the balance in silver, copper, and palladium, whereas the third of these alloys contains no platinum and higher amounts of silver. The last alloy shown in Table 9.18 contains no appreciable gold or platinum but consists of palladium and silver in approximately equal amounts with about 16 wt% copper. The Au-Ag-Cu-Pd wrought alloy (see Table 9.18) is similar to the Au-Cu-Ag-Pd-*II* casting alloy (see Table 9.5). These alloys differ only slightly in the gold/silver ratio. Other wrought alloys differ from the casting alloys primarily in their higher platinum contents and absence of iridium or ruthenium grain refiners. Platinum is added to increase the melting temperature of the alloys. The grain refinement is not necessary because these alloys are cold-worked into their final forms.

Properties

The properties of alloys used for wrought applications are shown in Table 9.19. The solidus (temperature at which the alloy is completely frozen) of these alloys ranges from 875°C for Au-Ag-Cu-Pd to 1500°C for Pt-Au-Pd. If the wrought form is to be cast to or soldered to, the solidus must be sufficiently high so the form does not melt or lose its fibrous structure during burnout or casting operations. The solidus required will depend on the metals to be joined, the solder, and the burnout and casting temperatures to be used. In general, alloys with high solidus temperatures also have higher recrystallization temperatures. These alloys are mostly white because of their high platinum and palladium contents. Exceptions are the Au-Pt-Ag-Cu and Au-Ag-Cu-Pd alloys, which are light yellow and yellow, respectively. Yield strength, elongation, and hardness are properties relevant to wrought alloys (see Table 9.19). The wrought form must generally have yield strength low enough to allow for adjustment (of a clasp or attachment) but be high enough that permanent distortion does not occur in service. Furthermore, the elongation must be sufficient to allow for adjustment without fracture. Three of the wrought alloys shown in Table 9.19 can be hardened by formation of ordered phases. The Au-Pt-Ag-Cu and Au-Ag-Cu-Pd alloys are hardened by an Au-Cu ordered phase, whereas the Pd-Ag-Cu alloys are hardened by a Pd-Cu ordered phase. As with the casting alloys, the ordered phase imparts significantly more strength and hardness to the alloy and lower elongation.

Wrought Stainless Steel Alloys

Steel is an iron-carbon alloy. The term *stainless steel* is applied to alloys of iron and carbon that contain chromium, nickel, manganese, and perhaps other metals to improve properties and give the stainless quality to the steel. Usually, stainless steel alloys are not cast, but instead are used in the wrought form in dentistry. As a result, the types of prostheses formed from these two materials differ. The most common applications of stainless steel for dental purposes at present are in the preparation of orthodontic appliances and fabrication of endodontic instruments, such as files and reamers. Some specialized applications of stainless steel exist for temporary space maintainers, prefabricated crowns, or other prostheses placed in the mouth, and for various clinical and laboratory instruments.

Composition

The various classes of stainless steel alloys are referred to as *ferritic*, *martensitic*, and *austenitic*, and they have different compositions, properties, and applications. The ferritic stainless steels are chromium steels employed in the manufacture of instruments or equipment parts in which some degree of tarnish resistance is desirable. A wide range of compositions is available in this group, in which chromium, the principal element contributing to stainless qualities, may vary from 15% to 25%. Elements such as carbon, silicon, and molybdenum are included but are all held within narrow limits.

The martensitic steels also are primarily chromium steels with a lower chromium content (about 12% to 18%). These steels can

TABLE 9.19 Properties of Typical Wrought Dental Alloys

	PROPERTY				
Alloy	Solidus (°C)	Color	0.2% Yield (Soft/Hard) (MPa)	Elongation (Soft/Hard) (%)	Vickers Hardness (Soft/Hard) (kg/mm^2)
Pt-Au-Pd	1500	White	750	14	270
Au-Pt-Pd	1400	White	450	20	180
Au-Pt-Cu-Ag	1045	White	400	35	190
Au-Pt-Ag-Cu	935	Light yellow	450/700	30/10	190/285
Au-Ag-Cu-Pd	875	Yellow	400/750	35/8	170/260
Pd-Ag-Cu	1060	White	515/810	20/12	210/300

be hardened to some degree by heat treatment, and they have a moderate resistance to tarnish. They are used chiefly in the manufacture of instruments and, to a limited degree, for orthodontic appliances.

The austenitic steels represent the alloys used most extensively for dental prostheses. The most common austenitic steel used in dentistry is 18–8 stainless steel, so named because it contains approximately 18% chromium and 8% nickel. The carbon content is between 0.08% and 0.20%, and titanium, manganese, silicon, molybdenum, niobium, and tantalum are present in minor amounts to give important modifications to the properties. The balance (≈72%) is iron.

Function of Alloying Elements and Chemical Resistance

The corrosion resistance of stainless steel is attributed largely to the presence of chromium in the alloy. Iron cannot be used without chromium additions because iron oxide (Fe_2O_3), or rust, is not adherent to the bulk metal. About 11% chromium is needed to produce corrosion resistance in pure iron, and the necessary proportion is increased with the addition of carbon to form steel. Chromium resists corrosion well because of the formation of a strongly adherent coating of oxide on the surface, which prevents further reaction with the metal below the surface. The formation of such an oxide layer is called *passivation.* The surface coating is not visible, even at high magnification, but the film adds to the metallic luster of the metal. The degree of passivity is influenced by a number of factors, such as alloy composition, heat treatment, surface condition, stress in the prosthesis, and the environment in which the prosthesis is placed. In dental applications, the stainless characteristics of the alloys can therefore be altered or lost by excessive heating during assembly or adaptation; using abrasives or reactive cleaning agents (specifically those containing chlorine), which can alter the surface conditions of the prosthesis; and even by poor oral hygiene practices over prolonged periods.

Of the stainless steel alloys in general use, the austenitic type of 18–8 stainless steel shows the greatest resistance to corrosion and tarnish. The chromium composition in these alloys must be between 13% and 28% for optimal corrosion resistance. If the chromium content is less than 13%, the adherent chromium oxide layer does not form. If there is more than 28% chromium, chromium carbides form at the grain boundaries, embrittling the steel. The amount of carbon must also be tightly controlled. If not, carbon will react with chromium, forming chromium carbides in the grain boundaries, which leads to depletion of chromium in the individual grains and decreases corrosion resistance in a process known as *sensitization.* Molybdenum increases the resistance to pitting corrosion.

The elements present in small amounts tend to prevent the formation of carbides between the carbon present in the alloy and the iron or chromium and, as a result, often are described as *stabilizing elements.* Some steels, termed *stabilized stainless steels,* contain titanium, niobium, or tantalum, so the carbides that do form are titanium carbides rather than chromium carbides.

The chemical resistance of stainless steel alloys is improved if the surface is clean, smooth, and polished. Irregularities promote electrochemical action on the surface of the alloy. Soldering operations on stainless steel with gold and silver solder may contribute to a reduction in stainless qualities because of electrogalvanic action between dissimilar metals or because of localized, improper composition of the stainless steel wire.

Stress-Relieving Treatments

The 18–8 alloys are not subject to an increase in properties by heat treatment, but they do respond to strain hardening as a result of cold work during adjustment or adaptation of the alloy to form the prosthesis. Heat treatment above 650°C results in recrystallization of the microstructure, compositional changes, and formation of chromium carbides, three factors that can reduce mechanical properties and corrosion resistance.

Prostheses formed from these alloys may, however, be subjected to a stress-relieving operation to remove the effects of cold working during fabrication, increase ductility, or produce some degree of hardening with some alloys. If heat treatment is to be performed, it should be held to temperatures between 400°C and 500°C for 5 to 120 seconds, depending on the temperature, type of prosthesis, and alloy being heated. A time of 1 minute at 450°C would represent an average treatment to be used on an orthodontic appliance. Keep in mind that temperatures above 650°C will soften or anneal the alloy, and the properties cannot be restored by further treatment. The main advantage of a low-temperature heat-treating operation is that it establishes a uniformity of properties throughout the prosthesis after adaptation and fabrication, which may reduce the tendency toward breakage in service. Factors affecting an alloy's ability to be heat treated and stress relieved include alloy composition, working history (i.e., fabrication procedure), and the duration, temperature, and atmosphere of the heat treatment.

A description of stainless steel orthodontic wires, wrought cobalt-chromium-nickel alloy, and other orthodontic wires can be found on the website http://evolve.elsevier.com/sakaguchi/restorative.

Wrought Nickel-Titanium Alloy

A wrought nickel-titanium alloy known as Nitinol is used as a wire for orthodontic appliances. Nitinol is characterized by its high resiliency, limited formability, and thermal memory. Other nickel-titanium alloys contain copper in small amounts to modify the temperature of the shape-memory effect described in the next section.

Composition and Shape-Memory Effect

The industrial alloy is 55% nickel and 45% titanium and possesses a temperature transition range (TTR). At temperatures below the TTR, the alloy can be deformed plastically. When the alloy is then heated from below to above the TTR, a temperature-induced crystallographic transformation from a martensitic to an austenitic microstructure occurs and the alloy returns to its original shape. Hence nickel-titanium is called a *shape-memory alloy.* The orthodontic alloy contains several percent cobalt to lower the TTR. A number of variations of the Ni-Ti alloy have been developed in dentistry. Compositional variations lead to changes in the martensitic and austenitic start and finish temperatures and mechanical properties. Only those wires with austenitic finish temperatures less than 37°C exhibit the property known as superelasticity, where the wire can be deformed dramatically without becoming strain hardened. For example, Fig. 9.13 illustrates the load-deflection curve for a nickel-titanium (Ni-Ti) orthodontic wire displaying superelasticity. Note that the loading (activation) portion of the curve is different from the unloading (deactivation) portion. This difference is called *hysteresis.*

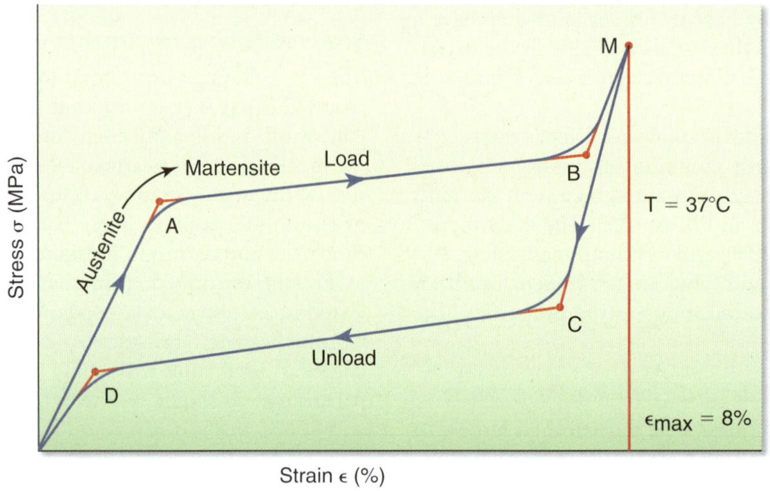

• **Fig. 9.13** Load-deflection curve for Ni-Ti orthodontic wire. Note that the loading (activation) portion of the curve is different from the unloading (deactivation) portion, indicating hysteresis in the material. *Ni-Ti*, Nickel-titanium.

TABLE 9.20 Properties of Orthodontic Wires in Tension, Bending, and Torsion

Property	18-8 Stainless Steel	Nickel-Titanium	Beta-Titanium
Tension			
Yield strength, 0.1% offset, MPa	1200	343	960
Elastic modulus, GPa	134	28.4	68.6
Springback (σ_s/E), 10^{-2}	0.89	1.40	1.22
Bending			
Yield strength, 2.9-degree offset, MPa	1590	490	1080
Elastic modulus, GPa	122	32.3	59.8
Spring rate, mm-N/degree	0.80	0.17	0.37
Torsion			
Spring rate, mm-N/degree	0.078	0.020	0.035

Values are for a 0.43 × 0.64-mm² rectangular wire.
(From Drake SR, Wayne DM, Powers JM, Asgar K. Mechanical properties of orthodontic wires in tension, bending, and torsion. *Am J Orthod.* 1982;82:206–210.)

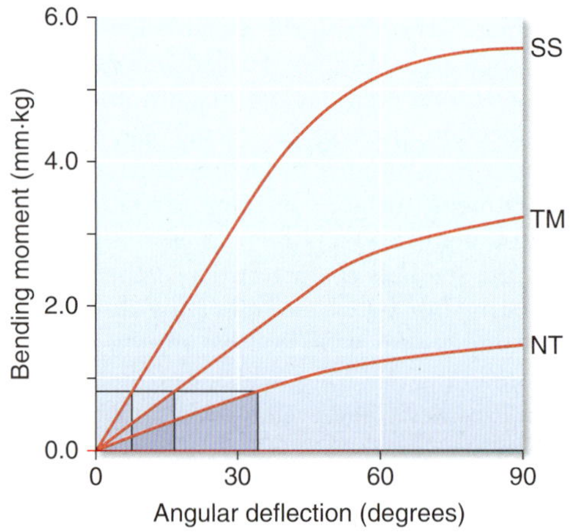

• **Fig. 9.14** Bending moment versus angular deflection. Stored energy at a fixed bending moment below the proportional limit for 0.48 × 0.64 mm wires of alloys stainless steel (*SS*), beta-titanium (*TM*), and nickel-titanium (*NT*). The stored energy is equal to the shaded areas under the curve for each wire. The spring rate is equal to the slope of each curve. (From Drake SR, Wayne DM, Powers JM, Asgar K. Mechanical properties of orthodontic wires in tension, bending, and torsion. *Am J Orthod.* 1982;82:206–210.)

Properties and Manipulation

Mechanical properties of an orthodontic nickel-titanium alloy are compared with those of stainless steel and a beta-titanium alloy in tension, bending, and torsion in Table 9.20. The nickel-titanium alloy has the lowest elastic modulus and yield strength but the highest springback (maximum elastic deflection). As shown in Figs. 9.14 and 9.15, nickel-titanium has the lowest spring rate but the highest resiliency in bending and torsion of the three alloys used for orthodontic wires. Clinically, the low elastic modulus and high resiliency mean that lower and more constant forces can be applied with activations and an increased working range. The high springback is important if large deflections are needed, such as with poorly aligned teeth. Nitinol wire requires special bending techniques and cannot be bent over a sharp edge or into a complete loop. Thus, the wire is more suited for use with pretorqued, preangulated brackets. The alloy is brittle and therefore cannot be soldered or welded, so wires must be joined mechanically.

A description of nickel-titanium endodontic instruments can be found on the website http://evolve.elsevier.com/sakaguchi/restorative.

Wrought Beta-Titanium Alloy

Composition and Microstructure

A titanium-molybdenum alloy known as *beta-titanium* is used as a wrought orthodontic wire. As discussed previously, CP Ti exists in a hexagonal, close-packed crystal lattice at temperatures below 883°C and in a body-centered cubic crystal lattice at higher temperatures. These structures are referred to as *alpha-titanium* and *beta-titanium*, respectively. The beta form of Ti can be stabilized at room temperature by alloying with certain elements.

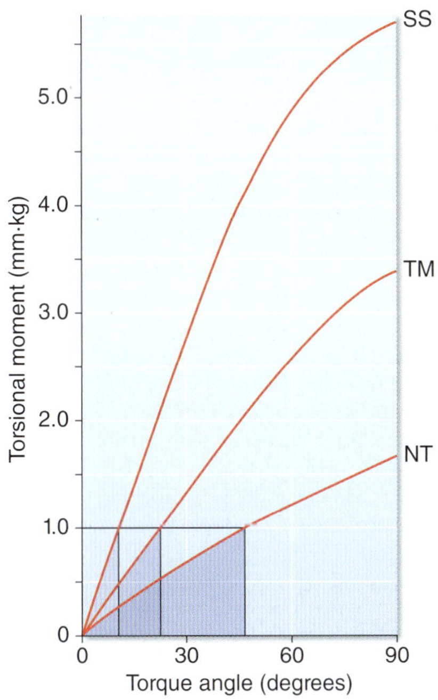

• **Fig. 9.15** Stored energy at a fixed torsional moment below the proportional limit for 0.48 × 0.64-mm wires of alloys stainless steel (*SS*), beta-titanium (*TM*), and nickel-titanium (*NT*). The stored energy is equal to the shaded area under the curve for each wire. The spring rate is equal to the slope of each curve. (From Drake SR, Wayne DM, Powers JM, Asgar K. Mechanical properties of orthodontic wires in tension, bending, and torsion. *Am J Orthod*. 1982;82:206–210.)

Beta titanium alloy for dental use has the composition of 78% titanium, 11.5% molybdenum, 6% zirconium, and 4.5% tin and is supplied as wrought wire.

Properties

Compared with stainless steel wires, beta-titanium wire has lower force magnitudes, a lower elastic modulus, higher springback (maximum elastic deflection), a lower yield strength, and good ductility, weldability, and corrosion resistance. The mechanical properties of beta-titanium alloy in tension, bending, and torsion are compared with stainless steel and nickel-titanium alloys in Table 9.20 and Fig. 9.15. Beta-titanium alloy has values of yield strength, modulus of elasticity, and springback intermediate to those of stainless steel and Nitinol. Its formability and weldability are advantages over Nitinol, and it has a larger working range than stainless steel wires.

Bibliography

Amalgam

Allan FC, Asgar K, Peyton FA. Micro-structure of dental amalgam. *J Dent Res*. 1965;44:1002.

Asgar K, Sutfin L. Brittle fracture of dental amalgam. *J Dent Res*. 1965;44:977.

Baran G, O'Brien WJ. Wetting of amalgam alloys by mercury. *J Am Dent Assoc*. 1977;94:898.

Boyer DB, Edie JW. Composition of clinically aged amalgam restorations. *Dent Mater*. 1990;6:146.

Branstromm M, Astrom A. The hydrodynamics of the dentine: its possible relationship to dentinal pain. *Int Dent J*. 1972;22:219.

Brockhurst PJ, Culnane JT. Organization of the mixing time of dental amalgam using coherence time. *Aust Dent J*. 1987;32:28.

Brown IH, Maiolo C, Miller DR. Variation in condensation pressure during clinical packing of amalgam restorations. *Am J Dent*. 1993;6:255.

Brown IH, Miller DR. Alloy particle shape and sensitivity of high-copper amalgams to manipulative variables. *Am J Dent*. 1993;6:248.

De Rossi SS, Greenberg MS. Intraoral contact allergy: a literature review and case reports. *J Am Dent Assoc*. 1998;129:1435.

Dunne SM, Gainsford ID, Wilson NH. Current materials and techniques for direct restorations in posterior teeth. Part 1: silver amalgam. *Int Dent J*. 1997;47:123.

Farah JW, Powers JM. Dental amalgam and mercury. *Dent Advis*. 1991;8(2):1.

Farah JW, Powers JM. High copper amalgams. *Dent Advis*. 1987;4(2):1.

Halbach S. Amalgam tooth fillings and man's mercury burden [Review]. *Human Exper Toxicol*. 1994;13:496.

Hero H. On creep mechanisms in amalgam. *J Dent Res*. 1983;62:44.

Jensen SJ, Jÿrgensen KD. Dimensional and phase changes of dental amalgam. *Scand J Dent Res*. 1985;93:351.

Kawakami M, Staninec M, Imazato S, et al. Shear bond strength of amalgam adhesives to dentin. *Am J Dent*. 1994;7:53.

Leinfelder KF. Dental amalgam alloys. *Curr Opin Dent*. 1991;1:214.

Lloyd CH, Adamson M. Fracture toughness (KIC) of amalgam. *J Oral Rehabil*. 1985;12:59.

Mahler DB, Adey JD, Marek M. Creep and corrosion of amalgam. *J Dent Res*. 1982;61:33.

Mahler DB, Adey JD, Marshall SJ. Effect of time at 37 degrees C on the creep and metallurgical characteristics of amalgam. *J Dent Res*. 1987;66:1146.

Mahler DB, Adey JD. Factors influencing the creep of dental amalgam. *J Dent Res*. 1991;70:1394.

Mahler DB, Marantz RL, Engle JH. A predictive model for the clinical marginal fracture of amalgam. *J Dent Res*. 1980;59:1420.

Mahler DB, Nelson LW. Factors affecting the marginal leakage of amalgam. *J Am Dent Assoc*. 1984;108:50.

Mahler DB, Nelson LW. Sensitivity answers sought in amalgam alloy microleakage study. *J Am Dent Assoc*. 1984;125:282.

Mahler DB, Terkla LG, van Eysden J, et al. Marginal fracture vs mechanical properties of amalgam. *J Dent Res*. 1970;49:1452.

Mahler DB, van Eysden J, Terkla LG. Relationship of creep to marginal fracture of amalgam. *J Dent Res*. 1975;54:183.

Mahler DB. Amalgam, a review. In: *International State-of-the-Art Conference on Restorative Dental Materials*. National Institute of Dental Research; 1986.

Mahler DB. Slow compressive strength of amalgam. *J Dent Res*. 1972;51:1394.

Mahler DB. The high-copper dental amalgam alloys. *J Dent Res*. 1997;76:537.

Martin JA, Bader JD. Five-year treatment outcomes for teeth with large amalgams and crowns. *Oper Dent*. 1997;22:72.

McCabe JF, Carrick TE. Dynamic creep of dental amalgam as a function of stress and number of applied cycles. *J Dent Res*. 1987;66:1346.

Mitchell RJ, Okabe T. Setting reactions in dental amalgam: part 1. Phases and microstructures between one hour and one week [Review]. *Crit Rev Oral Biol and Med*. 1996;7:12–22.

O'Brien WJ, Greener EH, Mahler DB. Dental amalgam. In: Reese JA, Valega TM, eds. *Restorative Dental Materials: An Overview*. Quintessence; 1985.

Ogura H, Miyagawa Y, Nakamura K. Creep and rupture of dental amalgam under bending stress. *Dent Mater J*. 1989;8:65.

Okabe T, Mitchell RJ. Setting reactions in dental amalgam: part 2. The kinetics of amalgamation [Review]. *Crit Rev Oral Biol Med*. 1996;7:23.

Osborne JW, Gale EN. Failure at the margin of amalgams as affected by cavity width, tooth position, and alloy selection. *J Dent Res*. 1981;60:681.

Powers JM, Farah JW. Apparent modulus of elasticity of dental amalgams. *J Dent Res*. 1975;54:902.

Ryge G, Telford RF, Fairhurst CW. Strength and phase formation of dental amalgam. *J Dent Res*. 1957;36:986.

Smales RJ, Hawthorne WS. Long-term survival of extensive amalgams and posterior crowns. *J Dent*. 1997;25:225.

Wilson NH, Wastell DC, Norman RD. Five-year performance of high-copper content amalgam restorations in a multiclinical trial of a posterior composite. *J Dent*. 1996;24:203.

Zardiackas LD, Anderson L Jr. Crack propagation in conventional and high copper dental amalgam as a function of strain rate. *Biomaterials*. 1986;7:259.

Bonding of Amalgam

Boyer DB, Roth L. Fracture resistance of teeth with bonded amalgams. *Am J Dent*. 1994;7:91.

Eakle WS, Staninec M, Yip RL, et al. Mechanical retention versus bonding of amalgam and gallium alloy restorations. *J Prosthet Dent*. 1994;72:351.

Hadavi R, Hey JH, Strasdin RB, et al. Bonding amalgam to dentin by different methods. *J Prosthet Dent*. 1994;72:250.

Staninec M. Retention of amalgam restorations: undercuts versus bonding. *Quint Int*. 1989;20:347.

Staninec M, Holt M. Bonding of amalgam to tooth structure: tensile, adhesion and microleakage tests. *J Prosthet Dent*. 1988;59:397.

Amalgam: Mercury and Biocompatibility Issues

Abraham JE, Svare EW. The effect of dental amalgam restorations on blood mercury levels. *J Dent Res*. 1984;63:71.

American Dental Association Council on Scientific Affairs. Dental amalgam—update on safety concerns. *J Am Dent Assoc*. 1998;129:494.

Arenholt-Bindslev D. Environmental aspects of dental filling materials. *Eur J Oral Sci*. 1998;106:713.

Berry TG, Nicholson J, Troendle K. Almost two centuries with amalgam: where are we today? *J Am Dent Assoc*. 1994;125:392.

Berry TG, Summitt JB, Chung AK, et al. Amalgam at the new millennium. *J Am Dent Assoc*. 1998;129:1547.

Burrows D. Hypersensitivity to mercury, nickel and chromium in relation to dental materials. *Int Dent J*. 1986;36:30.

Chang SB, Siew C, Gruninger SE. Factors affecting blood mercury concentrations in practicing dentists. *J Dent Res*. 1992;71:66.

Chew CL, Soh G, Lee AS, et al. Comparison of release of mercury from three dental amalgams. *Dent Mater*. 1989;5:244.

Craig RG. Biocompatibility of mercury derivatives. *Dent Mater*. 1986;2:91.

Fan PL, Arenholt-Bindslev D, Schmalz G, Halbach S, Berendsen H. Environmental issues in dentistry—mercury. FDI commission. *Int Dent J*. 1997;47:105–109.

Ferracane JL, Adey JD, Nakajima H, et al. Mercury vaporization from amalgams with varied alloy compositions. *J Dent Res*. 1995;74:1414.

Ferracane JL, Engle JH, Okabe T, et al. Reduction in operatory mercury levels after contamination or amalgam removal. *Am J Dent*. 1994;7:103.

Kaga M, Seale NS, Hanawa T, et al. Cytotoxicity of amalgams, alloys, and their elements and phases. *Dent Mater*. 1991;7:68.

Kingman A, Albertini T, Brown LJ. mercury concentrations in urine and whole blood associated with amalgam exposure in a US military population. *J Dent Res*. 1998;77:60.

Kurland LT, Faro SN, Siedler H. Minamata disease. *World Neurol*. 1960;1:370.

Mackert JR Jr. Dental amalgam and mercury. *J Am Dent Assoc*. 1991;122:54.

Mackert JR Jr, Berglund A. Mercury exposure from dental amalgam fillings: absorbed dose and the potential for adverse health effects. *Crit Rev Oral Biol Med*. 1997;8:410.

Mandel ID. Amalgam hazards: an assessment of research. *J Am Dent Assoc*. 1991;122:62.

Marek M. Corrosion test for dental amalgam. *J Dent Res*. 1980;59:63.

Marek M. Acceleration of corrosion of dental amalgam by abrasion. *J Dent Res*. 1984;63:1010.

Marek M. The release of mercury from dental amalgam: the mechanism and in vitro testing. *J Dent Res*. 1990;69:1167.

Marek M, Hockman RF, Okabe T. In vitro corrosion of dental amalgam phases. *J Biomed Mater Res*. 1976;10:789.

Marshall SJ, Lin JHC, Marshall GW. Cu_2O and $CuCl_2 \cdot 3Cu(OH)_2$ corrosion products on copper rich dental amalgams. *J Biomed Mater Res*. 1982;16:81.

Martin MD, Naleway C, Chou H-N. Factors contributing to mercury exposure in dentists. *J Am Dent Assoc*. 1995;126:1502.

Miller JM, Chaffin DB, Smith RG. Subclinical psychomotor and neuromuscular changes exposed to inorganic mercury. *Am Ind Hyg Assoc J*. 1975;36(10):725.

Okabe T, Ferracane J, Cooper C, et al. Dissolution of mercury from amalgam into saline solution. *J Dent Res*. 1987;66:33.

Okabe T, Yomashita T, Nakajima H, et al. Reduced mercury vapor release from dental amalgams prepared with binary Hg-In liquid alloys. *J Dent Res*. 1994;73:1711.

Olsson S, Bergman M. Daily dose calculations from measurements of intra-oral mercury vapor. *J Dent Res*. 1992;71:414.

Olstad ML, Holland RI, Pettersen AH. Effect of placement of amalgam restorations on urinary mercury concentration. *J Dent Res*. 1990;69:1607.

Pohl L, Bergman M. The dentist's exposure to elemental mercury vapour during clinical work with amalgam. *Act Odont Scand*. 1995;53:1023.

Powell LV, Johnson GH, Bales DJ. Effect of admixed indium on mercury vapor release from dental amalgam. *J Dent Res*. 1989;68:1231.

Powell LV, Johnson GH, Yashar N, et al. Mercury vapor release during insertion and removal of dental amalgam. *Oper Dent*. 1994;19:70.

Snapp KR, Boyer DB, Peterson LC, et al. The contribution of dental amalgam to mercury in blood. *J Dent Res*. 1989;68:780.

Veron C, Hildebrand HF, Martin P. Dental amalgams and allergy. *J Biol Buccale*. 1986;14:83.

Casting Alloys

Anusavice KJ, Shen C, Rawls HR. *Phillips' Science of Dental Materials*. 12th ed. Saunders; 2012.

Corso PP, German RM, Simmons HD. Corrosion evaluation of gold-based dental alloys. *J Dent Res*. 1985;64:854.

Council on Dental Materials. Instruments and equipment: classification system for cast alloys. *J Am Dent Assoc*. 1984;109:766.

Council on Dental Materials. Instruments and equipment: revised ANSI/ADA specification no. 5 for dental casting alloys. *J Am Dent Assoc*. 1989;118:379.

Federation Dentaire Internationale. Alternative casting alloys for fixed prosthodontics. *Int Dent J*. 1990;40:54.

German RM, Wright DC, Gallant RF. In vitro tarnish measurement on fixed prosthodontic alloys. *J Prosthet Dent*. 1982;47:399.

Gettleman L. Noble alloys in dentistry. *Curr Opin Dent*. 1991;2:218.

Givan DA. Precious metals in dentistry. *Dent Clin N Am*. 2007;51:591.

Glantz PO. Intraoral behaviour and biocompatibility of gold versus non precious alloys. *J Biol Buccale*. 1984;12:3.

Johansson BI, Lemons JE, Hao SQ. Corrosion of dental copper, nickel, and gold alloys in artificial saliva and saline solutions. *Dent Mater*. 1989;5:324.

Keller JC, Lautenschlager EP. Metals and alloys. In: von Recum AF, ed. *Handbook of Biomaterials Evaluation*. Macmillan; 1986.

Leinfelder KF. An evaluation of casting alloys used for restorative procedures. *J Am Dent Assoc*. 1997;128:37.

Leinfelder KF, Price WG, Gurley WH. Low-gold alloys: a laboratory and clinical evaluation. *Quint Dent Technol*. 1981;5:483.

Malhotra ML. Dental gold casting alloys: a review. *Trends Tech Contemp Dent Lab*. 1991;8:73.

Malhotra ML. New generation of palladium-indium-silver dental cast alloys: a review. *Trends Tech Contemp Dent Lab*. 1992;9:65.

Mezger PR, Stols AL, Vrijhoel MM, et al. Metallurgical aspects and corrosion behavior of yellow low-gold alloys. *Dent Mater*. 1989;5:350.

Moffa JP. Alternative dental casting alloys. *Dent Clin North Am*. 1983;27:733.

Morris HF, Manz M, Stoffer W, et al. Casting alloys: the materials and "The Clinical Effects". *Adv Dent Res.* 1992;6:28.

Powers JM, Wataha JC. *Dental Materials: Foundations and Applications.* 11th ed.. Elsevier; 2017.

Roberts HW, Berzins DW, Moore BK, Charlton DG. Metal-ceramic alloys in dentistry: a review. *J Pros.* 2009;18:188.

Stub JR, Eyer CS, Sarkar NK. Heat treatment, microstructure and corrosion of a low-gold casting alloy. *J Oral Rehabil.* 1986;13:521.

Vermilyea SG, Cai Z, Brantley WA, et al. Metallurgical structure and microhardness of four new palladium-based alloys. *J Prosthodont.* 1996;5:288.

Wataha JC. Biocompatibility of dental casting alloys: a review. *J Prosthet Dent.* 2000;83(2):223.

Wataha JC. Alloys for prosthodontic restorations. *J Prosthet Dent.* 2002;87:351.

Watanabe I, Watanabe E, Cai Z. Effect of heat treatment on mechanical properties of age-hardenable gold alloy at intraoral temperature. *Dent Mater.* 2001;17(5):388.

Wendt SL. Nonprecious cast metal alloys in dentistry. *Cur Opin Dent.* 1991;1:222.

Cast Base-Metal Alloys

Asgar K, Allan FC. Microstructure and physical properties of alloy for partial denture castings. *J Dent Res.* 1968;47:189.

Asgar K, Peyton FA. Effect of casting conditions on some mechanical properties of cobalt-base alloys. *J Dent Res.* 1961;40:73.

Asgar K, Peyton FA. Effect of microstructure on the physical properties of cobalt-based alloys. *J Dent Res.* 1961;40:63.

Baran GR. The metallurgy of Ni-Cr alloys for fixed prosthodontics. *J Prosthet Dent.* 1983;50:639.

Bates JF. Studies related to the fracture of partial dentures. *Br Dent J.* 1965;118:532.

Ben-Ur Z, Patael H, Cardash HS, et al. The fracture of cobalt-chromium alloy removable partial dentures. *Quint Int.* 1986;17:797.

Bumgardner JD, Lucas LC. Surface analysis of nickel-chromium dental alloys. *Dent Mater.* 1993;9:252.

Cecconi BT. Removable partial denture research and its clinical significance. *J Prosthet Dent.* 1978;39:203.

Council on Dental Materials. Instruments, and equipment: report on base metal alloys for crown and bridge applications: benefits and risks. *J Am Dent Assoc.* 1985;111:479.

Cunningham DM. Comparison of base metal alloys and Type IV gold alloys for removable partial denture frameworks. *Dent Clin North Am.* 1973;17:719.

Frank RP, Brudvik JS, Nicholls JI. A comparison of the flexibility of wrought wire and cast circumferential clasps. *J Prosthet Dent.* 1983;49:471.

Lucas LC, Lemons JE. Biodegradation of restorative metal systems. *Adv Dent Res.* 1992;65:32.

Mohammed H, Asgar K. New dental superalloy system: I. theory and alloy design. *J Dent Res.* 1973;52:136–144.

Morris HF, Asgar K. Physical properties and microstructure of four new commercial partial denture alloys. *J Prosthet Dent.* 1975;33:36.

Morris HF, Asgar K, Rowe AP, et al. The influence of heat treatments on several types of base-metal removable partial denture alloys. *J Prosthet Dent.* 1979;41:388.

Roach M. Base metal alloys used for dental restorations and implants. *Dent Clin N Am.* 2007;51:603.

Rowe AP, Bigelow WC, Asgar K. Effect of tantalum addition to a cobalt-chromium-nickel base alloy. *J Dent Res.* 1974;53:325.

Smith DC. Tissue reaction to noble and base metal alloys. In: Smith DC, William DF, eds. CRC Press; 1982. *Biocompatibility of Dental Materials.* 4.

Vallittu PK, Kokkonen M. Deflection fatigue of cobalt-chromium, titanium, and gold alloy cast denture clasps. *J Prosthet Dent.* 1995;74:412.

Wakasa K, Yamaki M. Corrosive properties in experimental Ni-Cu-Mn based alloy systems for dental purposes. *J Mater Sci Mater Med.* 1990;1:171.

Wakasa K, Yamaki M. Dental application of the 30Ni-30Cu-40Mn ternary alloy system. *J Mater Sci Mater Med.* 1990;1:44.

Wakasa K, Yamaki M. Tensile behaviour in 30Ni-30Cu-30Mn based alloys for a dental application. *J Mater Sci Mater Med.* 1991;2:71.

Wataha JC, Craig RG, Hanks CT. The release of elements of dental casting alloys into cell-culture medium. *J Dent Res.* 1991;70:1014.

Wataha JC, Craig RG, Hanks CT. The effects of cleaning on the kinetics of in vitro metal release from dental casting alloys. *J Dent Res.* 1992;71:1417.

Waterstrat RM. New alloys. *J Am Dent Assoc.* 1992;123:33.

Yong T, De Long B, Goodkind RJ, et al. Leaching of Ni, Cr and Be ions from base metal alloys in an artificial oral environment. *J Prosthet Dent.* 1992;68:692.

Wrought Base–Metal Alloys

Alapati SB, Brantley WA, Svec TA, et al. Scanning electron microscope observations of new and used nickel-titanium rotary files. *J Endod.* 2003;29:667.

Alapati SB, Brantley WA, Svec TA, et al. Observations of nickel-titanium rotary endodontic instruments that fractured during clinical use. *J Endod.* 2005;31:40.

Andreasen GF, Barrett RD. An evaluation of cobalt-substituted Nitinol wire in orthodontics. *Am J Orthod.* 1973;63:462.

Andreasen GF, Bigelow H, Andrews JG. 55 Nitinol wire: force developed as a function of "elastic memory". *Aust Dent J.* 1979;24:146.

Andreasen GF, Brady PR. A use hypothesis for 55 Nitinol wire for orthodontics. *Angle Orthod.* 1972;42:172.

Andreasen GF, Morrow RE. Laboratory and clinical analyses of Nitinol wire. *Am J Orthod.* 1978;73:142.

Brantley WA, Augat WS, Myers CL, et al. Bending deformation studies of orthodontic wires. *J Dent Res.* 1978;57:609.

Brantley WA, Svec TA, Iijima M, et al. Differential scanning calorimetric studies of nickel titanium rotary endodontic instruments. *J Endod.* 2002;28:567.

Brantley WA, Svec TA, Iijima M, et al. Differential scanning calorimetric studies of nickel-titanium rotary endodontic instruments after simulated clinical use. *J Endod.* 2002;28:774.

Burstone CJ, Goldberg AJ. Beta titanium: a new orthodontic alloy. *Am J Orthod.* 1980;77:121.

Chen R, Zhi YF, Arvystas MG. Advanced Chinese NiTi alloy wire and clinical observations. *Angle Orthod.* 1992;62:15.

Dolan DW, Craig RG. Bending and torsion of endodontic files with rhombus cross sections. *J Endod.* 1982;8:260.

Drake SR, Wayne DM, Powers JM, et al. Mechanical properties of orthodontic wires in tension, bending, and torsion. *Am J Orthod.* 1982;82:206.

Goldberg AJ, Burstone CJ, Hadjinikolaoa I, et al. Screening of matrices and fibers for reinforced thermoplastics intended for dental applications. *J Biomed Mater Res.* 1994;28:167.

Goldberg J, Burstone CJ. An evaluation of beta titanium alloys for use in orthodontic appliances. *J Dent Res.* 1979;58:593.

Ha'kel Y, Serfaty R, Bateman G, et al. Dynamic and cyclic fatigue of engine-driven rotary nickel-titanium endodontic instruments. *J Endod.* 1999;25:434.

Kapila S, Sachdeva R. Mechanical properties and clinical applications of orthodontic wires. *Am J Orthod Dentofac Orthop.* 1989;96:100.

Kusy RP. Comparison of nickel-titanium and beta titanium wire sizes to conventional orthodontic arch wire materials. *Am J Orthod.* 1981;79:625.

Neal RG, Craig RG, Powers JM. Cutting ability of K-type endodontic files. *J Endod.* 1983;9:52.

Neal RG, Craig RG, Powers JM. Effect of sterilization and irrigants on the cutting ability of stainless steel files. *J Endod.* 1983;9:93.

Newman JG, Brantley WA, Gorstein H. A study of the cutting efficiency of seven brands of endodontic files in linear motion. *J Endod.* 1983;9:316.

Peterson DS, Jubach TS, Katora M. Scanning electron microscope study of stainless steel crown margins. *ASDC J Dent Child.* 1978;45:376.

Schwaninger B, Sarkar NK, Foster BE. Effect of long-term immersion corrosion on the flexural properties of Nitinol. *Am J Orthod.* 1982;82:45.

Shastry CV, Goldberg AJ. The influence of drawing parameters on the mechanical properties of two beta-titanium alloys. *J Dent Res.* 1983;62:1092.

Stokes OW, Fiore PM, Barss JT, et al. Corrosion in stainless-steel and nickel-titanium files. *J Endod.* 1999;25:17.

Svec TA, Powers JM. A method to assess rotary nickel-titanium files. *J Endod.* 2000;26:517.

Svec TA, Powers JM. The deterioration of rotary nickel-titanium files under controlled conditions. *J Endod.* 2002;28:105.

Thompson SA. An overview of nickel-titanium alloys used in dentistry. *Int Endod J.* 2000;33:297.

Waters NE. Superelastic nickel-titanium wires. *Br J Orthod.* 1992;19:319.

Wilkinson JV. Some metallurgical aspects of orthodontic stainless steel. *Am J Orthod.* 1962;48:192.

Wilson DF, Goldberg AJ. Alternative beta-titanium alloys for orthodontic wires. *Dent Mater.* 1987;3:337.

Yoneyama T, Doi H. Superelasticity and thermal behaviour of NiTi orthodontic archwires. *Dent Mater.* 1992;11:1.

Titanium

Ducheyne P, Kohn D, Smith TS. Fatigue properties of cast and heat treated Ti-6Al-4V alloy for anatomic hip prostheses. *Biomaterials.* 1987;8:223.

Ida K, Tani Y, Tsutsumi S, et al. Clinical applications of pure titanium crowns. *Dent Mater J.* 1985;4:191.

Ida K, Togaya T, Tsutsumi S, et al. Effect of magnesia investments on the dental casting of pure titanium or titanium alloys. *Dent Mater J.* 1982;1:8.

Kohn DH, Ducheyne P. A parametric study of the factors affecting the fatigue strength of porous coated Ti-6Al-4V implant alloy. *J Biomed Mater Res.* 1990;24:1483.

Kohn DH, Ducheyne P. Microstructural refinement of beta-sintered and porous coated Ti-6Al-4V by temporary alloying with hydrogen. *J Mater Sci.* 1991;26:534.

Kohn DH, Ducheyne P. Tensile and fatigue strength of hydrogen treated Ti-6Al-4V alloy. *J Mater Sci.* 1991;26:328.

Lutjering G, Gysler A. Critical review-fatigue. In: Lutjering G, Zwicker U, Bunk W, eds. *Titanium, Science and Technology.* Deutsche Gesellschaft fur Metallkunde; 1985.

McCracken M. Dental implant materials: commercially pure titanium and titanium alloys. *J Prosthodont.* 1999;8(1):40.

Moser JB, Lin JH, Taira M, et al. Development of dental Pd-Ti alloys. *Dent Mater.* 1985;1:37.

Okabe T, Hero H. The use of titanium in dentistry. *Cells Mater.* 1995;5:211.

Szurgot KC, Marker BC, Moser JB, et al. The casting of titanium for removable partial dentures. *Dent Mater Sci QDT Yearbook.* 1988;171.

Taira M, Moser JB, Greener EH. Studies of Ti alloys for dental castings. *Dent Mater.* 1989;5:45.

Voitik AJ. Titanium dental castings, cold worked titanium restorations—yes or no? *Trends Tech Contemp Dent Lab.* 1991;8(10):23.

Waterstrat RM. *Comments on Casting of Ti-13Cu-4.5Ni Alloy*224. Department of Health, Education, and Welfare; 1977:224.

Yamauchi M, Sakai M, Kawano J. Clinical application of pure titanium for cast plate dentures. *Dent Mater J.* 1988;7:39.

10

Restorative Materials: Ceramics

YU ZHANG, ROBERT J. KELLY

CHAPTER OUTLINE

Ceramics

The term *ceramic* refers to any product made from a nonmetallic inorganic material usually processed by firing at a high temperature to achieve desirable properties. The more restrictive term *porcelain* refers to a specific compositional range of ceramic materials originally made by mixing feldspars (potassium and sodium aluminosilicates), quartz (silica), and kaolin (hydrated aluminosilicate) and firing at high temperatures. Dental ceramics for *metal-ceramic* restorations belong to this compositional range and are commonly referred to as *dental porcelains.*

The laboratory portion of ceramic restorations is usually made in a commercial dental laboratory by skilled technicians working with specialized equipment to shape and tint the restoration to the specifications provided by the dentist. Skilled technicians and artisans are also employed by the manufacturers of artificial denture teeth to produce the many forms, types, and shades necessary in this application of porcelain. However, a variety of machinable ceramics are also available for chair-side fabrication of all-ceramic restorations by computer-aided design/computer-aided manufacturing (CAD/CAM). A discussion of CAD/CAM systems is presented in Chapter 13.

Classification of Dental Ceramics

Dental ceramics can be classified according to their applications, fabrication method, or crystalline phase (Table 10.1).

Classification by Application

Ceramics have two major applications in dentistry: (1) ceramics for metal-ceramic crowns (Fig. 10.1, *right*) and fixed dental prostheses (FDPs); (2) all ceramic materials for crowns (Fig. 10.1, *left*), inlays, onlays, veneers, and FDPs. In addition, ceramic orthodontic brackets, ceramic denture teeth, and dental implants and abutments are available.

Classification by Fabrication Method

The classification by fabrication method is summarized in Table 10.1, which also includes examples of commercial ceramics and their manufacturers. The most common fabrication technique for metal-ceramic restorations is called *sintering.* Sintering is the process of firing the compacted ceramic powder at high temperatures to ensure optimal densification. This occurs by progressive pore elimination and viscous flow when the firing temperature is reached. All-ceramic restorations can also be produced by sintering, but they encompass a wider range of processing techniques, including slip casting, heat pressing, and CAD/CAM machining. Some of these techniques, such as machining and heat pressing, can also be combined to produce the final restoration.

Classification by Crystalline Phase

Regardless of their applications or fabrication technique, after firing, dental ceramics are composed of a glassy (or vitreous) phase and one or more crystalline phases, together with various amounts of porosity. Depending on the nature and amount of crystalline phase and porosity present, the mechanical and

TABLE 10.1 Classification of Dental Ceramic Materials With Examples of Products and Their Manufacturers

Application	Fabrication	Crystalline Phase	Products	Manufacturers
All-ceramic	Soft machined	Zirconia (3Y-TZP, tetragonal & cubic)	Cercon	Dentsply Sirona
			Lava	3M Company
			IPS e.max ZirCAD	Ivoclar Vivadent
			In-Ceram YZ	VITA Zahnfabrik
			Zpex	Tosoh Corporation
		Zirconia (3.7Y-PSZ, tetragonal & cubic)	KATANA ML	Kuraray Noritake
		Zirconia (4Y-PSZ, tetragonal & cubic)	Zpex 4	Tosoh Corporation
		Zirconia (4.8Y-PSZ, cubic & tetragonal)	KATANA STML	Kuraray Noritake
		Zirconia (5.3Y-PSZ, cubic & tetragonal)	Zpex Smile	Tosoh Corporation
		Zirconia (5.4Y-PSZ, cubic & tetragonal)	KATANA UTML	Kuraray Noritake
	Hard machined	Zirconia (3Y-TZP, tetragonal & cubic)	BruxZir NOW	Glidewell Laboratories
		Zirconia (4.7Y-PSZ, cubic & tetragonal)	BruxZir Esthetic NOW	Glidewell Laboratories
		Lithium disilicate ($Li_2Si_2O_5$)	IPS e.max CAD	Ivoclar Vivadent
		Lithium silicate (Li_2SiO_3)	Obsidian	Glidewell Laboratories
		Lithium disilicate/silicate ($Li_2Si_2O_5$ & Li_2SiO_3)	Vita Suprinity PC Celtra Duo	VITA Zahnfabrik Dentsply Sirona
		Lithium disilicate/aluminosilicate ($Li_2Si_2O_5$ & $LiAlSi_2O_6$)	N!CE	Institut Straumann
		Feldspar ($[Na, K]AlSi_3O_8$)	Vita Mark II	VITA Zahnfabrik
		Leucite ($KAlSi_2O_6$)	IPS Empress CAD	Ivoclar Vivadent
	Heat pressed	Leucite ($KAlSi_2O_6$)	IPS Empress	Ivoclar Vivadent
		Lithium disilicate ($Li_2Si_2O_5$)	IPS e.max Press	Ivoclar Vivadent
		Lithium disilicate ($Li_2Si_2O_5$)	Initial LiSi Press	GC Corporation
		Lithium disilicate/silicate ($Li_2Si_2O_5$ & Li_2SiO_3)	Celtra Press	Dentsply Sirona
		Fluorapatite ($Ca_5[PO_4]_3F$)	IPS e.max ZirPress	Ivoclar Vivadent
	Sintered	Leucite ($KAlSi_2O_6$)	IPS Empress layering ceramic	Ivoclar Vivadent
		Zirconia (ZrO_2)	All zirconia compositions	Various dental companies
		Alumina (Al_2O_3)	Procera AllCeram	Nobel Biocare
		Fluorapatite ($Ca_5[PO_4]_3F$)	IPS e.max Ceram layering ceramic	Ivoclar Vivadent
Metal-ceramic	Sintered	Leucite ($KAlSi_2O_6$)	VMK-95	VITA Zahnfabrik
Denture teeth	Manufactured	Feldspar	TruByte	Dentsply Sirona
		Feldspar	VITA LUMIN Vacuum	VITA Zahnfabrik

PSZ, Partially stabilized zirconia; *TZP*, tetragonal zirconia polycrystals.

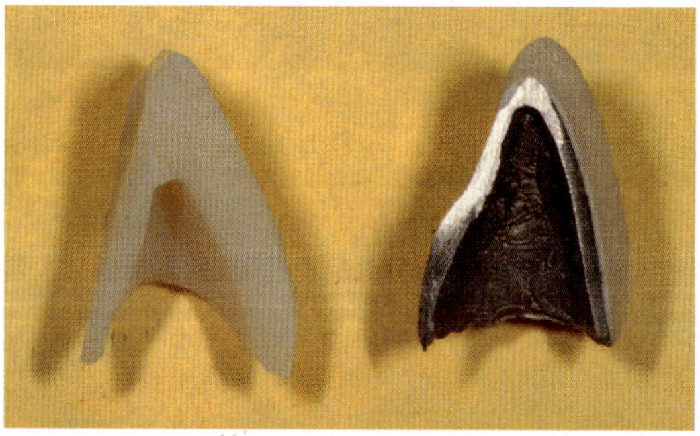

• **Fig. 10.1** Cutaways of all-ceramic crown *(left)* and porcelain fused to metal crown *(right)*. (Courtesy Dr. Charles Mark Malloy, Portland, OR.)

optical properties of dental ceramics vary widely. Increasing the amount of crystalline phase may lead to crystalline reinforcement and increase the resistance to crack propagation but also can decrease translucency. Materials for all-ceramic restorations have increased amounts of crystalline phase (between 35% for leucite-reinforced ceramics and up to 99% for polycrystalline zirconia ceramics such as 3Y-TZP, or 3 mol% yttria-stabilized tetragonal zirconia polycrystals) for better mechanical properties, but they are usually more opaque than dental porcelains and glass-ceramics with lower crystallinity. Table 10.1 lists the various combinations of fabrication techniques and crystalline phases found in dental ceramics.

General Applications of Ceramics in Prosthetic Dentistry

Ceramics represent the best material available for matching the aesthetics of a complex human tooth structure. Their applications in dentistry are steadily expanding as new materials and manufacturing techniques are being introduced. As mentioned earlier, they are used in single and multiunit metal-ceramic restorations. The applications of all-ceramic materials include inlays, onlays, veneers, and crowns. The development of high-strength zirconia-based systems has made possible the fabrication of FDPs, and dental implants and abutments. In addition, ceramics are still used to fabricate denture teeth. However, ceramics are brittle, weak in tension, and their performance is highly dependent on both their microstructure and the quality of the processing from the raw components to the final staining or glazing step.

Metal-Ceramic Crowns and Fixed Dental Prostheses

Ceramic is widely used as the veneering material in metal-ceramic crowns and FDPs. This development was the result of successfully matching the coefficients of thermal expansion of porcelain with that of metal alloys and achieving a proper metal-ceramic bond. The finished glazed restoration is color stable, tissue friendly, biologically inert, and chemically durable. Although progressively replaced with all-ceramic materials, metal-ceramic restorations are still widely used. However, although the survival rate of most all-ceramic crowns compares favorably to that of metal-ceramic crowns for single restorations, the *long-term* survival rate of multiunit all-ceramic FDPs remains lower.

All Ceramic Inlays, Onlays, Veneers, Crowns, and Fixed Dental Prostheses

Ceramics have been used to fabricate jacket crowns since the early 1900s, and at that time, feldspathic porcelains were the material of choice. Alumina-reinforced ceramics with improved mechanical properties were developed in the early 1960s. In the past 60 years, numerous novel materials and techniques for fabricating all-ceramic restorations have been introduced. As mentioned earlier, they include heat-pressed, slip-cast, and machined all-ceramic materials. These new materials and techniques have widened the range of applications of ceramics, and in general, made their processing easier and more reliable. Meanwhile, as technologies are constantly evolving, some techniques, such as slip casting, have been replaced by others, with increasing popularity for machined ceramics.

Ceramic inlays and onlays are becoming increasingly popular as an alternative to posterior resin composites. They have better abrasion resistance than posterior resin composites and therefore are more durable. However, occlusal adjustments are more difficult and can lead to subsequent wear of the opposing tooth if not properly polished. The marginal gap is clinically acceptable, yet greater than with gold inlays or onlays.

A ceramic aesthetic veneer (laminate veneer) is a layer of ceramic bonded to the facial surface of a prepared tooth often for cosmetic reasons. Ceramic veneers are custom made and fabricated in a dental laboratory. Initially, ceramic veneers were made of feldspathic porcelain and sintered. Currently, most ceramic veneers are fabricated by heat-pressing or machining, using either leucite-reinforced or lithia-based glass-ceramics. To obtain sufficient adhesion, the tooth enamel is etched with phosphoric acid, and the bonding surface of the ceramic is etched with 5% to 9% hydrofluoric acid gel and treated with a silane coupling agent. Resin composites specifically formulated for bonding to ceramic are used as the adhesive.

With the development of strong and aesthetic ceramic materials such as zirconia and lithia-based glass-ceramics, all ceramic FDPs and even full arch prostheses have been made available for oral rehabilitation. Ceramic FDPs take the form of either monolithic or veneered structures. They can be fabricated by machining (zirconia, lithia-based glass-ceramics) or by heat-pressing (lithia-based glass-ceramics), in a dental laboratory or a dentist's office.

Mechanical and Thermal Properties of Dental Ceramics

Toughening Mechanisms

Toughening mechanisms for glasses and ceramics are either "built-in" (intrinsic) to the material, relying on chemical composition or crystalline phases, or introduced by extrinsic processing steps. Crystalline reinforcement and transformation toughening are examples of "built-in" toughening mechanisms. Extrinsic processing steps, such as tempering, chemical strengthening, or glaze application, have also been used in the past to achieve strengthening.

The principle of toughening by crystalline reinforcement is to increase the resistance of the ceramic to crack propagation by introducing a dispersed crystalline phase with high toughness. Crystals can also act as crack deflectors when their coefficient of thermal expansion (CTE) is greater than that of the surrounding glassy matrix, placing them under tangential compressive stresses after the ceramic has been cooled to room temperature, as they contract more than the surrounding glassy matrix.

Stress-induced transformation toughening is obtained, for example, in ceramics consisting of partially stabilized tetragonal zirconia. Zirconia (ZrO_2) exists under several crystallographic forms. The monoclinic form is stable at all temperatures below 1170°C. The tetragonal form is stable between 1170° and up to 2370°C. The transformation from the tetragonal to the monoclinic form upon cooling is associated with a volume *increase* of the unit cell. This is the reason why compacts of pure unalloyed zirconia cannot be obtained at room temperature; the compact would spontaneously shatter upon cooling due to the transformation and volume increase. The tetragonal form can be partially stabilized to room temperature by doping with various oxides, such as yttrium oxide (Y_2O_3), cerium oxide (CeO_2), magnesium oxide (MgO), or calcium oxide (CaO). The strongest form of zirconia-based dental ceramics produced by machining followed by sintering at high temperature consists of tetragonal zirconia polycrystals, partially stabilized with 3 mole percent yttrium oxide (3Y-TZP). This partial stabilization or metastability of the tetragonal phase allows the transformation from tetragonal to monoclinic to occur under externally applied stresses. The transformation is also called *stress induced* and is accompanied by a volume increase with associated compressive stresses in the vicinity of the crack tip, eventually leading to closing and arrest of the crack in the transformed zone (Fig. 10.2). Transformation toughening is responsible for the excellent mechanical properties of 3Y-TZP. Fig. 10.3 shows a Vickers indentation in a 3Y-TZP dental ceramic under a 98.1-N load. Only one short crack can be seen emanating from one corner of the indentation, indicative of an excellent resistance to crack propagation.

Tempering and chemical strengthening are extrinsic strengthening techniques based on the creation of a compressive stress layer at the surface of a glass or a ceramic. Tempering is obtained

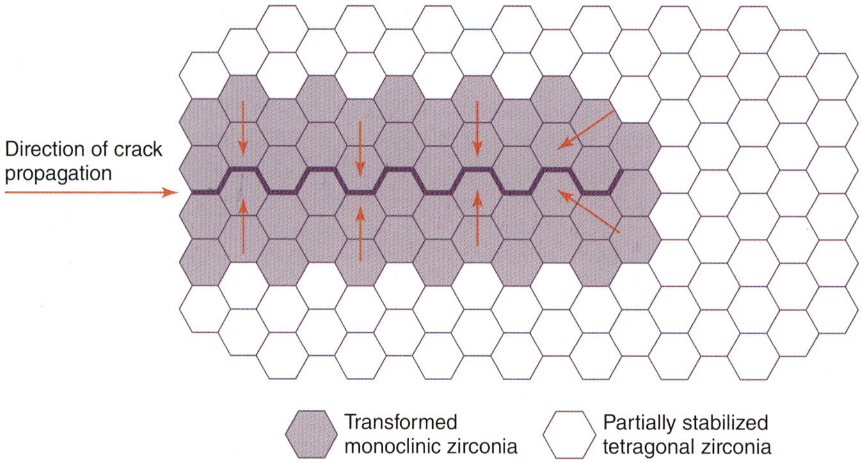

• **Fig. 10.2** Schematic of transformation toughening mechanism in partially stabilized zirconia.

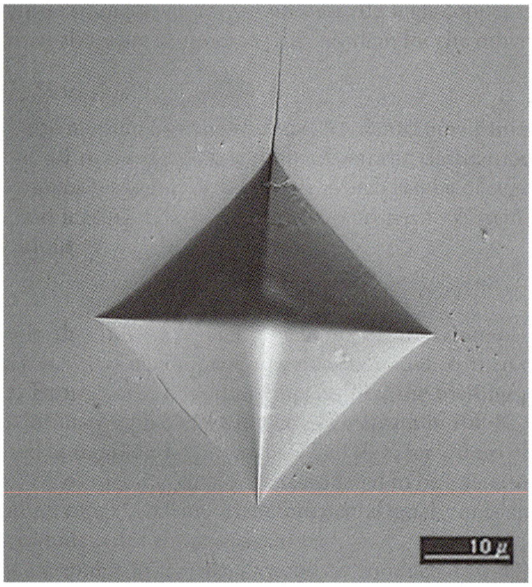

• **Fig. 10.3** Vickers indentation under a 98.1-N load on a zirconia-based dental ceramic.

by using rapid but controlled cooling rates, whereas chemical strengthening applies to glasses and ceramics with a large proportion of glassy matrix and relies on the replacement of small ions with larger ions within the matrix and above the glass transition temperature by diffusion from a molten salt bath in which the ceramic or glass is immersed. Although widely used in the glass industry, these techniques are no longer used for dental ceramics due to controllability issues, as well as potential elimination and benefit loss from grinding adjustments.

Glazing is the final step in the fabrication of metal-ceramic and porcelain-veneered all-ceramic restorations. This standard technique, also called *self-glazing*, does not significantly improve the flexural strength of feldspathic dental porcelains. However, a low-expansion glass called *glaze* can also be applied to the surface of the ceramic and then fired to high temperature. Upon cooling, this glaze layer is placed under compression from the greater contraction of the underlying ceramic. This layer is also known to reduce the depth and width of surface flaws, thereby improving the overall resistance of the ceramic to crack propagation.

Test Methods

Numerous test methods are available to evaluate the mechanical properties of ceramics. Studies of the influence of test method on the failure stress of brittle dental materials have shown that important test parameters are the specimen thickness, contact zone at loading, homogeneity and porosity of the material, and loading rate. For this reason, discrepancies exist among the published values of mechanical properties for a given ceramic. Manufacturers evaluate dental ceramics using a standard (ISO 6872) published and regularly revised by the International Organization for Standardization. Set protocols are proposed to quantify radioactivity, flexural strength, linear CTE, glass transition temperature, and chemical solubility.

Sometimes, researchers use testing protocols and fixtures aimed at simulating dental morphology. However, the experimental variables can become extremely complex and difficult to reproduce in this type of testing. Finite element analysis constitutes another approach to the simulation of clinical conditions. Failure predictions for ceramic inlays by the finite element analysis technique have successfully matched fractographic analyses of clinically failed restorations. Fractography is well established as a failure-analysis technique for glasses and ceramics. It has been recognized as a powerful analytical tool in dentistry. The in vivo failure stress of clinically failed all-ceramic crowns may be estimated using fractography (see more discussion in the online chapter on Testing).

Comparative Data

Representative flexural strength data for dental ceramics are summarized in Table 10.2. Feldspathic porcelains for metal-ceramic restorations have a mean flexural strength between 60 and 80 MPa. This value is lower than those listed for all-ceramic materials; however, because metal-ceramic restorations are supported by a metallic framework, their long-term probability of survival is usually higher than that of leucite-reinforced or lithia–based glass-ceramics.

Among the currently available all-ceramic materials, tetragonal zirconia (3Y-TZP) ceramics exhibit the highest flexure strength values (900–1500 MPa), followed by recently introduced translucent zirconia ceramics with higher cubic contents (450–900 MPa), and lithia–reinforced glass-ceramics (210–620 MPa). The flexural strength of leucite-reinforced ceramics is around 120 to 140 MPa. As mentioned previously, the nature and amount of the crystalline phase present in the ceramic material strongly influences the mechanical properties of the final product. The shear strength

TABLE 10.2 Flexural Strength of Selected Dental Ceramics

Processing Technique	Crystalline Phase	Flexural Strength (MPa)	Percent Crystallinity
Soft machined	Zirconia (3Y-TZP, tetragonal + cubic)	1087 ± 173	Highly crystalline
	Zirconia (4Y-PSZ, tetragonal + cubic)	831 ± 43	Highly crystalline
	Zirconia (5Y-PSZ, cubic + tetragonal)	609 ± 30	Highly crystalline
Hard machined	Feldspar ([Na, K]$AlSi_3O_8$)	122 ± 13	≈30
	Lithium disilicate ($Li_2Si_2O_5$)	462 ± 34	70
	Lithium disilicate/silicate ($Li_2Si_2O_5$ + Li_2SiO_3)	210 ± 35	51
	Leucite ($KAlSi_2O_6$)	≈160[a]	≈35
Heat pressed	Leucite ($KAlSi_2O_6$)	106 ± 17	35
	Lithium disilicate ($Li_2Si_2O_5$)	445 ± 47	61
	Lithium disilicate/silicate ($Li_2Si_2O_5$ + Li_2SiO_3)	624 ± 106	45
Sintered	Leucite ($KAlSi_2O_6$)	104	35–40
	Fluorapatite ($Ca_5[PO_4]_3F$)	≈80[a]	10
Sintered metal-ceramic	Leucite ($KAlSi_2O_6$)	61 ± 5	15–25

[a]Data from manufacturer.

Data from Zhang Y, Vardhaman S, Rodrigues CS, Lawn BR. A critical review of dental lithia-based glass-ceramics. *J Dent Res.* 2023;102(3):245–253; Zhang Y, Lawn BR. Novel zirconia materials in dentistry. *J Dent Res.* 2018;97(2):140–147; Guazzato M, Albakry M, Ringer SP, Swain MV. Strength, fracture toughness, and microstructure of a selection of all-ceramic materials. Part I. Pressable and alumina glass-infiltrated ceramics. *Dent Mater.* 2004;20:441–448; Guazzato M, Albakry M, Ringer SP, Swain MV. Strength, fracture toughness, and microstructure of a selection of all-ceramic materials. Part II. Zirconia-based dental ceramics. *Dent Mater.* 2004;20:449–456; Denry IL, Holloway JA, Tarr LA. Effect of heat treatment on microcrack healing behavior of a machinable dental ceramic. *J Biomed Mater Res.* 1999;48:791–796; Della Bona A, Mecholsky JJ Jr, Anusavice KJ. Fracture behavior of lithia disilicate- and leucite-based ceramics. *Dent Mater.* 2004;20:956–962; Höland W, Beall G. *Glass-Ceramic Technology.* The American Ceramic Society; 2002.

of feldspathic porcelain is 110 MPa, and the diametral tensile strength is lower at 34 MPa. The compressive strength is about 172 MPa, and the Knoop hardness is 460 kg/mm^2.

Fracture toughness is another important property of ceramics; it measures the resistance to brittle fracture when a crack is present. The fracture toughness of conventional feldspathic porcelains is very similar to that of soda lime glass (0.78 MPa · m$^{0.5}$). Leucite-reinforced ceramics exhibit slightly higher fracture toughness values (1.2 MPa · m$^{0.5}$), followed by lithia–reinforced glass-ceramics (1.4–2.4 MPa · m$^{0.5}$). 3Y-TZP ceramics have the highest fracture toughness of all-ceramic materials (up to 6.0 MPa · m$^{0.5}$).

The elastic constants of dental ceramics are needed in the calculations of both flexural strength and fracture toughness. Poisson's ratio ranges between 0.21 and 0.33 for dental ceramics. The modulus of elasticity is about 70 GPa for feldspathic porcelain, 100 GPa for lithia-based glass-ceramics, 210 GPa for 3Y-TZP ceramics (which is similar to steel), and up to 380 GPa for alumina-based ceramics.

Sintering of structural ceramics is associated with shrinkage as porosity is eliminated by firing at high temperatures. Shrinkage remains an issue for all-ceramic materials with the exception of ceramics machined from fully sintered ceramic blocks and heat-pressed ceramics. Shrinkage of the veneering ceramics applied on all-ceramic cores has to be carefully compensated for during porcelain buildup. The large shrinkage of machined zirconia restorations (about 25%) during sintering at high temperatures is compensated for at the design stage by computerized enlargement of the restorations.

The density of fully sintered feldspathic porcelain is around 2.45 g/cm^3 and decreases as the amount of porosity increases. The density of ceramic materials also depends on the amount and nature of crystalline phase present. The theoretical density of 3Y-TZP dental ceramics is 6.08 g/cm^3, assuming that the material is pore-free. A density greater than 98.7% of the theoretical density is required for medical-grade 3Y-TZP ceramics. All currently used dental zirconia ceramics, including 3Y-TZP, 4Y-PSZ (partially stabilized zirconia), and 5Y-PSZ have a density that meets this standard requirement.

The thermal properties of feldspathic porcelain include a conductivity of 0.0030 cal/s/cm^2 (°C/cm), a diffusivity of 0.64 mm^2/s, and a linear CTE of about 12.0 × 10^{-6}/°C between 25°C and 500°C. The CTE is about 10 × 10^{-6}/°C for aluminous ceramics and lithium disilicate ceramics, 10.5 × 10^{-6}/°C for zirconia-based ceramics (3Y, 4Y, 5Y-PSZ), and 14 to 18 × 10^{-6}/°C for leucite-reinforced ceramics. The low thermal conductivity of zirconia-based ceramics was responsible for early issues of chipping and delamination of the veneering porcelain when fast heating and cooling rates were used. These issues have been addressed by strict recommendations regarding firing schedules for veneering porcelains on zirconia, including slower heating and cooling rates.

Optical Properties of Dental Ceramics

Shade matching is a critical problem in replacing natural teeth. In addition, porcelain, being mostly amorphous in structure, cannot match the optical properties of crystalline enamel completely. As a result, ultraviolet (UV) and visible light rays are reflected, refracted, and absorbed unevenly by the combination of dentin/enamel, compared with porcelain. As a consequence, restorations viewed from one incidence angle may not appear the same as they do when viewed from a different incidence angle. The cementing medium is an important factor in the final appearance of an all-ceramic restoration. Zirconia-based all-ceramic materials are not etchable due to the absence of a glassy phase, but their opacity may permit cementation with various luting agents without

TABLE 10.3 Percent Light Transmission of 1-mm Thick Dentin Porcelains

Shade	Ceramco	Vita	Neydium	Will-Ceram	Steeles
59	29.97	22.66	31.93	26.06	27.23
62	27.85	—	—	27.88	—
65	23.31	20.39	35.39	33.50	22.10
67	26.32	18.04	23.58	19.03	23.42
91	31.81	—	38.41	—	—

Modified from Brodbelt RHW, O'Brien WJ, Fan PL. Translucency of dental porcelains. *J Dent Res.* 1980;59:70–75.

the need for specific shade matching. However, more translucent all-ceramic restorations, such as leucite-reinforced heat-pressed or machined inlays, crowns, or veneers, usually require the use of color-matched resin cements that are available in different shades.

The shades of commercial premixed dental porcelain powders are in the yellow to yellow-red range. Because the range of shades existing in natural teeth is much greater than the range available in a kit of premixed porcelains, modifier porcelains are also available for precise shade adjustments. These modifiers are strongly pigmented porcelains usually supplied in blue, yellow, pink, orange, brown, and gray. The dental technician may add the modifier porcelain to the opaque and body porcelains during the building of the crown. Extrinsic surface staining is another way of changing the appearance of a ceramic crown. It involves the application of highly pigmented glazes. The main disadvantages of surface staining compared with intrinsic staining are limited durability (a result of solubility) and the reduction of translucency.

Translucency is another critical property of dental ceramics. The translucency of opaque, dentin (body), and enamel (incisal) porcelains differs considerably. By design, opaque porcelains have very low translucency, allowing them to efficiently mask metal substructure surfaces. Tin oxide (SnO_2) and titanium oxide (TiO_2) are important opacifying oxides for opaque porcelains. Dentin porcelain translucency values range between 18% and 38% (Table 10.3). Enamel porcelains have the highest values of translucency, ranging between 45% and 50%. The translucency of materials for all-ceramic restorations varies with the nature and amount of the reinforcing crystalline phase. Alumina- and zirconia-based ceramics are more opaque, whereas leucite-reinforced and lithia–based ceramics are more translucent. Recently, zirconia ceramics with increased translucency have become available. Greater translucency is obtained by either decreasing the amount of alumina additive in the 3Y-TZP composition or using higher amounts of yttrium oxide stabilizer to increase the amount of the more translucent cubic phase. To mimic the optical properties of human enamel, opalescence is also a desirable optical property. Opalescence is a form of light scattering and occurs when the size of crystalline phase particles is equal to or shorter than the wavelength of light. An opalescent glass appears reddish-orange in transmitted light and blue in reflected or scattered light. Both zirconium oxide and yttrium oxide have been shown to increase opalescence in base dentin ceramics due to their light-scattering effect.

Dental enamel also exhibits fluorescence. This characteristic is achieved in dental porcelains by adding rare earth oxides (such as cerium oxide). Because the outer layers of a ceramic crown are translucent, the apparent color is affected by reflectance from the inner opaque or core ceramic. For metal-ceramic restorations, shade mixing results from combining the light reflected from the inner, opaque porcelain surface and the light transmitted through the body porcelain. The thickness of the body porcelain layer determines the final shade obtained with a given opaque porcelain.

All-Ceramic Restorations

Materials for all-ceramic restorations use a wide variety of crystalline phases as reinforcing agents and contain up to 99% by volume of crystalline phase. The nature, amount, and particle size distribution of the crystalline phase directly influences the mechanical, thermal, and optical properties of the ceramic material. The match between the refractive indexes of the crystalline phase and glassy matrix is an important factor for controlling the translucency of porcelain and glass ceramics.

As mentioned earlier, several processing techniques are available for fabricating all-ceramic restorations: sintering, heat pressing, slip casting, and CAD/CAM. Fig. 10.1, *left,* illustrates the cross section of an all-ceramic crown.

Sintered All-Ceramic Materials

Although dental ceramics have been around for over two centuries, until the 1960s their clinical indications had been limited to dentures, inlays, onlays, and porcelain veneers for anterior teeth. The role of ceramics in dentistry began to become more prominent with the development of resilient metal copings and strong ceramic materials, both associated with sintered ceramic materials. Two main types of ceramic materials are available for the sintering technique: zirconia-based ceramics and leucite-reinforced ceramics.

Zirconia-Based Ceramics

Zirconia was introduced to dentistry in the late 1990s. The first generation of dental zirconia was fabricated from 3 mol% (or 5.8 wt%) yttrium oxide stabilized zirconia powder doped with 0.25 wt% alumina as a sintering aid. The microstructure of these polycrystalline 3Y-TZP ceramics consists mainly of densely packed tetragonal zirconia grains with a mean grain size of 0.2 to 1.0 μm, depending on sintering temperature and duration (Fig. 10.4E), which can vary from 1350°C to 1600°C and 2 to 6 hours, respectively, depending on the manufacturer. This first-generation zirconia exhibits the highest flexural strength (900 to 1500 MPa) and highest fracture toughness (up to 6 MPa · $m^{0.5}$) of all currently available dental ceramics. However, that material is predominantly opaque. Thus it is primarily used as a strong

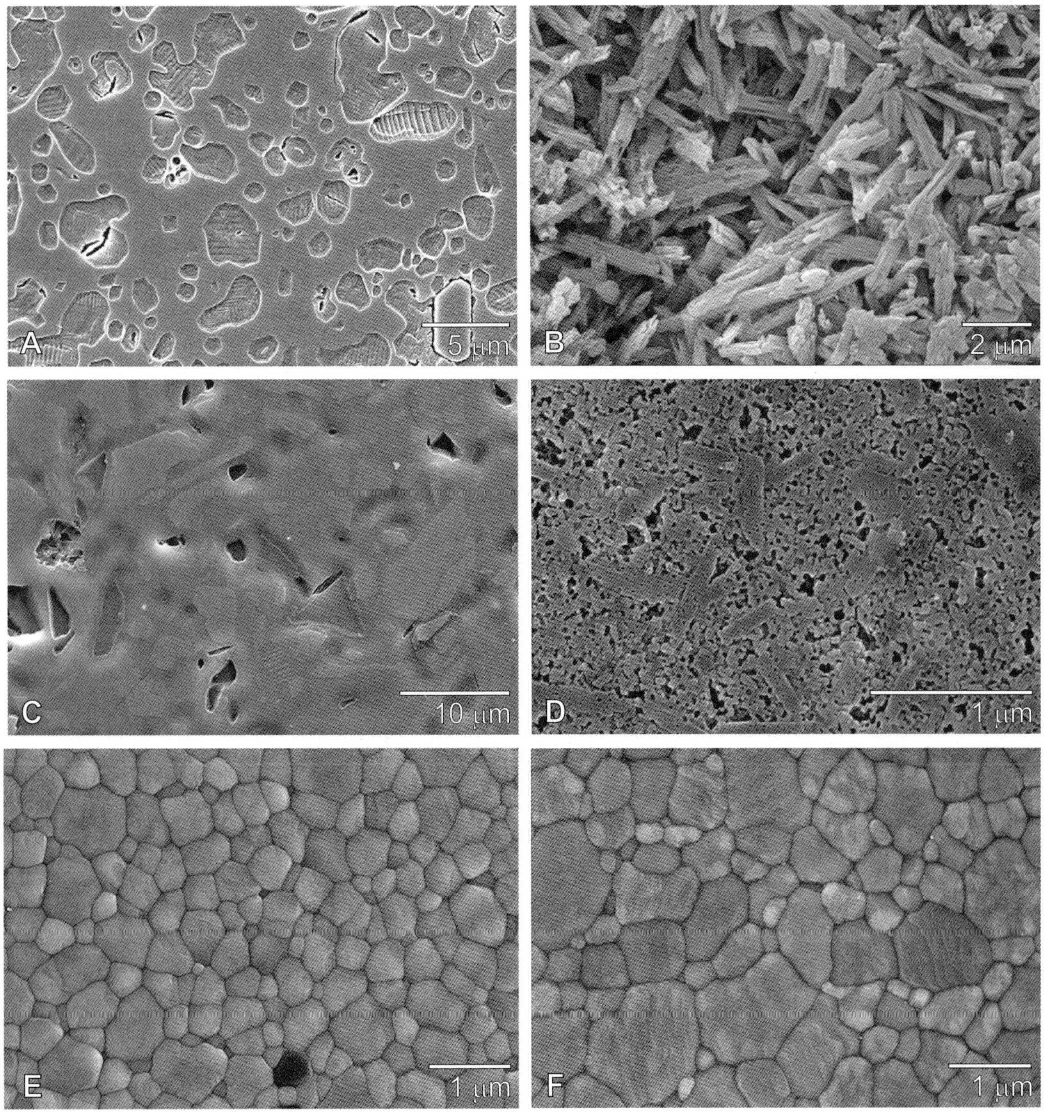

• **Fig. 10.4** Scanning electron micrographs showing the microstructure of selected all-ceramic materials (polished and etched surfaces). (A) Leucite-reinforced heat-pressed ceramic; (B) lithium disilicate heat-pressed ceramic; (C) feldspar-based machinable ceramic; (D) zirconia lithium silicate machinable ceramic; (E) soft-machined sintered zirconia ceramic (3Y-TZP); (F) soft-machined sintered high-translucency zirconia ceramic (cubic and tetragonal).

framework to support weak but aesthetic porcelain veneers. Clinical studies have revealed that while zirconia frameworks are very fracture resistant, chipping, fracture, and delamination of porcelain veneers is a frequent problem. These findings have been explained by the fact that both veneering porcelain and zirconia cores exhibit low thermal conductivity and that thermal gradients may develop when fast heating or cooling rates are used, leading to transient stresses and microcracking.

To improve zirconia translucency and aesthetics, so as to circumvent issues with veneer chipping and fracture, four successive generations have been developed. The increase in translucency is obtained either by decreasing the amount of alumina present to 0.05 wt% or less (second-generation) or by adding higher amounts of yttria (up to 6 mol%, third-generation) to stabilize the cubic polymorph of zirconia as a major crystalline phase. Cubic zirconia is more translucent due to its isotropic crystal symmetry, compared with tetragonal zirconia, which is anisotropic and birefringent. The retention of cubic zirconia at room temperature is also accompanied with a substantial increase in grain size (see Fig. 10.4F). The cubic form of zirconia is not transformable and exhibits lower fracture toughness. This is reflected in the lower mechanical properties of the high cubic content zirconia formulations, with a reported flexural strength of 609 MPa and a fracture toughness of 2.4 MPa · $m^{0.5}$. More recently, in order to further enhance the aesthetics of zirconia restorations, polychromatic multilayered structures (fourth-generation) and graded compositions and shades (fifth-generation) have been introduced.

The microstructures of these variants come in different forms, depending on the cubic phase content (5% to 80%) and grain size (0.2 µm to 5 µm). Measured strengths vary from 450 to 1500 MPa. Appearance varies from predominantly opaque to substantially translucent. In general, increasing yttria content yields an increase in translucency but a decrease in strength. Consequently, modern zirconia-based materials have a wide range of clinical indications, including single crowns, multiunit FDPs, frameworks for porcelain-veneered restorations, inlays, onlays, veneers, and implants and abutments.

Leucite-Reinforced Ceramic

Leucite-reinforced ceramics containing up to 45% by volume of tetragonal leucite were used for the fabrication of all-ceramic sintered restorations. Leucite acts as a reinforcing phase; the greater leucite content (compared with conventional feldspathic porcelain for metal-ceramic restorations) leads to higher flexural strength (104 MPa) and compressive strength. The large amount of leucite in the material also contributes to a high thermal contraction coefficient. In addition, the large mismatch in thermal contraction between leucite ($20–25 \times 10^{-6}/°C$) and the glassy matrix ($8 \times 10^{-6}/°C$) results in the development of tangential compressive stresses in the glassy matrix surrounding the leucite crystals upon cooling, because the crystals contract more than the surrounding glassy matrix. These stresses can act as crack deflectors and contribute to increased resistance of the ceramic to crack propagation (fracture toughness).

Heat-Pressed All-Ceramic Materials

Heat pressing relies on the application of external pressure at high temperatures to sinter and shape the ceramic. Heat pressing is used in dentistry to produce all-ceramic crowns, inlays, onlays, veneers, and more recently, FDPs. During heat pressing, ceramic ingots are brought to high temperature in a phosphate-bonded investment mold produced by the lost wax technique. The heat-pressing temperature is chosen near the softening point of the ceramic. A pressure of 0.3 to 0.4 MPa is then applied through a refractory plunger. This allows filling of the mold with the softened ceramic. The high temperature is held for durations between 10 and 20 minutes. Heat-pressing requires a specially designed automated pressing furnace (Fig. 10.5) and classically promotes a good dispersion of the crystalline phase within the glassy matrix. The mechanical properties of heat-pressed ceramics are therefore maximized compared with their sintered counterparts.

Leucite-Based Ceramic

First-generation heat-pressed ceramics contain tetragonal leucite ($KAlSi_2O_6$ or $K_2O \cdot Al_2O_3 \cdot 4SiO_2$) as a reinforcing phase, in amounts varying from 35% to 55% by volume. Heat-pressing temperatures for this system are between 1150°C and 1180°C with a dwell at each temperature of about 20 minutes. The ceramic ingots are available in a variety of shades. The final microstructure of these heat-pressed ceramics consists of leucite crystals, 1 to 5 μm, dispersed in a glassy matrix (Fig. 10.4A). The amount of porosity in the heat-pressed ceramic is 9 vol%. Two techniques are available: a staining technique and a layering technique involving the application of veneering ceramic. The two techniques lead to comparable mean flexural strength values for the resulting ceramic. To ensure compatibility with the thermal expansion coefficient of the veneering ceramic, the thermal expansion coefficient of the core material for the veneering technique ($14.9 \times 10^{-6}/°C$) is lower than that of the core material for the staining technique ($18 \times 10^{-6}/°C$). The flexural strength of these ceramics (120 MPa) is almost double that of conventional feldspathic porcelains. This increase in strength can be explained by the fact that these ceramics possess a higher crystallinity and that the heat-pressing process generates an excellent dispersion of these fine leucite crystals. In addition, as mentioned earlier, residual thermal stresses around the leucite crystals promote crack deflection and contribute to improved mechanical performance. The main advantages of leucite-reinforced ceramics are their excellent aesthetics and translucency, whereas their limitations lie in their modest mechanical properties restricting their use to anterior single-unit restorations.

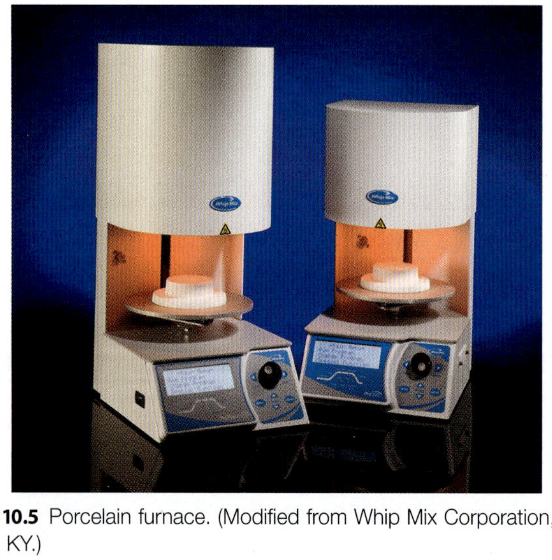

• **Fig. 10.5** Porcelain furnace. (Modified from Whip Mix Corporation, Louisville, KY.)

Lithia–Based Ceramic

The second generation of heat-pressed ceramics contains lithium disilicate ($Li_2Si_2O_5$) as a major crystalline phase. Heat pressing takes place in the 910°C to 920°C temperature range, using the same equipment as for the leucite-based ceramics. Heat-pressed restorations are later veneered with ceramics of matching thermal expansion or stained. The final microstructure consists of about 65% by volume of highly interlocking prismatic lithium disilicate crystals (2–5 μm in length, 0.8 μm in diameter) dispersed in a glassy matrix (Fig. 10.4B). The amount of porosity after heat pressing is about 1 vol%. Compared with first-generation leucite-based ceramics, the main advantage of lithium disilicate–based ceramics is their enhanced flexural strength (445 MPa) and fracture toughness ($2.25\ MPa \cdot m^{0.5}$). This can be explained by a higher crystallinity and a "logs-on-the-river" microstructure consisting of elongated, highly interlocked, and needle-shaped lithium disilicate crystals. In addition, the thermal expansion mismatch between the lithium disilicate crystals and the glassy matrix leads to compressive residual stresses which, combined with multiple crystal orientations, is efficient in promoting multiple crack deflections, thereby increasing the resistance to crack propagation. Finally, several studies have reported that heat pressing promotes crystal alignment along the direction of pressing because of the high aspect ratio of the crystals. This leads to an even higher resistance to crack propagation in the direction perpendicular to crystal alignment. The enhanced mechanical properties of these second-generation heat-pressed ceramics have extended their range of dental applications, making possible the fabrication of multiunit FDPs.

Prompted by the clinical success of the second generation of heat-pressed lithium disilicate glass-ceramic materials, a battery of pressable lithia-based glass-ceramics has been developed by various manufacturers. The composition of these materials varies from lithium disilicate to lithium silicate to biphasic lithium disilicate/lithium silicate. The crystalline content varies from 40% to 75% by volume. Measured flexure strength varies from 360 to 630 MPa and fracture toughness from 1.8 to 2.4 $MPa \cdot m^{0.5}$. In general, a larger crystal size with a higher aspect ratio yields both a higher strength and toughness.

Machinable All-Ceramic Materials

All-ceramic materials can be machined in the fully sintered state. This is termed *hard machining*, and restorations produced in this way are machined directly to final size. Some all-ceramic materials also can be machined in a soft, partially sintered state and later fully sintered. This is called *soft machining*. The latter technique requires milling of enlarged restorations to compensate for sintering shrinkage and is well adapted to ceramics that are difficult to machine in the fully sintered state, such as alumina and zirconia.

Hard Machining

Machinable ceramics can be milled to form inlays, onlays, veneers, and crowns using the CAD/CAM technology to produce restorations in one office visit. After the tooth is prepared, the preparation is optically scanned and the image is digitized. The restoration is designed with the aid of a computer, as shown in Fig. 10.6. The restoration is then machined from ceramic blocks by a computer-controlled milling machine. The milling process varies from several minutes for sintered feldspathic ceramics to 45 minutes for densely sintered zirconia, depending on the strength and hardness of the ceramic milling blocks. Restorations are bonded to the tooth preparation with resin cements. The most recent versions of intraoral scanners combined with digital impression reconstruction software allow complete tridimensional visualization of the projected restoration with *virtual seating* capabilities. The various

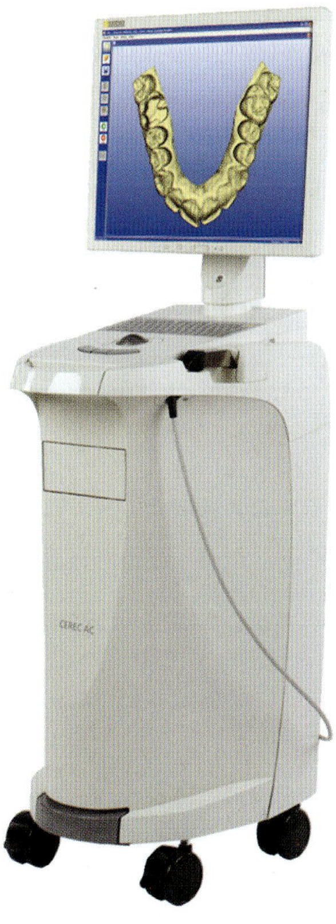

• **Fig. 10.6** Chair-side computer-aided design system for all-ceramic restoration fabrication. (Courtesy Sirona Dental Systems, LLC, Charlotte, NC.)

surfaces of the virtual restoration can be modified in all three dimensions prior to machining. Further information on digital impression systems can be found in Chapter 13.

Several machinable feldspathic ceramics, glass-ceramics, and zirconia are presently available for hard machining. The feldspathic ceramic contains approximately 30 vol% feldspar ([Na, K] $AlSi_3O_8$) as a major crystalline phase, dispersed in a glassy matrix (see Fig. 10.4C). Its flexural strength is ranked as moderate (120 MPa). Several brands of leucite- and lithia-reinforced glass-ceramic blocks, and a 3Y-TZP and a 4.7Y-PSZ fully sintered block from Glidewell labs are also available for hard machining by CAD/CAM. The leucite-reinforced ceramic blocks are similar in microstructure and mechanical properties to the first-generation heat-pressed, leucite-reinforced ceramics. The original type of lithium disilicate glass-ceramic blocks are machined in a partially crystallized state, which corresponds to a softer and easier-to-machine material compared to that in the fully crystallized state. In the partially crystallized (nucleated) state, the glass-ceramic contains crystal nuclei of both lithium metasilicate (Li_2SiO_3) and lithium disilicate ($Li_2Si_2O_5$). By controlling the nucleation and crystallization heat treatment, the number of nucleation sites, crystal size, and nature of the crystalline phases can be adjusted to modulate the translucency of this glass-ceramic. Low-, medium-, and high-translucency blocks are proposed for CAD/CAM machining. After the restorations are machined, a heat treatment at 850°C for 10 minutes is performed to complete the crystallization process and ensure that the glass-ceramic possesses optimized mechanical properties prior to glazing and cementation. Depending on the translucency, the microstructure will be slightly different, with the high-translucency glass-ceramic exhibiting lithium disilicate crystals (1.5 × 0.8 μm) in a glassy matrix, and the low-translucency ceramic exhibiting a larger number of smaller (0.8 × 0.2 μm) interlocked lithium disilicate crystals. The flexural strength after completion of the crystallization heat treatment is between 360 and 480 MPa, according to manufacturer data.

Another lithia–based glass-ceramic was recently introduced, in which about 10 wt% zirconium dioxide is added to a lithium silicate glass composition and remains in solution in the glassy matrix. This modification leads to a larger amount of glassy matrix in the precrystallized (nucleated) state, with ease of machining due to the presence of lithium metasilicate crystals. The final microstructure after completion of the crystallization heat treatment (840°C for 8 minutes) consists of lithium silicate (0.1 to 0.2 μm platelets) interlocked with lithium disilicate crystals (0.5 to 0.8 μm long prisms), leading to a glass ceramic with excellent translucency and mechanical properties comparable to those of lithium disilicate glass ceramics (see Fig. 10.4D).

Soft Machining Followed by Sintering

In 2002, the first zirconia-based ceramic for soft machining was introduced on the dental market. The material consists of predominantly tetragonal zirconia polycrystals partially stabilized by the addition of 3 mole percent yttrium oxide (3Y-TZP). Single or multiunit restorations are produced by direct ceramic machining (DCM) of pre-sintered 3Y-TZP blocks. These blocks are relatively soft and easy to mill, thus leading to substantial savings in time and tool wear compared with fully sintered zirconia. The process involved the fabrication of a full contour wax-up of the restoration that was later digitized with a laser scanner. Restorations were oversized at the design and machining stages, to compensate for the large shrinkage (20–25%) that occurs during the sintering process at high temperatures (1350°C for 2 hours).

Since the introduction of the DCM technique, a wide variety of partially sintered 3Y-TZP blocks have become available for soft machining by CAD/CAM. In this case, the wax-up step is eliminated, a digital impression of the preparation is made, and the restoration design is accomplished with a computer. Similar to the DCM technique, machined restorations are fully sintered at high temperatures.

The metastability of 3Y-TZP ceramics should be kept in mind when surface-altering treatments such as grinding or air abrasion are performed. Given the fact that transformability increases with grain size, such treatments have the potential to trigger the tetragonal to monoclinic transformation with the immediate beneficial consequence of producing surface compressive stresses. However, long-term effects may be detrimental due to the combination of defects produced by the surface treatment and the presence of underlying tensile stresses. This is why extreme care should be taken to follow the manufacturer's instructions when working with partially stabilized zirconia-based ceramics.

Hard-machining techniques make it possible to fabricate the restoration chairside in one office visit. However, all-ceramic materials available with these techniques either exhibit low to moderate strength (e.g., feldspathic ceramics and glass-ceramics) or are very difficult and time-consuming to mill (i.e., fully sintered zirconia), thus their clinical applications are restricted to single-unit restorations or short-span FDPs.

The benefit of fabricating the restoration in one office visit is lost with soft-machining techniques because restorations require sintering at high temperatures for several hours after they are machined. To overcome this drawback, high-speed sintering protocols using an induction furnace have been developed. Zirconia restorations can now be sintered within 15 to 30 minutes. Studies from the dental literature have reported a nonuniform microstructure along with a small amount of porosity within the speed-sintered parts, which significantly compromises the zirconia's translucency and, to a lesser degree, its strength. This has prompted most dental clinics and labs to only use 4Y-PSZ for high-speed sintering. Thus the chairside treatment option for zirconia restorations is primarily limited to single crowns due to the relatively low strength of 4Y-PSZ and challenges in uniformly speed sintering thick sections of restoration, such as connectors and pontics of multiunit FDPs. High-speed sintering is a technology in progress.

Metal-Ceramic Restorations

Metal-ceramic restorations consist of a cast metallic framework on which at least two layers of ceramic are baked (Fig. 10.7). The first layer applied is a thin opaque layer, consisting of porcelain modified with opacifying oxides. Its role is to mask the dark-gray appearance of the oxidized metal framework to permit the achievement of adequate esthetics. This thin opaque layer also establishes the metal-ceramic bond. The next step is the buildup of dentin and enamel (most translucent) porcelains to obtain an esthetic appearance similar to that of a natural tooth. Dentin and enamel porcelain powders are mixed with modeling liquid (mainly distilled water) to a creamy consistency and applied to the opaque layer. The porcelain is then condensed by vibration and removal of the excess water with absorbent tissue. The porcelain buildup has to be oversized to compensate for the large shrinkage (25–30%) associated with the sintering process. After building up of the porcelain powders, metal-ceramic restorations are slowly dried to allow for adequate water diffusion and evaporation, and sintered

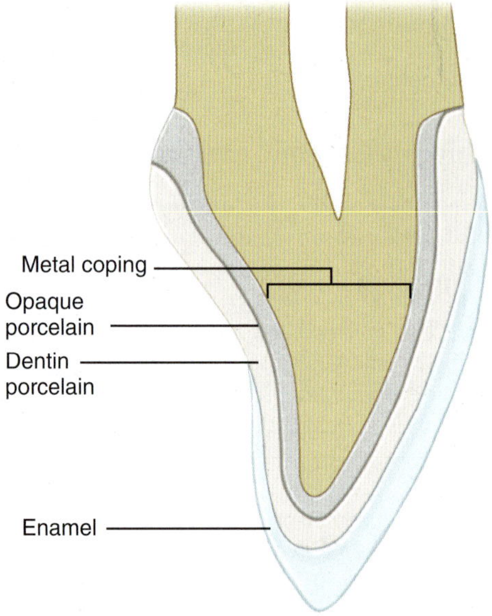

• **Fig. 10.7** Cross section of a metal-ceramic crown showing metal coping, opaque porcelain layer, dentin, and enamel porcelain layers.

under vacuum in a porcelain furnace. Sintering under vacuum helps eliminate pores. As the furnace door closes, the pressure is lowered to 0.01 MPa (0.1 atmosphere). The temperature is raised until the sintering temperature is reached, the vacuum is then released, and the furnace pressure returns to 0.1 MPa (1 atmosphere). In combination with viscous flow at high temperatures, the increase in pressure helps close residual pores. The result is a dense, relatively pore-free porcelain, as illustrated in Fig. 10.8. Studies have shown that sintering under vacuum reduces the amount of porosity from 5.6% in air-fired porcelains to 0.56%. This decrease in porosity is noticeable by the associated increase in translucency. Opaque, dentin, and enamel porcelains are available in various shades.

Fig. 10.9 shows two three-unit metal-ceramic FDPs. When fabricated by skilled technicians, these restorations provide excellent esthetics, along with adequate strength because of the metal framework support. The alloys used for casting the substructure are usually gold-based containing tin and indium.

It is essential that the CTE of the veneering porcelain be slightly lower than that of the alloy to ensure that the ceramic is in slight compression after cooling. This will prevent microcrack formation in the porcelain and enhance long-term clinical performance.

Requirements for a Metal-Ceramic System

1. The alloy must have a high melting temperature. The melting range must be substantially higher (greater than 100°C) than the firing temperature of the veneering porcelain and solders used to join segments of an FDP.
2. The veneering porcelain must have a low fusing temperature so that no creep, sag, or distortion of the framework takes place during sintering.
3. The porcelain must wet the alloy readily when applied as a slurry to prevent voids forming at the metal-ceramic interface. In general, the contact angle should be 60 degrees or less.
4. A strong bond between the ceramic and metal is essential and is achieved by the chemical reaction of the opaque porcelain

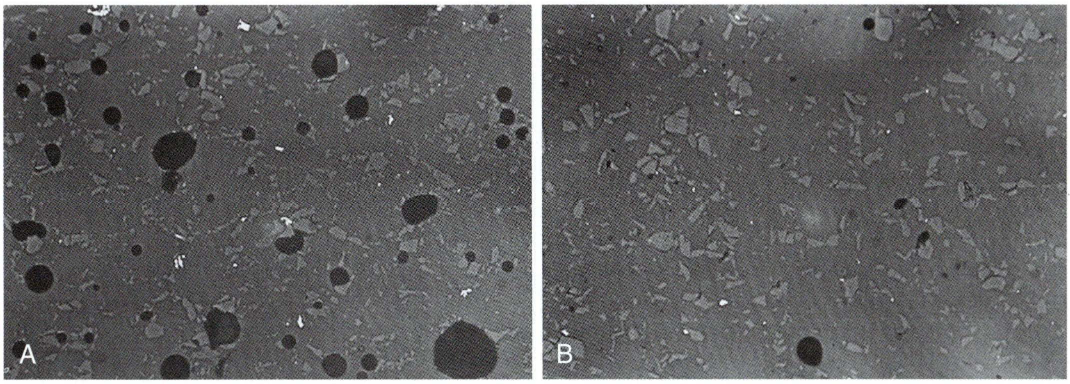

• **Fig. 10.8** Air-fired and vacuum-fired porcelain. (A) Optical micrograph of air-fired porcelain, showing porosity. (B) Optical micrograph of vacuum-fired porcelain showing minimal porosity. (Courtesy J.O. Semmelman, York, PA, 1959, Dentsply International.)

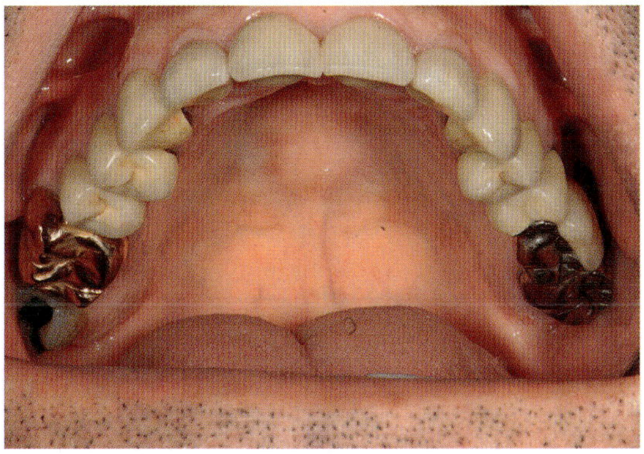

• **Fig. 10.9** View of metal-ceramic fixed dental prostheses. (Courtesy Dr. Charles Mark Malloy, Portland, OR.)

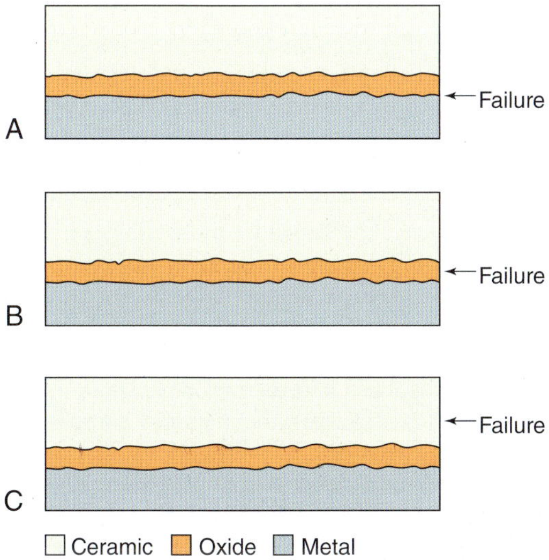

• **Fig. 10.10** Diagram showing three observed types of bond failure in metal-ceramic systems. (A) Metal-metal oxide (adhesive); (B) metal oxide-metal oxide (cohesive); and (C) ceramic-ceramic (cohesive). Note: The dimensions of the layers are not to scale.

with metal oxides on the surface of metal (Fig. 10.10) and by mechanical interlocking made possible by roughening of the metal coping.

5. CTEs of the porcelain and metal must be compatible so that the veneering porcelain never undergoes tensile stresses, which would lead to cracking. Metal-ceramic systems are therefore designed so that the CTE of the metal is slightly higher than that of the porcelain, thus placing the veneering porcelain in compression (where it is stronger) following cooling (see Fig. 9.9). This is assuming that linear coefficients of thermal expansion of both porcelain and metal are identical to linear coefficients of thermal contraction.
6. Adequate stiffness and strength of the metal framework are especially important for FDPs and posterior crowns. High stiffness of the metal reduces tensile stresses in the porcelain by limiting deflection amplitude and deformation (strain). High strength is essential in the interproximal connector areas of FDPs.
7. High resistance to deformation at high temperatures is essential. Metal copings are relatively thin (0.4 to 0.5 mm); no distortion should occur during firing of the porcelain or the fit of the restorations would be compromised.
8. Adequate design of the restoration is critical. The preparation should provide for adequate thickness of the metal coping, as well as enough space for an adequate thickness of the porcelain to yield an aesthetic restoration. During the preparation of the metal framework, prior to porcelain application, it is important that all sharp angles be eliminated and rounded to later avoid stress concentration in the porcelain. If full porcelain coverage is not used (e.g., a metal occlusal surface), the position of the metal-ceramic junction should be located at least 1.5 mm from all centric occlusal contacts.

Metal-Ceramic Bonding

The bond strength between porcelain and metal is an important requirement for good long-term performance of metal-ceramic restorations. In general, the bond is a result of chemisorption by diffusion between the surface oxide layer on the alloy and the porcelain. For metal alloys that do not oxidize easily, this oxide layer is formed during a special firing cycle prior to opaque porcelain application. For metal alloys that do oxidize easily, the oxide layer is formed during wetting of the alloy by the porcelain and subsequent firing cycle. The most common mechanical failure for metal-ceramic restorations is debonding of the porcelain from the metal. Many factors control metal-ceramic adhesion: the formation of strong chemical bonds, mechanical interlocking between the two materials, and thermal residual stresses. In addition, as noted earlier, the porcelain must be wet and fuse to the surface to form a uniform interface with no voids. These factors are also important for ceramic coatings on metallic implants.

From a practical standpoint, the surface roughness at the metal-ceramic interface has a large effect on the quality of the metal-ceramic bond. Airborne particle abrasion is routinely used on metal frameworks for metal-ceramic restorations to produce a clean surface with controlled roughness. During the firing cycle, the porcelain softens, its viscosity decreases, and the porcelain first wets the metal surface before the interlocking between porcelain and metal is created. The increased area of the rough metal surface also permits the formation of a greater density of chemical bonds. The contact angle between the porcelain and metal is a measure of the wetting and, to some extent, the quality of the bond that forms. Low contact angles are indicative of good wetting. The contact angle of porcelain on a gold (Au) alloy is about 60 degrees. A scanning electron micrograph of the oxidized surface of a gold (Au)-platinum (Pt)-palladium (Pd) 98% noble alloy is shown in Fig. 9.8. However, rough surfaces can reduce adhesion if the porcelain does not wet the surface and voids are present at the interface.

The formation of an oxide layer at the surface of the metal has been shown to be the key to an adequate metal-ceramic bond. Noble metal alloys, which are resistant to oxidizing, usually have other more easily oxidized elements added, such as indium (In) and tin (Sn), to form an oxide layer and improve the bond. The oxide layer is formed during a special firing cycle prior to porcelain application. Some noble alloys containing silver have been shown to lead to porcelain discoloration or greening, explained by ionic diffusion of silver in the porcelain. Base-metal alloys contain elements, such as nickel (Ni) and chromium (Cr), that oxidize easily, and care must be taken to avoid the formation of too thick an oxide layer. Manufacturers specify firing conditions for the formation of an optimal oxide layer and often indicate the color of the oxide. Oxides rich in nickel (NiO) tend to be dark gray, whereas those rich in chromium (Cr_2O_3) are greenish. If firing recommendations are not followed, these oxides may dissolve in the porcelain during firing, leading to discoloration visible in areas where the porcelain is thinnest; for example, near the gingival margin of the restoration. Some alloys form oxide layers rich in Cr_2O_3, which do not bond or adhere well to the alloy. These alloys typically require the application of a bonding agent to the alloy surface to modify the type of oxide formed. In some cases, manufacturers recommend an oxidation firing under reduced pressure to limit the thickness of the oxide layer. An oxidation firing in air may lead to a thicker oxide layer.

High thermal residual stresses between the metal and porcelain can lead to failure. If the metal and ceramic have largely different thermal expansion coefficients, the two materials will contract at different rates during cooling and large thermal residual stresses will form along the metal-ceramic interface. If these stresses are very high (whether tensile or compressive), the porcelain will crack and/or delaminate from the metal. Even if these stresses do not cause immediate failure, they can still weaken the bond, and lead to delayed failure. To avoid these problems, porcelains and alloys are formulated to have adequately matched thermal expansion coefficients. Most porcelains have coefficients of thermal expansion between 13.0 and 14.0×10^{-6}/°C, and metals between 13.5 and 14.5×10^{-6}/°C. The difference of 0.5×10^{-6}/°C in thermal contraction between metal and porcelain causes the metal to contract slightly more than the ceramic during cooling. This condition places the porcelain under slight residual compression, which makes it less sensitive to the tensile stresses induced by mechanical loading.

A metal-ceramic bond may fail in any of three possible locations (see Fig. 10.10). Knowing the location of failure provides considerable information on the quality of the bond. The highest bond strength leads to failure within the porcelain when tested (see Fig. 10.10C); this is observed with some alloys that were properly prepared with excellent wetting by the porcelain and is also called a *cohesive failure*. Testing these high-strength specimens using the push-through shear test shows that the bond strength is approximately the same as the shear strength of the porcelain. Another possible cohesive failure is within the oxide layer (see Fig. 10.10B). Failures occurring at the interface between metal and oxide layer (see Fig. 10.10A) are called *adhesive failures* and are commonly observed with metal alloys that are resistant to forming surface oxides, such as pure gold or platinum, and exhibit poor bonding. Base-metal alloys commonly exhibit failures within the oxide layer if an excessively thick oxide layer is present.

Ceramics for Metal-Ceramic Restorations

Ceramics for metal-ceramic restorations must fulfill five requirements: (1) they must simulate the appearance of natural teeth, (2) they must fuse at relatively low temperatures, (3) they must have thermal expansion coefficients compatible with alloys used for metal frameworks, (4) they must age well in the oral environment, and (5) they must have low abrasiveness. Porcelains are carefully formulated to achieve these requirements. These ceramics are composed of a crystalline phase (leucite) dispersed in a glassy (amorphous) matrix. Their chemical composition includes silica (SiO_2), alumina (Al_2O_3), sodium oxide (Na_2O), and potassium oxide (K_2O) (Table 10.4). Opacifiers (TiO_2, ZrO_2, SnO_2), various heat-stable coloring oxides, and small amounts of fluorescing oxides (CeO_2) are added to match the appearance of the dentin-enamel complex structure. The presence of a large amount of glassy phase in dental porcelains (80–90 vol%) permits a translucency similar to that of enamel. Coloring oxides and opacifiers allow fine tuning of the final appearance and shade control. Porcelain is supplied as a fine powder of controlled granulometry.

Dental Porcelain

Composition

The quality of any ceramic depends on the choice of components, correct proportioning of each component, and control of the firing procedure. High-purity components are used in the manufacture of dental porcelains because of the stringent requirements of optical properties and chemical inertness, combined with adequate strength, toughness, and thermal expansion.

In its mineral state, feldspar, the main raw component of dental porcelains for metal-ceramic restorations, is crystalline and opaque. Chemically, it is designated as potassium aluminosilicate, with a composition of $KAlSi_3O_8$ or $K_2O \cdot Al_2O_3 \cdot 6SiO_2$. Feldspar melts incongruently at about 1150°C, forming various silicate minerals, possibly leucite ($KAlSi_2O_6$ or $K_2O \cdot Al_2O_3 \cdot 4SiO_2$), and molten glass.

Manufacture

Many dental porcelain manufacturers buy feldspar as powder already screened and cleaned from impurities to their specifications. Other raw materials used in the manufacture of dental porcelains are various types of silica (SiO_2) in the form of fine powder, alumina (Al_2O_3), as well as alkali and alkaline earth carbonates as fluxes. During the manufacturing process, the ground components are carefully mixed together and heated to about 1200°C in

TABLE 10.4 Composition of Dental Ceramics for Fusing to High-Temperature Alloys

Compound	Biodent Opaque BG 2 (%)	Ceramco Opaque 60 (%)	V.M.K. Opaque 131 (%)	Biodent Dentin BD 27 (%)	Ceramco Dentin T 69 (%)
SiO_2	52.0	55.0	52.4	56.9	62.2
Al_2O_3	13.55	11.65	15.15	11.80	13.40
CaO	—	—	—	0.61	0.98
K_2O	11.05	9.6	9.9	10.0	11.3
Na_2O	5.28	4.75	6.58	5.42	5.37
TiO_2	3.01	—	2.59	0.61	—
ZrO_2	3.22	0.16	5.16	1.46	0.34
SnO_2	6.4	15.0	4.9	—	0.5
Rb_2O	0.09	0.04	0.08	0.10	0.06
BaO	1.09	—	—	3.52	—
ZnO	—	0.26	—	—	—
UO_3	—	—	—	—	—
B_2O_3, CO_2, and H_2O	4.31	3.54	3.24	9.58	5.85

From Nally JN, Meyer JM. Experimental study on the nature of the ceramic-metallic bonding. *SSO Schweiz Monatsschr Zahnheilkd.* 1970;80(3):250–278. [Article in French].

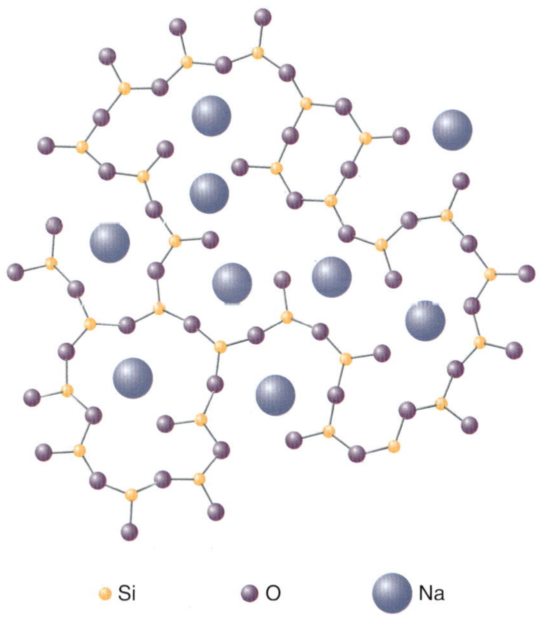

• **Fig. 10.11** Two-dimensional structure of sodium silicate glass. *Na*, Sodium; *O*, oxygen; *Si*, silicon. (Modified from Warren BE, Biscoe J. Fourier analysis of x-ray patterns of soda-silica glass. *J Am Ceram Soc.* 1938;21(7):259–265.)

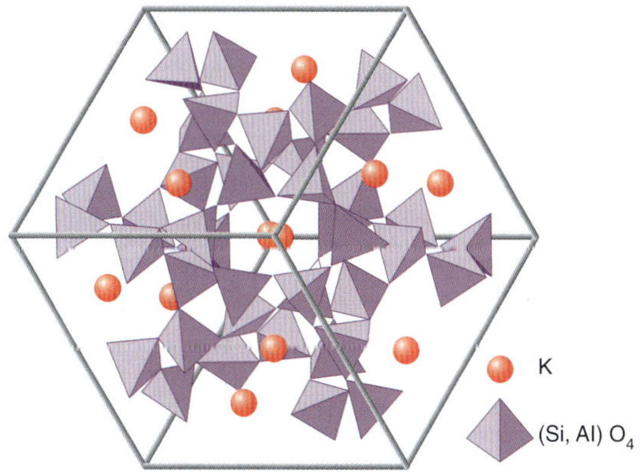

• **Fig. 10.12** Three-dimensional structure of leucite ($KAlSi_2O_6$). *Al*, Aluminum; *K*, potassium; *O*, oxygen; *Si*, silicon.

large crucibles. As mentioned earlier, feldspar melts incongruently at about 1150°C to form a glassy phase with an amorphous structure, as illustrated in Fig. 10.11, and crystalline phases, possibly consisting of leucite, a potassium aluminosilicate ($KAlSi_2O_6$).

The mix is then cooled very rapidly (quenched) in water causes the mass to shatter into small fragments. The product obtained, called a *frit,* is ball milled to achieve proper particle size distribution. Coloring pigments in small quantities are added at this stage to obtain the delicate shades necessary to mimic natural teeth. The metallic pigments include titanium oxide for yellow-brown shades, manganese oxide for lavender, iron oxide for brown, cobalt oxide for blue, copper or chromium oxides for green, and nickel oxide for brown. In the past, uranium oxide was used to provide fluorescence; however, because of the small amount of radioactivity, lanthanide oxides (such as cerium oxide) have been substituted for this purpose. Tin, titanium, and zirconium oxides are used as opacifiers.

After the manufacturing process is completed, feldspathic dental porcelain consists of a glassy (or amorphous) phase and leucite ($KAlSi_2O_6$) as a crystalline phase. The glassy phase formed during the manufacturing process has properties typical of glass, such as low toughness and strength, and high translucency. The crystalline structure of leucite is tetragonal at room temperature (Fig. 10.12). Leucite undergoes a reversible crystallographic phase transformation at 625°C, a temperature above which its structure becomes cubic. This transformation is accompanied by a thermal expansion resulting in a 1.2 vol% increase of the unit cell. This explains the high thermal expansion coefficient associated with tetragonal leucite (greater than 20×10^{-6}/°C). As a result, the amount of leucite present (10–20 vol%) controls the thermal expansion coefficient of the porcelain so that it is adequately matched to that of dental alloys.

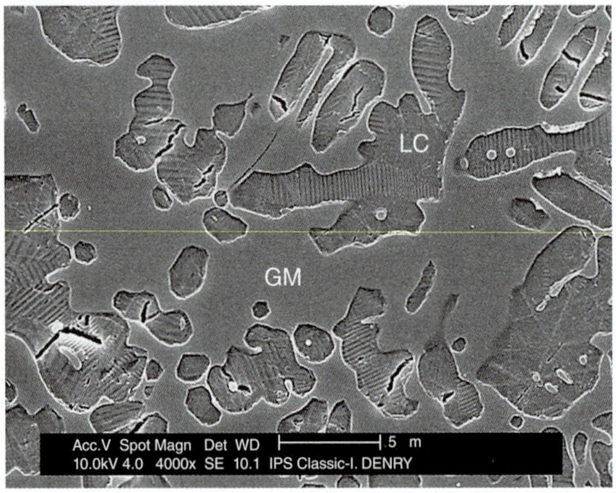

• **Fig. 10.13** Scanning electron micrograph showing the microstructure of feldspathic porcelain for metal-ceramic restorations. *GM*, Glassy matrix; *LC*, leucite crystal.

The microstructure of conventional feldspathic porcelain is shown in Fig. 10.13; the glassy phase has been lightly acid-etched to reveal the leucite crystals. Typical compositions for opaque and dentin porcelain powders are given in Table 10.4.

Feldspathic porcelains have other qualities that make them well suited for metal-ceramic restorations. They fuse at lower temperatures than do many other ceramic materials, lessening the potential for distortion of the metal coping. This is made possible by the presence of alkali oxides (Na_2O and K_2O) in the glassy matrix; these oxides are responsible for the creation of nonbridging oxygens in the glass network, thereby lowering the fusing temperatures to the range 930°C to 980°C. Porcelains having an even lower fusing temperature (760°C–780°C) and high CTE (15.8×10^{-6}/°C) are also available. These porcelains are designed to be compatible with bonding to yellow high-Au alloys, which have coefficients of thermal expansion between 16.1 and 16.8×10^{-6}/°C. They can, however, be abrasive to opposing teeth because of their hardness; this becomes a significant problem if the porcelain surface is roughened by occlusal adjustments.

Effect of Design on Metal-Ceramic Restorations

Because ceramics are weak in tension and can withstand very little strain before fracturing, the metal framework must be rigid to minimize deformation of the porcelain. However, copings should be as thin as possible to allow space for the porcelain to mask the metal framework without overcontouring the porcelain. This consideration is especially true for alloys that appear gray. This might lead to the conclusion that nickel-chromium (Ni-Cr) or cobalt-chromium (Co-Cr) alloys would be superior to the noble alloys because their moduli of elasticity (stiffness) are 1.5 to 2 times greater and the thickness of the coping could be halved. However, loading the restoration places it in bending, and the bending deflection is a function of only the first power of the modulus, whereas it is a function of the cube of the thickness. It can be shown that for a typical dental metal-ceramic restoration, the thickness of a base-metal coping can be reduced only about 7% because of the higher modulus of elasticity. Thus the advantage of the higher modulus for the base-metal alloys is minimal.

The labial margin of metal-ceramic prostheses is a critical area regarding design because there is little porcelain thickness at the margin to mask the appearance of the metal coping and to resist fracture. Recommended margin designs include a 90-degree shoulder, a 120-degree shoulder, or a shoulder bevel. Provided that the shoulder depth is at least 1.2 mm, these designs should all provide sufficient porcelain thickness to minimize the risk of porcelain fracture.

When using partial porcelain coverage, such as when a metal occlusal surface is desired, the position of the metal-ceramic joint is critical. Because of the large difference in modulus of elasticity between porcelain and metal, stresses occur at the interface when the restoration is loaded. These stresses should be minimized by placing the metal-ceramic junction at least 1.5 mm from centric occlusal contacts.

The geometry of the interproximal connector area between abutment crown and pontic is critical in the design of a metal-ceramic FDP. The inciso-cervical thickness of the connector should be large enough to prevent deformation or fracture because deflection is decreased as the cube of the thickness; greater thickness will minimize deflection of the framework, which may lead to debonding or fracture of the porcelain. It should be noted that an FDP is not a uniform beam; maximum deflection on loading will occur at the thinnest cross section, which is the interproximal connector area. However, connector thickness cannot impinge on gingival tissues or restrict access to oral hygiene procedures.

Failure and Repair of Metal-Ceramic Restorations

Metal-ceramic restorations remain a viable material combination selected for crown and bridge applications and have a 10-year success rate of about 95%. The majority of retreatments are due to biological failures, such as tooth fracture, periodontal disease, and secondary caries. Prosthesis fracture and esthetic failures account for only 20% of retreatment cases for single-unit restorations. For metal-ceramic FDPs, prosthesis fracture is the most common reason for retreatment, with long-span FDPs (five or more units) having approximately twice the incidence of failure compared with short-span FDPs.

When metal-ceramic prosthesis fails, it is often due to adhesive failure between porcelain and metal or cohesive failure within the ceramic near the metal-ceramic interface. Ideally, the prosthesis should be retrieved, metal surfaces should be cleaned, and a new oxide layer should be formed on the exposed area of metal prior to porcelain application and firing. However, this cannot be achieved intraorally, and removal of the prosthesis is both unpleasant for the patient and time consuming. Thus a variety of techniques have been developed for porcelain repair using resin composites. All of these techniques present the challenge of bonding chemically dissimilar materials. When porcelain fragments are available and no functional loading is exerted on the fracture site, silane coupling agents can be used to achieve good adhesion between the composite and porcelain; however, comparable bonding agents are not as available for metal alloys and this type of repair is considered only temporary. Systems are available for coating the metal surface with silica particles through airborne particle abrasion. The particles are embedded in the metal surface upon impact, then a silane coupling agent can be applied. Alternatively, base metal alloys can be coated with tin followed by the application of an acidic primer. Both methods achieve adequate bond strength and may delay the eventual need for remaking the prosthesis.

For a discussion of porcelain application and properties of porcelain denture teeth, please go to the website http://evolve.elsevier.com/sakaguchi/restorative.

Bibliography

Albakry M, Guazzato M, Swain MV. Influence of hot pressing on the microstructure and fracture toughness of two pressable dental glass–ceramics. *J Biomed Mater Res*. 2004;71B:(1):99–107.

Ban S. Reliability and properties of core materials for all-ceramic dental restorations. *Japan Dent Sci Rev*. 2008;44(1):3–21.

Baran GR, O'Brien WJ, Tien TY. Colored emission of rare-earth ions in a potassium feldspar glass. *J Dent Res*. 1977;56(11):1323–1329.

Benetti P, Kelly JR, Sanchez M, Della Bona A. Influence of thermal gradients on stress state of veneered restorations. *Dent Mater*. 2014;30(5):554–563.

Brodbelt RH, O'Brien WJ, Fan PL. Translucency of dental porcelains. *J Dent Res*. 1980;59(1):70–75.

Chevalier J, Grémillard L, Virkar AV, et al. The tetragonal-monoclinic transformation in zirconia: lessons learned and future trends. *J Am Ceram Soc*. 2009;92(9):1901–1920.

Della Bona A, Mecholsky JJ Jr, Anusavice KJ. Fracture behavior of lithia disilicate- and leucite-based ceramics. *Dent Mater*. 2004;20(10):956–962.

Denry I, Holloway J. Ceramics for dental applications: a review. *Materials*. 2010;3(1):351–368.

Denry I, Kelly JR. Emerging ceramic-based materials for dentistry. *J Dent Res*. 2014;93(12):1235–1242.

Denry I, Kelly JR. State of the art of zirconia for dental applications. *Dent Mater*. 2008;24(3):299–307.

Denry IL, Holloway JA, Colijn HO. Phase transformations in a leucite-reinforced pressable dental ceramic. *J Biomed Mater Res*. 2001;54(3):351–359.

Denry IL, Holloway JA, Tarr LA. Effect of heat treatment on microcrack healing behavior of a machinable dental ceramic. *J Biomed Mater Res*. 1999;48(6):791–796.

Dong JK, Luthy H, Wohlwend A. Heat-pressed ceramics: technology and strength. *Int J Prosthodont*. 1992;5(1):9–16.

Filser F, Kocher P, Gauckler LJ. Net-shaping of ceramic components by direct ceramic machining. *Assembly Autom*. 2003;23(4):382–390.

Garvie RC, Hannink RH, Pascoe RT. Ceramic steel? *Nature*. 1975;258:703–704.

Gray HS. The porcelain jacket crown. *N Z Dent J*. 1963:283–287.

Guazzato M, Albakry M, Ringer SP, Swain MV. Strength, fracture toughness and microstructure of a selection of all-ceramic materials. Part II. Zirconia-based dental ceramics. *Dent Mater*. 2004;20(5):449–456.

Hannink RHJ, Kelly PM, Muddle BC. Transformation toughening in zirconia-containing ceramics. *J Am Ceram Soc*. 2000;83(3):461–487.

Heffernan MJ, Aquilino SA, Diaz-Arnold AM, et al. Relative translucency of six all-ceramic systems. Part I: core materials. *J Prosthet Dent*. 2002;88(1):4–9.

Heffernan MJ, Aquilino SA, Diaz-Arnold AM, et al. Relative translucency of six all-ceramic systems. Part II: core and veneer materials. *J Prosthet Dent*. 2002;88(1):10–15.

Höland W, Apel E, van't Hoen C, et al. Studies of crystal phase formations in high-strength lithium disilicate glass-ceramics. *J Non-Cryst Solids*. 2006;352(38-39):4041–4050.

Höland W, Beall G. *Glass-Ceramic Technology*. The American Ceramic Society; 2002.

International Organization for Standardization (ISO). *ISO/FDIS 6872: Dentistry—Ceramic materials*; 2024.

Kelly JR, Campbell SD, Bowen HK. Fracture surface analysis of dental ceramics. *J Prosthet Dent*. 1989;62(5):536–541.

Kelly JR, Denry I. Stabilized zirconia as a structural ceramic: an overview. *Dent Mater*. 2008;24(3):289–298.

Kelly JR, Tesk JA, Sorensen JA. Failure of all-ceramic fixed partial dentures in vitro and in vivo: analysis and modeling. *J Dent Res*. 1995;74(6):1253–1258.

Kingery WD, Bowen HK, Uhlmann DR. *Introduction to Ceramics*. John Wiley & Sons; 1976.

Kosmac T, Oblak C, Jevnikar P, et al. Strength and reliability of surface treated Y-TZP dental ceramics. *J Biomed Mater Res*. 2000;53(4):304–313.

Kruger S, Deubener J, Ritzberger C, Höland W. Nucleation kinetics of lithium metasilicate in ZrO_2-bearing lithium disilicate glasses for dental application. *Int J Appl Glass Sci*. 2013;4(1):9–19.

Lawn BR, Pajares A, Zhang Y, et al. Materials design in the performance of all-ceramic crowns. *Biomaterials*. 2004;25(14):2885–2892.

McLean JW. Alumina reinforced porcelain jacket crown. *J Am Dent Assoc*. 1967;75(3):621–628.

Meyer JM, O'Brien WJ, Cu Y. Sintering of dental porcelain enamels. *J Dent Res*. 1976;55(4):696–699.

Morena R, Lockwood PE, Fairhurst CW. Fracture toughness of commercial dental porcelains. *Dent Mater*. 1986;2(2):58–62.

Paravina R, Powers J. *Esthetic Color Training in Dentistry*. Mosby; 2004.

Piche PW, O'Brien WJ, Groh CL, et al. Leucite content of selected dental porcelains. *J Biomed Mater Res*. 1994;28(5):603–609.

Sailer I, Feher A, Filser F, et al. Five-year clinical results of zirconia frameworks for posterior fixed partial dentures. *Int J Prosthodont*. 2007;20(4):383–388.

Shiraishi T, Wood DJ, Shinozaki N, van Noort R. Optical properties of base dentin ceramics for all-ceramic restorations. *Dent Mater*. 2011;27(2):165–172.

Spear F, Holloway J. Which all-ceramic system is optimal for anterior esthetics? *J Am Dent Assoc*. 2008;139:19S–24S.

Tholey MJ, Swain MV, Thiel N. SEM observations of porcelain Y-TZP interface. *Dent Mater*. 2009;25(7):857–862.

Thompson JY, Anusavice KJ, Naman A, et al. Fracture surface characterization of clinically failed all-ceramic crowns. *J Dent Res*. 1994;73(12):1824–1832.

Tinschert J, Zwez D, Marx R, et al. Structural reliability of alumina-, feldspar-, leucite-, mica- and zirconia-based ceramics. *J Dent*. 2000;28(7):529–535.

Vines R, Semmelman J. Densification of dental porcelain. *J Dent Res*. 1957;36(6):950–956.

Von Steyern PV, Carlson P, Nilner K. All-ceramic fixed partial dentures designed according to the DC-Zircon® technique. A 2-year clinical study. *J Oral Rehabil*. 2005;32(3):180–187.

Weinstein M, Weinstein LK, Katz S, et al. *Fused porcelain-to-metal teeth, U.S. Patent No. 3,052,982, United States Patent Office*; 1962.

Zhang Y, Lawn BR. Long term strength of ceramics for biomedical applications. *J Biomed Mater Res*. 2004;69B(2):166–172.

Zhang Y. Making yttria-stabilized tetragonal zirconia translucent. *Dent Mater*. 2014;30(10):1195–1203.

Metal Ceramic Systems

Anusavice KJ, Hojjatie B. Stress distribution in metal-ceramic crowns with a facial porcelain margin. *J Dent Res*. 1987;66(9):1493–1498.

Anusavice KJ, Ringle RD, Fairhurst CW. Bonding mechanism evidence in a ceramic non-precious alloy system. *J Biomed Mater Res*. 1977;11(5):701–709.

Anusavice KJ, Ringle RD, Fairhurst CW. Identification of fracture zones in porcelain-veneered-to-metal bond test specimens by ESCA analysis. *J Prosthet Dent*. 1979;42(4):417–421.

Anusavice KJ, Ringle RD, Morse PK, et al. A thermal shock test for porcelain metal systems. *J Dent Res*. 1981;60(9):1686–1691.

Anusavice KJ. Reducing the failure potential of ceramic-based restorations. Part 1: metal-ceramic crowns and bridges. *Gen Dent*. 1996;44(6):492–494.

Council on Dental Materials and Devices. How to avoid problems with porcelain-fused-to-metal restorations. *J Am Dent Assoc*. 1977;95(4):818–822.

Dent RJ, Preston JD, Moffa JP, et al. Effect of oxidation on ceramometal bond strength. *J Prosthet Dent*. 1982;47(1):59–62.

Donovan T, Prince J. An analysis of margin configurations for metal-ceramic crowns. *J Prosthet Dent*. 1985;53(2):153–157.

Eden GT, Franklin OM, Powell JM, et al. Fit of porcelain fused-to-metal crown and bridge casting. *J Dent Res*. 1979;58(12):2360–2368.

Fairhurst CW, Anusavice KJ, Hashinger DT, et al. Thermal expansion of dental alloys and porcelains. *J Biomed Mater Res*. 1980;14(4):435–446.

Farah JW, Craig RG. Distribution of stresses in porcelain-fused-to-metal and porcelain jacket crowns. *J Dent Res*. 1975;54(2):255–261.

Faucher RR, Nicholls JI. Distortion related to margin design in porcelain-fused-to-metal restorations. *J Prosthet Dent*. 1980;43(2):149–155.

Haselton DR, Diaz-Arnold AM, Dunne JT. Shear bond strengths of 2 intraoral porcelain repair systems to porcelain or metal substrates. *J Prosthet Dent*. 2001;86(5):526–531.

Heintze SD, Rousson V. Survival of zirconia- and metal-supported fixed dental prostheses: a systematic review. *Int J Prosthodont*. 2010;23(6):493–502.

Johnson T, van Noort R, Stokes CW. Surface analysis of porcelain fused to metal systems. *Dent Mater*. 2006;22(4):330–337.

Jones DW. Coatings of ceramics on metals. In: Ducheyne P, Lemons JE, eds.*Bioceramics: Materials Characteristics Versus in Vivo Behavior*. vol. 523. New York Academy of Science; 1988.

Kànànen M, Kivilahti J. Bonding of low-fusing dental porcelain to commercially pure titanium. *J Biomed Mater Res*. 1994;28(9):1027–1035.

Lautenschlager EP, Greener EH, Elkington WE. Microprobe analysis of gold-porcelain bonding. *J Dent Res*. 1969;48(6):1206–1210.

Leibrock A, Degenhart M, Behr M, et al. In vitro study of the effect of thermo- and load-cycling on the bond strength or porcelain repair systems. *J Oral Rehabil*. 1999;26(2):130–137.

Lenz J, Schwarz S, Schwickerath H, et al. Bond strength of metal-ceramics systems in three-point flexure bond test. *J Appl Biomater*. 1955;6(1):55–64.

Lubovich RP, Goodkind RJ. Bond strength studies of precious, semiprecious, and non-precious metal-ceramic alloys with two porcelains. *J Prosthet Dent*. 1977;37(3):288–299.

Mackert Jr JR, Twiggs SW, Evans-Williams AL. Isothermal anneal effect on leucite content in dental porcelains. *J Dent Res*. 1995;74(6):1259–1265.

Malhotra ML, Maickel LB. Shear bond strength of porcelain-fused-to-alloys of varying noble metal contents. *J Prosthet Dent*. 1980;44(4):405–412.

Nally JN, Meyer JM. Experimental study on the nature of the ceramic-metallic bonding. *Schweiz Monatsschr Zahnheilked*. 1970;80(3):250–278.

Nâpânkangas R, Salonen-Kemppi MA, Raustia AM. Longevity of fixed metal ceramic bridge prostheses: a clinical follow-up study. *J Oral Rehabil*. 2002;29(2):140–145.

Özcan M, Niedermeier W. Clinical study on the reasons for and location of failures of metal-ceramic restorations and survival of repairs. *Int J Prosthodont*. 2002;15(3):299–302.

Ringle RD, Fairhurst CW, Anusavice KJ. Microstructures in non-precious alloys near the porcelain-metal interaction zone. *J Dent Res*. 1979;58(10):1987–1993.

Robin C, Scherrer SS, Wiskott HWA, et al. Weibull parameters of composite resin bond strengths to porcelain and noble alloy using the Rocatec system. *Dent Mater*. 2002;18(5):389–395.

Shell JS, Nielsen JP. Study of the bond between gold alloys and porcelain. *J Dent Res*. 1962;41(6):1424–1437.

Shimoe S, Tanoue N, Yanagida H, et al. Comparative strength of metal-ceramic and metal-composite bonds after extended thermocycling. *J Oral Rehabil*. 2004;31(7):689–694.

Walton TR. A 10-year longitudinal study of fixed prosthodontics: clinical characteristics and outcome of single-unit metal-ceramic crowns. *Int J Prosthodont*. 1999;12(6):519–526.

Zarone F, Russo S, Sorrentino R. From porcelain-fused-to-metal to zirconia: clinical and experimental considerations. *Dent Mater*. 2011;27(1):83–96.

11

Impression and Casting Materials

DESPOINA BOMPOLAKI

CHAPTER OUTLINE

Impression materials are used to register or reproduce the form and spatial relationship of the teeth and oral tissues. Hydrocolloids and synthetic elastomeric polymers are among the materials most commonly used to make impressions of various areas of the dental arch. Each of these classes of materials has certain advantages and disadvantages, as well as specific indications. Therefore an understanding of the physical characteristics and the limitations of each material is necessary for their successful use in clinical dentistry. Digital impressions are described in Chapter 13. Impression materials and techniques are discussed on the website http://evolve.elsevier.com/sakaguchi/restorative.

Clinical Use of Impression Materials

Impression materials are used to create a negative reproduction of the hard and soft oral tissues. The area involved may vary from a single tooth to the whole arch, either dentate or edentulous. The impression (negative) can be poured with dental stone or other model material; once the model material has been set, it can be separated from the impression. The resulting product is the cast (positive). An impression and a stone cast made from the impression are shown in Fig. 11.1. Casts of the oral cavity are used to evaluate the orthodontic, occlusal, or other anatomical features of the mouth. In addition, casts are the connective link between the clinical and the laboratory portion during fabrication of various types of oral prostheses.

Impression materials are carried to the mouth in an unset (flowable) condition using a tray. When the impression material has set, the tray is removed from the mouth with a quick and steady motion. The cast is made by filling the impression with dental stone or other cast material or by scanning the impression and printing a plastic model from the digitized impression (see Chapter 13). The accuracy, detail, and quality of this final replica are of greatest importance. When the positive reproduction takes the form of the tissues of the maxilla or mandible and serves for the fabrication of oral prostheses, such as dentures, crowns, or fixed dental prostheses, (such as a bridge), it is described as a *cast.* The positive reproduction of the form of a prepared tooth constitutes a *die* for the fabrication of fixed dental prostheses such as crowns or onlays. When a positive likeness of the arch or certain teeth is reproduced for orthodontic treatment, it is sometimes described as a *model*, although *cast* is the more proper term. On other occasions and in other branches of dentistry, these terms are used interchangeably. Sometimes impression materials are used to duplicate a cast or model that has been formed when more than one positive reproduction is required. Such impression materials are referred to as *duplicating* materials (for additional information refer to the website http://evolve.elsevier.com/sakaguchi/restorative).

A variety of impression trays are used to make impressions. Examples of typical impression trays are shown in Fig. 11.2. The tray is positioned intraorally so the material is supported and brought into contact with the oral tissues, and then held without movement until the impression material has fully set. The tray with the impression material is then removed from the mouth, and the impression is disinfected and subsequently poured with cast material to make a positive replica. The clinical impression

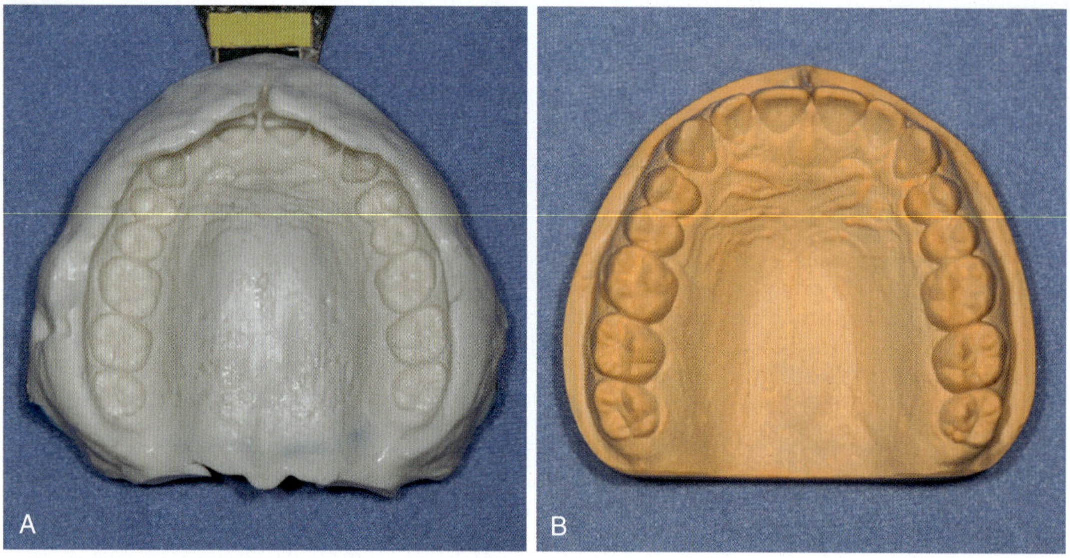

• **Fig. 11.1** Alginate impression (A) and gypsum stone cast (B). (Courtesy Dr. Charles Mark Malloy and Dr. Kyle Malloy, Portland, OR).

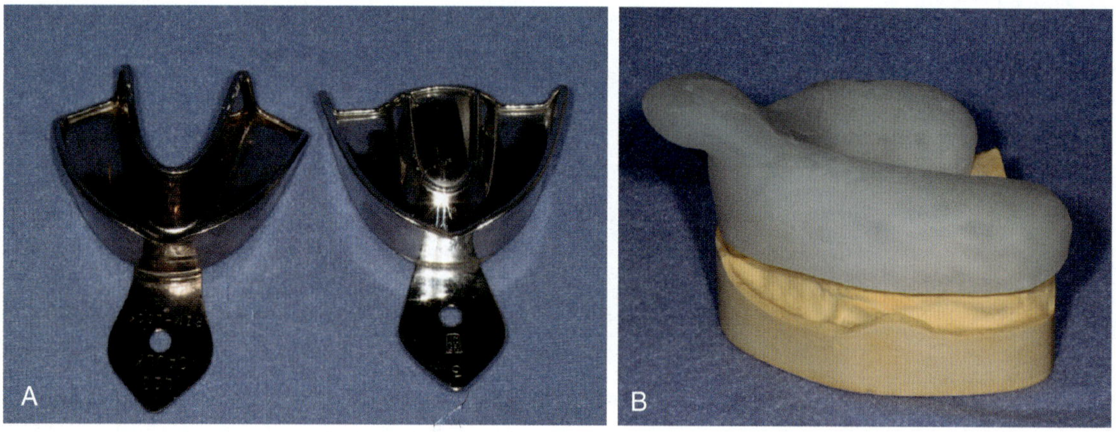

• **Fig. 11.2** (A) Mandibular and maxillary rim-lock impression trays. (B) Custom impression tray. (Courtesy Dr. Charles Mark Malloy, Portland, OR).

technique and the production of the cast can vary depending on the impression material that was utilized.

Desirable Qualities of Impression Materials

Affording safe contact with intraoral tissues and having the ability to fulfill the needs of clinical procedures are critical requirements that dictate the physical properties of dental impression materials. No impression material fulfills every requirement, and selection of the material best suited for a particular clinical situation and technique rests with the dentist. The desirable properties of an impression can be summarized briefly as follows:

1. A pleasant odor and taste
2. Absence of toxic or irritant constituents
3. Adequate shelf life for requirements of storage and distribution
4. Economically commensurate with the results obtained
5. Easy to use, with minimum additional equipment needs
6. Setting time that meets clinical requirements
7. Satisfactory consistency and texture
8. Wettability of oral tissues
9. Elastic properties that allow easy removal of the set material from the mouth as well as good elastic recovery
10. Adequate strength to avoid breaking or tearing upon removal from the mouth
11. Dimensional stability over temperature and humidity conditions that are normally encountered during clinical and laboratory procedures, for a period long enough to permit the production of a cast or die
12. Compatibility with cast and die materials
13. Accuracy and ability to reproduce fine detail
14. Ability to be disinfected without loss of accuracy
15. No release of gas or other by-products during the setting of the impression or cast and die materials

Types of Impression Materials

Alginate hydrocolloid and elastomeric impression materials are the most widely used today. Elastomeric impression materials have replaced rigid setting materials such as plaster, impression compound, and zinc oxide-eugenol for recording soft-tissue and occlusal relationships. Information on plaster, impression compound, and zinc oxide-eugenol impression materials can be found on the website http://evolve.elsevier.com/sakaguchi/restorative.

Alginate Hydrocolloids

Dental alginate impression materials change from the sol phase to the gel phase as part of a chemical reaction. Once gelation is completed, the material cannot be re-dissolved to a sol phase. These hydrocolloids are called *irreversible* to distinguish them from the agar reversible hydrocolloids. Agar impression materials are described on the website http://evolve.elsevier.com/sakaguchi/restorative. Alginate impressions are widely used to create study casts for diagnostic and treatment planning purposes, monitoring of tooth and tissue movement, and fabrication of various types of dental prostheses.

Alginate impression products have acceptable elastic properties. Preparation for use requires only the mixing of measured quantities of powder and water. The resulting paste flows well and registers acceptable anatomical detail. Gypsum casts are made by pouring dental stone into the impression; no separating medium is necessary. The powder is supplied in bulk containers along with suitable measures for dispensing the correct quantities of powder and water. The powder is also available in sealed premeasured pouches, containing a quantity suitable for a single impression and ready for mixing with a measured quantity of water. These methods of packaging, together with the measuring devices supplied by the manufacturer, are shown in Fig. 11.3.

Composition and Chemistry

Potassium and sodium salts of alginic acid have properties that make them suitable for compounding a dental impression material. Alginic acid, which is prepared from a marine plant, is a high-molecular-weight block copolymer, as shown in the top part of the formula for alginate mentioned later. The properties of alginate raw material depend largely on the degree of polymerization and the ratio of the different types of blocks in the polymeric molecules. The final product can vary from strong and brittle gels to weaker and more flexible gels.

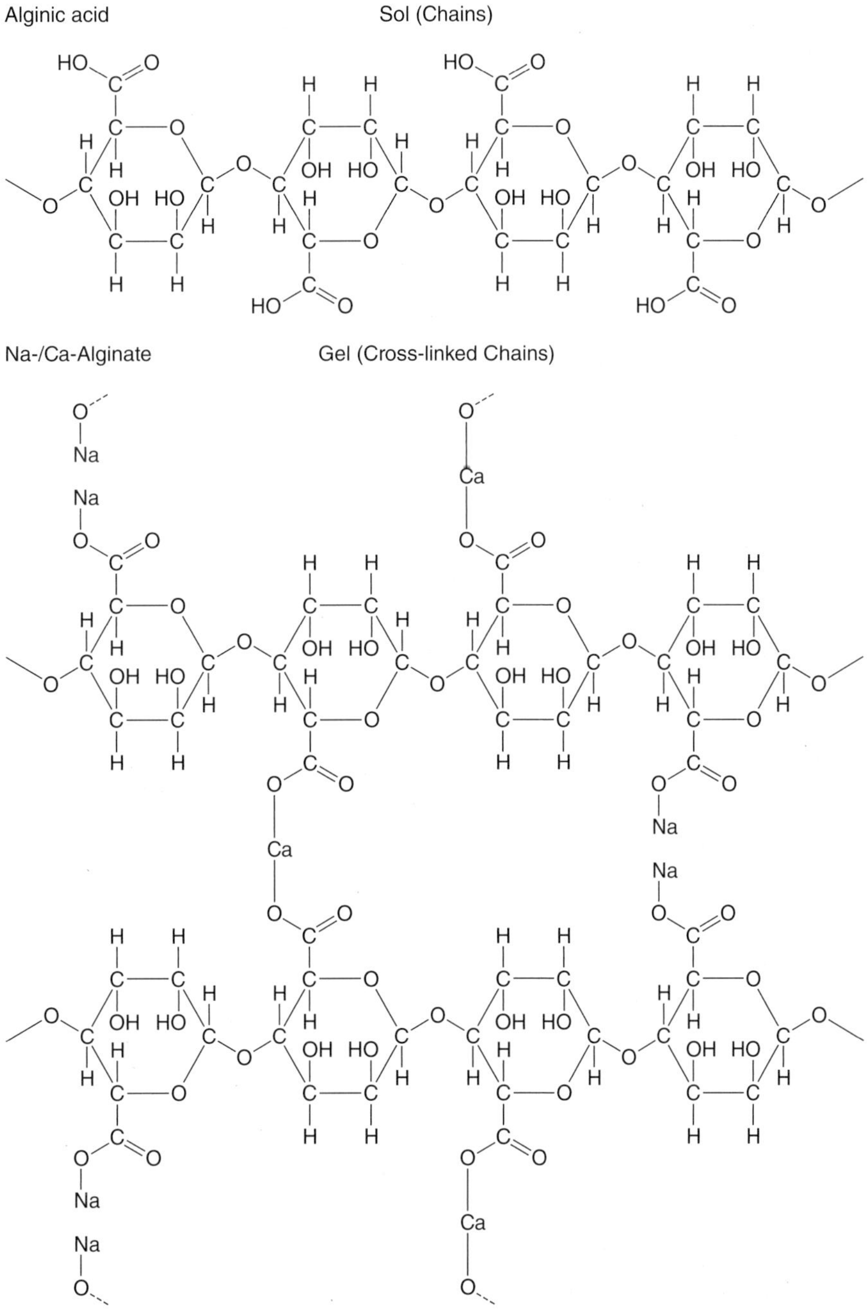

$$CaSO_4 - 2H_2O(s) \longrightarrow Ca^{2+}(aq) + SO_4^{2-}(aq)$$
$$Na - Alginate(s) \longrightarrow Na^{+}(aq) + Alginate^{-}(aq)$$
$$Na_4P_2O_7(s)\ (retarder) \longrightarrow 4Na^{+}(aq) + P_2O_7^{4-}(aq)$$
$$2Ca^{2+}(aq) + P_2O_7^{4-}(aq) \longrightarrow Ca_2P_2O_7(s)$$

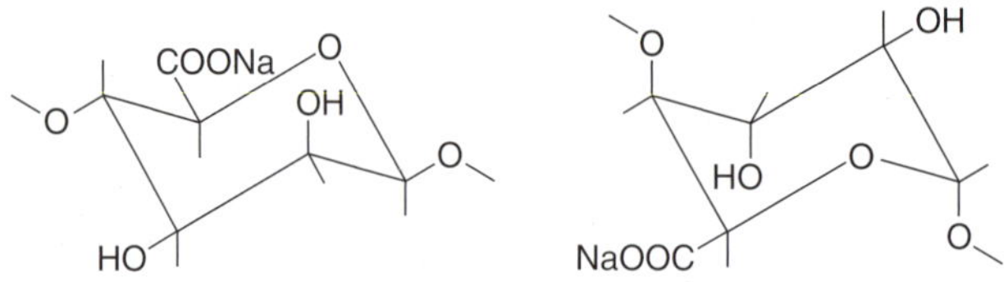

Mannuronate Guluronate

Sol

↓

$$Ca^{2+}(aq) + Alginate^{-}(aq) \longrightarrow Ca - Alginate^{+}$$

↓

Gel network

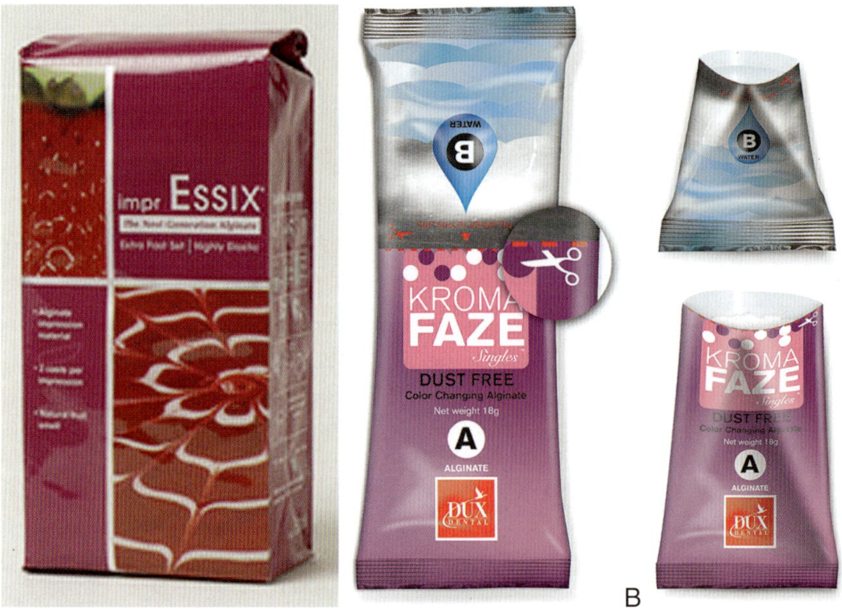

A B

• **Fig. 11.3** Alginate impression products. (A) imprESSIX (Courtesy DENTSPLY Raintree Essix, Bradenton, FL). (B) Kromafaze (Courtesy DUX Dental, Oxnard, CA).

Solutions of these soluble salts, when reacted with calcium salt, produce an insoluble flexible gel commonly called *calcium alginate*; the structures are shown in the schemes above. Upon mixing with water, the alginate impression material first forms a sol. Following the chemical reaction described previously a gel is formed to create the set impression material. The concept of sols and gels is presented in the discussion of colloids in Chapter 4.

This chemical reaction described in this chapter using the sodium salt. The equally common potassium salt reacts similarly. In an alginate impression compound, the calcium sulfate dihydrate, soluble alginate, and sodium phosphate are included in the powder. When water is added to the powder, compounds disassociate. Calcium ions from the calcium sulfate dihydrate react preferentially with phosphate ions from the sodium phosphate and pyrophosphate to form insoluble calcium phosphate. Calcium phosphate is formed rather than calcium alginate because it has a lower solubility. Thus the sodium phosphate is called a *retarder* and prolongs the working time for the mixed alginate.

After the phosphate ions are depleted, the calcium ions react with the soluble alginate to form the insoluble calcium alginate,

TABLE 11.1 Ingredients in an Alginate Impression Powder and Their Functions

Ingredient	Weight (%)	Function
Potassium alginate	18	To dissolve in water and react with calcium ions
Calcium sulfate dihydrate	14	To react with potassium alginate to form an insoluble calcium alginate gel
Potassium sulfate, potassium zinc	10	To counteract the inhibiting effect of the hydrocolloid on the fluoride, silicates, or borates setting of gypsum, giving a high-quality surface to the die
Sodium phosphate	2	To react preferentially with calcium ions to provide working time before gelation
Diatomaceous earth or silicate	56	To control the consistency of the mixed alginate and the powder flexibility of the set impression
Organic glycols	Small	To make the powder dustless
Wintergreen, peppermint, anise	Trace	To produce a pleasant taste
Pigments	Trace	To provide color
Disinfectants (e.g., quaternary ammonium salts and chlorhexidine)	1–2	To help in the disinfection of viable organisms

which together with water forms the insoluble calcium alginate gel. This reaction is irreversible; it is not possible to convert the calcium alginate to a sol after it has set.

To meet the critical requirements of dental impression material, this reaction must be controlled to attain the desirable properties of consistency, working time, setting time, strength, flexibility, elastic quality, and smooth, hard surfaces on gypsum casts. These requirements are achieved by adding agents to control the rate of the reaction, develop strength and elasticity in the gel, and counteract the delaying effect of alginate on the setting of gypsum products. The incorporation of suitable fillers in correct quantities produces a consistency that is suitable for various clinical uses.

The composition of a typical alginate impression material and the function of its ingredients are shown in Table 11.1. Manufacturers adjust the concentration of sodium phosphate to produce regular- and fast-set alginates. They also adjust the concentration of filler to control the flexibility of the set impression material from soft-set to hard-set. Although alginate impressions are usually made in a tray, injection types are much more fluid after mixing and more flexible after setting. Manufacturers add organic glycols to the alginate powder to reduce dust. Diatomaceous earth or fine siliceous particles are used as fillers. Because these particles can be a respiratory irritant, inhalation of the dust should be minimized. Impressions should be disinfected with a spray solution after removal from the mouth and before pouring with a cast material. Other ingredients in some products include antimicrobial agents and pH indicator dyes that change color when setting has occurred to provide a visual indication of working time and setting time. More recent alginate formulations have increased dimensional stability on storage, allowing impressions to be poured at a later time.

Proportioning and Mixing

The proportioning of the powder and water before mixing is critical to obtaining consistent results. Changes in the water-to-powder (W/P) ratio will alter the consistency and setting times of the mixed material and also the strength and quality of the set impression. Usually the manufacturers provide suitable containers for proportioning the powder and water by volume, and these are sufficiently accurate for clinical use.

The mixing time for regular-set alginate is 1 minute. This time should be carefully followed, because both undermixing and overmixing are detrimental to the strength of the set impression. Fast-set alginates should be mixed with water for 45 seconds. The powder and water are best mixed vigorously in a flexible rubber bowl with an alginate spatula or a spatula of the type used for mixing plaster and stone. Mechanical mixing devices that minimize air entrapment during mixing and produce a more consistent mix are also available.

Properties

Some typical properties of a tray-type alginate impression material are listed in Table 11.2.

Working Time

The fast-set materials have working times of 1.25 to 2 minutes, whereas working time of the regular-set materials is usually 3 minutes, but may be as long as 4.5 minutes. With a mixing time of 45 seconds for the fast-set types, 30 to 75 seconds of working time remain before the impression is set. For the regular-set materials, a mixing time of 60 seconds leaves 2 to 3.5 minutes of working time. In both cases, the mixed alginate must be promptly loaded into the tray and fully seated intraorally.

Setting Time

Setting times range from 1 to 5 minutes. The American National Standards Institute/American Dental Association (ANSI/ADA) specification No. 18 (International Organization for Standardization [ISO] 1563) requires that it be at least that value listed by the manufacturer and at least 15 seconds longer than the stated working time. Lengthening the setting time is better accomplished by reducing the temperature of the water used with the mix than by reducing the proportion of powder. Altering the W/P ratio reduces the strength and accuracy of the alginate. Selecting an alginate with a different setting time is a better alternative than changing the W/P ratio.

TABLE 11.2 Typical Properties of Alginate and Heavy-Bodied Agar Hydrocolloid Impression Materials

	Working Time (min)	Setting Time (min)	Gelation (°C)	Recovery[a] (%)	Flexibility[b] (%)	Compressive Strength[c] (MPa)	Tear Strength[d] (kN/m)
Alginate	1.25–4.5	1.5–5.0	—	98.2	8–15	0.49–0.88	0.4–0.7
Agar	—	—	37–45	99.0	4–15	0.78	0.8–0.9

[a]At 10% compression for 30 seconds.
[b]At a stress of 1000 g/cm^2.
[c]At a loading rate of 10 kg/min.
[d]ASTM Tear Die C at 25 cm/min.

The setting reaction is a typical chemical reaction, and the rate can be approximately doubled by a temperature increase of 10°C. However, using water that is cooler than 18°C or warmer than 24°C is not advisable, as the temperature of the water also affects the comfort of the patient. The clinical setting time is detected by a loss of surface tackiness. If possible, the impression should be left in place 2 to 3 minutes after the loss of tackiness, because the tear strength and elastic recovery (recovery from deformation) increase significantly during this period.

Elastic Recovery

A typical alginate impression is compressed about 10% in areas of undercuts during removal. The actual magnitude depends on the extent of the undercuts and the space between the tray and the teeth. The ANSI/ADA specification requires that the elastic recovery be more than 95% when the material is compressed 20% for 5 seconds at the time it would normally be removed from the mouth. As indicated in Table 11.2, a typical value for elastic recovery is 98.2%. The corresponding permanent deformation is 1.8%.

The permanent deformation (or lack of elastic recovery), indicated as percent compression set, is a function of percent compression, time under compression, and time after removal of the compressive load, as illustrated in Fig. 11.4. Note that permanent deformation is a time-dependent property. Lower permanent deformation (higher elastic recovery) occurs (1) when the percent compression is lower, (2) when the impression is under compression for a shorter time, and (3) when the recovery time is longer, up to about 8 minutes after the release of the load. Clinically these factors translate into requirements for a reasonable bulk of alginate between the tray and the teeth, appropriate retention of the alginate in the tray, and rapid removal of the impression from the mouth. The usual procedures followed to disinfect the impression and produce gypsum cast provide adequate time for any recovery that might occur.

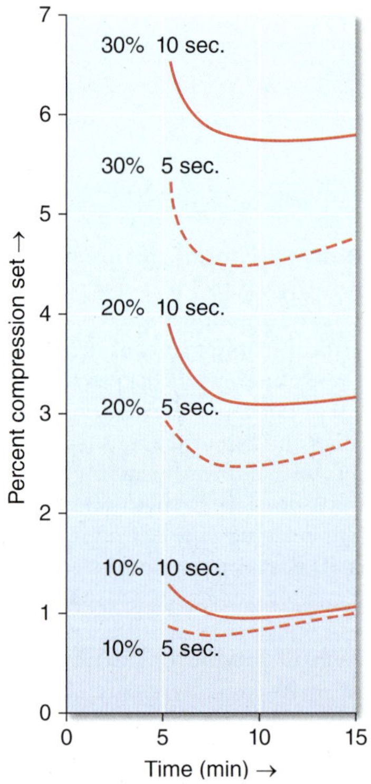

• **Fig. 11.4** Variation of compression set with time of an alginate impression material at strains of 10%, 20%, and 30% applied for 5 and 10 seconds. (Modified from Wilson HJ. Elastomeric impression materials. 1. The setting material. *Br Dent J.* 1966;121(6):277–283).

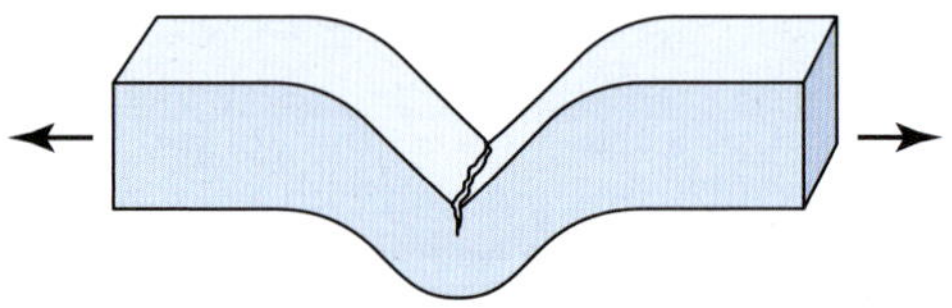

• **Fig. 11.5** Sketch of tear strength specimen with load applied in the directions of the *arrows*; the specimen tears at the V-notch.

Flexibility

The ANSI/ADA specification permits a range of 5% to 20% at a stress of 0.1 MPa, and most alginates have a typical value of 14%. However, some of the hard-set materials have values from 5% to 8%. What is critical is that some flexibility is required for ease of removal of the impression.

Strength

The compressive and tear strengths of alginates are listed in Table 11.2. Both properties are time dependent, with higher values obtained at higher rates of loading. Compressive strengths range from approximately 0.5 to 0.9 MPa. The ANSI/ADA specification requires that certified products have a compressive strength of at least 0.35 MPa. Tear strengths vary from 0.4 to 0.7 kN/m, and this property is probably more important than compressive strength. The tear strength is a measure of the force-to-thickness ratio needed to initiate and continue tearing and is often determined on a specimen of the shape shown in Fig. 11.5. Tearing occurs in the thin sections of the impression, and the probability

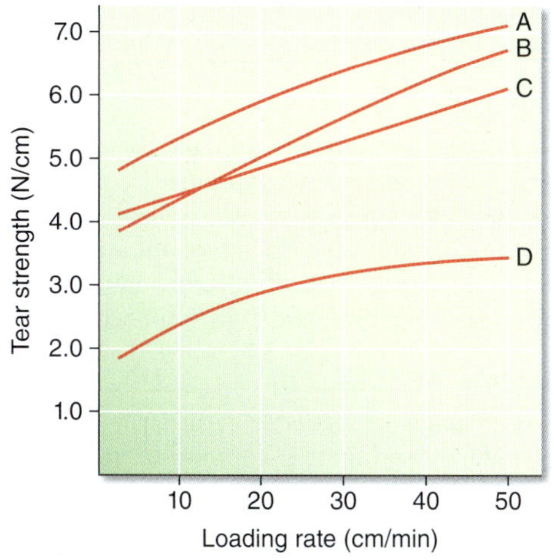

• **Fig. 11.6** Tear strength (N/cm) of alginate impression materials as a function of rate of loading (cm/min). Materials *A, B,* and *C* are designed to be used in a tray; *D* is a syringe material. (Modified from MacPherson GW, Craig RG, Peyton FA. Mechanical properties of hydrocolloid and rubber impression materials. *J Dent Res*. 1967;46(4):714–721).

of tearing decreases with increasing rates of removal. The effect of loading rate on the tear strength of several alginates is shown in Fig. 11.6. Values for tray materials range from 0.38 to 0.48 N/mm at 20 mm/min to 0.6 to 0.7 N/mm at 500 mm/min. The greater strength at faster load rates provides the rationale to remove the impression from the mouth with a quick motion. The lower tear strength at corresponding rates for the syringe materials reflects the decreased alginate content in the syringe material.

Compatibility with Gypsum

The selection of an alginate–gypsum combination that produces good surface quality and detail is highly important. The surface quality and ability of alginate–gypsum combinations to reproduce fine V-shaped grooves are shown in Fig. 11.7A and B. A type III model plaster was poured against an alginate in Fig. 11.7A, and type IV dental stone was poured against the same alginate in Fig. 11.7B. The finest groove was 0.025 mm wide in each instance. The combination in Fig. 11.7B was not as compatible as the one in Fig. 11.7A with respect to either surface quality or detail. For purposes of comparison, in Fig. 11.7C, the same type IV dental stone used in Fig. 11.7B was poured against a polysulfide impression, showing enhanced detail.

The impression must be rinsed well in cold water to remove saliva and any blood and then disinfected. Next, all free surface water should be removed before pouring the impression. Saliva and blood interfere with the setting of stone, and if free water accumulates, it tends to collect in the deeper parts of the impression, such as the areas corresponding to the cusp tips, and dilute the gypsum model material, yielding a soft, chalky surface at the critical occlusal portion of the cast. The excess surface water has been removed when the reflective surface becomes dull. If the alginate impression is stored for 30 minutes or more before being poured, it should be rinsed with cool water to remove any exudate on the surface caused by syneresis of the alginate gel; exudate will retard (inhibit/delay) the setting of the gypsum. Thereafter, it should be wrapped loosely in a moist paper towel and sealed in a plastic bag to avoid moisture loss.

The set stone cast should not remain in contact with the alginate impression for extended periods of time (i.e., over an hour), because contact of the slightly soluble calcium sulfate dihydrate with the alginate gel containing a significant amount of water is detrimental to the surface quality of the stone cast.

Dimensional Stability

Alginate impressions lose water by evaporation and shrink when exposed to air. Impressions left on the bench for as short as 30 minutes may become inaccurate enough to require remaking the impression. Even if the impression stored for more than 30 minutes in air was immersed in water, it would not be feasible to determine whether the correct amount of water had been absorbed, and in any case, the previous dimensions would not be reproduced. For maximum accuracy, the cast material should be poured into the alginate impression as soon as possible. If for some reason the

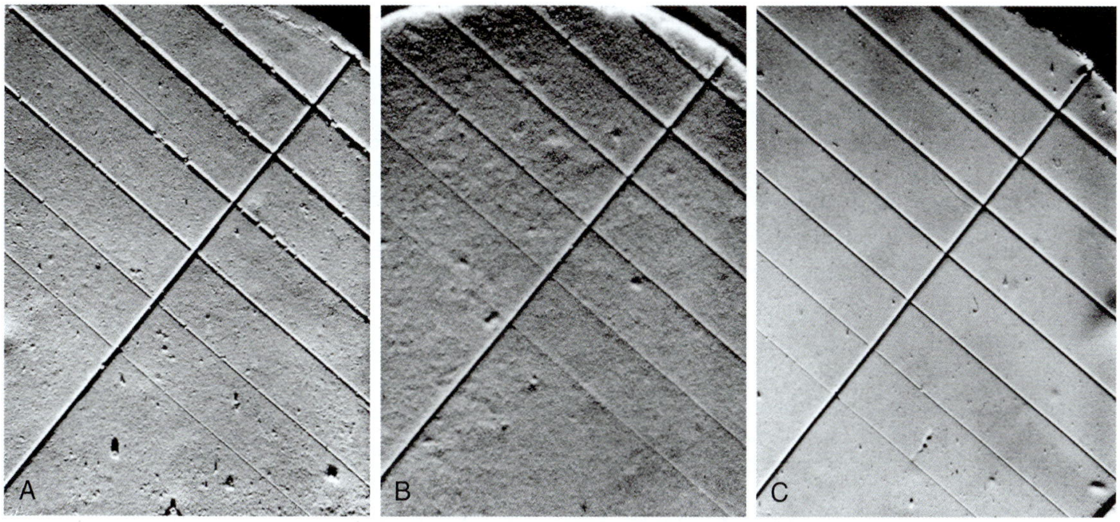

• **Fig. 11.7** Surface quality and reproduction using model plaster and dental stone. (A) Model plaster poured against alginate; (B) dental stone poured against the same alginate; and (C) the same dental stone poured against polysulfide. It should be emphasized that another alginate with the same plaster and stone could yield opposite results. (From Craig RG, MacPherson GW. *Ann Arbor: University of Michigan School of Dentistry*; 1965).

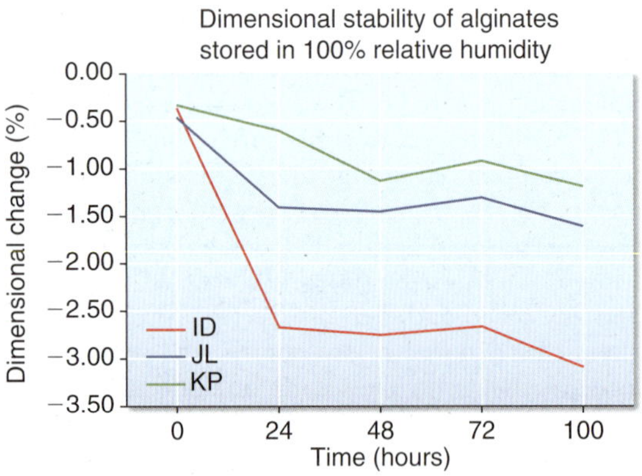

• **Fig. 11.8** Dimensional change of alginate impression materials stored in 100% relative humidity. (Modified from Lu H, Frey GN, Powers JM. unpublished data).

casts cannot be prepared directly, the impressions should be stored in 100% relative humidity in a plastic bag or wrapped in a damp (but not wringing-wet) paper towel. There is a greater chance for distortion the longer the impression is stored (Fig. 11.8). New alginates have improved long-term storage ranging from 48 to 120 hours when stored in a plastic bag. When longer storage or transportation times are expected, alternate impression methods (such as digital acquisition) are preferred, to eliminate the issue of physical distortion.

Disinfection

Disinfection of impressions is a concern with respect to viral diseases, such as hepatitis B, acquired immunodeficiency syndrome, and herpes simplex, because the viruses may be transferred to stone casts and present a risk to dental laboratory and operating personnel.

All alginate impressions should be disinfected before being poured with stone. The most common form of disinfection is spraying, but studies have shown that alginate impressions can also be immersed in disinfectant. The effect of disinfection in 1% sodium hypochlorite or 2% potentiated glutaraldehyde solutions on accuracy and surface quality has been measured after 10- to 30-minute immersion. Statistically significant dimensional changes were observed; however, the changes were on the order of 0.1% and the quality of the surface was not impaired. Such changes would be insignificant for clinical applications such as the preparation of diagnostic and definitive casts. In another study, immersion disinfection of alginates demonstrated little effect on accuracy and surface quality, but it was shown that one alginate product was best immersed in iodophor and another brand in glyoxal glutaraldehyde.

Elastomeric Impression Materials

Four types of synthetic elastomeric impression materials are available to record dental impressions: polysulfides, condensation silicones, addition silicones polyvinylsiloxanes (PVS), and polyethers. Polysulfides were the first synthetic elastomeric impression material introduced (1950). Condensation silicones were made available to dentists in 1955, polyether in 1965, and addition silicones in 1975. Polysulfide and condensation silicone impression materials are described on the website http://evolve.elsevier.com/sakaguchi/restorative. PVS and polyethers form the vast majority of elastomeric impressions used worldwide today. Hybrids of PVS and polyethers are also available. Changes in recent years have provided greater choice of consistency and new mixing techniques.

Consistencies

Elastomeric impression materials are typically supplied in several consistencies (viscosities) to accommodate a range of impression techniques. Addition silicones are available in extra-low, low (syringe or wash), medium (regular), monophase, high (tray), and putty (extra-high) consistencies. Polyether impression materials are available in low, medium, and high consistencies.

Mixing Systems

Two types of systems are available to mix the catalyst and base thoroughly before making the impression: static (*automixing*) and dynamic (*mechanical*) mixing. A very popular means of mixing the catalyst and base is with a so-called *automixing system*, in which the base and catalyst materials are packaged in separate cylinders of a plastic cartridge. The cartridge is placed in a mixing gun containing two plungers that are advanced by a ratchet mechanism to extrude equal quantities of base and catalyst through the static-mixing tip containing a stationary plastic internal spiral; the two components are folded over each other many times as they are pushed through the spiral, resulting in a uniform mix at the tip end. Because one cylinder may be filled slightly more than the other, the first part of the mix from a new cartridge should be discarded. In addition, care must be taken to ensure that the cartridge tips are not occluded before attaching the mixing tip.

The mixed material can be extruded directly into an injection syringe or into the impression tray. Intraoral delivery tips can be placed on the end of the static mixing tip, and the mixed material can be injected around the tooth preparation. The tip can be removed, and additional mixed material can be extruded into the impression tray. The automixing systems have been shown to result in mixes with many fewer voids than hand mixes, which used to be done on a waxy paper pad using a mixing spatula. Although for each mix the material left in the mixing tip is wasted, the average loss is only 1 to 2 mL, depending on the manufacturer's tip, whereas three to four times this much is wasted in a hand mix as a result of overestimating the amount needed for the impression. Initially, automixing was used for low consistencies, but new designs of guns and mixing tips allow all consistencies except putty to be used with this system. Static mixing, or automixing, is available for addition silicones and polyethers.

The second system is a mechanical mixer, illustrated in Fig. 11.9. The catalyst and base are supplied in large foil bags housed in a cartridge, which is inserted into the top compartment of the mixing machine. A new, plastic mixing tip is placed on the

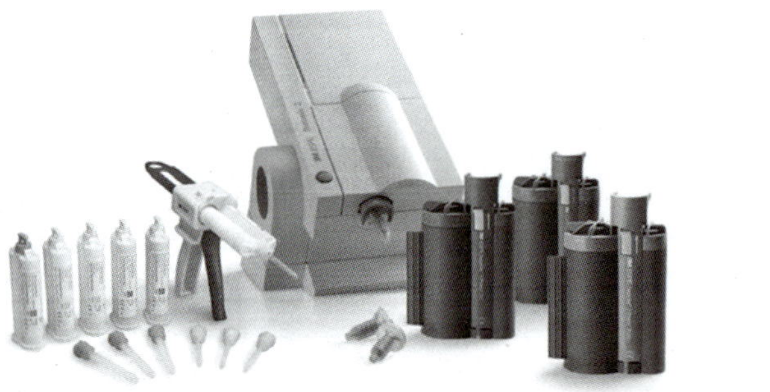

• **Fig. 11.9** Addition-silicone impression materials packaged with automixed cartridges, mixing gun, static mixing tips, and dynamic mechanical mixer. (Courtesy 3M Company, St. Paul, MN.)

front of the machine, and when the button is depressed to activate the system, parallel plungers push against the collapsible foil bags, thereby opening the bags and forcing material into the dynamic mixing tip. This mixing tip differs from automixing in that the internal spiral is motor driven, so it rotates. Therefore mixing is accomplished by this rotation combined with the forward motion of the material through the spiral. In this manner, thorough mixing can be ensured and higher viscosity material can be mixed with ease. The advantage of this system is ease of use, speed, and thoroughness of mixing, but requires a larger investment for the initial purchase of the system compared with hand and automixing. In addition there is slightly more material retained in the mixing tip compared to automixing, but still less than the material that is wasted during hand mixing. Dynamic, or mechanical, mixing is available for addition silicones and polyethers.

One variation in mixing is with the two-putty addition-silicone systems mixed by hand. Scoops are supplied by the manufacturer for dispensing, and the putties are most often kneaded with fingers until free from streaks. The putty materials that have a liquid catalyst are initially mixed with a spatula until the catalyst is reasonably incorporated, and mixing is completed by hand. It should also be noted that latex gloves may interfere with setting of addition-silicone impression materials, as discussed later.

Impression Techniques

Three common methods for making impressions for fixed restorations are 1. simultaneous, dual-viscosity technique; 2. single-viscosity or monophase technique; and 3. putty-wash technique. In nearly all cases, impression material is injected directly onto the prepared teeth and a tray containing the bulk of the impression material is seated intraorally thereafter. After the impression material is set, the tray is removed.

The simultaneous, dual-viscosity technique is one in which low-consistency material is injected with a syringe into critical areas and the high-consistency material is mixed and placed in an impression tray. After injecting the low-viscosity material, the tray containing the higher-viscosity material is seated intraorally. In this manner, the more viscous tray impression material forces the lower-viscosity material to flow into fine aspects of the areas of interest. Because they are both mixed at nearly the same time, the materials join, bond, and set together. After the materials have set, the tray and the impression are removed. An example of an impression using this procedure is shown in Fig. 11.10.

In the single-viscosity or monophase technique, impressions are often taken with medium-viscosity impression material. Addition-silicone and polyether impression materials are well suited for this technique because both have a capacity for shear thinning. As described in Chapter 4, pseudoplastic materials demonstrate decreased viscosity when subjected to high shear rates such as those occurring during mixing and syringing. When the medium viscosity material is forced through an impression syringe, the viscosity is reduced, whereas the viscosity of the same material residing in the tray is unaffected. In this manner, such materials can be used for syringing and for trays, as previously described for the simultaneous, dual-viscosity technique. The mechanism for shear thinning is also discussed in the later section on the viscosity of impression materials.

The putty-wash technique is a two-step impression procedure whereby a preliminary impression is taken in high- or putty-consistency material before the tooth preparation is completed. Space is provided for a low-consistency material by a variety of techniques, and after tooth preparation, a low-consistency material

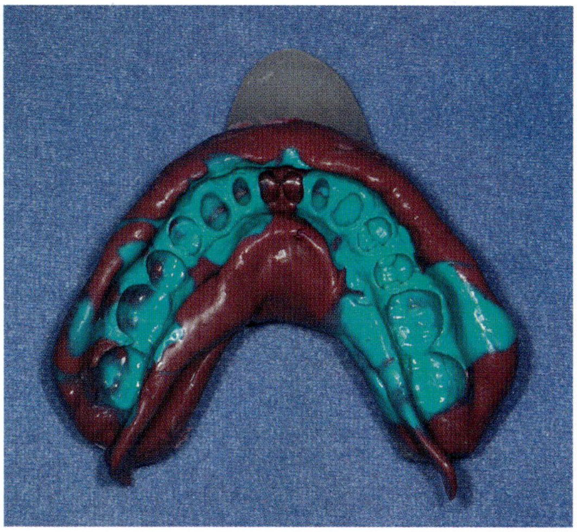

• **Fig. 11.10** An elastomeric addition-silicone impression. Turquoise material is of a low or injection consistency, and maroon material is of a high or tray consistency. (Courtesy Dr. Charles Mark Malloy, Portland, OR).

is syringed into the area and the preliminary impression is reinserted. The low- and high-consistency materials bond, and after the low-consistency material sets, the impression is removed. This procedure is sometimes called a *wash technique*. The putty-consistency materials and this impression technique were developed for condensation silicones, in order to minimize the effects of dimensional change during polymerization. Most of the polymerization shrinkage occurs within the putty material when the preliminary impression is made, confining final shrinkage to the thin wash portion of the impression. In addition, because the putty material has a much higher filler content, it inherently shrinks less than the low viscosity, low filler content wash material. Therefore by making the majority of the impression with the putty material the overall shrinkage is significantly decreased. Care must be taken so the wash material can freely escape via vents in the putty material when the wash impression is made. If not, the wash material can compress the putty in the second-stage impression, inducing permanent distortion and inaccuracies in the impression. The putty-wash technique was extended to addition silicones after their introduction, even though their polymerization shrinkage is significantly lower.

Manufacturers add coloring agents to the accelerator or base as an aid in determining the thoroughness of the mix. Normally a different color is used for each consistency of a particular product line so one can distinguish the wash (low) consistency from the tray consistency in the set impression. Retarders may be added as well to control working and setting time of the products. Some manufacturers have added flavors to addition silicones.

Composition and Reactions

The next two sections describe the general composition and setting reactions of addition-silicone and polyether impression materials. The following section describes their physical properties, permitting a more direct comparison of the various types.

Addition Silicone

Addition silicone (also called polyvinylsiloxane or PVS) is available in extra low, low, medium, heavy, and very heavy (putty) consistencies. A representative product line of addition silicones is shown in Fig. 11.11. The base paste of this class of impression materials contains a moderately low-molecular-weight polymer

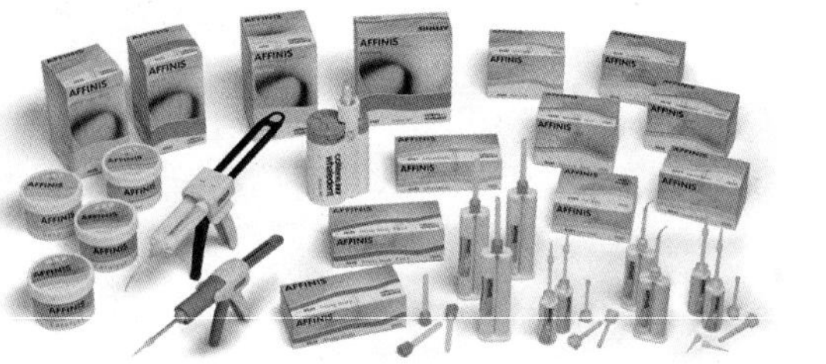

• **Fig. 11.11** Various consistencies and types of packaging of an addition-silicone impression material. (Courtesy Coltene/Whaledent Inc, Cuyahoga Falls, OH).

(polymethylhydrosiloxane) with more than three and up to ten pendant or terminal hydrosilane groups per molecule (see formulas below and addition-silicone formula 1 [AS1]). The base also contains filler.

Pendant hydrosilane groups Terminal hydrosilane groups

Polymethylhydrosiloxane

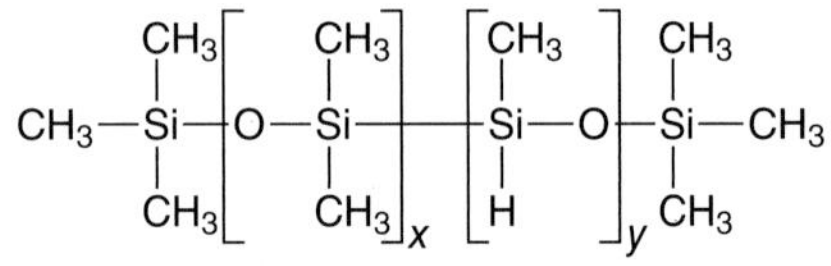

AS1 Vinylpolysiloxane

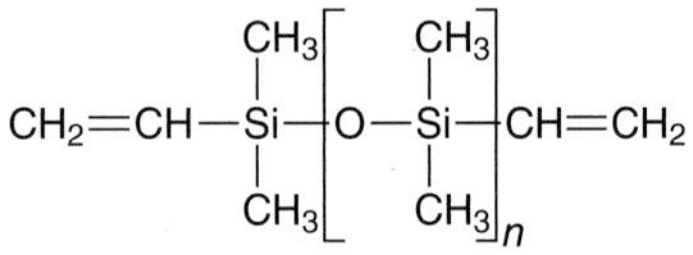

The accelerator (catalyst) and the base paste contain a dimethylsiloxane polymer with vinyl terminal groups, plus filler. The accelerator also contains a platinum catalyst of the so-called *Karstedt type*, which is a complex compound consisting of platinum and 1,3-divinyltetramethyldisiloxane. Unlike the condensation type, the addition reaction does not normally produce a low-molecular-weight by-product, as indicated in the reaction shown below (AS2).

A secondary reaction can occur, however, with the production of hydrogen gas if –OH groups are present. The gas forms bubbles on the surface of the impression. The most important source of –OH groups is water (H–OH), the reaction of which under consumption of Si–H units is illustrated earlier (AS3). Another possible source of hydrogen gas is a side reaction of the Si–H units of the polymethylhydrosiloxane with each other, under the influence of the platinum catalyst, also shown earlier (AS3).

Not all addition-silicone impression materials release hydrogen gas, and because it is not known which ones do, it is recommended that at least 30 minutes are allowed for the setting reaction to be completed before the impression is poured with stone. Epoxy dies should not be poured until the impression has stood overnight. The difference in the delay with stone and epoxy is that stone products have much shorter setting times than epoxy die materials. Some products contain a hydrogen absorber such as palladium, and gypsum and epoxy die materials can be poured against them as soon as practical. Examples of high-strength stone poured after 15 minutes against addition silicone, with and without a hydrogen absorber, are shown in Fig. 11.12.

Latex gloves have been shown to adversely affect the setting of addition-silicone impressions. Sulfur compounds that are used in the vulcanization of latex rubber gloves can migrate to the surface of stored gloves. These compounds can be transferred onto the prepared teeth and adjacent soft tissues during tooth preparation and also during placement of tissue retraction cord. They can also be incorporated directly into the impression material when mixing two putties by hand. These compounds can poison the platinum-containing catalyst, which results in retarded or no polymerization in the contaminated area of the impression. Thorough

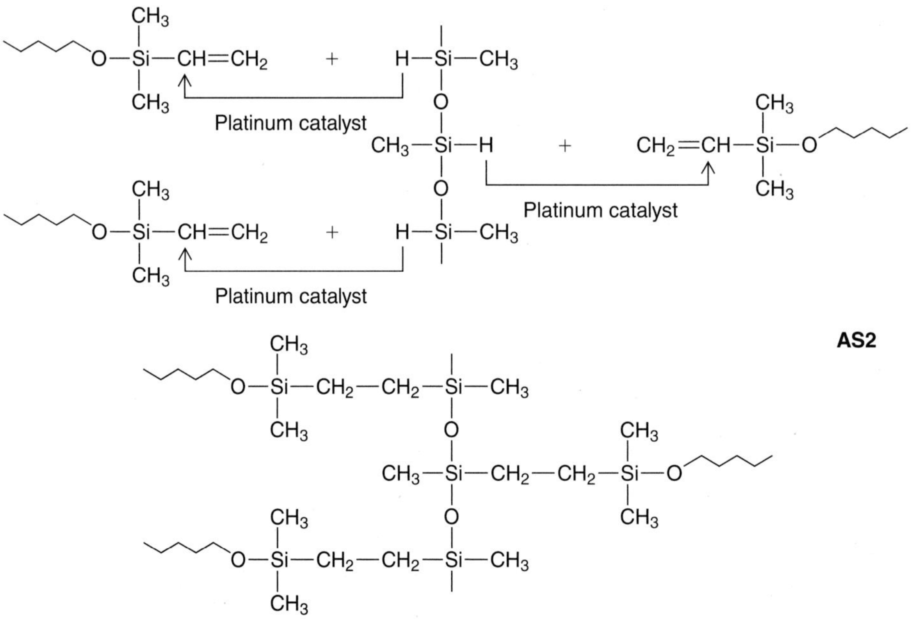

AS2

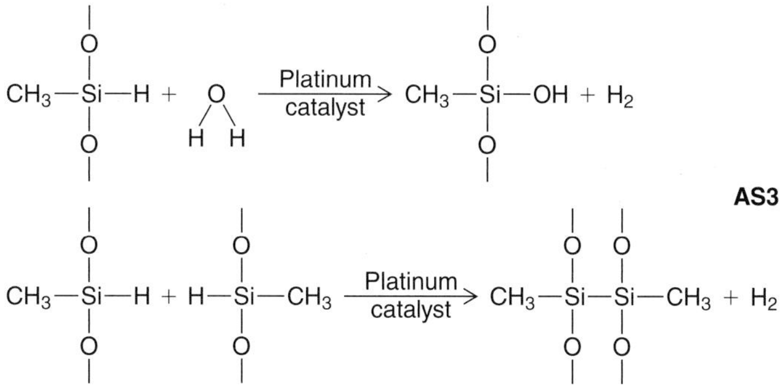

AS3

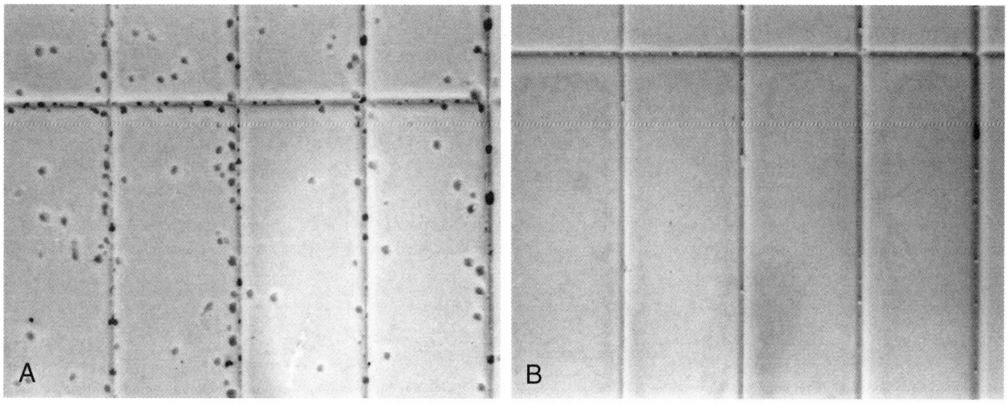

• **Fig. 11.12** Addition-silicone impressions poured into high-strength stone at 15 minutes. (A) Bubbles are caused by the release of hydrogen. (B) No bubbles are apparent because palladium hydrogen absorber is included in the impression material.

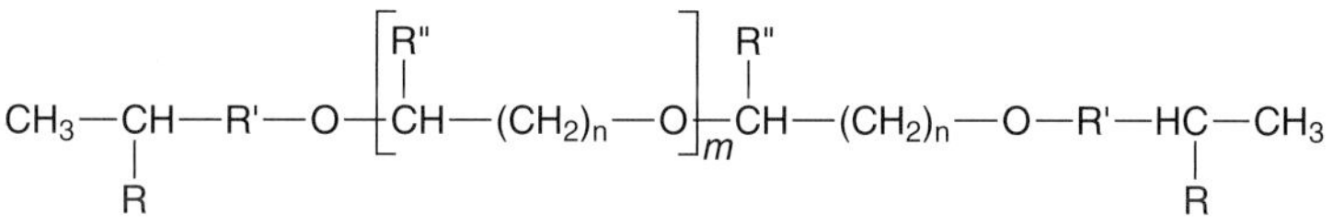

PE1

washing of the gloves with detergent and water just before mixing may minimize this effect, and some brands of gloves interfere with the setting more than others. Vinyl and nitrile gloves do not have such an effect. Residual monomer in acrylic provisional restorations and resin composite cores has a similar inhibiting effect on the setting of addition-silicone materials. The preparation and adjacent soft tissues can also be cleaned with 2% chlorhexidine to remove contaminants.

Polyether

Polyethers are supplied in low-, medium-, and heavy-body consistency. The base paste consists of a long-chain polyether copolymer with alternating oxygen atoms and methylene groups (O–[CH_2]n) and reactive terminal groups (see polyether 1 [PE1]). Also incorporated are a silica filler, compatible plasticizers of a non-phthalate type, and triglycerides. In the catalyst paste, an aliphatic cationic starter serves as a cross-linking agent. The catalyst also includes silica filler and plasticizers. Coloring agents are added to base and catalyst to aid in the recognition of different material types. Examples of polyether impression materials are shown in Fig. 11.9.

The reaction mechanism is shown (PE2) in a simplified form. The elastomer is formed by cationic polymerization by opening of the reactive terminal rings. The backbone of the polymer is believed to be a copolymer of ethylene oxide and tetramethylene oxide units. The reactive terminal rings open under the influence of the cationic initiator of the catalyst paste and can then, as a cation itself, attack and open additional rings. Whenever a ring is

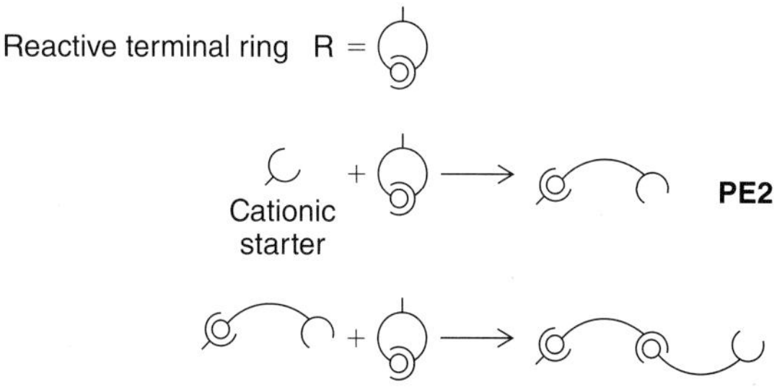

PE2

PE3

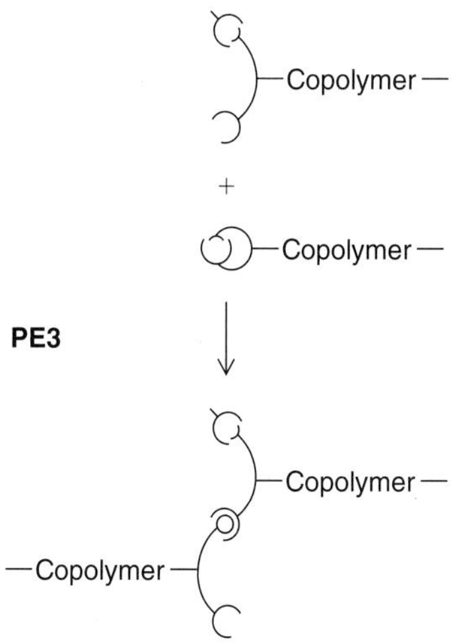

TABLE 11.3 **Setting Properties of Elastomeric Impression Materials**

Material	Consistency	Temperature Rise (°C)	Viscosity 45 s after Mixing (cp)	Working Time (min)	Setting Time (min)	Dimensional Change at 24 h (%)
Polysulfides						
	Low	3.4	60,000	4–7	7–10	−0.40
	Medium		110,000	3–6	6–8	−0.45
	High		450,000	3–6	6–8	−0.44
Silicones						
Condensation	Low	1.1	70,000	2.5–4	6–8	−0.60
	Very high			2–2.5	3–6	−0.38
Addition	Low			2–4	4–6.5	−0.15
	Medium		150,000	2–4	4–6.5	−0.17
	High			2.5–4	4–6.5	−0.15
	Very high			1–4	3–5	−0.14
Polyethers						
	Low	4.2		3	6	−0.23
	Medium		130,000	2.5–3	6	−0.24
	High			2.5	5.5	−0.19

opened, the cation function remains attached, thus lengthening the chain (see PE3). Because of the identical chemical base, all polyether consistencies can be freely combined with each other. A chemical bond between all materials develops during curing.

Setting Properties

Typical values of the setting properties of elastomeric impression materials are presented in Table 11.3. The temperature rise in typical mixes of impression materials was pointed out in the previous section, but Table 11.3 illustrates that the temperature rise is small and of no clinical concern.

Viscosity

The viscosity of materials 45 seconds after mixing is listed in Table 11.3. As expected, the viscosity increases for the same type of material from low to high consistencies. Viscosity is a function of time after the start of mixing.

A shearing force can affect the viscosity of polyether and addition-silicone impression materials, as was mentioned in the section on impression techniques. This effect is called *shear thinning* or *pseudoplasticity.* For impression materials possessing this characteristic, the viscosity of the unset material diminishes with an increasing outside force or shearing speed. When the influence is discontinued, the viscosity immediately increases. This property is very important for the use of monophase impression materials and is illustrated for polyether in Fig. 11.13. In the case of polyether, shear-thinning properties are influenced by a weak network of triglyceride crystals. The crystals align when the impression material is sheared, as occurs when mixed or flowing through a syringe tip. The microcrystalline triglyceride network ensures that the polyether remains viscous in the tray or on the tooth but flows under pressure. This allows a single or monophase material to be used as a low- and medium-consistency material. Cooling of the pastes results in substantial viscosity increase. Before using, pastes have to be brought to room temperature.

The effect of shear rate (rotational speed of the viscometer) on the viscosity of single-consistency (monophase) addition silicones is shown in Fig. 11.14. Although all products showed a decrease in viscosity with increasing shear rate, the effect was much more pronounced for two products, Ba and Hy, with about an eight- to eleven-fold decrease from the lowest to the highest shear rate. The substantial decrease in viscosity at high shear stress, which is comparable with the decrease during syringing, permits the use of a single mix of material, with a portion to be used as syringe material and another portion to be used as tray material in the syringe-tray technique.

Working and Setting Times

The working and setting times of addition-silicone and polyether impression materials are listed in Table 11.3. In general, for a given class of elastomeric impression materials by a specific manufacturer, the working and setting times decrease as the viscosity increases from low to high. Polyethers show a clearly defined working time with a sharp transition into the setting phase. This behavior is often called *snap-set.* This transition from plastic condition into elastic properties is rather short compared with older addition silicones, which was shown in investigations of rheological properties of setting materials (Fig. 11.15).

Note that the working and setting times of the elastomeric impression materials are shortened by increases in temperature and humidity; on hot, humid days this effect should be considered in the clinical application of these materials. Similarly, if longer working times are desired, such as in cases where multiple tooth preparations need to be captured in the impression, previous refrigeration of the impression material can be considered.

The initial (or working) and final setting times can be determined fairly accurately by using a penetrometer with a needle and weight selected to suit these materials. The Vicat penetrometer, as shown in Fig. 11.16, with a 3-mm-diameter needle and a total weight of 300 g, has been used by a number of investigators. A

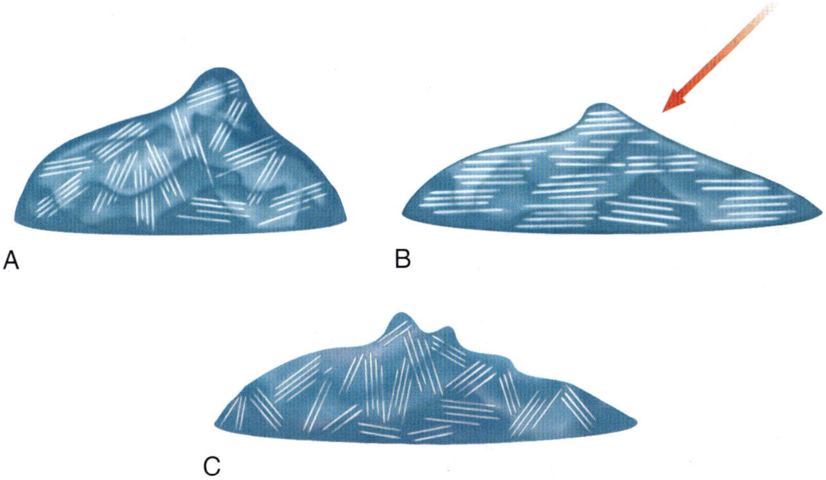

• **Fig. 11.13** Demonstration of the mechanism for the property of shear thinning or pseudoplasticity in polyethers. The triglyceride network (A) within the impression material aligns when sheared as with syringing, and (B) to achieve a lower viscosity. Once the shear force is removed, the viscosity increases with randomization of the triglyceride network (C).

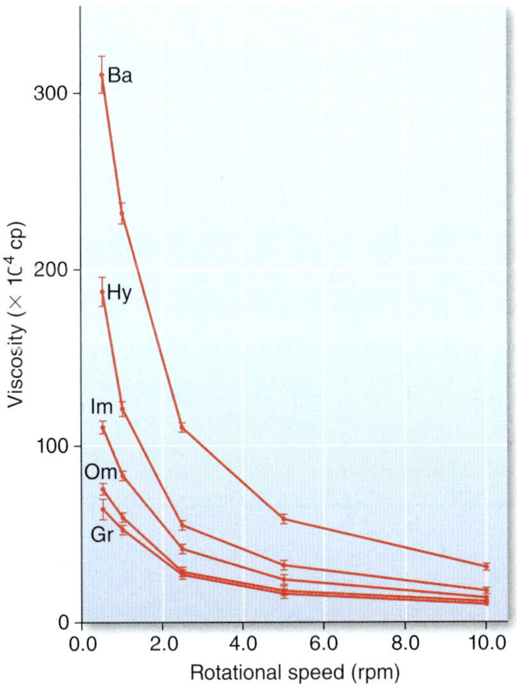

• **Fig. 11.14** Viscosity in centipoise as a function of shear rate (rotational speed of the viscometer) for five single-consistency addition-silicone impression materials. A rotational speed of 0.5 rpm would represent a shear rate comparable with that observed when placing the material in a tray, and a speed of 10 rpm would represent a shear rate comparable with that experienced when syringing the material. (Data from Kim KN, Craig RG, Koran A 3rd. Viscosity of monophase addition silicones as a function of shear rate. *J Prosthet Dent*. 1992;67(6):794–798).

metal ring, 8 mm high and 16 mm in diameter is filled with freshly mixed material and placed on the penetrometer base. The needle is applied to the surface of the impression material for 10 seconds, and a reading is taken. This is repeated every 30 seconds. The initial set is that time at which the needle no longer completely penetrates the specimen to the bottom of the ring. The final set is the time of the first of three identical non-maximum penetration

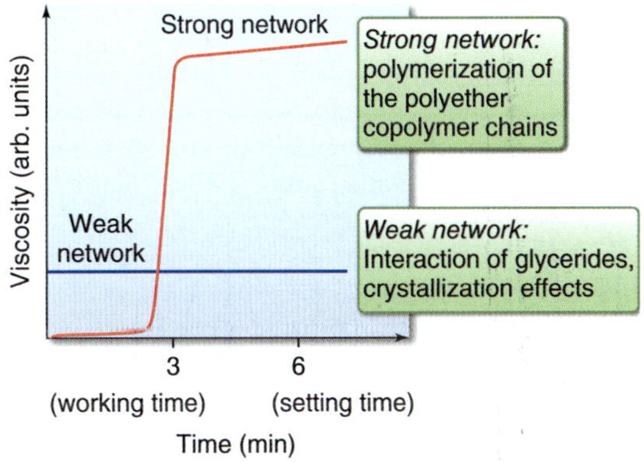

• **Fig. 11.15** Illustration of the snap-set of polyether. The initial viscosity of the unset material is influenced by the structural triglycerides, whereas the polymerization of copolymer chains thereafter provides a quick increase in viscosity as the material sets.

readings. When the material is set, the elasticity still allows penetration of the needle, but it is the same at each application.

Dimensional Change on Setting

The impression material undergoes a dimensional change in setting. The major factor for contraction during setting is cross-linking and rearrangement of bonds within and between polymer chains. Impressions can expand if water sorption takes place and an impression can be distorted if seated after the material has set to any degree. Finally, distortion or creep will occur if the material does not recover elastically when the set impression is removed from undercuts. Imbibition is discussed in the section on disinfecting impressions, and creep-induced distortion is discussed under elastic recovery.

Addition-silicone and polyether impression materials undergo shrinkage due to polymerization. The linear dimensional change between a die and the impression after 24 hours is listed in Table 11.3. The addition silicones have the smallest change of about –0.15%, followed by the polyethers at about –0.2%. The contraction is low for these two products because there is no loss of by-products.

The rate of shrinkage of elastomeric impression materials is not uniform during the 24 hours after removal from the mouth. In

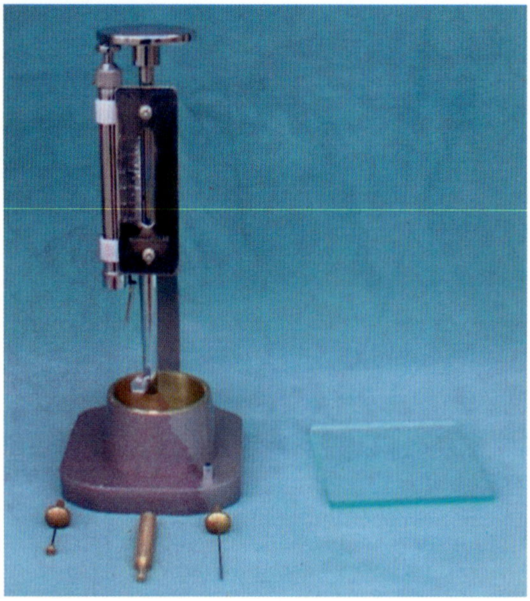

• **Fig. 11.16** Vicat penetrometer used to determine setting time of impression materials and other restorative materials.

general, about half the shrinkage observed at 24 hours occurs during the first hour after removal; therefore for greatest accuracy, the casts and dies should be prepared promptly, although in air the elastomeric impression materials are much more stable than hydrocolloid products.

Mechanical Properties

Typical mechanical properties of elastomeric impression materials are listed in Table 11.4. The permanent deformation (in the current specification, elastic recovery, which is 100% minus the permanent deformation), strain in compression, and dimensional change are properties used in ANSI/ADA specification No. 19 (ISO 4823) to classify elastomeric impression materials as low, medium, high, or very high viscosity types. The requirements for these properties are given in Table 11.5. Further requirements of the specification for elastomeric impression materials are indicated in Table 11.6. The consistency diameter is used to classify viscosity by measuring the diameter of the disk formed when 0.5 mL of mixed material is subjected to a 5.6-N weight at 1.5 minutes after mixing for 12 minutes. Because the setting times of elastomeric impression materials vary, the consistency diameter is affected not only by the viscosity but also by the setting time. The classification of a material by the consistency diameter may be different from that by a true viscosity measurement.

Elastic Recovery

The order in which the permanent deformation of the elastomeric impression materials is listed in Table 11.4 demonstrates that addition silicones have the best elastic recovery during removal from the mouth, followed by polyethers. A material with a permanent deformation of 1% has an elastic recovery of 99%.

Strain in Compression

The strain in compression under a stress of 0.1 MPa is a measure of the flexibility of the material. Table 11.4 illustrates that, in general, the low-consistency materials of each type are more flexible than the high-consistency elastomeric impressions. For a given consistency, polyethers are generally the stiffest, followed by addition silicones.

Flow

Flow is measured on a cylindrical specimen 1 hour old, and the percent flow is determined 15 minutes after a load of 1 N is

TABLE 11.4 Mechanical Properties of Elastomeric Impression Materials

Material	Consistency	Permanent Deformation[a] (%)	Strain in Compression (%)	Flow (%)	Shore A Hardness	Tear Strength (kN/m)
Polysulfides						
	Low	3–4	14–17	0.5–2	20	2.5–7.0
	Medium	3–5	11–15	0.5–1	30	3.0–7.0
	High	3–6	9–12	0.5–1	35	—
Silicones						
Condensation	Low	1–2	4–9	0.05–0.1	15–30	2.3–2.6
	Very high	2–3	2–5	0.02–0.05	50–65	—
Addition	Low	0.05–0.4	3–6	0.01–0.03	35–55	1.5–3.0
	Medium	0.05–0.3	2–5	0.01–0.03	50–60	2.2–3.5
	High	0.1–0.3	2–3	0.01–0.03	60–70	2.5–4.3
	Very high	0.2–0.5	1–2	0.01–0.1	50–75	—
Polyethers						
	Low	1.5	3	0.03	35–40	1.8
	Medium	1–2	2–3	0.02	40–60	2.8–4.8
	High	2	3	0.02	40–50	3.0

[a]Elastic recovery from deformation is 100% minus the percent permanent deformation.

TABLE 11.5 Elastic Recovery, Strain in Compression, and Dimensional Change Requirements for Elastomeric Impression Materials

		STRAIN IN COMPRESSION (%)		
Viscosity Type	Minimum Elastic Recovery (%)	Minimum	Maximum	Maximum Dimensional Change in 24 h (%)
Low	96.5	2.0	20	1.5
Medium	96.5	2.0	20	1.5
High	96.5	0.8	20	1.5
Very high	96.5	0.8	20	1.5

TABLE 11.6 Requirements by ANSI/ADA Specification No. 19 (ISO 4823) for the Various Viscosities of Elastomeric Impression Materials

			DIAMETER OF CONSISTENCY DISK (mm)		REPRODUCTION OF DETAIL	
Viscosity	Maximum Mixing Time (min)	Minimum Working Time (min)	Minimum	Maximum	Line Width in Impression (mm)	Line Width in Gypsum (mm)
Low	1	2	36	—	0.020	0.020
Medium	1	2	31	41	0.020	0.020
High	1	2	—	35	0.050	0.050
Very High	1	2	—	35	0.075	0.075

ADA, American Dental Association; *ANSI*, American National Standards Institute; *ISO*, International Organization for Standardization.

applied. As seen in Table 11.4, silicones and polyethers have low values of flow.

Typical elastomeric impression materials easily meet the mechanical property requirements of ANSI/ADA specification No. 19 (see Table 11.6). Although the flow, hardness, and tear strengths of elastomeric impression materials are not mentioned in the specification, these are also important properties and are listed in Table 11.4.

Hardness

The Shore A hardness increases from low to high consistency. When two numbers are given, the first represents the hardness 1.5 minutes after removal from the mouth, and the second represents the hardness after 2 hours. The low-, medium-, and high-viscosity addition silicones do not change hardness significantly with time, whereas the hardness of polyethers does increase with time. In addition, the hardness and strain in compression affect the force necessary to remove the impression from the mouth. Clinically, low flexibility and high hardness can be compensated for by providing more space for the impression material between the tray and the teeth. This can be accomplished with the addition of block-out material for custom trays or by selecting a larger tray when using stock trays.

A new variation in polyether provides less resistance to deformation during removal of the impression from the mouth and the gypsum cast from the impression. To achieve this, the filler content was reduced from 14 to 6 parts per unit, thereby reducing the Shore A hardness from 46 to 40 after 15 minutes, and from 61 to 50 after 24 hours. The ratio of high-viscous softener to low-viscous softener was changed to achieve a consistency similar to that of the conventional monophase polyether.

Tear Strength

Tear strength is important because it indicates the ability of a material to withstand tearing in thin interproximal areas and margins of periodontally involved teeth. The tear strengths listed in Table 11.4 are a measure of the force needed to initiate and continue tearing a specimen of unit thickness. As the consistency of the impression type increases, tear strength undergoes a small increase, but most of the values are between 2.0 and 3.9 kN/m. Values for very high consistency types are not listed because this property is not important for these materials. Higher tear strengths for elastomeric impression materials are desirable, and compared with the values for hydrocolloid impression materials of 0.3 to 0.7 kN/m, they demonstrate a major improvement.

Creep Compliance

Elastomeric impression materials are viscoelastic, and their mechanical properties are time dependent. For example, the higher the rate of deformation, the higher the tear strength; and the longer the impressions are deformed, the higher the permanent deformation. As a result, plots of creep compliance versus time describe the properties of these materials better than stress-strain curves. Creep-compliance time curves for low-consistency polysulfide, condensation silicone, addition silicone, and medium-consistency polyether are shown in Fig. 11.17. The initial creep compliance illustrates polysulfide is the most flexible and polyether is the least flexible. The flatness or parallelism of the curves with respect to the time axis indicates low permanent deformation and excellent recovery from deformation during the removal of an impression; addition silicones and polyethers have the best elastic recovery.

The recoverable viscoelastic quality of the materials is indicated by differences between the initial creep compliance and the creep

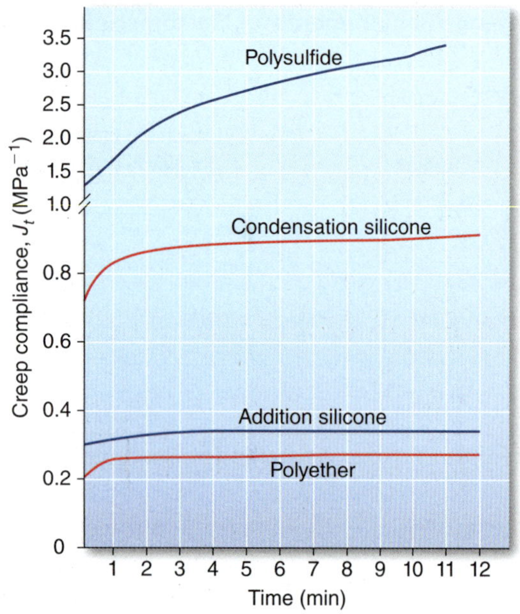

• **Fig. 11.17** Creep compliance of elastomeric impression materials at the time recommended for removal from the mouth. (Data from Tolley LG, Craig RG. Viscoelastic properties of elastomeric impression materials: polysulphide, silicone and polyether rubbers. *J Oral Rehabil*. 1978;5:121–128).

compliance value obtained by extrapolation of the linear portion of the curve to zero time. As a result, addition silicones have the lowest viscoelastic quality and require less time to recover viscoelastic deformation, followed by polyethers.

Detail Reproduction

The requirements of elastomeric impression materials are listed in Table 11.6. Except for the very high-viscosity products, all should reproduce a V-shaped groove and a 0.02-mm wide line in the elastomeric. The impression should be compatible with gypsum products so the 0.02-mm line is transferred to gypsum die materials. Low-, medium-, and high-viscosity elastomeric impression materials have little difficulty meeting this requirement.

Wettability of Elastomeric Impression Materials

Wettability may be assessed by measuring the advancing contact angle of water on the surface of the set impression material or by using a tensiometer to measure forces as the material is immersed and removed (Wilhelmy technique). The advancing contact angles for elastomeric impression materials are listed in Table 11.7. Of all the impression materials discussed in this chapter, only alginates can be considered truly hydrophilic. All of the elastomeric impression materials possess advancing and receding contact angles greater than 45 degrees. There are, however, differences in wetting among and within types of elastomeric impression materials. Traditional addition silicone is not as wettable as polyether. When mixes of gypsum products are poured into hydrophobic addition silicone, high contact angles are formed, making the preparation of bubble-free casts difficult.

Surfactants have been added to addition silicones by manufacturers to reduce the contact angle, improve wettability, and simplify the pouring of gypsum casts. This class with improved wetting characteristics is most accurately called *hydrophilized addition silicone*. Most commonly, nonionic surfactants have gained importance in this area. These molecules consist of an oligoether

TABLE 11.7 Wettability of Elastomeric Impression Materials

Material	Advancing Contact Angle of Water (degrees)	Castability of High-Strength Dental Stone (%)
Polysulfide	82	44
Condensation silicone	98	30
Addition silicone		
Hydrophobic	98	30
Hydrophilic	53	72
Polyether	49	70

or polyether substructure as the hydrophilic part and a silicone-compatible hydrophobic part (Fig. 11.18A). The mode of action of these wetting agents is believed to be a diffusion-controlled transfer of surfactant molecules from the polyvinylsiloxane into the aqueous phase, as shown, thereby altering the surface tension of the surrounding liquid. As a result, a reduction in surface tension and therefore greater wettability of the polyvinylsiloxane is observed (Fig. 11.18B). This mechanism differs from polyethers, which possess a high degree of wettability because their molecular structure contains polar oxygen atoms, which have an affinity for water. Because of this affinity, polyether materials flow onto hydrated intraoral surfaces and are therefore cast with gypsum more easily than are addition silicones. This affinity also allows polyether impressions to adhere quite strongly to soft and hard tissues.

By observing water droplets on impression surfaces, it has been shown that hydrophilized addition silicones and polyethers are wetted the best, and condensation silicones and conventional addition silicones the least. Wettability was directly correlated to the ease of pouring high-strength stone casts of an extremely critical die, as shown in Table 11.7. Using a tensiometer to record forces of immersed impression specimens, polyether was shown to wet significantly better than hydrophilized addition silicones for both advancing (74 degrees vs. 108 degrees) and receding contact angles (50 degrees vs. 81 degrees).

To evaluate the ability of impression materials to reproduce detail under wet and dry surface conditions, impressions were made of a standard wave pattern used to calibrate surface analyzers. The surfaces of impressions were scanned for average roughness (Ra) after setting to determine their ability to reproduce the detail of the standard, the value of which is shown with a *double line* in Fig. 11.19. From a clinical standpoint, most impression materials produced acceptable detail under wet and dry conditions. Polyethers produced slightly better detail than did addition silicones and were generally unaffected by the presence of moisture, whereas detail decreased for some addition silicones under wet conditions, even if hydrophilized.

Disinfection of Elastomeric Impressions

All impressions should be disinfected upon removal from the mouth to prevent contamination of gypsum casts and laboratory personnel. Several studies confirm that addition-silicone and polyether impressions can be disinfected by immersion in several different disinfectants for up to 18 hours without a loss of surface quality and accuracy.

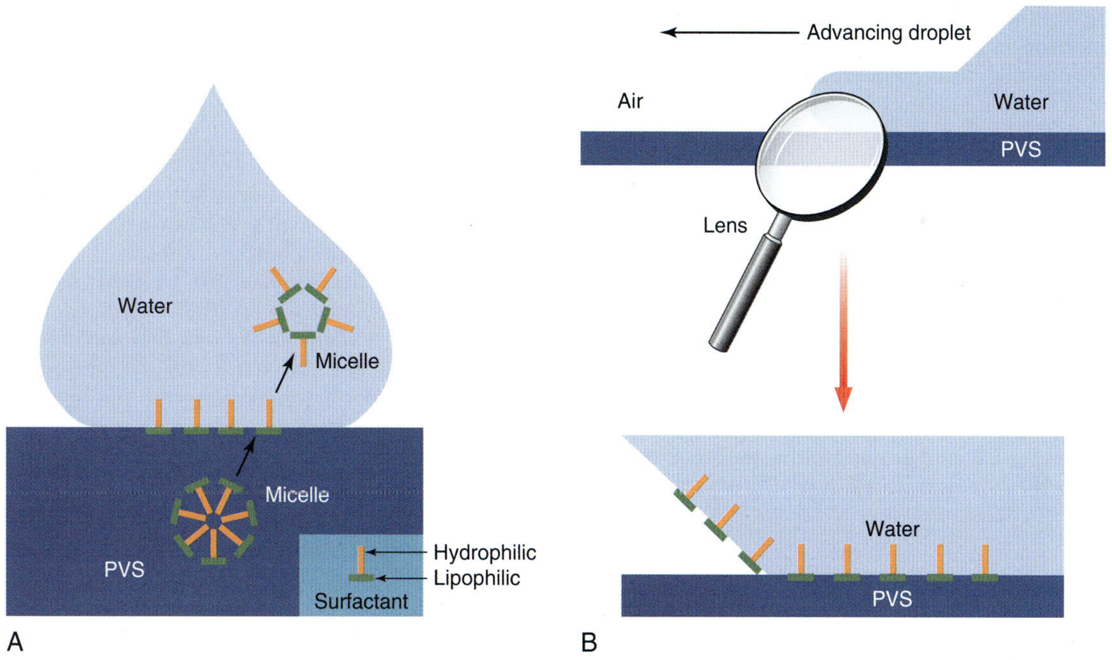

• **Fig. 11.18** Hydrophilization of addition silicones. (A) The hydrophilization of addition silicones is gained with the incorporation of nonionic surfactants shown as micelles. These molecules consist of a hydrophilic part and a silicone-compatible hydrophobic part. The mode of action of these surfactants is thought to be a diffusion-controlled transfer of surfactant molecules from the polyvinylsiloxane into the aqueous phase, as shown. In this manner, the surface tension of the surrounding liquid is altered. (B) This increased wettability allows the addition silicone to spread more freely along the surface. *PVS*, Polyvinylsiloxane.

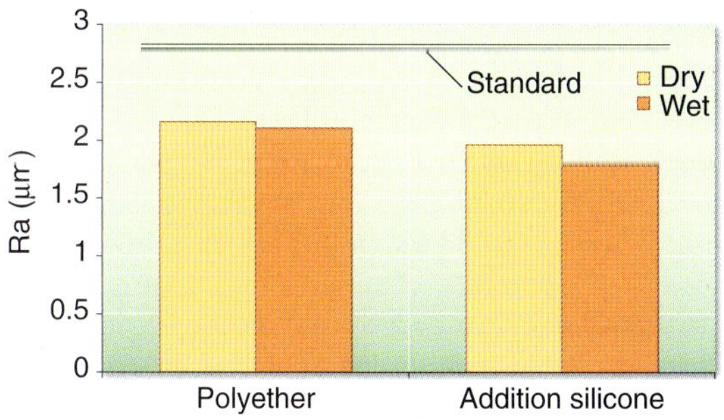

• **Fig. 11.19** Ability of polyether and hydrophilized addition-silicone materials to reproduce detail under dry and wet conditions. The average roughness, Ra, of the standard from which impressions were made is shown *(double line).* Polyethers produced the best detail and were unaffected by moisture. The detail captured by addition silicones decreased slightly in the presence of moisture. (Data from Johnson GH, Lepe X, Berg JC. Effect of moisture on the quality of crown and bridge impressions. *J Dent Res.* 1998;77(Spec Issue B);798).

Relationship of Properties and Clinical Application

Accuracy, the ability to record detail, ease of handling, and setting characteristics are of prime importance in dental impressions. Silicones generally have shorter working times than polysulfides but somewhat longer times than polyethers. Single-mix materials have some advantages because, due to shear thinning, they have low viscosities when mixed or syringed but higher viscosities when inserted in a tray. The time of placement of an elastomeric impression material is critical because viscosity increases rapidly with time as a result of the polymerization reaction. If the material is placed in the mouth after the consistency or viscosity has increased via polymerization, internal stresses induced in the impression are released after the impression is removed from the mouth, resulting in an inaccurate impression.

Thorough mixing is essential; otherwise portions of the mix could contain insufficient accelerator to polymerize thoroughly or may not set at the same rate as other portions of the impression. In this event, removal of the impression would cause less elastic recovery and result in an inaccurate impression. Automixing and mechanical mixing systems save time in mixing and result in a more bubble-free impression.

Polymerization of elastomeric impression materials continues after the material has set, and the mechanical properties improve with time. Premature removal may result in high permanent deformation; however, excessively long times in the mouth are unacceptable to the patient. The manufacturer usually recommends a minimum time for leaving the impression in the mouth, and this minimum is used for testing the materials according to ANSI/ADA specification No. 19.

Dimensional changes in setting can be compensated for by use of a double-impression or putty-wash technique, as described earlier. The double-impression technique is suitable for use with a stock impression tray because the preliminary impression serves as a custom tray. With the monophase and simultaneous dual-viscosity technique, a slight improvement in accuracy results when a custom-made tray is used because it provides a uniform thickness of impression material. Several studies have shown, however, that relatively stiff stock plastic or metal trays yield nearly the same accuracy.

Clinical studies have shown that the viscosity of the impression material is the most important factor in producing impressions and dies with minimal bubbles and maximum detail. As a result, the syringe-tray technique produced superior clinical results in the reproduction of fine internal detail of proximal boxes or grooves.

The accuracy of the impression may be affected when the percentage of deformation and the time involved in removing the impression are increased. In both instances, permanent deformation increases, the amount depending on the type of elastomeric impression material.

Because elastomeric impressions recover from deformation for a period after their removal, some increase in accuracy can be expected during this time. However, polymerization shrinkage is also occurring, and the overall accuracy is determined by a combination of these two effects. Insignificant elastic recovery occurs after 20 to 30 minutes; therefore dies should be prepared promptly after that time for greatest accuracy. Addition silicones that release hydrogen are an exception to this guideline.

Second pours of gypsum products into addition-silicone impressions produce dies that are not quite as accurate as the first because the impression can be deformed during the removal of the first die; however, they are usually sufficiently accurate to be used as a working die.

Occlusal Registration Materials

The majority of currently available occlusal registration products are addition silicones or polyethers, and most are supplied in automix cartridges. Their properties are listed in Table 11.8. These materials are characterized by short working times and the length of time left in the mouth compared with typical elastomeric impression materials. They are also noted for their high stiffness, indicated by the low percent strain in compression, and for their low flow and dimensional change even after 7 days. The property that distinguishes addition silicones from polyethers is their lower dimensional change after removal; however, either is superior to the stability of waxes for making occlusal records.

Impression Trays

Impression materials can be carried using either prefabricated (stock) or custom impression trays. Both types of trays require the use of a tray adhesive, which must be allowed to dry before placing the impression material in the tray.

Stock trays vary considerably between manufacturers. When a stock tray is chosen, care must be taken to ensure that the tray is well adapted to the tissues and is adequately reinforced to prevent flexing during impression fabrication and removal. Stock trays can be either metal or plastic; metal trays are indicated for use with alginate, whereas plastic trays are more suitable for elastomeric materials.

Custom impression trays provide uniform clearance between the tray and the tissues, allowing a more even distribution of the impression material during the impression procedure, and improved accuracy. Custom trays are indicated when the impression needs to capture more than one tooth preparation, or when a stock tray is not compatible with the patient's arch form or size. Light-activated and vacuum-formed polymers are used more frequently than chemically accelerated acrylic to produce custom impression trays because of the volatility of the acrylic monomer and sensitivity to the monomer reported by dental staff. Vacuum-formed polystyrene is popular with commercial laboratories for its ease of fabrication. These trays must be handled carefully because they are more flexible than acrylic trays and can be deformed easily by the application of heat.

Light-activated tray materials have many advantages over chemically accelerated acrylic. They are similar to light-activated denture base materials but are of a different color. The trays are strong, easy to make, contain no methyl methacrylate, and have negligible polymerization shrinkage in the light chamber. They can be used soon after processing because there is no clinically significant dimensional change after polymerization.

Cast or Die Materials

Dental stones, plaster, epoxy resin, and refractory materials are some of the materials used to make casts or dies from dental impressions. The selection of one of these is determined by the particular impression material in use and by the purpose for which the die or cast is to be used.

Impressions in alginate hydrocolloids can be used only with a gypsum material, such as plaster, stone, or casting investment. Various elastomeric impression materials can be used to prepare gypsum or epoxy dies. Impression materials can also be digitally scanned to produce printed plastic casts or dies (see Chapter 13).

Desirable Qualities of a Cast or Die Material

Cast and die materials must reproduce an impression accurately and remain dimensionally stable under normal conditions of use and storage. Setting expansion, contraction, and dimensional variations in response to changes in temperature must be held to a minimum. Not only should the cast be accurate, but it should also satisfactorily reproduce fine detail and have a smooth, hard surface. Such an accurate cast or die must also be strong and durable and withstand the subsequent manipulative procedures without fracture or abrasion of the surface. Qualities of strength, resistance to shearing forces or edge strength, and abrasion resistance are therefore important and are required in varying degrees, according to the purpose for which the cast or die is to be used. For example, since a study cast will not be subjected to much stress in use, it might be formed from stone or plaster in which the aforementioned qualities are at a minimum. However, an elastomeric impression used to produce an indirect inlay could be poured in high-strength stone or epoxy, thereby producing a die in which these qualities are sufficient to withstand the carving and finishing procedures that are a part of this technique.

TABLE 11.8 Properties of Elastomeric Impression Materials Used for Occlusal Registrations

					DIMENSIONAL CHANGE		
Material	Mixing Type	Working Time (min)	Time in Mouth (min)	Strain in Compression (%)	Flow (%)	1 Day (%)	7 Days (%)
Addition silicone	Automix	0.5–3.0	1.0–3.0	1.0–2.9	0.0–0.01	0.0 to −0.15	−0.04 to −0.20
Addition silicone	Hand mix	1.4	2.5	0.92	0.0	−0.06	−0.08
Polyether	Hand mix	2.1	3.0	1.97	0.0	−0.29	−0.32

The color of a cast or die can facilitate manipulative procedures, such as waxing inlay patterns, by presenting a contrast in color to the inlay wax. The ease with which the material can be adapted to the impression and the time required before the cast or die is ready for use are of considerable practical significance.

Gypsum Products

Gypsum products include dental plaster, stone, high-strength/high-expansion stone, and casting investments, and are used for several different purposes. For example, impression plaster is used to make impressions of edentulous mouths or to mount casts, whereas dental stone is used to form a die that duplicates the oral anatomy when poured into any type of impression. Gypsum products are also used as a binder for silica in gold alloy casting investments, soldering investments, and investment for low-melting-point nickel–chromium alloys. High-strength dental stones make excellent casts or dies, readily reproduce the fine detail of a final impression, are dimensionally stable over long periods, and can withstand most of the manipulative procedures involved in the production of appliances and restorations.

The main reason for such diversified use is that the properties of gypsum materials can be easily modified by physical and chemical means.

The dihydrate form of calcium sulfate, called *gypsum*, usually appears white to milky yellowish and is found in a compact mass in nature. The mineral gypsum has commercial importance as a source of plaster of Paris. The term *plaster of Paris* was given to this product because it was obtained by burning the gypsum from deposits near Paris, France. Deposits of gypsum, however, are found in most countries.

Chemical and Physical Nature of Gypsum Products

Most gypsum products are obtained from natural gypsum rock. Because gypsum is the dihydrate form of calcium sulfate ($CaSO_4 \cdot 2H_2O$), on heating, it loses three-fourths of its H_2O and is converted to calcium sulfate hemihydrate ($CaSO_4 \cdot \frac{1}{2}H_2O$), sometimes written $(CaSO_4)_2 \cdot H_2O$. When calcium sulfate hemihydrate is mixed with water, the reverse reaction takes place, and the calcium sulfate hemihydrate is converted back to calcium sulfate dihydrate. Therefore partial dehydration of gypsum rock and rehydration of calcium sulfate hemihydrate constitute a reversible reaction. Chemically, the exothermic reaction is expressed as follows:

$$\underset{\text{Plaster of Paris}}{CaSO_4 \cdot \tfrac{1}{2}H_2O} + \underset{\text{Water}}{1\tfrac{1}{2}H_2O} \rightarrow \underset{\text{Gypsum}}{CaSO_4 \cdot 2H_2O} + 3900\,\text{cal/g mol}$$

This chemical reaction takes place regardless of whether the gypsum material is used as an impression material, a die material, or a binder in casting investment.

Manufacture of Dental Plaster, Stone, and High-Strength Stone

Three types of base raw materials are derived from partial dehydration of gypsum rock, depending on the nature of the dehydration process. *Plasters* are fluffy, porous, and least dense, whereas the *hydrocal* variety has a higher density and is more crystalline. *Densite* is the densest of the raw materials. These three types of raw materials are used to formulate the four types of relatively pure gypsum products used in dentistry. They are classified as plasters (model and laboratory), low- to moderate-strength dental stones, high-strength/low-expansion dental stones, and high-strength/high-expansion dental stones, or alternatively as types 2, 3, 4, and 5 in ANSI/ADA specification No. 25 (ISO 6873).

Although these types have identical chemical formulas of calcium sulfate hemihydrate, $CaSO_4 \cdot \frac{1}{2}H_2O$, they possess different physical properties, which makes each of them suitable for a different dental purpose. All four forms are derived from natural gypsum deposits, with the main difference being the manner of driving off part of the water of the calcium sulfate dihydrate. Synthetic gypsum can also be used to formulate some products but is less popular because of higher manufacturing costs.

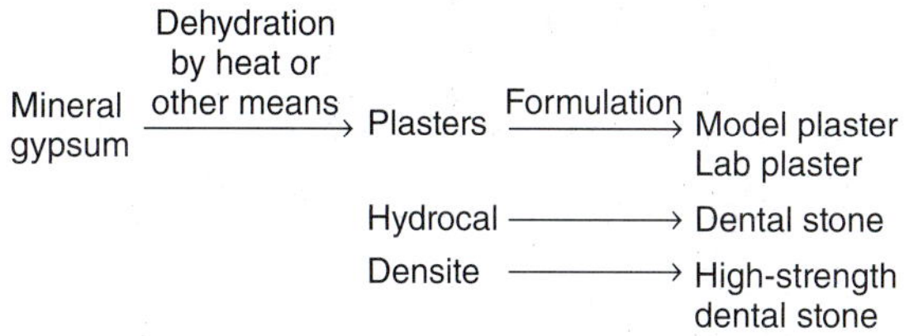

Plasters are produced when the gypsum mineral is heated in an open kettle at a temperature of about 110°C to 120°C. The hemihydrate produced is called *β-calcium sulfate hemihydrate.* Such a powder is known to have a somewhat irregular shape and is porous in nature. These plasters are used in formulating models and lab plasters. Crystals of model plaster are shown in Fig. 11.20.

If gypsum is dehydrated under pressure and in the presence of water vapor at about 125°C, the product is called *hydrocal.* The powder particles of this product are more uniform in shape and denser than the particles of plaster. Crystals of a dental stone are shown in Fig. 11.21. The calcium sulfate hemihydrate produced in

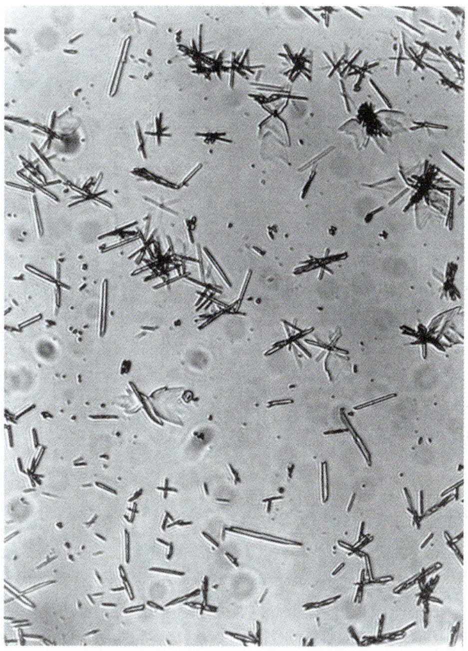

• **Fig. 11.20** Crystals of model plaster.

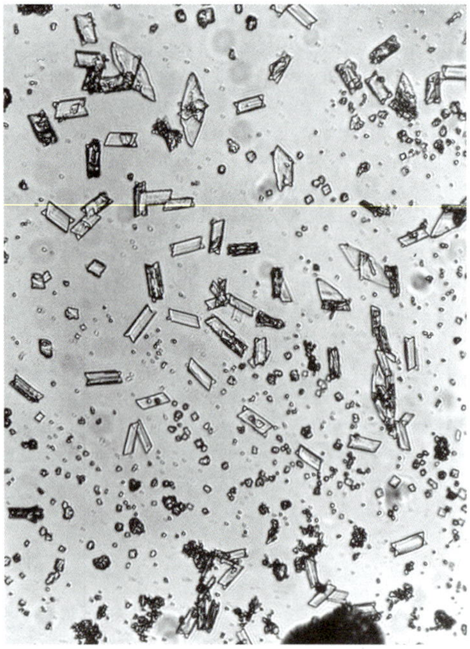

• **Fig. 11.21** Crystal structure typical of dental stone.

this manner is designated as α-*calcium sulfate hemihydrate*. Hydrocal is used in making low- to moderate-strength dental stones.

Types 4 and 5 high-strength dental stones are manufactured with a high-density raw material called *densite*. This variety is made by boiling gypsum rock in a 30% calcium chloride solution, after which the chloride is washed away with hot water (100°C) and the material is ground to the desired fineness. The powder obtained by this process is the densest of the types. These materials are generally formulated as high-strength/low-expansion dental stones or high-strength/high-expansion dental stones.

Gypsum products may be formulated with chemicals that modify their handling characteristics and properties. Potassium sulfate, K_2SO_4, and terra alba (set calcium sulfate dihydrate) are effective accelerators. Sodium chloride in small amounts shortens the setting reaction but increases the setting expansion of the gypsum mass. Sodium citrate and Borax, $Na_2B_4O_7$, are dependable retarders. A mixture of calcium oxide (0.1%) and gum arabic (1%) reduces the amount of water necessary to mix gypsum products, resulting in improved properties. Type 4 gypsum differs from type 5 in that type 4 contains extra salts to reduce its setting expansion.

Chemical Reaction

The chemical reaction that takes place during the setting of gypsum products determines the quantity of H_2O needed for the reaction. For example, 100 g of plaster requires 18.6 g of water to form 118 g of calcium sulfate dihydrate. As seen in practice, however, model plaster cannot be mixed with such a small amount of water and still develop a mass suitable for manipulation. Table 11.9 shows the recommended mixing water, required water, and excess water for model plaster, dental stone, and high-strength dental stone.

For example, to mix 100 g of model plaster to a usable flowable consistency, use 45 g of water. Note that only 18.6 g of 45 g of water reacts with the 100 g of model plaster; the excess (45 g −18.6 g = 26.4 g) is distributed as free water in the set mass without taking part in the chemical reaction. When the set material is dried, the excess water evaporates and leaves porosity in the structure, weakening it. Therefore set model plaster is weaker than dental stone, which in turn is weaker than high-strength dental stone. If 100 g of model plaster is mixed with 50 g of water, the resultant mass is thinner and mixes and pours easily into a mold, but the quality of the set gypsum is inferior and weaker than when 45 g of water is used. When model plaster is mixed with a lesser amount of water, the mixed mass is thicker, is more difficult to handle, and traps air bubbles easily when it is poured into a mold, but the set gypsum is usually stronger. Thus careful control of the proper amount of water in the mix is necessary for proper manipulation and quality of the set mass.

Water-to-Powder Ratio of Dental Stone and High-Strength Dental Stone

The reason for the differences among the recommended amounts of mixing water for model plaster, dental stone, and high-strength dental stone is in the shape and form of the calcium sulfate hemihydrate crystals. Some calcium sulfate hemihydrate crystals are comparatively irregular in shape and porous in nature, as are the crystals in model plaster, whereas the crystals of dental stone and the two high-strength dental stones are dense and more regular in shape, as shown in Figs. 11.20 and 11.21. This difference in the physical shape and nature of the crystals makes it possible to obtain the same consistency with less excess water with dental stone and high-strength dental stones than with model plaster.

When mixed with water, model plaster, dental stone, or high-strength dental stones set to a hard mass of gypsum. The gypsum products known as high-strength dental stones (types 4 and 5) are the strongest, the mass produced as model plaster is the weakest, and dental stone produces an intermediate-strength material. As noted before, all gypsum products have the same chemical formula, and the chemical nature of the masses produced by mixing them with water is also identical; the differences among them are primarily in their physical properties.

Mechanism of Setting

The most important and well-recognized theory for the mechanism of the setting is the crystalline theory. It was originated in 1887 by Henry Louis Le Chatelier, a French chemist. The theory

TABLE 11.9 Required and Excess Water for Gypsum Materials[a]

Gypsum	Mixing Water (mL/100 g of Powder)	Required Water (mL/100 g of Powder)	Excess Water (mL/100 g of Powder)
Model plaster	37–50	18.6	18–31
Dental stone	28–32	18.6	9–13
High-strength dental stone	19–24	18.6	0–5

[a]Water-to-powder ratio varies with each product.

received the full support of Jacobus Henricus van 't Hoff, a famous Dutch chemist in Berlin at the turn of the century. According to the explanation of van 't Hoff, the setting reaction of water with calcium sulfate hemihydrate to form calcium sulfate dihydrate is caused by the difference in solubility between these two components. Calcium sulfate dihydrate is less soluble than the hemihydrate form. When the hemihydrate dissolves in water, the dihydrate, having lower solubility, is then supersaturated and precipitates out of solution from points of nucleation in the form of needle-like crystals. Bonding between contacting crystals results in the final cohesive structure.

Volumetric Changes During Setting

Stoichiometrically, calcium sulfate hemihydrate should contract volumetrically during the setting process by about 7%. However, experiments have determined that all gypsum products expand linearly during setting. According to the crystalline theory of Le Chatelier and van 't Hoff, the expansion results from the thrusting action of gypsum crystals, $CaSO_4 \cdot 2H_2O$, during their growth from a supersaturated solution. The combination of the stoichiometric (chemical) contraction of calcium sulfate hemihydrate being transformed into the dihydrate with the linear expansion of the outer dimensions caused by the growth of calcium sulfate dihydrate, leads to overall expansion, a characteristic of porous materials.

Effect of Spatulation

The mixing process, called *spatulation*, has a definite effect on the setting time and setting expansion of the material. Within practical limits, an increase in the amount of spatulation (either speed of spatulation, or time of spatulation, or both) shortens the setting time. As soon as the powder is placed in water, the chemical reaction starts, and some calcium sulfate dihydrate is formed. During spatulation the newly formed calcium sulfate dihydrate breaks down to smaller crystals and starts new centers of nucleation, from which the calcium sulfate dihydrate can be precipitated. Because an increased amount of spatulation causes more nuclei centers to be formed, the conversion of calcium sulfate hemihydrate to dihydrate is accelerated.

Effect of Temperature

The temperature of the water used for mixing, as well as the temperature of the environment, both have a significant effect on the setting reaction of gypsum products. One of the consequences of increasing temperature is a change in the relative solubilities of calcium sulfate hemihydrate and calcium sulfate dihydrate, which alters the rate of the reaction. The ratio of the solubilities of calcium sulfate hemihydrate and calcium sulfate dihydrate at 20°C is about 4.5 (Table 11.10). As the temperature increases, the solubility ratios decrease, until 100°C is reached and the ratio becomes 1. As the ratio of the solubilities becomes lower, the reaction is slowed, and the setting time is increased. Another consequence of increasing temperature is the change in ion mobility. In general, as the temperature increases, the mobility of the calcium and sulfate ions increases, which tends to increase the rate of the reaction and shorten the setting time. The effects of these two phenomena are superimposed, and the practical outcome is that increasing the temperature from room temperature of 20°C to body temperature of 37°C increases the rate of the reaction slightly and shortens the setting time.

Effect of Humidity

When the relative humidity increases to 70% and above, moisture in the air can cause some conversion of hemihydrate to dihydrate.

TABLE 11.10 Solubility of Calcium Sulfate Hemihydrate and Calcium Sulfate Dihydrate at Different Temperatures

Temperature (°C)	$CaSO_4 \cdot {}^1/_2H_2O$ (g/100 g Water)	$CaSO_4 \cdot 2H_2O$ (g/100 g Water)
20	0.90	0.200
25	0.80	0.205
30	0.72	0.209
40	0.61	0.210
50	0.50	0.205
100	0.17	0.170

Because dihydrate crystals can accelerate the reaction by providing more nuclei for crystallization, the initial result is acceleration of setting. However, further contamination by moisture can reduce the amount of hemihydrate remaining to form gypsum, and retardation of setting will occur. Therefore all gypsum products should be kept in a closed container and well protected from moisture in the air.

Effect of Colloidal Systems and pH

Colloidal systems such as agar and alginate retard the setting of gypsum products. If these materials are in contact with $CaSO_4 \cdot ½H_2O$ during setting, a soft, easily abraded surface is obtained. Accelerators such as potassium sulfate are added to improve the surface quality of the set $CaSO_4 \cdot 2H_2O$ against agar or alginate.

These colloids do not retard the setting by altering the solubility ratio of the hemihydrate and dihydrate forms, but rather by being adsorbed on the hemihydrate and dihydrate nucleation sites, thus interfering in the hydration reaction. The adsorption of these materials on the nucleating sites retards the setting reaction more effectively than adsorption on the calcium sulfate hemihydrate. Liquids with low pH, such as saliva, also retard the setting reaction. Liquids with high pH accelerate setting.

Properties

The important properties of gypsum products include quality, fluidity at pouring time, setting time, linear setting expansion, compressive strength, hardness and abrasion resistance, and reproduction of detail. Some of these property requirements, described by ANSI/ADA specification No. 25 (ISO 6873), are summarized in Table 11.11.

Setting Time

Definition and Importance

The time required for the reaction to be completed is called the *final setting time.* If the rate of the reaction is too fast or the material has a short setting time, the mixed mass may harden before the operator can manipulate it properly. By contrast, if the rate of reaction is too slow, an excessively long time is required to complete the operation. Therefore a proper setting time is one of the most important characteristics of gypsum materials.

The chemical reaction is initiated at the moment the powder is mixed with water, but at the early stage, only a small portion of the hemihydrate is converted to gypsum. The freshly mixed mass has a semifluid consistency and can be poured into a mold of any

TABLE 11.11 **Property Requirements for Gypsum Materials**

Type	Setting Time (min)	Setting Expansion Range (%)	COMPRESSIVE STRENGTH (MPa) Minimum	Maximum	Reproduction of Detail (µm)
1. Impression plaster	2.5–5.0	0–0.15	4.0	8.0	75 ± 8
2. Model plaster	±20%[a]	0–0.30	9.0	—	75 ± 8
3. Dental stone	±20%	0–0.20	20.0	—	50 ± 8
4. High-strength/ low-expansion dental stone	±20%	0–0.15	35.0	—	50 ± 8
5. High-strength/ high-expansion dental stone	±20%	0.16–0.30	35.0	—	50 ± 8

[a]Setting time shall be within 20% of value claimed by manufacturer.

shape. As the reaction proceeds, however, more and more calcium sulfate dihydrate crystals are produced. The viscosity of the mixed mass increases, and the mass can no longer flow easily into the fine details of the mold. This time is called the *working time*.

The final setting time is defined as the time at which the material can be separated from the impression without distortion or fracture. The initial setting time is the time required for gypsum products to reach a certain arbitrary stage of firmness in their setting process. In the normal case, this arbitrary stage is represented by a semi-hard mass that has passed the working stage but is not yet completely set. At final setting, the conversion of calcium sulfate hemihydrate to calcium sulfate dihydrate is virtually completed.

Measurement

The initial setting time is usually measured arbitrarily by some form of penetration test, although occasionally other types of test methods have been designed. For example, the loss of gloss from the surface of the mixed mass of model plaster or dental stone is an indication of this stage in the chemical reaction and is sometimes used to indicate the initial set of the mass. Similarly, the setting time may be measured by the temperature rise of the mass, because the chemical reaction is exothermic.

The Vicat apparatus shown in Fig. 11.16 is commonly used to measure the initial setting time of gypsum products. It consists of a rod weighing 300 g with a needle of 1 mm diameter. A ring container is filled with the mix, the setting time of which is to be measured. The rod is lowered until it contacts the surface of the material, then the needle is released and allowed to penetrate the mix. When the needle fails to penetrate to the bottom of the container, the material has reached the Vicat or the initial setting time. Other types of instruments, such as Gillmore needles, can be used to obtain the initial and final setting times of gypsum materials.

Control of Setting Time

Methods for controlling setting time have been discussed previously. Initially the manufacturer can add various components that act as either accelerators or retarders. The operator can alter setting time by changing the temperature of the mix water and by changing the degree of spatulation. The W/P ratio can also affect setting time; using more water in the mix can prolong the setting time as shown in Table 11.12. However, this method should never be employed, as it would compromise mechanical properties. The effect of spatulation on setting time of model plaster and dental stone is shown in Table 11.13. Increased spatulation shortens the setting time. Properties of a high-strength dental stone mixed by hand and by a power-driven mixer with vacuum are shown in Table 11.14. The setting time is usually shortened for power mixing compared with hand mixing.

TABLE 11.12 **Effect of Water-to-Powder Ratio on Setting Time**

Material	W/P Ratio (mL/g)	Spatulation Turns	Initial (Vicat) Setting Time (min)
Model plaster	0.45		8
	0.50	100	11
	0.55		14
Dental stone	0.27		4
	0.30	100	7
	0.33		8
High-strength dental stone	0.22		5
	0.24	100	7
	0.26		9

W/P ratio, Water-to-powder ratio.

TABLE 11.13 **Effect of Spatulation on Setting Time**

Material	W/P Ratio (mL/g)	Spatulation Turns	Setting Time (min)
Model plaster	0.50	20	14
	0.50	100	11
	0.50	200	8
Dental stone	0.30	20	10
	0.30	100	8

W/P ratio, Water-to-powder ratio.

TABLE 11.14 Properties of a High-Strength Dental Stone Mixed by Hand and by a Power-Driven Mixer with Vacuum

	Hand Mix	Power-Driven Mix with Vacuum
Setting time	8.0	7.3
Compressive strength at 24 h (MPa)	43.1	45.5
Setting expansion at 2 h (%)	0.045	0.037
Viscosity, centipoise (cp)	54,000	43,000

TABLE 11.15 Viscosity of Several High-Strength Dental Stones and Impression Plaster

Material	Viscosity (cp)[b]
High-Strength Dental Stone[a]	
A	21,000
B	29,000
C	50,000
D	54,000
E	101,000
Impression plaster	23,000

[a]Stones were mixed with 1% sodium citrate solution to retard setting.
[b]Viscosity was measured 4 minutes from the start of mixing.

The easiest and most reliable way to change the setting time is to add different chemicals. Potassium sulfate, K_2SO_4, is known as an effective accelerator, and the use of a 2% aqueous solution of this salt rather than water reduces the setting time of model plaster from approximately 10 minutes to about 4 minutes. By contrast, sodium citrate is a dependable retarder. The use of a 2% aqueous solution of borax to mix with the powder may prolong the setting time of some gypsum products to a few hours.

If a small amount of set calcium sulfate dihydrate is ground and mixed with model plaster, it provides nuclei of crystallization and acts as an accelerator. The set gypsum used as an accelerator is called *terra alba*, and it has a pronounced effect at lower concentrations. Manufacturers usually take advantage of this fact and add about 1% terra alba to plaster.

Viscosity

The viscosities of several high-strength dental stones and impression plaster are listed in Table 11.15. A range of viscosities from 21,000 to 101,000 centipoises (cp) was observed for five different high-strength stones. More voids were observed in casts made from the stones with the higher viscosities. Impression plaster is used infrequently, but it has a low viscosity, which makes it possible to take impressions with a minimum of force on the soft tissues (mucostatic technique).

Compressive Strength

When set, gypsum products show relatively high values of compressive strength. The compressive strength is inversely related to the W/P ratio of the mix. The more water used to make the mix, the lower the compressive strength.

Model plaster has the greatest quantity of excess water, whereas high-strength dental stone contains the least excess water. The excess water is uniformly distributed in the mix and contributes to the volume but not to the strength of the material. Set model plaster is more porous than set dental stone, causing the apparent density of model plaster to be lower. Because high-strength dental stone is the densest, it shows the highest compressive strength, with model plaster being the most porous and thus the weakest.

The 1-hour compressive strength values are about 12.5 MPa for model plaster, 31 MPa for dental stones, and 45 MPa for high-strength dental stones. These values are representative of the normal mixes, but they vary as the W/P ratio is increased or decreased. The effect of the W/P ratio on the compressive strength of these materials is given in Table 11.16. As shown in Table 11.14, the compressive strength of a high-strength dental stone is improved slightly by vacuum mixing. Evidently, when stone is mixed with the same W/P ratio as model plaster, the compressive strength of dental stone is almost the same as that of model plaster. Similarly, the compressive strength of high-strength dental stone with W/P ratios of 0.3 and 0.5 is similar to the normal compressive strength of dental stone and model plaster.

At 1 or 2 hours after the final setting time, the hardened gypsum material appears dry and seems to have reached its maximum strength. However, this is not the case. The wet strength is the strength of gypsum materials with some or all of the excess water present in the specimen. The dry strength is the strength of the gypsum material with all of its excess water driven out. The dry compressive strength is usually about twice that of the wet strength. It should be noted that as the hardened mass slowly loses its excess water, the compressive strength of the material does not increase uniformly. The effect of drying on the compressive strength of dental stone is shown in Fig. 11.22. Theoretically, about 8.8% of excess water is in the hardened mass of the stone. As the mass loses up to 7% of the water, no appreciable change develops in the compressive strength of the material. When the mass loses 7.5% of the excess water, however, the strength increases sharply, and

TABLE 11.16 Effect of Water-to-Powder Ratio on the Compressive Strength of Model Plaster, Dental Stone, and High-Strength Dental Stone[a]

Material	W/P Ratio (mL/g)	Compressive Strength (MPa)
Model plaster	0.45	12.5
	0.50	11.0
	0.55	9.0
Dental stone	0.27	31.0
	0.30	20.5
	0.50	10.5
High-strength dental stone	0.24	38.0
	0.30	21.5
	0.50	10.5

W/P ratio, Water-to-powder ratio.
[a]All mixes spatulated 100 turns and tested 1 hour after the start of mixing.

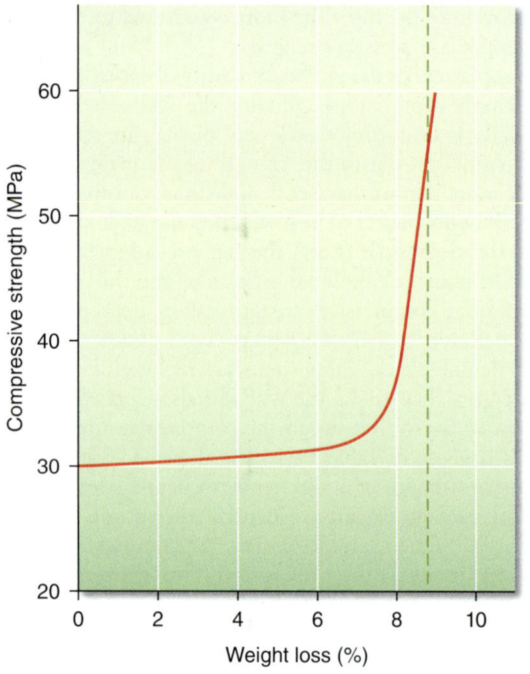

• **Fig. 11.22** Effect of loss of excess water on compressive strength of dental stone.

when all of the excess (8.8%) is lost, the strength of the material is over 55 MPa.

The drying time for gypsum materials varies according to the size of the gypsum mass and the temperature and humidity of the storage atmosphere. At room temperature and average humidity, about 7 days are necessary for an average denture flask filled with gypsum materials to lose the excess water.

Surface Hardness and Abrasion Resistance

The surface hardness of unmodified gypsum materials is related in a general way to their compressive strength. A high compressive strength of the hardened mass corresponds to a high surface hardness. After the final setting occurs, the surface hardness remains practically constant until most excess water is evaporated from the surface, after which its increase is similar to the increase in compressive strength. The surface hardness increases at a faster rate than the compressive strength because the surface of the hardened mass reaches a dry state earlier than the inner portion of the mass.

Attempts have been made to increase the hardness of gypsum products by impregnating the set gypsum with epoxy or methyl methacrylate monomer that is allowed to polymerize. Increases in hardness were obtained for model plaster but not for dental stone or high-strength dental stone. Increases in scratch resistance of 15% to 41% were observed for a high-strength dental stone impregnated with epoxy resins or a light-cured dimethacrylate resin. In general, impregnating set gypsum with resin increases abrasion resistance, but decreases compressive strength and surface hardness.

The idea of drying molds, casts, or dies in an oven to obtain a quick, dry compressive strength and dry surface hardness of a material is not practical because the gypsum would be dehydrated, which would reduce the strength instead of increasing it. Soaking the gypsum dies or casts in glycerin or different oils does not improve the surface hardness but rather makes the surface smoother so that a wax carver or other instrument will not cut the stone as it slides over the surface. Mixing high-strength dental stone with a commercial hardening solution containing colloidal silica (about 30%) improves the surface hardness of the set gypsum. The Knoop hardness of two commercial high-strength dental stones was 54 and 77 kg/mm^2 when mixed with water. When the hardening solution was used, these values increased to 62 and 79 kg/mm^2, respectively. Increased surface hardness does not necessarily mean improved abrasion resistance because hardness is only one of many factors that can affect wear resistance. Gypsum dies abrade more readily than epoxy dies, even though the gypsum dies are harder. Two-body abrasion studies suggest that commercial hardening solutions do not improve the abrasion resistance of high-strength dental stones. However, the clinical relevancy of the two-body abrasion test on gypsum has not been established.

Although the use of disinfectant chemicals on gypsum dies effectively destroys potentially dangerous organisms, some can damage the surface of a die. Surfaces can be eroded, and the surface hardness can be adversely affected by treatment with some commonly used disinfectants. Other disinfectants, including sodium hypochlorite solutions, have very little effect on the surfaces of gypsum dies.

Reproduction of Detail

American National Standards Institute/American Dental Association specification No. 25 requires that types 1 and 2 reproduce a groove 75 µm in width, whereas types 3, 4, and 5 reproduce a groove 50 µm in width (see Table 11.11). Gypsum dies do not reproduce surface detail as well as electroformed or epoxy dies because the surface of the set gypsum is porous on a microscopic level (Fig. 11.23). Air bubbles are often formed at the interface of the impression and gypsum cast because freshly mixed gypsum does not wet some elastomeric impression materials (condensation silicones) well. The incorporation of nonionic surfactants in silicone impression materials improves the wetting of the impression by slurry water. The use of vibration during the pouring of a cast reduces the presence of air bubbles. Contamination of the impression in which the gypsum die is poured by saliva or blood can also affect the detail reproduction. Rinsing the impression and blowing away excess water can improve the detail recorded by the gypsum die material.

Setting Expansion

When set, all gypsum products show a measurable linear expansion. The percentage of setting expansion, however, varies from one

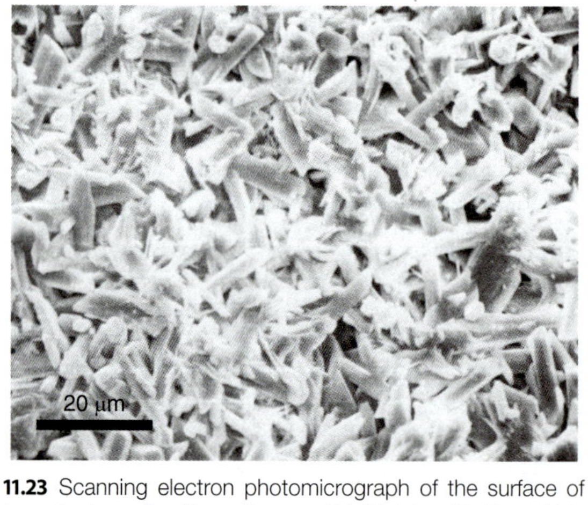

• **Fig. 11.23** Scanning electron photomicrograph of the surface of a set high-strength stone die. (From Powers JM, Wataha JC. *Dental Materials: Foundations and Applications*. 11th ed. Elsevier; 2017).

type of gypsum material to another. Under ordinary conditions, plasters have 0.2% to 0.3% setting expansion, low- to moderate-strength dental stones about 0.15% to 0.25%, and high-strength dental stones only 0.08% to 0.10%. The setting expansion of high-strength/high-expansion dental stones ranges from 0.10% to 0.20%. Typically over 75% of the expansion observed at 24 hours occurs during the first hour of setting.

The setting expansion may be controlled by different manipulative conditions and by the addition of some chemicals. Mechanical mixing decreases setting expansion. As shown in Table 11.14, a vacuum-mixed high-strength stone expands less at 2 hours than when mixed by hand. Power mixing appears to cause a greater initial volumetric contraction than is observed for hand mixing. The W/P ratio of the mix also has an effect, with an increase in the ratio reducing the setting expansion. The addition of different chemicals not only affects the setting expansion of gypsum products but may also change other properties. For example, the addition by the manufacturer of sodium chloride (NaCl) in a small concentration increases the setting expansion of the mass and shortens the setting time. The addition of 1% potassium sulfate, by contrast, decreases the setting time but has no effect on the setting expansion.

If the gypsum materials are immersed in water during the setting process, the setting expansion increases. This is called *hygroscopic expansion.* A typical, high-strength dental stone has a setting expansion of about 0.08%, which increases to 0.10% with water immersion. Increased expansion is observed when dental stone hardens as it comes in contact with a hydrocolloid impression. A more detailed explanation of hygroscopic expansion is presented later under casting investments with a gypsum binder.

Manipulation

When any gypsum product is mixed with water, it should be spatulated properly to obtain a smooth mix. Water is dispensed into a mixing bowl of an appropriate size and design (Fig. 11.24). The powder is added and allowed to settle into the water for about 30 seconds. This technique minimizes the amount of air incorporated into the mix during initial spatulation by hand. Spatulation can be continued by hand using a spatula with a stiff blade (Fig. 11.25) with the bowl on a vibrator (see Fig. 11.25) or a power-driven mechanical spatulator (Fig. 11.26). A summary of the effect of various manipulative variables on the properties of gypsum products is presented in Table 11.17.

Spatulation by hand involves stirring the mixture vigorously while wiping the inside surfaces of the bowl with the spatula. Spatulation to wet and mix the powder uniformly with the water requires about 1 minute at 2 revolutions per second.

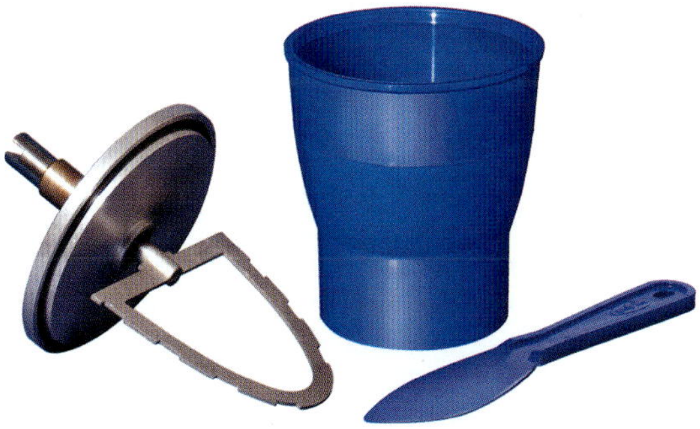

• **Fig. 11.24** Flexible rubber mixing bowl and metal spatula with a stiff blade. (Courtesy Whip Mix Corporation, Louisville, KY).

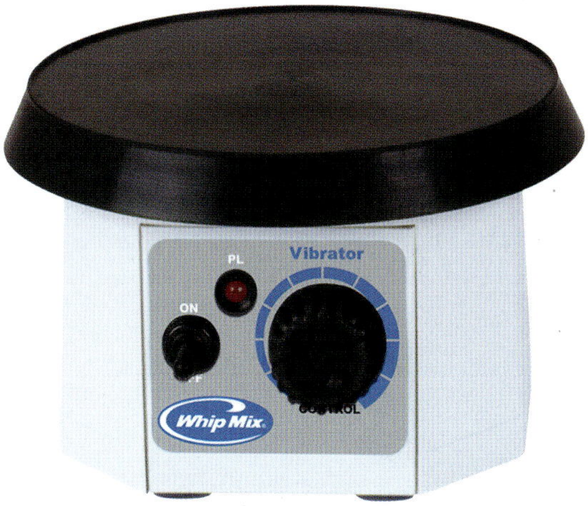

• **Fig. 11.25** A vibrator is designed to promote the release of bubbles in the gypsum mix and to facilitate pouring of the impression. (Courtesy Whip Mix Corporation, Louisville, KY).

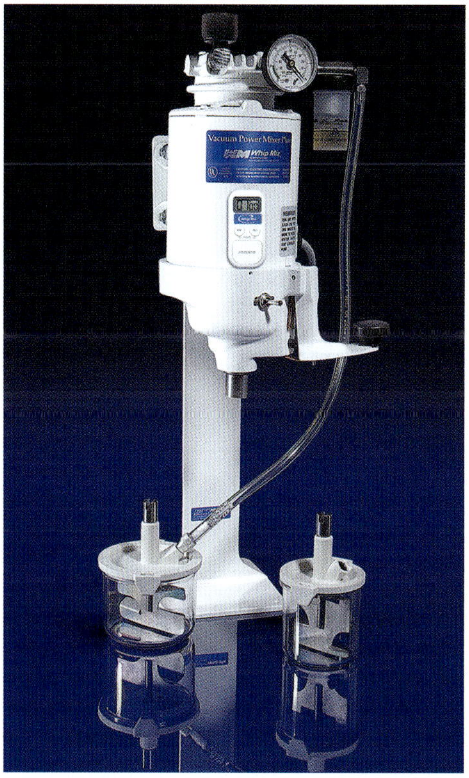

• **Fig. 11.26** Power-driven mechanical spatulator with a vacuum attachment. (Courtesy Whip Mix Corporation, Louisville, KY).

Spatulation with a power-driven mechanical spatulator requires that the powder initially be wet by the water as with hand mixing. The mix is then spatulated for 20 seconds on the low-speed drive of the mixer. Vacuuming during mixing reduces the air entrapped in the mix. Vibration immediately after mixing and during pouring of the gypsum minimizes air bubbles in the set mass.

Pouring an impression with gypsum requires care to avoid trapping air in critical areas. The mixed gypsum should be added slowly to the impression with a small instrument such as a wax spatula. The mass should run into the rinsed impression under vibration in such a manner that it pushes air ahead of itself as it fills the impressions of the teeth. Commonly the teeth of a cast are

TABLE 11.17 Summary of Effect of Manipulative Variables on Properties of Gypsum Products

Manipulative Variable	Setting Time	Consistency	Setting Expansion	Compressive Strength
Increase water-to-powder ratio	Increase	Increase	Decrease	Decrease
Increase rate of spatulation	Decrease	Decrease	Increase	No effect
Increase temperature of mixing water from 23° to 30°C	Decrease	Decrease	Increase	No effect

W/P ratio, Water-to-powder ratio.

poured in dental stone or high-strength dental stone, whereas the base is poured in model plaster for easier trimming.

Once poured, the gypsum material should be allowed to harden for 45 to 60 minutes before the impression and cast are separated and disinfected. Models can be disinfected by immersion in 1:10 dilution of sodium hypochlorite for 30 minutes or with a spray of iodophor following manufacturer's instructions.

Epoxy Die Materials

In the past, epoxy materials were supplied in the form of a paste to which a liquid activator (amine) was added to initiate hardening. Nowadays fast-setting epoxy materials are supplied in automixing systems similar to those described for automixing addition silicones. The epoxy resin is in one cartridge, and the catalyst is in the other. Forcing the two pastes through the static mixing tip thoroughly mixes the epoxy material, which can be directly injected into an elastomeric impression. If desired, a small intraoral delivery tip may be attached to the static mixing tip for injecting into detailed areas of the impression. The fast-setting epoxy hardens rapidly, so dies can be waxed 30 minutes after injection. Because water retards the polymerization of resin, epoxy resins cannot be used with water-containing agar and alginate impression materials, and thus are limited to use with elastomeric impression materials.

Comparison of Impression and Die Materials

High-strength stone dies may be from 0.35% larger to 0.25% smaller than the original, depending on the location of the measurement and the impression material used. In general, occlusogingival (vertical) changes are greater than buccolingual or mesiodistal (horizontal) changes. The shrinkage of the impression material toward the surfaces of the tray in the horizontal direction usually results in dimensions larger than the original. In the vertical direction, shrinkage is away from the free surface of the impression and toward the tray, and dimensions smaller than the original are obtained.

All epoxy dies exhibit some polymerization shrinkage, with values ranging from 0.1% to 0.3%, and as a result, the dies are undersized. Ranking materials by the ability of an impression-die combination to reproduce surface detail produces different results than does ranking by dimensional change values. If a release agent is not needed on the surface of the impression, epoxy dies are best for reproducing detail (10 µm), followed by high-strength stone dies (170 µm). The silicone-epoxy combination produces the sharpest detail, although not all epoxy die materials are compatible with all silicone impression materials.

Resistance to abrasion and scraping should also be considered. Epoxy dies have high resistance whereas high-strength stone dies have the least resistance.

Casting Investments

The adoption of the casting practice in dentistry for making gold alloy inlays, crowns, bridges, and other restorations represents one of the major advances in restorative dentistry. Alloys with higher melting points, such as palladium and base-metal alloys, have been cast into fixed and removable dental prostheses by using the same lost-wax technique used for gold alloys. All such casting operations involve (1) a wax pattern of the object to be reproduced; (2) a suitable mold material, known as investment, which is placed around the pattern and permitted to harden; (3) suitable furnaces for burning out the wax patterns and heating the investment mold; and (4) proper facilities to melt and cast the alloy. An *investment* can be described as a ceramic material that is suitable for forming a mold into which a metal or alloy is cast. The operation of forming the mold is described as *investing*. Details of the casting technique are described on the website http://evolve.elsevier.com/sakaguchi/restorative.

Properties Required of an Investment

1. Easily manipulated: Not only should it be possible to mix and manipulate the mass of the investment readily and to paint the wax pattern easily, but it should also harden within a relatively short time.
2. Sufficient strength at room temperature: The investment should permit ease in handling and provide enough strength at higher temperatures to withstand the impact force of the molten metal. The inner surface of the mold should not break down at a high temperature.
3. Stability at higher temperatures: The investment should not decompose to give off gases that could damage the surface of the alloy.
4. Sufficient expansion: The investment should expand enough to compensate for shrinkage of the wax pattern and metal that takes place during the casting procedure.
5. Beneficial casting temperatures: Preferably the thermal expansion versus temperature curve should have a plateau of the thermal expansion over a range of casting temperatures.
6. Porosity: The investment should be porous enough to permit the air or other gases in the mold cavity to escape easily during the casting procedure.
7. Smooth surface: Fine detail and margins on the casting should be preserved.

8. Ease of divestment: The investment should break away readily from the surface of the metal and should not have reacted chemically with it.
9. Inexpensive.

These requirements describe an ideal investment. No single material is known that completely fulfills all these requirements. However, by blending different ingredients, an investment that possesses most of the required qualities can be developed. These ideal qualities are the basis for considering the behavior and characteristics of casting investments.

Composition

In general, an investment is a mixture of three distinct types of materials: refractory material, binder material, and other chemicals.

Refractory Material

Refractory material is usually a form of silicon dioxide, such as quartz, tridymite, cristobalite, or a mixture of these. Refractory materials are contained in all dental investments, whether for casting gold or high-melting-point alloys.

Binder Material

Because the refractory materials alone do not form a coherent solid mass, some kind of binder is needed. The common binder used for dental casting gold alloy is α-calcium sulfate hemihydrate. Phosphate, ethyl silicate, and other similar materials also serve as binders for high-temperature casting investments. These latter investments are described later in conjunction with investment for casting high-melting-point alloys.

Other Chemicals

Usually a mixture of refractory materials and a binder alone is not enough to produce all the desirable properties required of an investment. Other chemicals, such as sodium chloride, boric acid, potassium sulfate, graphite, copper powder, or magnesium oxide, are often added in small quantities to modify various physical properties. For example, small amounts of chlorides or boric acid enhance the thermal expansion of investments bonded by calcium sulfate.

Calcium Sulfate-Bonded Investments

In general, the investments suitable for casting gold alloys contain 65% to 75% quartz or cristobalite, or a blend of the two, in varying proportions; 25% to 35% of α-calcium sulfate hemihydrate; and about 2% to 3% chemical modifiers. With the proper blending of these basic ingredients, the manufacturer is able to develop an investment with an established set of physical properties that are adequate for dental gold casting practices. A list of specific compositions is of little value, however, because the final product's properties are influenced by both the ingredients present in the investment and the manner in which the mass is manipulated and used in making the mold.

Investments with calcium sulfate hemihydrate as a binder are relatively easy to manipulate. The calcium sulfate–bonded investment is usually limited to gold castings and is not heated above 700°C. The calcium sulfate portion of the investment decomposes into sulfur dioxide and sulfur trioxide at temperatures over 700°C, tending to embrittle the casting metal. Therefore the calcium sulfate type of binder is usually not used in investments for making castings of high-melting-point metals such as palladium or base-metal alloys.

Properties of Calcium Sulfate-Bonded Investments

American National Standards Institute/American Dental Association specification No. 126 (ISO 7490) for gypsum-bonded casting investments applies to two different types of investments suitable for casting dental restorations of gold alloys:

Type 1: For casting inlays and crowns
Type 2: For casting complete denture and removable partial denture frameworks

Both types have calcium sulfate as a binder material. The physical properties included in this specification are appearance of powder, fluidity at working time, setting time, compressive strength, linear setting expansion, and linear thermal expansion. The values allowed for these properties are summarized in the specifications. The manipulation of investments in the inlay casting procedure is discussed in detail on the website http://evolve.elsevier.com/sakaguchi/restorative.

Effect of Temperature on Investment

In casting with the lost-wax process, the wax pattern is invested and placed in an oven at a temperature that melts and removes the wax from the investment, thereby leaving a mold cavity into which the molten metal is cast. This oven temperature varies from one technique to another, but in no case is it lower than 550°C or higher than 700°C for calcium sulfate-bonded investments. During the heating process, the refractory material is affected differently by the thermal changes than is the gypsum binder.

Effect of Temperature on Silicon Dioxide Refractories

Each of the polymorphic forms of silica (quartz, tridymite, and cristobalite) expands when heated, but the percentage of expansion varies from one type to another. Pure cristobalite expands by 1.6% at 250°C, whereas quartz expands about 1.4% at 600°C, and the thermal expansion of tridymite at 600°C is less than 1%. The percentage of expansion of the three types of silica versus temperature is shown in Fig. 4.41. None of the three forms of silica expands uniformly; instead they all show a break (nonlinearity) in their thermal expansion curves. In the case of cristobalite, the expansion is somewhat uniform up to about 200°C. At this temperature, its expansion increases sharply from 0.5% to 1.2%, and then above 250°C it again becomes more uniform. At 573°C quartz also shows a break in the expansion curve, and tridymite shows a similar break at a much lower temperature.

The breaks on the expansion versus temperature curves indicate that cristobalite and quartz each exist in two polymorphic forms, one of which is more stable at a higher temperature and the other at a lower temperature. The form that is more stable at room temperature is called the α-form, and the one that is more stable at higher temperatures is designated as the β-form. Tridymite has three stable polymorphic forms. Therefore the temperatures of 220°C for cristobalite, 573°C for quartz, and 105° and 160°C for tridymite are displacive transition temperatures. A displacive change involves expansion or contraction in the volume of the mass without breaking any bonds. In changing from the α-form (which is the more stable form at room temperature) to the β-form (which is stable at higher temperatures), all three forms of silica expand. The amount of expansion is highest for cristobalite and lowest for tridymite.

The quartz form of silica is found abundantly in nature, and it can be converted to cristobalite and tridymite by being heated through a reconstructive transition during which bonds are broken and a new crystal structure is formed. The α-quartz is converted to β-quartz at a temperature of 573°C. If the β-quartz is heated to 870°C and maintained at that temperature, it is converted to β-tridymite. From β-tridymite, it is possible to obtain either α-tridymite or β-cristobalite. If β-tridymite is cooled rapidly to 120°C and held at that temperature, it is changed to α-tridymite, which is stable at room temperature. By contrast, if β-tridymite is heated to 1475°C and held at that temperature, it is converted to β-cristobalite. Further heating of β-cristobalite produces fused silica, but if it is cooled to 220°C and held at that temperature, α-cristobalite is formed. These transitions are shown in the following equation.

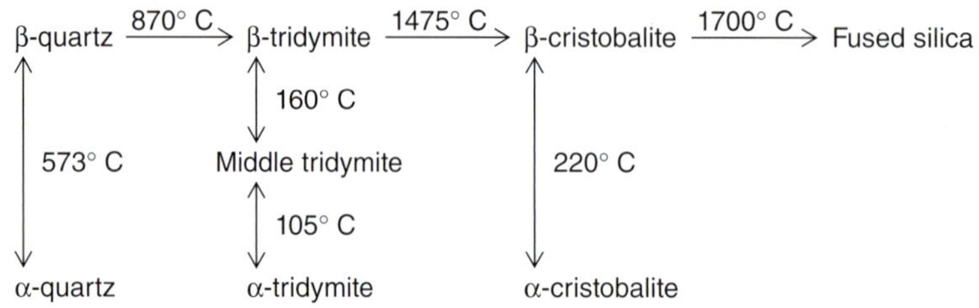

All forms of silica are in their α-forms in the investment, and during the heating process, they are converted completely or in part to their corresponding β-forms. This transition involves an expansion of the mass, which helps compensate for the casting shrinkages.

Effect of Temperature on Calcium Sulfate Binders

The binder used for gold alloy casting investments in dentistry is α-calcium sulfate hemihydrate. During the investing process, some of the water mixed with the investment reacts with the hemihydrate and is converted to calcium sulfate dihydrate, whereas the remainder of the water is uniformly distributed in the mix as excess water. During the early stages of heating, the excess water evaporates. As the temperature rises to about 105°C, calcium sulfate dihydrate starts losing water. The investment mass is then heated further to the proper temperature for casting the metal. In this way, anhydrous calcium sulfate, silica, and certain chemical additives remain to form the mold into which the gold alloy is cast.

It has been observed experimentally that investment expands when it is first heated from room temperature to about 105°C, then contracts slightly or remains unchanged up to about 200°C, and between 200°C and 700°C it registers varying degrees of expansion, depending on its silica composition. These properties are explained as follows: up to about 105°C, ordinary thermal expansion occurs. Above 105°C, the calcium sulfate dihydrate is converted to anhydrous calcium sulfate. Dehydration of the dihydrate and a phase change of the calcium sulfate anhydrite cause a contraction. However, the α-form of tridymite (which might be present as an impurity) is expanding and compensates for the contraction of the calcium sulfate sufficiently to prevent the investment from registering significant contraction. At elevated temperatures, the α-forms of silica present in the investment are converted to the β-forms, which cause some additional expansion.

The thermal expansion curves for a currently available hygroscopic type of investment containing quartz *(A)* and a thermal expansion type of investment containing cristobalite *(B)* are shown in Fig. 11.27, which illustrates the expected degree of expansion at different temperatures. The expansion of the silica content of the investment not only must be sufficiently high to overcome all the contraction but should also take place at temperatures close to the temperature at which contraction of the hemihydrate occurs.

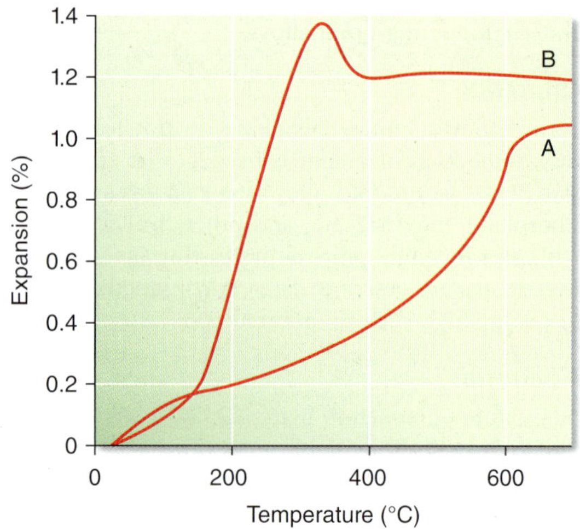

• **Fig. 11.27** Thermal expansion curves for calcium sulfate–bonded investments. (A) Hygroscopic type; (B) thermal expansion type. (Modified from Asgar K. Casting restorations. In: Clark JW, ed. *Clinical Dentistry*. vol. 4. Harper & Row; 1976).

Cooling of the Investment

When the investment cools, the refractory and binder contract according to a thermal contraction curve that is different from the thermal expansion curve of the investment (Fig. 11.28). Upon cooling to room temperature, the investment exhibits an overall contraction compared to its initial dimensions. On reheating to the temperature previously attained, the investment does not expand thermally to the previous level; moreover, the process of cooling and reheating causes internal cracks in the investment that can affect the quality of the casting.

Setting Expansion of Calcium Sulfate-Bonded Investment

All the calcium sulfate-bonded investments currently available for casting gold alloys have both setting and thermal expansion. The sum of these two expansions results in a total dimensional change that is an essential property of dental casting investments because it provides compensation for the casting shrinkage of the casting alloys. The setting expansion of an investment, like that of other gypsum products discussed earlier in this chapter, is the linear expansion that takes place during the setting of the investment.

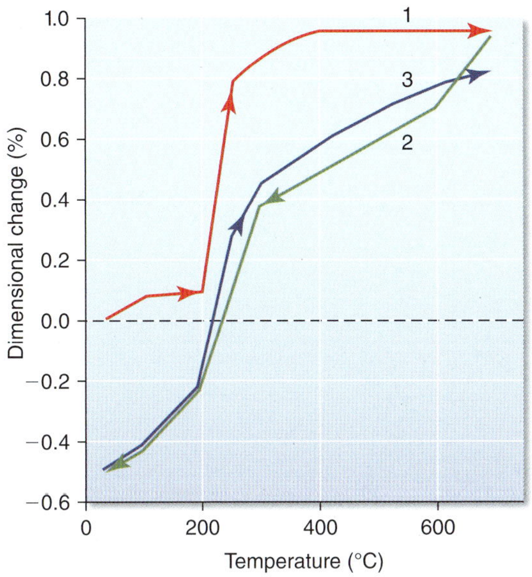

• **Fig. 11.28** Thermal expansion and contraction curves for calcium sulfate–bonded investment (thermal expansion type). *Curve 1* is first heating, *curve 2* is cooling, and *curve 3* is reheating.

If the investment is setting surrounded by air, the expansion is referred to as *normal setting expansion*. On the other hand, if the mixed investment is setting in contact with water, the expansion is substantially greater and is called *hygroscopic setting expansion*. Such contact with water can be achieved in the commonly used casting techniques of (1) placing a wet liner inside the casting ring in which the investment is poured, or (2) if after investing, the casting ring is placed in a water bath. The presently accepted mechanism for hygroscopic setting expansion also relates to the normal setting expansion that occurs when the investment mix sets in contact with air. The basis for this mechanism lies in the role played by the surface tension of the mix water and can be described as follows. After the investment is mixed, water surrounds the components of the setting investment. As the reaction of the calcium sulfate binder progresses, the surrounding water is reduced and growing gypsum crystals impinge on the surface of the remaining water whose surface tension inhibits outward crystal growth. When the water needed for the reaction is used up and the reaction is virtually completed, the growth of gypsum crystals stops in its inhibited form.

If the investment is poured into a casting ring having a water-filled liner, the gypsum crystals can grow further, but only until the new water surface provided by the additional water in the liner is reached; surface tension then inhibits further growth. If water is supplied to the mixed investment mass by immersing the invested ring in a water bath, no new surface is close enough to provide inhibition of crystal growth. The resulting hygroscopic setting expansion for complete immersion as measured in an unconfined trough (ANSI/ADA specification No. 126) is more than twice that of normal expansion. However, when the investment is setting in a confined ring, hygroscopic expansion is limited by the confinement of the ring. For hygroscopic expansion, the additional water provided must be presented to the investment during setting. This is significantly different than adding more water to the premixture components (i.e., increasing the W/P ratio). Another requirement for hygroscopic expansion is that the additional water be presented before the observed loss of gloss, that is, when the setting reaction has not reached completion and the mix water can still be observed on the surface of the setting investment. This allows the additional water to join the remaining mix water and extend the water surface so that the action of surface tension is either delayed or inactive.

Particle Size of Silica

The particle size of calcium sulfate hemihydrate has little effect on hygroscopic expansion, whereas the particle size of silica has a significant effect. Finer silica produces higher settings and hygroscopic expansions.

Silica-to-Binder Ratio

Investments usually contain 65% to 75% silica, 25% to 35% calcium sulfate hemihydrate (stone), and about 2% to 3% of some additive chemicals to control the different physical properties and to color the investments. If the silica/stone ratio is increased, the hygroscopic expansion of the investment also increases, but the strength of the investment decreases.

Water-to-Powder Ratio

As with the setting expansion of gypsum products, the more water in the mix (the thinner the mix or the higher the W/P ratio), the less the normal and hygroscopic setting expansions. Less thermal expansion is also obtained with a thinner mix.

Spatulation

The effect of spatulation on the setting and hygroscopic expansion of the investment is similar to that on the setting expansion of all gypsum products.

Age of Investment

Investments that are 2 or 3 years old do not expand as much as freshly prepared investments. For this reason, the containers of investment must be kept tightly closed as much as possible, especially if the investment is stored in a humid atmosphere.

Water-Bath Temperature

For the water-bath immersion technique, the temperature of the water bath has a measurable effect on the wax pattern. At higher water-bath temperatures, the wax pattern expands, requiring less expansion of the investment to compensate for the total casting shrinkage. In addition, higher water-bath temperatures soften the wax. The softened wax then provides less resistance to the expansion of the investment, thus making the setting expansion more effective. The net effect is higher expansion of the mold with higher water-bath temperatures.

Thermal and Hygroscopic Casting Investment

Casting techniques involving gypsum-bonded investments are often classified as thermal or hygroscopic techniques. The thermal technique directs placing the invested ring after setting into the burnout oven set for a relatively high temperature (649°C), whereas the hygroscopic technique directs immersing the invested ring before setting in a water bath and then, after setting, placing the ring into the burnout oven set for relatively low temperature (482°C). Although all gypsum-bonded investments exhibit both thermal and hygroscopic setting expansion, the relative proportion of these two expansions can vary. Investments used in the thermal technique usually contain cristobalite as the refractory ingredient, which has a high thermal expansion. Investments used in the hygroscopic technique usually contain quartz or tridymite, which have lower thermal expansions but higher hygroscopic setting expansions.

Investment for Casting High-Melting-Point Alloys

Most palladium and base-metal alloys used for removable partial denture frameworks and ceramic-metal restorations have high melting temperatures. They should be cast at a mold temperature greater than 700°C. For this reason, calcium sulfate-bonded investments are usually not used for casting these alloys. Only one base-metal alloy for dental applications possesses a low enough melting point to be cast into a mold at 700°C with a calcium sulfate binder. This alloy is an exception because base-metal alloys are usually cast into molds at 850°C to 110°C. To withstand these high temperatures, the molds require different types of binders, such as silicate and phosphate compounds. This type of investment usually has less than 20% binder, and the remainder of the investment is quartz or another form of silica.

Phosphate-Bonded Investment

The most common type of investment for casting high-melting point alloys is the phosphate-bonded investment. This type of investment consists of three different components. One component contains a water-soluble phosphate ion. The second component reacts with phosphate ions at room temperature. The third component is a refractory, such as silica. Different materials can be used in each component to develop different physical properties.

The binding system of a typical phosphate-bonded investment undergoes an acid-base reaction between acid monoammonium phosphate ($NH_4H_2PO_4$) and basic magnesia (MgO). The soluble phosphate in water reacts with the sparingly soluble magnesia at its surface, forming a binding medium with filler particles embedded in the matrix. The chemical reaction at room temperature can be expressed simply as follows:

$$NH_4H_2PO_4 + MgO + H_2O \rightarrow NH_4MgPO_4 \cdot 6H_2O + H_2O$$

The water produced by this reaction at room temperature lowers the viscosity of the mix as spatulation continues.

As the reaction takes place, colloidal particles are formed with a strong interaction among the particles. During setting and burnout, the sequence of chemical and thermal reactions causes various phase changes, providing room-temperature strength (green strength) and high-temperature strength that enable the investment to withstand the impact of high-melting-point alloys. Phases formed at high temperatures include $Mg_2P_2O_7$ and subsequently $Mg_3(PO_4)_2$. To produce higher expansion, a combination of different particle sizes of silica is used.

These investments can be mixed with water or with a special liquid supplied by the manufacturer. The special liquid is a form of silica sol in water. As shown in Fig. 11.29, phosphate-bonded investments possess higher setting expansion when they are mixed with the silica sol than when mixed with water. With a mix containing silica sol, the investment mass is capable of expanding hygroscopically, whereas if the mix is only water, the hygroscopic expansion of such an investment is negligible. Not all phosphate-bonded investments, however, can expand hygroscopically. Using silica sol instead of water with phosphate-bonded investment also increases its strength considerably. Fig. 11.30 shows thermal expansion curves of two commercial phosphate-bonded investments mixed according to the manufacturers' recommended liquid-to-powder ratio. Both the setting and thermal expansions must be considered in selecting these investments.

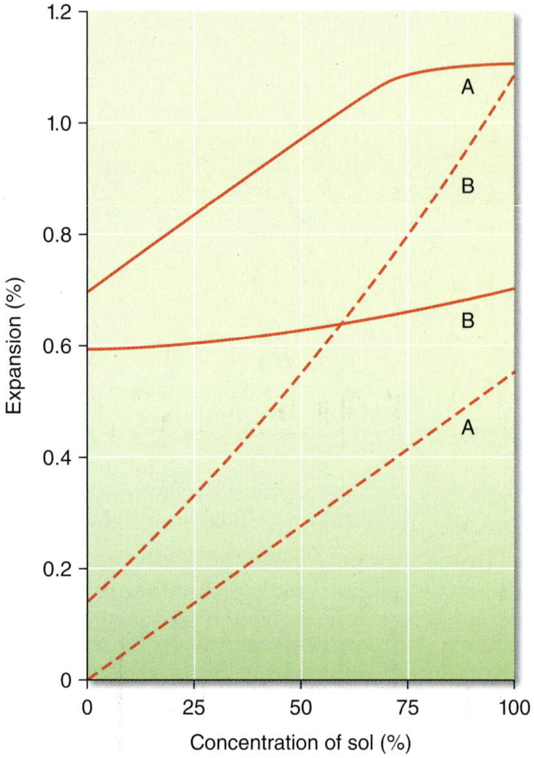

• **Fig. 11.29** Effect of silica sol concentration on thermal expansion *(solid lines)* at 800°C and setting expansion *(dotted lines)* of two phosphate-bonded investments. *A*, Thermal expansion type; *B*, hygroscopic expansion type. (Data from Zarb GA, Bergman G, Clayton JA, MacKay HF, eds. *Prosthodontic Treatment for Partially Edentulous Patients*. Mosby; 1978).

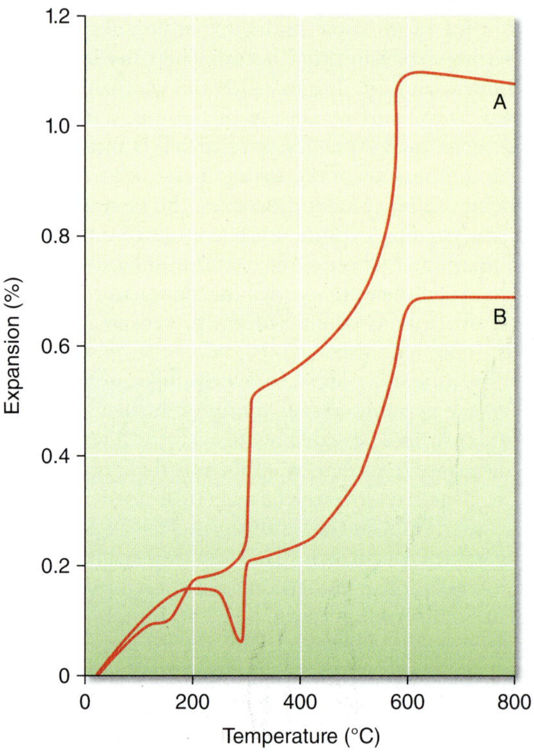

• **Fig. 11.30** Thermal expansion curves of two phosphate-bonded investments mixed at recommended liquid-to-powder ratios. *A*, Thermal expansion type; *B*, hygroscopic expansion type. (Data from Zarb GA, Bergman G, Clayton JA, MacKay HF, eds. *Prosthodontic Treatment for Partially Edentulous Patients*. Mosby; 1978).

American National Standards Institute/American Dental Association specification No. 126 (ISO 9694) for dental phosphate-bonded casting investments specifies two types of investments for alloys having a solidus temperature above 1080°C:

Type 1: For inlays, crowns, and other fixed restorations
Type 2: For removable partial denture frameworks

The following properties and their specified values are described by the specification: fluidity, initial setting time, compressive strength, and linear thermal expansion. The setting time must not differ by more than 30% from the time stated by the manufacturer. The compressive strength at room temperature shall not be less than 2.5 MPa for type 1 investments and 3.0 MPa for type 2 investments. The linear thermal expansion must not differ by more than 15% from the time stated by the manufacturer.

Silica-Bonded Investment

Another type of binding material for investments used with casting high-melting-point alloys is a silica-bonding ingredient. This type of investment may derive its silica bond from ethyl silicate, an aqueous dispersion of colloidal silica, or from sodium silicate. One such investment consists of silica refractory, which is bonded by the hydrolysis of ethyl silicate in the presence of hydrochloric acid. The product of the hydrolysis is a colloidal solution of silicic acid and ethyl alcohol, which can be written as follows:

$$Si(OC_2H_5)_4 + 4H_2O \xrightarrow{HCl} Si(OH)_4 + 4C_2H_5OH$$

In practice, however, the reaction is more complicated, and instead of tetra silicic acid, which is converted into $SiO_2 \cdot 2H_2O$, a polymerized compound of silicon is formed with the following structure:

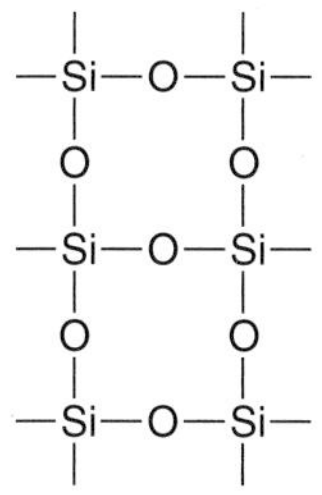

This material has an even higher silica content and better refractory properties than the $SiO_2 \cdot 2H_2O$.

Ethyl silicate has the disadvantage of giving off flammable components during processing, and the method is expensive; thus other techniques and methods have been developed to reduce the use of this material. Sodium silicate and colloidal silica are more common binders of the silica type.

Today this investment is usually supplied with two bottles of special liquid, instead of water, with which the investment powder should be mixed. In one of the bottles the manufacturer usually supplies a properly diluted water-soluble silicate solution. The other bottle usually contains a properly diluted acid solution, such as a solution of hydrochloric acid. The contents of each bottle can be stored almost indefinitely. Before use, an equal volume from each bottle is mixed and allowed to stand for a prescribed time, according to the manufacturer's instructions, so hydrolysis can take place and freshly prepared silicic acid forms.

American National Standards Institute/American Dental Association specification No. 126 (ISO 11246) for ethyl silicate casting investments specifies setting time, compressive strength, and linear thermal expansion. The setting time must not differ by more than 30% from the time stated by the manufacturer. The compressive strength at room temperature shall not be less than 1.5 MPa. The linear thermal expansion must not differ by more than 15% from the time stated by the manufacturer.

Brazing Investment

When brazing (soldering) the parts of a restoration, such as clasps on a removable partial denture framework, the parts must be surrounded with a suitable ceramic or investment material before the heating operation. The assembled parts are temporarily held together with sticky wax until they are surrounded with the appropriate investment material, after which the wax is softened and removed. The portion to be soldered is left exposed and free from investment to permit wax removal and effective heating before it is joined with solder.

American National Standards Institute/American Dental Association specification No. 126 (ISO 11244) for dental brazing investments defines two types of investment:

Type 1: Gypsum-bonded dental brazing investments
Type 2: Phosphate-bonded dental brazing investments

The specification specifies quality, fluidity, setting time, compressive strength, linear thermal expansion, and linear setting expansion. The setting time must not differ by more than 30% from the time stated by the manufacturer. The compressive strength shall be in the range of 2.0 to 10 MPa. The linear setting and thermal expansions must not differ by more than 15% from the time stated by the manufacturer.

The investment for soldering low-melting-point alloys is similar to casting investments containing quartz and a calcium sulfate hemihydrate binder. For high-melting-point alloys, a phosphate-bonded investment is used.

Soldering investments are designed to have lower setting and thermal expansions than casting investments, a feature that is desirable so the assembled parts do not shift in position during the setting and heating of the investment. Soldering investments are often made of ingredients that do not have as fine a particle size as the casting investment because the smoothness of the mass is less important.

Investments for All-Ceramic Restorations

Two types of investment materials have been developed for producing all-ceramic restorations. The first type is used for the cast glass technique. This investment is provided by the manufacturer of the glass casting equipment and is composed of phosphate-bonded refractories. The second type of all-ceramic investment is the refractory die type of material, which is used for all-ceramic veneers, inlays, and crowns. Refractory dies are made by pouring the investment into impressions. When the investment is set, the die is removed and is heated to remove gases that may be detrimental to the ceramic (degassing). A refractory die spacer may be added to the surface. Next, porcelain or other ceramic powders are added to the die surface and fired. These materials must accurately reproduce the impression, remain undamaged during the porcelain firing, and have a thermal expansion compatible with that of the ceramic (otherwise the ceramic could crack during cooling). These materials are also phosphate-bonded, and they generally contain fine-grained refractory fillers to allow accurate reproduction of detail. ANSI/ADA specification No. 126 (ISO 11245) for phosphate-bonded refractory die materials describes the required properties.

Bibliography

Review Articles: Impression Materials

Allen EP, Bayne SC, Becker IM, et al. Annual review of selected dental literature: report of the committee on scientific investigation of the American Academy of Restorative Dentistry. *J Prosthet Dent.* 1999;82(1):27–66.

Allen EP, Bayne SC, Donovan TE, et al. Annual review of selected dental literature. *J Prosthet Dent.* 1996;76(1):56–93.

Craig RG. Review of dental impression materials. *Adv Dent Res.* 1988;2(1):51–64.

Donovan TE, Chee WW. A review of contemporary impression materials and techniques. *Dent Clin North Am.* 2004;48(2):vi–vii, 445–470.

Jendresen MD, Allen EP, Bayne SC, et al. Annual review of selected dental literature: report of the committee on scientific investigation of the American Academy of Restorative Dentistry. *J Prosthet Dent.* 1998;80:81–120.

Whitters CJ, Strang R, Brown D, et al. Dental materials: 1997 literature review. *J Dent.* 1999;27:401–435.

Punj A, Bompolaki D, Garaicoa J. Dental impression materials and techniques. *Dent Clin North Am.* 2017;61(4):779–796. doi: 10.1016/j.cden.2017.06.004 28886768.

Agar and Alginate Hydrocolloids

Bergman B, Bergman M, Olsson S. Alginate impression materials, dimensional stability and surface detail sharpness following treatment with disinfectant solutions. *Swed Dent J.* 1985;9:255–262.

Buchan S, Peggie RW. Role of ingredients in alginate impression compounds. *J Dent Res.* 1966;45:1120–1129.

Cserna A, Crist R, Adams A, et al. Irreversible hydrocolloids: a comparison of antimicrobial efficacy. *J Prosthet Dent.* 1994;71:387–389.

Ellis B, Lamb DJ. The setting characteristics of alginate impression materials. *Br Dent J.* 1981;151:343–346.

Fish SF, Braden M. Characterization of the setting process in alginate impression materials. *J Dent Res.* 1964;43:107–117.

Ghani F, Hobkirk JA, Wilson M. Evaluation of a new antiseptic-containing alginate impression material. *Br Dent J.* 1990;169:83–86.

Hall BD, Munoz-Viveros CA, Naylor WP, et al. Effects of a chemical disinfectant on the physical properties of dental stones. *Int J Prosthodont.* 2004;17:65–71.

Hilton T, Schwartz R, Bradley D. Immersion disinfection of irreversible hydrocolloid impressions. Part II: effects on gypsum casts. *Int J Prosthodont.* 1994;7:424–433.

Hutchings MI, Vanderwalle K, Schwartz R, et al. Immersion disinfection of irreversible hydrocolloid impressions in pH-adjusted sodium hypochlorite. Part 2: effect on gypsum casts. *Int J Prosthodont.* 1996;9:223–229.

Johnson GH, Chellis KD, Gordon GE, et al. Dimensional stability and detail reproduction of alginate and elastomeric impressions disinfected by immersion. *J Prosthet Dent.* 1998;79:446–453.

MacPherson GW, Craig RG, Peyton FA. Mechanical properties of hydrocolloid and elastomeric impression materials. *J Dent Res.* 1967;46:714–721.

Miller MW. Syneresis in alginate impression materials. *Br Dent J.* 1975;139:425–430.

Murata H, Kawamura M, Hamada T, et al. Physical properties and compatibility with dental stones of current alginate impression materials. *J Oral Rehabil.* 2004;31:1115–1122.

Peutzfeldt A, Asmussen E. Effect of disinfecting solutions on accuracy of alginate and elastomeric impressions. *Scand J Dent Res.* 1989;97:470–475.

Peutzfeldt A, Asmussen E. Effect of disinfecting solutions on surface texture of alginate and elastomeric impressions. *Scand J Dent Res.* 1990;98:74–81.

Schwartz R, Bradley D, Hilton T, et al. Immersion disinfection of irreversible hydrocolloid impressions. Part I: microbiology. *Int J Prosthodont.* 1994;7:418–423.

Vanderwalle K, Charlton D, Schwartz R, et al. Immersion disinfection of irreversible hydrocolloid impressions with sodium hypochlorite. Part II: effect on gypsum. *Int J Prosthodont.* 1994;7:315–322.

Wanis TM, Combe EC, Grant AA. Measurement of the viscosity of irreversible hydrocolloids. *J Oral Rehabil.* 1993;20:379–384.

Wilson HJ. Elastomeric impression materials. 1. The setting material. *Br Dent J.* 1966;121:277–283.

Woodward JD, Morris JC, Khan Z. Accuracy of stone casts produced by perforated trays and nonperforated trays. *J Prosthet Dent.* 1985;53:347–350.

Properties and Use of Elastomeric Impression Materials

Baumann MA. The influence of dental gloves on the setting of impression materials. *Br Dent J.* 1995;179:130–135.

Boening KW, Walter MH, Schuette U. Clinical significance of surface activation of silicone impression materials. *J Dent.* 1998;26:447–452.

Chai J, Pand IC. A study of the thixotropic property of elastomeric impression materials. *Int J Prosthodont.* 1994;7:155–158.

Chen SY, Liang WM, Chen FN. Factors affecting the accuracy of elastometric impression materials. *J Dent.* 2004;32:603–609.

Cho GC, Chee WW. Distortion of disposable plastic stock trays when used with putty vinyl polysiloxane impression materials. *J Prosthet Dent.* 2004;92:354–358.

Chong YH, Soh G. Effectiveness of intraoral delivery tips in reducing voids in elastomeric impressions. *Quint Int.* 1991;22:897–900.

Cook WD. Permanent set and stress relaxation in elastomeric impression materials. *J Biomed Mater Res.* 1981;15:449–463.

Cook WD. Rheological studies of the polymerization of elastomeric impression materials. I. Network structure of the set state. *J Biomed Mater Res.* 1982;16:315–330.

Cook WD. Rheological studies of the polymerization of elastomeric impression materials. II. Viscosity measurements. *J Biomed Mater Res.* 1982;16:331–344.

Cook WD. Rheological studies of the polymerization of elastomeric impression materials. III. Dynamic stress relaxation modulus. *J Biomed Mater Res.* 1982;16:345–357.

Cook WD, Liem F, Russo P, et al. Tear and rupture of elastomeric dental impression materials. *Biomaterials.* 1984;5:275–280.

Craig RG. Evaluation of an automatic mixing system for an addition silicone impression material. *J Am Dent Assoc.* 1985;110:213–215.

Craig RG, Sun Z. Trends in elastomeric impression materials. *Oper Dent.* 1994;19:138–145.

Craig RG, Urquiola NJ, Liu CC. Comparison of commercial elastomeric impression materials. *Oper Dent.* 1990;15:94–104.

Gordon GE, Johnson GH, Drennon DG. The effect of tray selection on the accuracy of elastomeric impression materials. *J Prosthet Dent.* 1990;63:12–15.

Herfort TW, Gerberich WW, Macosko CW, et al. Viscosity of elastomeric impression materials. *J Prosthet Dent.* 1977;38:396–404.

Herfort TW, Gerberich WW, Macosko CW, et al. Tear strength of elastomeric impression materials. *J Prosthet Dent.* 1978;39:59–62.

Hondrum S. Tear and energy properties of three impression materials. *Int J Prosthodont.* 1994;7:517–521.

Idris B, Houston F, Claffey N. Comparison of the dimensional accuracy of one-step techniques with the use of putty/wash addition silicone impression materials. *J Prosthet Dent.* 1995;74:535–541.

Inoue K, Wilson HJ. Viscoelastic properties of elastomeric impression materials. II. Variation of rheological properties with time, temperature and mixing proportions. *J Oral Rehabil.* 1978;5:261–267.

Johansson EG, Erhardson S, Wictorin L. Influence of stone mixing agents, impression materials and lubricants on surface hardness and dimensions of a dental stone die material. *Acta Odontol Scand.* 1975;33:17–25.

Johnson GH, Craig RG. Accuracy of four types of rubber impression materials compared with time of pour and a repeat pour of models. *J Prosthet Dent.* 1985;53:484–490.

Johnson GH, Craig RG. Accuracy of addition silicones as a function of technique. *J Prosthet Dent.* 1986;55:197–203.

Kim KN, Craig RG, Koran A 3rd. Viscosity of monophase addition silicones as a function of shear rate. *J Prosthet Dent.* 1992;67:794–798.

Koran A, Powers JM, Craig RG. Apparent viscosity of materials used for making edentulous impressions. *J Am Dent Assoc.* 1977;95:75–79.

Lampe I, Marton S, Hegedus C. Effect of mixing technique on shrinkage rate of one polyether and two polyvinyl siloxane impression materials. *Int J Prosthodont.* 2004;17:590.

Laufer BZ, Baharav H, Ganor Y, et al. The effect of marginal thickness on the distortion of different impression materials. *J Prosthet Dent.* 1996;76:466–471.

Lee IK, Delong R, Pintado MR, et al. Evaluation of factors affecting the accuracy of impressions using quantitative surface analysis. *Oper Dent.* 1995;20:246–252.

Lepe X, Johnson GH, Berg JC, et al. Effect of mixing technique on surface characteristics of impression materials. *J Prosthet Dent.* 1998;79:495–502.

Lorren RA, Salter DJ, Fairhurst CW. The contact angles of die stone on impression materials. *J Prosthet Dent.* 1976;36:176–180.

Lu H, Nguyen B, Powers JM. Mechanical properties of 3 hydrophilic addition silicone and polyether elastomeric impression materials. *J Prosthet Dent.* 2004;92:151–154.

Mansfield MA, Wilson HJ. Elastomeric impression materials: a comparison of methods for determining working and setting times. *Br Dent J.* 1972;132:106–110.

McCabe JF, Arikawa H. Rheological properties of elastomeric impression materials before and during setting. *J Dent Res.* 1998;77:1874–1880.

McCabe JF, Bowman AJ. The rheological properties of dental impression materials. *Br Dent J.* 1981;151:179–183.

McCabe JF, Storer R. Elastomeric impression materials. The measurement of some properties relevant to clinical practice. *Br Dent J.* 1980;149:73–79.

Michalakis KX, Pissiotis A, Anastasiadou V, et al. An experimental study on particular physical properties of several interocclusal recording media. Part III: resistance to compression after setting. *J Prosthodont.* 2004;13:233–237.

Neissen LC, Strassler H, Levinson PD, et al. Effect of latex gloves on setting time of polyvinylsiloxane putty impression material. *J Prosthet Dent.* 1986;55:128–129.

Norling BK, Reisbick MH. The effect of nonionic surfactants on bubble entrapment in elastomeric impression materials. *J Prosthet Dent.* 1979;42:342–347.

Ohsawa M, Jorgensen KD. Curing contraction of addition-type silicone impression materials. *Scand J Dent Res.* 1983;91:51–54.

Pang IC, Chai J. The effect of a shear load on the viscosities of ten vinyl polysiloxane impression materials. *J Prosthet Dent.* 1994;71:177–182.

Pratten DH, Craig RG. Wettability of a hydrophilic addition silicone impression material. *J Prosthet Dent.* 1989;61:197–202.

Rueda LJ, Sy-Munoz JT, Naylor WP, et al. The effect of using custom or stock trays on the accuracy of gypsum casts. *Int J Prosthodont.* 1996;9:367–373.

Salem NS, Combe EC, Watts DC. Mechanical properties of elastomeric impression materials. *J Oral Rehabil.* 1988;15:125–132.

Sandrik JL, Vacco JL. Tensile and bond strength of putty-wash elastomeric impression materials. *J Prosthet Dent.* 1983;50:358–361.

Schelb E, Cavazos E Jr, Troendle KB, et al. Surface detail reproduction of type IV dental stones with selected polyvinyl siloxane impression materials. *Quint Int.* 1991;22:51–55.

Sneed WD, Miller R, Olean J. Tear strength of ten elastomeric impression materials. *J Prosthet Dent.* 1983;49:511–513.

Stackhouse JA Jr. The accuracy of stone dies made from rubber impression materials. *J Prosthet Dent.* 1970;24:377–386.

Stackhouse Jr JA. Relationship of syringe-tip diameter to voids in elastomeric impressions. *J Prosthet Dent.* 1985;53:812–815.

Tolley LG, Craig RG. Viscoelastic properties of elastomeric impression materials. *J Oral Rehabil.* 1978;5:121–128.

Vermilyea SG, Huget EF, de Simon LB. Apparent viscosities of setting elastomers. *J Dent Res.* 1980;59:1149–1151.

Williams JR, Craig RG. Physical properties of addition silicones as a function of composition. *J Oral Rehabil.* 1988;15:639–650.

Disinfection of Elastomeric Impression Materials

Bergman M, Olsson S, Bergman B. Elastomeric impression materials: dimensional stability and surface sharpness following treatment with disinfection solutions. *Swed Dent J.* 1980;4:161–167.

Drennon DG, Johnson GH. The effect of immersion disinfection of elastomeric impressions on the surface detail reproduction of improved gypsum casts. *J Prosthet Dent.* 1990;63:233–241.

Drennon DG, Johnson GH, Powell GL. The accuracy and efficacy of disinfection by spray atomization on elastomeric impressions. *J Prosthet Dent.* 1989;62:468–475.

Johnson GH, Drennon DG, Powell GL. Accuracy of elastomeric impressions disinfected by immersion. *J Am Dent Assoc.* 1988;116:525–530.

Lepe X, Johnson GH. Accuracy of polyether and addition silicone after long-term immersion disinfection. *J Prosthet Dent.* 1997;78:245–249.

Lepe X, Johnson GH, Berg JC. Surface characteristics of polyether and addition silicone impression materials after long term disinfection. *J Prosthet Dent.* 1995;74:181–186.

Morgano SM, Rios MP, Stein RS, et al. Effects of chemical disinfectant solutions on the stability and accuracy of the dental impression complex. *J Prosthet Dent.* 1996;76:356–362.

Storer R, McCabe JF. An investigation of methods available for sterilising impressions. *Br Dent J.* 1981;151:217–219.

Thouati A, Deveraux E, Lost A, et al. Dimensional stability of seven elastomeric impression materials immersed in disinfectants. *J Prosthet Dent.* 1996;76:8–14.

Tray Materials

Carrotte PV, Johnson A, Winstanley RB. The influence of the impression tray on the accuracy of impressions for crown and bridge work—an investigation and review. *Br Dent J.* 1998;185:580–585.

Martinez LJ, von Fraunhofer JA. The effects of custom try material on the accuracy of master casts. *J Prosthodont.* 1998;7:106–110.

Millstein P, Maya A, Segura C. Determining the accuracy of stock and custom tray impression/casts. *J Oral Rehabil.* 1998;25:645–648.

Pagniano RP, Scheid RC, Clowson RL, et al. Linear dimensional change of acrylic resins used in the fabrication of custom trays. *J Prosthet Dent.* 1982;47:279–283.

Dental Plaster and Stone

Chong JA, Chong MP. Docking AR. The surface of gypsum cast in alginate impression. *Dent Pract.* 1965;16:107–109.

Docking AR. Some gypsum precipitates. *Aust Dent J.* 1965;10:428–430.

Earnshaw R. The consistency of gypsum products. *Aust Dent J.* 1973;18:33–37.

Earnshaw R, Smith DC. The tensile and compressive strength of plaster and stone. *Aust Dent J.* 1966;11:415–422.

Fairhurst CW. Compressive properties of dental gypsum. *J Dent Res.* 1960;39:812–824.

Fan PL, Powers JM, Reid BC. Surface mechanical properties of stone, resin, and metal dies. *J Am Dent Assoc.* 1981;103:408–411.

Garber DK, Powers JM, Brandau HE. Effect of spatulation on the properties of high-strength dental stones. *J Mich Dent Assoc.* 1985;67:133–136.

Hollenback GM, Smith DD. A further investigation of the physical properties of hard gypsum. *J Calif Dent Assoc.* 1967;43:221–227.

Mahler DB. Hardness and flow properties of gypsum materials. *J Prosthet Dent.* 1951;1:188–195.

Mahler DB, Asgarzadeh K. The volumetric contraction of dental gypsum material on setting. *J Dent Res.* 1953;32:354–361.

Sanad ME, Combe EC, Grant AA. The use of additives to improve the mechanical properties of gypsum products. *J Dent Res.* 1982;61:808–810.

Sarma AC, Neiman R. A study on the effect of disinfectant chemicals on physical properties of die stone. *Quint Int.* 1990;21:53–59.

Stern MA, Johnson GH, Toolson LB. An evaluation of dental stones after repeated exposure to spray disinfectants. Part I: abrasion and compressive strength. *J Prosthet Dent.* 1991;65:713–718.

Torrance A, Darvell BW. Effect of humidity on calcium sulphate hemihydrate. *Aust Dent J.* 1990;35:230–235.

von Fraunhofer JA, Spiers RR. Strength testing of dental stone: a comparison of compressive, tensile, transverse, and shear strength tests. *J Biomed Mater Res*. 1983;17:293–299.

Wiegman-Ho L, Ketelaar JA. The kinetics of the hydration of calcium sulfate hemihydrate investigated by an electric conductance method. *J Dent Res*. 1982;61:36–40.

Williams GJ, Bates JF, Wild S. The effect of surface treatment of dental stone with resins. *Quint Dent Technol*. 1983;7:41–45.

Casting Investments

Anderson JN. *Applied Dental Materials*. 5th ed. Blackwell Scientific; 1976.

Asgar K. Casting restorations. In: Clark JW, ed. *Clinical Dentistry*. vol. 4. Harper & Row; 1976.

Asgarzadeh K, Mahler DB, Peyton FA. The behavior and measurement of hygroscopic expansion of dental casting investment. *J Dent Res*. 1954;33:519–530.

Chew CL, Land MF, Thomas CC, et al. Investment strength as a function of time and temperature. *J Dent*. 1999;27:297–302.

Docking AR, Chong MP. The hygroscopic setting expansion of dental casting investments. IV. *Aust J Dent*. 1949;53:261–267.

Eames WB, Edwards CR Jr, Buck WH Jr. Scraping resistance of dental die materials: a comparison of brands. *Oper Dent*. 1978;3:66–72.

Earnshaw R. The effect of restrictive stress on the thermal expansion of gypsum-bonded investments. I. Inlay casting investments, "thermal expansion" type. *Aust Dent J*. 1966;11:345–350.

Earnshaw R. The effects of additives on the thermal behaviour of gypsum-bonded casting investments. I. *Aust Dent J*. 1975;20:27–31.

Earnshaw R, Morey EF, Edelman DC. The effect of potential investment expansion and hot strength on the fit of full crown castings made with phosphate-bonded investment. *J Oral Rehabil*. 1997;24:532–539.

Higuchi T. Study of thermal decomposition of gypsum bonded investment. I. Gas analysis, differential thermal analysis, thermobalance analysis, x-ray diffraction. *Kokubyo Gakkai Zasshi*. 1967;34:217–224.

Jones DW. Thermal analysis and stability of refractory investments. *J Prosthet Dent*. 1967;18:234–241.

Jones DW, Wilson HJ. Setting and hygroscopic expansion of investments. *Br Dent J*. 1970;129:22–26.

Luk HW-K, Darvell BW. Strength of phosphate-bonded investments at high temperature. *Dent Mater*. 1991;7:99–102.

Luk HW-K, Darvell BW. Effect of burnout temperature on strength of phosphate-bonded investments. *J Dent*. 1997;25:153–160.

Luk HW-K, Darvell BW. Effect of burnout temperature on strength of phosphate-bonded investments—part II: effect of metal temperature. *J Dent*. 1997;25:423–430.

Lyon HW, Dickson G, Schoonover IC. Effectiveness of vacuum investing in the elimination of surface defects in gold castings. *J Am Dent Assoc*. 1953;46:197–198.

Miyaji T, Utsumi K, Suzuki E, et al. Deterioration of phosphate-bonded investment on exposure to 100% relative humidity atmosphere. *Bull Tokyo Med Dent Univ*. 1982;29:53–62.

Mori T. Thermal behavior of the gypsum binder in dental casting investments. *J Dent Res*. 1986;65:877–884.

Neiman R, Sarma AC. Setting and thermal reactions of phosphate investments. *J Dent Res*. 1980;59:1478–1485.

O'Brien WJ, Nielsen JP. Decomposition of gypsum investment in the presence of carbon. *J Dent Res*. 1959;38:541–547.

Phillips RW. Relative merits of vacuum investing of small castings as compared to conventional methods. *J Dent Res*. 1947;26:343–352.

Ryge G, Fairhurst CW. Hygroscopic expansion. *J Dent Res*. 1956;35:499–508.

Schilling ER, Miller BH, Woody RD, et al. Marginal gap of crowns made with a phosphate-bonded investment and accelerated casting method. *J Prosthet Dent*. 1999;81:129–134.

Shell JS, Hollenback GM. Setting and thermal investment expansion in longitudinal and transverse directions. *J Calif Dent Assoc*. 1965;41:511–514.

Tiara M, Okazaki M, Takahashi J, et al. Effects of four mixing methods on setting expansion and compressive strength of six commercial phosphate-bonded silica investments. *J Oral Rehabil*. 2000;27:306–311.

Weinstein LJ. Composition for dental molds. *U.S. Patent.*. 1929;1:708436.

Zarb GA, Bergman B, Clayton JA, MacKay HF, eds. *Prosthodontic Treatment for Partially Edentulous Patients*. Mosby; 1978.

12 Cementation

ROBERTO R. BRAGA

CHAPTER OUTLINE

Cementation is one of the final steps in the sequence of clinical procedures for indirect restorations. There are two objectives for the cementation, or luting, procedure: to help retain the restoration in place and to maintain the integrity of the remaining tooth structure. Retention is achieved by friction (or micromechanical interlocking), by an adhesive joint consisting of the prepared tooth, the cement, and the restoration, or a combination of both mechanisms. An effective interfacial seal depends on the ability of the cement to fill the irregularities between the tooth and the restoration and to resist the action of the oral environment, short and long term. Adhesion is also important in this context because a strong bond between the luting agent and the dental substrates may help prevent bacteria from colonizing the interface and minimizing the transit of fluids that may cause dentin hypersensitivity.

This chapter describes the composition, properties, manipulation, and indications for use of acid-base and resin-based cements. Acid-base cements are easy to use and, when correctly indicated, provide good long-term clinical service. Some release fluoride and chemically bond to tooth structures. Resin cements have a chemistry based on resin composites. They show high bond strengths to tooth structures. Some products also contain monomers that are compatible with primers that enable bonding to metal alloys and ceramics. In general, resin cements have better mechanical properties than acid-base cements, but the cementation process is more technique-sensitive.

The fundamental technologies and chemistries used to formulate the various types of adhesives and luting cements are derived from their corresponding restorative materials. However, in most cases, modifications have been made to create formulations suitable for a particular clinical application in terms of viscosity and handling characteristics.

Different clinical situations require different luting agents and no one material is recommended for every case. Therefore it is important to differentiate luting cements based on their mechanical properties and overall characteristics to identify the best options available for each clinical situation.

Classification and Characteristics of Luting Agents

Classification

Luting agents can be classified according to the length of time they are expected to stay in function as provisional or definitive. Provisional (temporary) cements are recommended for fixation of temporary restorations used between the clinical appointments necessary to finish the definitive restoration. Because temporary restorations often need to be removed during treatment, provisional cements must have a relatively low strength and be easily handled. Also, they must not irritate the pulp. Examples of temporary luting agents are zinc oxide–eugenol and non-eugenol cements and calcium hydroxide pastes. Definitive cements must remain in function for the longest time possible and, as such, must have sufficient properties to withstand masticatory loads.

According to the setting mechanism, luting agents are divided into categories: those presenting an acid-base reaction (which include glass-ionomer, resin-modified glass ionomer, zinc oxide–eugenol, zinc polycarboxylate, and zinc phosphate), those that set by dissolution and reprecipitation in aqueous medium (calcium aluminate cements) and those setting by polymerization (resin cements, compomers, and self-adhesive resin cements). In some cases, this classification refers to the predominant setting mechanism because resin-modified glass ionomers also contain polymerizable groups, whereas compomers and self-adhesive resin cements also may have an acid-base reaction. A summary of the main classes of luting agents is shown in Table 12.1.

TABLE 12.1 Summary of Basic Composition (liquid in the row and powder in the column) and Resulting Luting Agents

	Phosphoric Acid	Eugenol	Polyacrylic Acid*	Resin Monomers
Zinc oxide	Zinc phosphate	Zinc oxide–eugenol	Zinc polycarboxylate	–
Silicate glass	Silicate cement	–	Glass ionomers (can be resin-modified)	Resin cements (can be acidic*)

The asterisk (*) indicates that the material may chemically bond to the tooth structure.

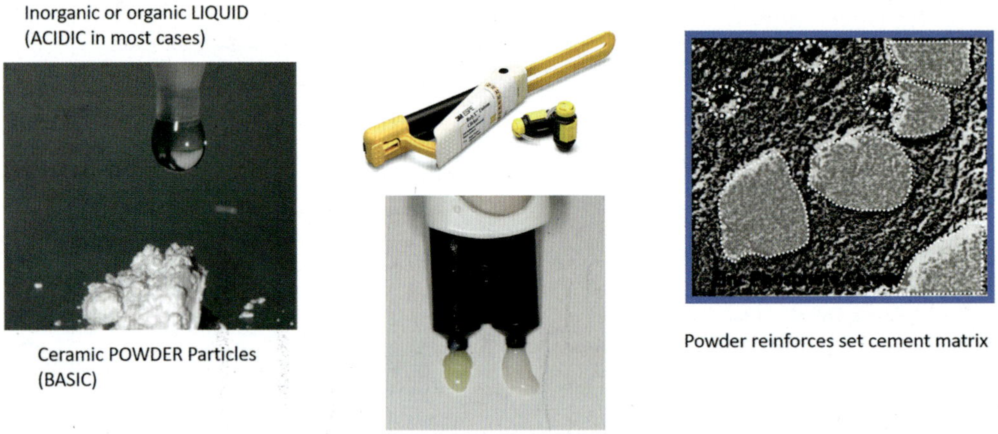

• **Fig. 12.1** Commercial presentation of luting agents (powder/liquid pairs or paste/paste pairs), being comprised essentially of a powder/filler-reinforced matrix.

• BOX 12.1 ISO Standards for Dental Cements

ISO 3107:2004 (zinc oxide–eugenol and non-eugenol cements)
ISO 9917-1:2007 (powder:liquid acid-base cements)
ISO 9917-2:2010 (resin-modified cements)
ISO 4049:2009 (polymer-based cements)

The physical requirements of luting cements are described in the following standards from the International Association for Standardization: ISO 3107:2004 (zinc oxide–eugenol and non-eugenol cements), ISO 9917-1:2007 (powder/liquid acid-base cements), ISO 9917-2:2010 (resin-modified cements), and ISO 4049:2009 (polymer-based cements) standards (Box 12.1). Those requirements, along with other important characteristics are described below.

Biocompatibility

Luting agents are often placed in contact with large areas of exposed dentin. Also, remaining dentin thickness can be insufficient to protect the pulp tissue from external stimuli. The majority of the luting agents show cytotoxicity in vitro, to different degrees. Histological studies also show early inflammatory reactions to cements placed close to connective tissue. Such responses are usually associated with the initial low pH of some acid-base cements, self-etch resin cements, or monomers present in resin-modified glass ionomers and resin cements.

Interfacial Sealing and Anticariogenic Activity

The sealing of the tooth/restoration interface is important to prevent bacteria penetration that may lead to secondary caries and also, when dentin is involved, prevent excessive fluid movement in the dentinal tubules that may cause hypersensitivity. Sealing is related to the ability of the cement to penetrate the irregularities of both substrates and establish an intimate contact with them. Ideally, luting cements should not shrink upon setting, or voids may develop at the interface. Adhesion also contributes to good interfacial sealing. Fluoride-containing cements are used in an attempt to inhibit bacterial activity; however, the clinical significance of fluoride release from luting cements is yet to be confirmed.

Adhesion

Lack of retention is a common cause of failure of indirect restorations. The use of adhesive materials may reduce the risk of displacement. In some instances (e.g., porcelain crowns), bonding may reduce the risk of restoration fracture. Adhesion may also help improve interfacial sealing. Adhesion may occur by chemical or physical bonding, micromechanical interlocking, or friction. Some acid-base cements and self-adhesive resin cements bond to dental tissues by chelation involving metal ions and carboxylic or phosphate groups. Resin cements require the use of adhesive systems to establish a strong bond to dentin and enamel.

Mechanical Properties

In general, luting agents are comprised of a filler-reinforced matrix, formed either by a powder/liquid pair or a paste/paste pair (Fig. 12.1). Mechanically, luting cements are described in terms of strength (usually in compression or in flexure), elastic modulus, fatigue resistance, fracture toughness, and wear. Wear is less of a problem, as long as the cement line is not exposed directly to masticatory forces (e.g., a full crown). Fatigue strength is usually considered more representative of the type of loading cements must endure in the clinic. However, fatigue tests are a lot more time-consuming than static strength tests (see Online Chapter 1). Elastic modulus expresses the amount of elastic (recoverable) deformation the cement presents relative to a stress state caused by external loading. Fracture toughness describes the resistance to unstable crack propagation that will cause catastrophic failure of the material.

Permanent luting cements must have high strength (both static and fatigue), fracture toughness, and good wear resistance. Ideal values for elastic modulus are debatable, and values can vary substantially even among permanent cements. Temporary cements, on the other hand, must have a relatively low strength; otherwise, the removal of the temporary restoration can become a difficult task.

Handling Properties and Radiopacity

Ease of use, long working time, and short setting time are desirable characteristics of luting cements. Along with powder and liquid materials, recent products are encapsulated or presented as two-paste, self-dispensing systems, which makes proportioning and mixing faster and less prone to error. A long working time is important to make sure the cement presents low viscosity while the restoration is seated. Otherwise, adaptation may be compromised. For some materials (e.g., resin cements), removal of excess cement also needs to be done before setting. Radiopacity is important to allow the excess cement to be diagnosed radiographically.

Viscosity and Film Thickness

Low film thickness is important to allow for the correct seating of the restoration. Film thickness is usually determined by the cement's average particle size and its viscosity. Some cements are pseudoplastic, behaving excessively thick at the end of the mixing period, but flowing well under a force. Overall, if handled properly and applied within the recommended working time, all currently available materials are able to reach a thickness below that required by the ISO standards (i.e., 25 μm). However, some cements may show a sudden increase in viscosity and film thickness if they continue to be manipulated after the end of the recommended working time.

Solubility

Solubility refers to the resistance to disintegration and dissolution when the cement is immersed in water or other solutions, such as saliva. It affects the marginal integrity of the indirect restoration, which may increase plaque accumulation. Resin-based cements present much lower solubility than acid-base cements.

Aesthetics

When used with translucent materials or when restoration margins are exposed, shade and translucency of the cement are important aspects to be considered because they may affect the final aesthetic result of the restoration. This is particularly critical with ceramic laminate veneers. Resin cements are the most aesthetic luting materials available. Glass ionomer, resin-modified glass ionomer, compomer, and self-adhesive resin cements also have good aesthetics. Zinc polyacrylate, zinc oxide–eugenol, and zinc phosphate are opaque.

Acid-Base Cements

Zinc Oxide–Eugenol and Non-eugenol Cements

The reaction between zinc oxide and eugenol has several applications in dentistry, such as endodontic sealers and root-end filling materials, periodontal dressing, inelastic impression materials, cavity bases, and temporary restorations. For luting purposes, different formulations of zinc oxide–eugenol (ZOE) cements are available for both temporary cementation and permanent fixation of metallic and metalloceramic crowns and bridges. Due to the inhibitory effect of eugenol on polymerization of methacrylate-based resins and luting composites, temporary cements using nonphenolic components are often preferred over conventional formulations. Their popularity is justified by their ease of use, antibacterial action, and anodyne effect (sedative) on the dental pulp. A video showing zinc-oxide eugenol (ZOE) cements as provisional materials is available online.

Composition

The powder is mainly composed of zinc oxide, with up to 8% of other zinc salts (acetate, propionate, or succinate) as accelerators. Rosin (abietic acid) is added to reduce brittleness and increase working time and strength. The liquid contains eugenol (4 allyl 2 methoxy phenol), a weak acid (Fig. 12.2). Acetic acid (up to 2%) is added as accelerator. In two-paste materials used for temporary cementation, one paste contains zinc oxide mixed with mineral or vegetable oils, whereas fillers are incorporated into eugenol to form the other paste. Non-eugenol materials use long-chain aliphatic acids or aryl-substituted butyric acid to react with zinc oxide particles. Other oils can be added to adjust paste consistency.

An important improvement of ZOE cements was the development of materials in which the liquid is a mixture of 2-ethoxybenzoic acid (EBA) and eugenol, roughly in a 2:1 ratio. Rather than forming a stronger matrix, the addition of EBA allows for the use of very high powder:liquid ratios (6:1), which intrinsically increases the strength of the set cement. In these materials, alumina (30%) was added to the powder as a reinforcing agent. The incorporation of 20% particulate poly(methyl methacrylate) is also used to improve mechanical properties in some products.

Setting Reaction and Structure

The reaction of zinc oxide with eugenol results in the formation of a zinc eugenolate chelate, that is, a complex in which one zinc (Zn) atom binds to two eugenolate molecules (Fig. 12.2). As the dissociation constant of eugenol is small, the reaction rate is increased with the use of more reactive oxides, along with the presence of accelerators. The acid-base reaction does not take place in an aqueous medium; however, water plays a very important role in the reaction because it reacts with zinc oxide forming $ZnOH^+$ ions that dissociate into Zn^{2+} and OH^-. The zinc cations then react with the eugenolate, whereas the hydroxyl anions react with the H^+ forming water. Because water is present both as a reagent and as a final product, the reaction is autocatalytic. The presence of acetic acid eliminates the need for water to initiate the reaction.

The structure of the set cement is represented by zinc oxide particles dispersed within an amorphous zinc eugenolate matrix. EBA also forms a chelate with zinc oxide, and crystalline phases have been identified within the matrix of EBA-eugenol cements.

Manipulation considerations for this material can be found on the book's website http://evolve.elsevier.com/sakaguchi/restorative

Properties

ZOE cements are considered biocompatible because of their neutral pH, antibacterial action, and anodyne effect on hyperemic pulpal tissue. Their antibacterial activity in vitro was shown to be more efficient than that displayed by conventional or resin-modified glass ionomers. That characteristic associated with good marginal sealing favors the recovery of the pulp. Eugenol released

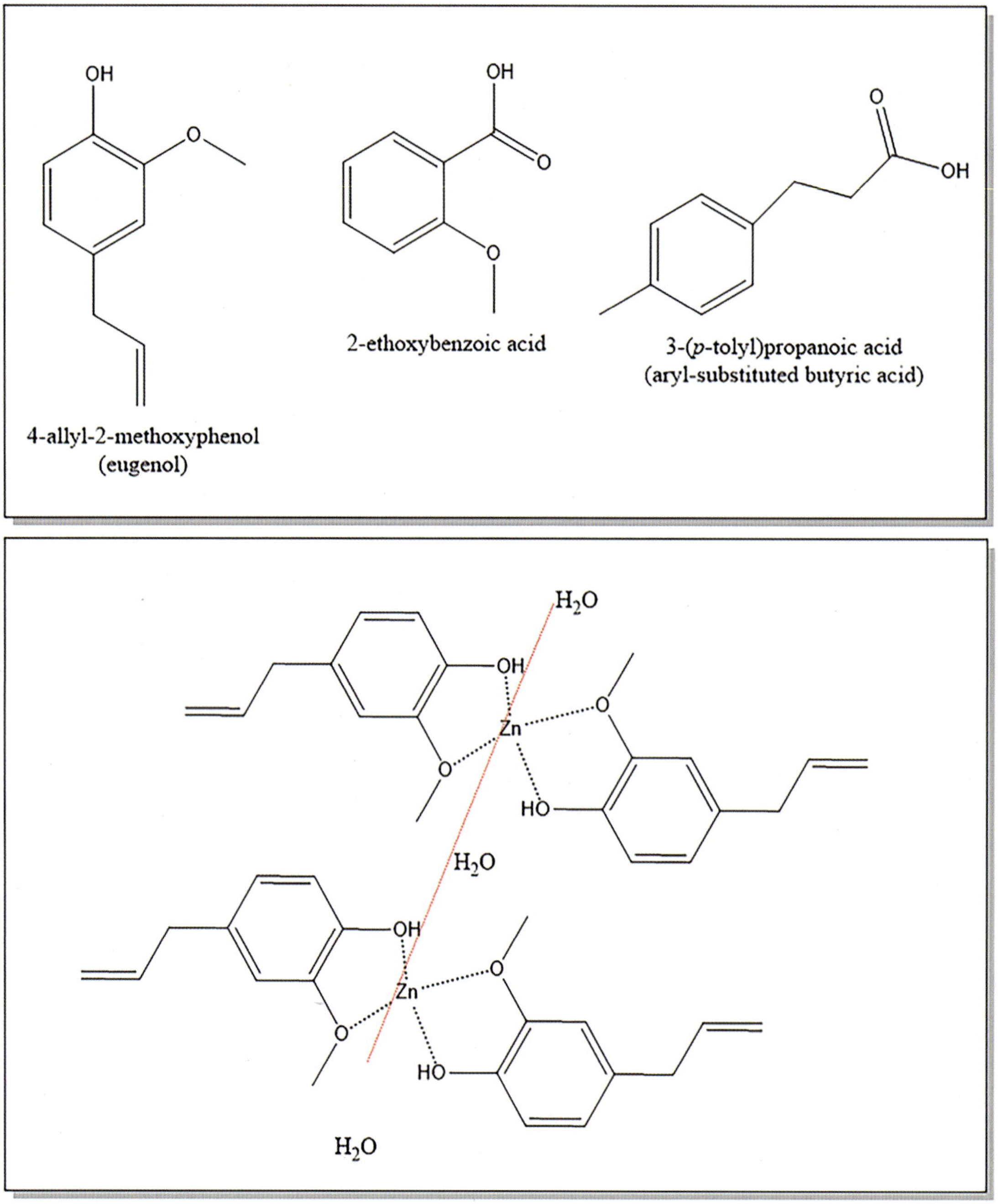

• **Fig. 12.2** Molecular structures for eugenol (4-allyl-2-methoxy phenol) and Aryl-substituted butyric acid molecule, used to replace eugenol in "non-eugenol" formulations. Also depicted: 2-ethoxybenzoic acid (EBA), used in association with eugenol in some reinforced ZOE formulations; zinc eugenolate structure, a chelate, product of the acid-base reaction between zinc hydroxide and eugenol.

from the salt matrix may contribute to pain relief in preparations with little remaining dentin thickness. However, in high concentrations, or when placed directly in contact with connective tissue, it may increase the inflammatory response because of its cytotoxicity.

The low strength displayed by ZOE cements makes them a suitable material for temporary cementation. The ISO 3107 standard (2004) establishes a maximum 24-hour compressive strength of 35 MPa for type 1 materials (i.e., those intended for temporary cementation). An important aspect related to the mechanical behavior of ZOE cements is that their properties are very sensitive to temperature. For example, compressive strength at 37°C may represent only 20% of what is present at 23°C. EBA-eugenol cements can be several times stronger than the basic formulation (72 MPa versus 26 MPa, in compression at room temperature). EBA-alumina cements can present 20% higher strength compared to EBA-eugenol materials. Though these values are above the minimum compressive strength required for type 2 materials (i.e., permanent luting cements) of 35 MPa, both reinforced ZOE cements are the weakest among luting agents used for permanent cementation. The elastic modulus of EBA-eugenol cements (determined at room temperature) is only 3 GPa.

Set ZOE cements present significant plasticity and flow under load. Plastic strain at fracture was shown to be above 15% at 37°C, as compared with a maximum value of 4% for other acid-base and resin cements. Creep behavior may explain the good marginal seal achieved with these materials, even considering their setting shrinkage. Linear shrinkage values of wet samples after 24 hours were shown to be 0.31% for the basic ZOE formulation, 0.38% for EBA-eugenol, and 0.12% for EBA-eugenol/alumina cements.

Film thickness measured according to the ISO standard ranges between 16 and 28 µm for EBA/alumina materials; therefore it is close to the maximum value allowed. Simulated crowns cemented with a basic formulation and an EBA-eugenol cement showed similar film thicknesses at the occlusal surface (20–25 µm), whereas film thickness was higher (57 µm) for the EBA-alumina cement.

The zinc eugenolate matrix chelate is very unstable in water. Its hydrolysis forms eugenol and zinc hydroxide, releasing the zinc oxide particles exposed in the process. In vitro studies showed that zinc 2-ethoxybenzoate matrix formed in EBA-eugenol cements is even more prone to hydrolysis than the zinc eugenolate. In vivo, material loss after 6 months was three to seven times higher for an EBA-alumina compared to other acid-base cements. Clinically, fixed prostheses cemented with EBA-alumina cement showed a success rate of 92% after 2.5 years, whereas for zinc polycarboxylate, it was 95%. Zinc phosphate, for many decades the "gold standard" for permanent luting agents, showed a success rate of 98%.

The inhibitory effect of methoxyphenols such as eugenol on the polymerization of methacrylate resins is of clinical importance. Eugenol is considered a *free-radical scavenger*, due to the presence of the allyl group in its structure acting as a degradative chain-transfer agent (i.e., when activated, it preferably undergoes primary radical termination, rather than propagation). Temporary cements containing eugenol may negatively affect the polymerization of methyl methacrylate used in provisional restorations. If the final restoration will be bonded to the prepared tooth, the polymerization of both the adhesive system and the resin cement may be inhibited, increasing the risk of debonding, or even fracture in case of low-strength ceramic or indirect composite restorations. In fact, in ZOE cement/composite interfaces, composite mechanical properties were reduced up to 100 µm away from the interface, which may be relevant if the resin cement is applied to a eugenol-contaminated surface. However, several in vitro investigations have shown that bond strength to dentin is not adversely affected if the surface is thoroughly cleaned prior to adhesive application.

Glass Ionomer

Glass-ionomer (or glass polyalkeonate) cement is arguably one of the most popular materials for permanent cementation used in the clinic, along with resin cements. The chemistry that is the basis for these cements is similar to that in glass-ionomer restorative, lining, and preventive materials (see Chapter 6), although there are some important differences in working and setting behavior to fit the needs of luting agents, which will be discussed later. Besides good physical properties, glass ionomers adhere to the tooth structure and metals and, most importantly, release significant amounts of fluoride, which increase the resistance of enamel and dentin to acid dissolution and act as a bacteriostatic agent. Fluoride release makes this material the first choice for cementation of orthodontic bands. It is indicated for cementation of metallic and metal-ceramic restorations, as well as high-strength ceramic crowns and fixed prostheses. Its setting reaction is sensitive to moisture conditions, and for this reason, it is extremely important to protect the cement against gain (imbibition) and loss (syneresis) of water during the first 24 hours.

Composition

Details of chemical composition and setting reaction are provided in Chapter 6. Briefly, the powder is a calcium fluoroaluminosilicate glass with maximum particle size of 15 µm. Other glasses can be formulated in which calcium is replaced by strontium or lanthanum to increase radiopacity. The basic character of the glass is defined by its alumina:silica ratio, which must exceed 1:2 by mass in order to react with acids. Large amounts of fluoride are incorporated in the glass by adding calcium and sodium fluoride to the other oxides. Fluoride is an important component because it lowers the melting point and enhances the translucency of the powder, and improves the consistency of the mixed paste and the strength of the set material. The presence of electropositive ions, such as Ca^{2+} and Na^+, is important to balance the electrical charges in the basic aluminosilicate lattice. Zinc oxide and barium glasses can be added to the powder to increase radiopacity.

The liquid contains homopolymers of acrylic acid or copolymers of acrylic, itaconic, maleic, and tricarboxylic acids. Overall, high molecular weights and increased acid concentrations improve physical properties of the set cement, but they also increase the viscosity of the liquid. Therefore commercial materials usually employ polyacids with average molecular weight of 10,000 g/mol and concentrations around 45% by mass. Dextrotartaric, or (+)-tartaric, acid (around 5% by mass) is an important component of the liquid because it accelerates the setting without shortening working time. Its presence increases cement strength and allows for the use of glasses with higher fluoride content and therefore higher translucency.

To avoid the increase in viscosity of the liquid after prolonged storage, some products contain the polyacid in freeze-dried form, added to the powder. In this case, the powder is mixed with distilled water or a tartaric acid solution. Such presentation adds the advantage of allowing the use of polyacids with higher molecular weight and in higher concentrations, which increases the strength of the set material.

Setting Reaction and Structure

When the powder is brought in contact with the acid solution, H^+ from the acid attacks the glass, releasing metal ions (Al^{3+}, Ca^{2+}, Na^+, and F^-) and silicic acid (general formula: $[SiO_x\{OH\}_{4-2x}]_n$). More details on the composition can be found in Chapter 6, and a schematic of the setting events is shown in Fig. 12.3. The silicic acid

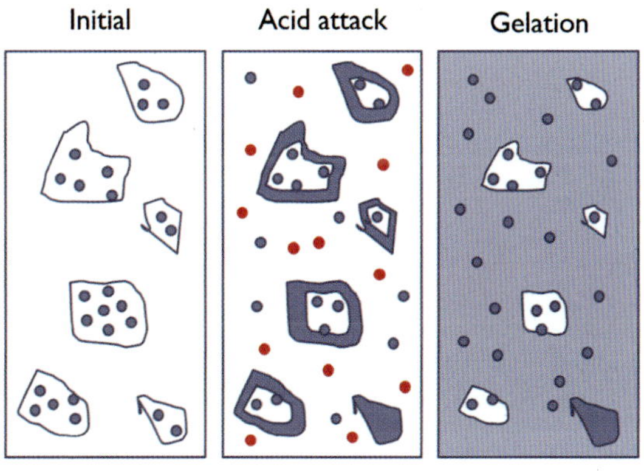

• **Fig. 12.3** Setting phases of a glass-ionomer cement.

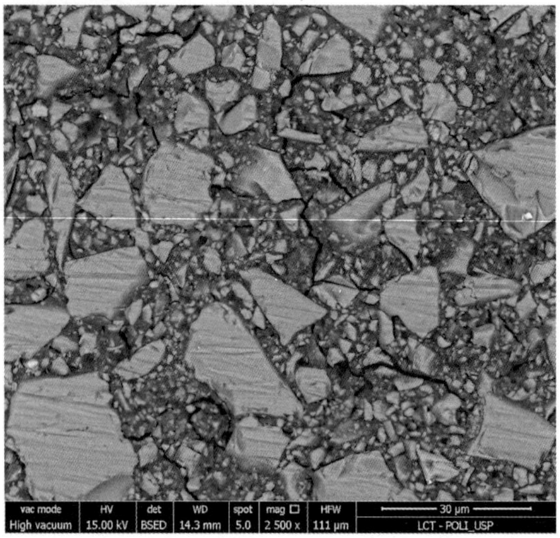

• **Fig. 12.4** Scanning electron microscope image of a conventional glass-ionomer cement microstructure. The unreacted glass particles are surrounded by calcium, aluminum, and fluoroaluminum polyacrylates. (Image courtesy of Dr. Handially Vilela).

condenses on the ion-depleted outer layer of the particle forming a layer of silica gel. Calcium ions are preferentially released from the glass. As the concentration of ions in the solution increases, the pH rises and metal ions begin to condense among the poly(acrylic acid) chains precipitating the polyacrylate salts, initially in a sol state (initial set) and later turning into a gel. The precipitation of aluminum salts initiates after a few hours into the reaction because it is released from the glass as a strong complex with fluoride. The reaction continues until all the ions are bound to the polyacrylate. From a clinical standpoint, the fact that ions remain in solution for extended periods of time before reacting with the polyanions, even after the initial set, is critical. If ions are washed out from the cement, the structure of the polysalt matrix is irreversibly compromised. Also, calcium polyacrylate is more vulnerable to dissolution in water than aluminum polyacrylate formed at later stages. On the other hand, water plays a very important role in the reaction and in the set cement because it remains tightly bound to the cement structure, hydrating the silica gel layer and involving the cation-polyacrylate bonds. Therefore a high relative humidity (approximately 80%) is the ideal condition for the setting reaction to take place.

The (+)-tartaric acid is a stronger acid than poly(acrylic acid) and therefore reacts first with the glass and can form complexes with metal cations at lower pH. Its presence extends working time by delaying the formation of calcium polyacrylate, and upon gelation, it accelerates the setting by increasing the deposition rate of aluminum polyacrylate.

The set cement is constituted by a hydrogel of calcium, aluminum, and fluoroaluminum polyacrylates involving the unreacted glass particles sheathed by a weakly bonded siliceous hydrogel layer (Fig. 12.4). About 20% to 30% of the glass is dissolved in the reaction. Smaller glass particles may be entirely dissolved and replaced by siliceous hydrogel particles containing fluorite crystallites. The stability of the matrix derives from the association of chain entanglements, weak ionic cross-linking, and hydrogen bonding.

Manipulation considerations can be found on the book's website http://evolve.elsevier.com/sakaguchi/restorative

Properties

Glass-ionomer cements are considered mild to the pulp compared to their predecessors, such as zinc phosphate, which used phosphoric acid solutions. However, inflammatory response is more intense than that associated with ZOE cements. In fact, the biocompatibility of glass ionomers is controversial, and in vitro results seem to vary according to the commercial brand tested. In general, there is some consensus regarding the fact that freshly mixed cements may present different degrees of cytotoxicity and cause a mild transient inflammatory response when placed in contact with pulpal connective tissue, but such response is greatly attenuated if at least 1-mm thickness of dentin is present. Besides a low remaining dentin thickness, the risk of postoperative sensitivity increases if a faulty technique is used. Thin mixtures seem to increase the risk of sensitivity. Rather than pulpal irritation, it is possible that postoperative pain may be related to the hydrostatic pressure exerted by the cement through the dentin tubules during placement of the restoration.

Glass-ionomer cements release significant amounts of fluoride, both in the short and long term, which was shown to have an important anticariogenic effect. Fluoride release increases the resistance of enamel to acid dissolution, inhibits bacterial growth, and interferes with the metabolism of the dental plaque. The use of glass ionomer for orthodontic bonding reduced the risk of white spot formation almost by half compared to resin cement. However, when patients were exposed to fluoride-containing toothpaste, no differences in enamel or dentin demineralization under accumulated plaque were observed in the short term between an ionomeric and a resin cement. It must be emphasized that the surface area of the luting cement exposed to the oral environment is small. Therefore the amount of fluoride released to the adjacent structures, as well as the fluoride recharging ability of the cement layer may be less clinically relevant compared to direct glass-ionomer restorations.

Bonding to tooth structures is one of the most advantageous features of glass ionomers. It helps enhance the marginal sealing of the restoration compared to nonadhesive cements but is not high enough to significantly increase retention. The proposed adhesion mechanism is twofold: it occurs by the displacement of phosphate ions from the hydroxyapatite by carboxylate ions pendant from the polyacid chains, and/or by the incorporation of these carboxylate groups into the hydroxyapatite structure. Either mechanism is aided by micromechanical interlocking achieved by a shallow hybridization of the partially demineralized dentin (Fig. 12.5). Dentin surface treatment with 10% to 20% polyacrylic acid for 5 to 20 seconds (shorter times for higher concentrations) significantly increases bond strength by removing the smear layer, partially demineralizing the surface creating microporosities for micromechanical interlocking, and enhancing the chemical interaction of poly(alkenoic acid) with the hydroxyapatite. A solution containing 3% to 10% citric acid is also effective because Fe^{3+} ions deposited on the dentin surface increase the interaction with the cement. Bond strength of glass ionomer to dentin and enamel varies according to commercial product tested, but when loaded in shear it is around 2 to 5 MPa. Glass-ionomer cements bond well to stainless steel, noble, and non-noble alloys and titanium, but not to ceramics.

The mechanical properties of glass ionomers are superior to those of other acid-base cements and increase significantly over long periods. Compressive strength is between 100 and 150 MPa; therefore it is far beyond the minimum of 70 MPa specified in the ISO 9917 standard. These cements are much weaker in tension because of their brittle nature, with diametral tensile strengths of about 6 MPa. Elastic modulus is around 15 GPa. Film thickness is below the maximum allowed by the ISO standard (25 µm) and should not prevent the correct seating of the restoration if the cement is properly handled.

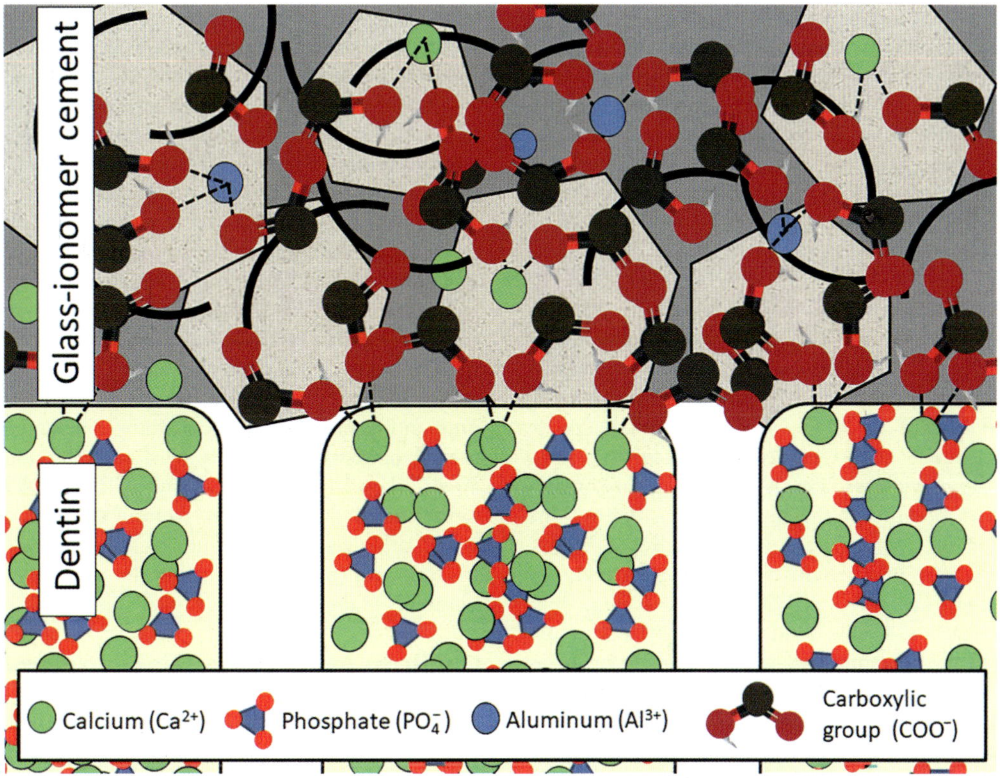

• **Fig. 12.5** Proposed adhesion mechanism to tooth structure for glass-ionomer cements. Ionized carboxylate groups displace phosphate ions from the hydroxyapatite and are incorporated into the hydroxyapatite structure.

Erosion tests in vitro using citric acid showed that the fully set glass ionomers are more resistant than nonadhesive acid-base luting cements and erode in levels similar to those shown by enamel and dentin. Such behavior may be related to the silica gel layer that envelopes the glass particles.

Resin-Modified Glass Ionomer

Resin-modified (or hybrid) glass ionomers set by both an acid-base and a polymerization reaction. The technology was originally developed for direct restoratives, but as with resin cements, the chemistry was adapted to formulate luting cements. Although details of chemistry and setting reactions of resin-modified glass-ionomer systems are provided in Chapter 6, this section gives a brief overview pertinent to luting cements. This class of cements does not show the early sensitivity to moisture conditions presented by conventional glass ionomers because of the presence of a polymeric phase, which prevents the loss of water and metal ions from the immature polysalt matrix. Available as a powder-liquid, paste-paste, or capsule system, self-cured resin-modified glass-ionomer luting cements are recommended for permanent cementation of ceramic-metal crowns and fixed prostheses; metal inlays, onlays, and crowns; prefabricated or cast posts; high-strength core ceramics; and luting of orthodontic appliances. A light-cured version recommended for orthodontic bracket bonding was also developed. One commercial example is shown in Fig. 12.6. One example of resin-modified glass ionomer cement used to cement a zirconia crown can be found online.

Composition

The chemistry of resin-modified glass ionomers is more complex than that of conventional glass ionomers (see Chapter 6).

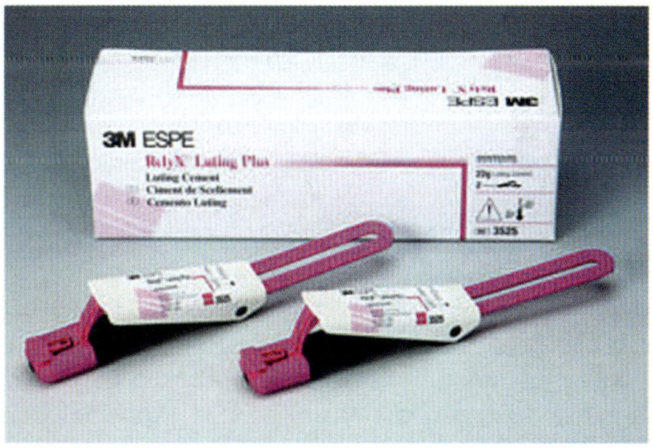

• **Fig. 12.6** Commercial example of a resin-modified glass-ionomer cement.

In powder-liquid systems, the powder contains fluoroaluminosilicate glass particles similar in composition to those found in conventional glass ionomers. Catalysts for the self-cure (redox) polymerization are added to the powder. The liquid may contain poly(acrylic acids) modified with pendant methacrylate groups replacing a small part of the carboxylic radicals, 2-hydroxyethyl methacrylate (HEMA), water, and tartaric acid. HEMA replaces part of the water and is a small molecule (molecular weight: 130 g/mol) soluble in water due to the presence of a hydroxyl group in its structure. Another liquid formulation contains similar concentrations (around 25–30% each) of a copolymer of poly(acrylic acid), HEMA, and water, and smaller amounts of low-viscosity dimethacrylate resins (such as urethane or triethyleneglycol dimethacrylates). Initiators for the light-cured polymerization, if present, are found in the liquid.

Formulations of paste-paste materials are brand-specific. Basically, one of the pastes contains the glass particles, HEMA, and a dispersing agent. Water and the reducing agent of the self-cure activation may be present, as well as possibly a urethane dimethacrylate. The other paste contains the modified poly(acrylic acid), water, the oxidizing agent of the activation system, and fillers and may contain HEMA or a high-viscosity dimethacrylate monomer, such as biphenol A glycidyl methacrylate (Bis-GMA).

Setting Reaction and Structure

The setting reaction of resin-modified glass-ionomer cement comprises two different mechanisms. The initial set is the result of either a light-cured or self-cured polymerization reaction of the methacrylate groups, present as pendant groups on the poly(acrylic acid) chain, in the HEMA molecule, or in the dimethacrylate monomers. Refer to reactions in Chapter 6. The acid-base reaction, described in the previous section, is slower than in conventional glass ionomers because of the lower water content. The HEMA polymer and the polysalt are linked by hydrogen bonds. However, phase separation between the two matrices formed may occur. The use of a modified poly(acrylic acid) prevents phase separation, because the carbon double bond in the HEMA structure may polymerize with the pendant methacrylate from the polyacid chain. As a result, the cement matrix is formed by both ionic and covalent crosslinks. For further discussion, refer to Chapter 6.

Manipulation considerations can be found on the book's website http://evolve.elsevier.com/sakaguchi/restorative

Properties

Resin-modified glass ionomers are considered less biocompatible than conventional glass ionomers because of the presence of HEMA. Besides its allergenic effect, it is a potential source of adverse reactions in the pulp. The largest amounts of HEMA are released in the first 24 hours, but release continues for several days. When resin-modified glass ionomer was placed in direct contact with human pulpal connective tissue, inflammatory responses from mild to severe and a large necrotic area were observed after almost 1 year. The liquid has low vapor pressure, so there is risk of inhalation and eye irritation. The release of free HEMA from the cement is higher in under-cured materials. Therefore the correct mixing technique must be used to optimize the polymerization. In light-cured materials, the recommended exposure conditions must be followed.

In vitro fluoride release by conventional and resin-modified luting glass ionomers was found to be similar over a 28-day period, ranging from 30 to 198 ppm, depending on the product and testing conditions. Mineral loss and lesion depth around orthodontic brackets in vitro were significantly lower with resin-modified glass ionomers, compared to one resin cement and one luting compomer. Fluoride release is higher after 24 hours, stabilizing at a much lower level after 2 weeks.

Resin-modified glass-ionomer cements show shear bond strength to conditioned dentin (10% citric acid, 2% ferric chloride for 20 seconds) or enamel (10% polyacrylic acid solution for 20 seconds) in the range of 8 to 12 MPa. The bonding mechanisms are the same as described for conventional glass ionomers. The lower bond strength to enamel compared to resin cements may actually facilitate orthodontic bracket debonding. They bond to metal alloys and high-strength ceramics, with initial shear bond strengths of 2 to 5 MPa. Bond strength to metal alloy is significantly increased with the use of metal primers. Because of the presence of methacrylate groups, these cements bond well to resin composites. Retention of metal-ceramic crowns to prepared teeth may vary significantly between the two-paste and the powder: liquid versions of the same product, and it is usually higher in the latter.

In terms of mechanical properties, resin-modified glass-ionomer cements show compressive strength similar to conventional glass ionomers, between 90 and 140 MPa, and lower elastic modulus (3 to 6 GPa). Flexural strength may vary between 15 and 30 MPa. Film thickness determined at room temperature 2 minutes after the start of mixing may vary between 9 and 25 μm. However, film thickness may increase substantially if the restoration is not placed within the recommended working time.

The presence of HEMA increases the water sorption of resin-modified glass ionomers, compared to conventional glass ionomers and resin cements. In fact, some manufacturers do not recommend its use for luting low-strength ceramic crowns because of the risk of fracture caused by swelling of the cement. Water uptake after 7 days measured according to ISO 4049 may be three to nine times higher compared to resin cements. Solubility in water is also about two to four times higher compared to resin cements. In lactic acid (pH = 4), the solubility of some resin-modified glass ionomers is about 10 times higher than resin cements.

Calcium Aluminate/Glass-Ionomer Cement

This material contains a mixture of monocalcium aluminate ($CaOAl_2O_3$), inert glasses, and, in some cases, glass-ionomer particles. The liquid can be either a polycarboxylic acid solution or a mixture of polyacrylic, tartaric, and neutral polycarboxylic acids. This material does not set solely by acid-base reaction, but also by dissolution and reprecipitation of the monocalcium aluminate particles. In contact with water, the monocalcium aluminate dissolves and reprecipitates as katoite ($Ca_3Al_2[SiO_4]_{1.5}[OH]_6$) and aluminum hydroxide ($Al[OH]_3$, or gibbsite). The new crystals attach to the tooth structure, which, combined with its alkaline pH, could reduce the risk of postoperative sensitivity. Due to its calcium content and high pH, these cements were shown to promote hydroxyapatite precipitation in vitro. The performance in terms of mechanical properties and crown retention (metal and ceramic) is similar to self-adhesive cements. Because the aluminum hydroxide initially forms as an amorphous gel, removal of excess cement is facilitated.

Resin-Based Cements

Resin Cements

Overview

Resin cements are low-viscosity composite materials with filler distribution and initiator content adjusted to allow for a low film thickness and suitable working and setting times. They have a wide range of applications, from inlays to fixed bridges, prefabricated posts, and orthodontic appliances (commercial examples shown in Fig. 12.7). They are mandatory materials for luting low-strength ceramic and laboratory-processed composite restorations, but can also be used with cast restorations, particularly in cases where extra retention is needed. The ISO specification 4049 (2009) classifies resin cements according to curing mode as class 1 (self-cured), class 2 (light-cured), or class 3 (dual-cured). Most of the commercial products are dual-cured, combining chemical and light-activation mechanisms. These materials show a comfortable working time and the same "cure on command"

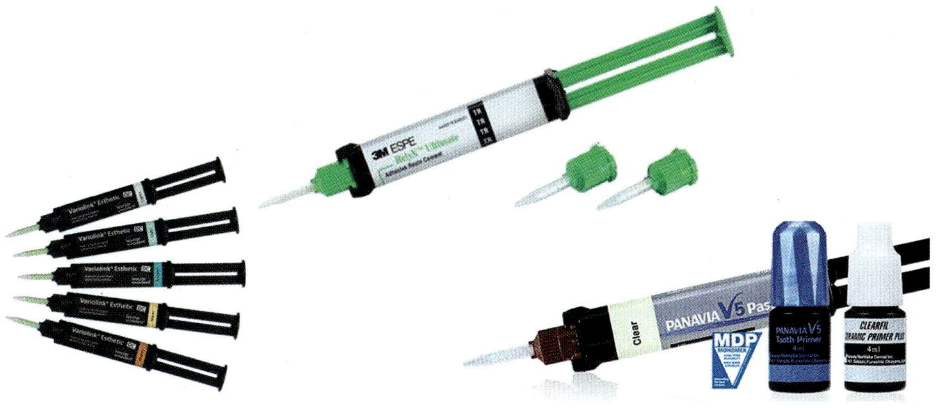

• **Fig. 12.7** Commercial examples of resin cements.

characteristic of light-cured composites, and also the security of high degrees of conversion even in areas not exposed to the light. Class 1 and class 3 materials are typically hand- or automixed two-paste systems (base and catalyst). Self-cured and dual-cured materials can be opaque or translucent, and those indicated for cementation of ceramic restorations are usually provided in several shades. Light-cured materials are indicated for bonding laminated ceramic veneers (aesthetic cements) or orthodontic brackets. Some aesthetic resin cements used for cementation of veneers include glycerin-based, water-soluble "try-in" pastes to help with shade selection. One example of a resin cement used to cement Lithium-disilicate restorations can be found online.

Composition

Most resin cements share a very similar composition to that of restorative composites, which are described in Chapter 8. The organic matrix contains dimethacrylate monomers and oligomers. High-molecular-weight molecules such as Bis-GMA (Mw = 512 g/mol), urethane dimethacrylate (UDMA, Mw = 480 g/mol), and ethoxylated Bis-GMA (Bis-EMA Mw = 540 g/mol) are combined with smaller molecules usually derived from ethylene glycol dimethacrylates (DEGDMA, Mw = 242 g/mol, and TEGDMA, Mw = 286 g/mol) to achieve a high degree of conversion with relatively low volumetric shrinkage. The filler fraction may vary between 30% and 66% by volume and comprises silanated radiopaque glasses such as barium, strontium, or zirconia, along with silica particles. Average filler size may vary between 0.5 and 8.0 µm. Microfilled cements are also available, with an average filler size of 40 nm. Pigments and opacifiers are also present in both pastes.

Some adhesive resin cements contain acidic monomers. One example combines 10-methacryloyloxydecyl dihydrogen phosphate (10-MDP), a polymerizable phosphoric acid ester, with Bis-GMA. Another product contains 4-methacryloxyethyl-trimellitic anhydride (4-META) and methylmethacrylate in the liquid, poly(methyl methacrylate) in the powder, and tri-n-butylborane (TBB) as catalyst.

Camphorquinone and a tertiary amine are present in one of the pastes to initiate the light-activated reaction. Benzoyl peroxide, the self-cure activator, is present in the catalyst paste. The amine functions as a proton donor and is considered an accelerator of free-radical production. Aromatic amines (such as ethyl 4-dimethylaminobenzoate [EDMAB]) are considered more efficient than aliphatic amines (such as 2-[dimethylamino]ethyl methacrylate [DMAEMA]). The presence of amine in the composite matrix poses some clinically relevant concerns. First, amines are known to degrade over time, producing colored products that alter the shade of the cement. Second, they become inactive when in contact with acidic adhesive systems, and when cement polymerization takes place in the absence of light activation, the deleterious effect on degree of conversion may increase the risk of restoration debonding. It is important to point out that the relative amounts of self-cure and light-cure initiators vary a lot among commercial brands. Consequently, some materials are more dependent on light activation to achieve a high degree of conversion. Likewise, some commercial materials cure more promptly in the absence of light than others.

Setting Reaction and Structure

Resin cements are set by free-radical polymerization resulting in the formation of a densely cross-linked structure involving the filler particles. Free radicals are generated by light activation, in which camphorquinone in the excited state combines with two amine molecules to generate two free radicals. In the absence of light, free radicals are formed by redox reaction of the amine-peroxide system. A crosslink is formed when a propagating chain encounters an unreacted carbon double bond in a different polymer chain. Polymerization proceeds until the mobility of the reactive species becomes restricted by the increasing viscosity of the material and free radicals cannot propagate further, becoming entrapped in the polymer. Final degree of conversion is around 70% and depends on matrix formulation, initial viscosity, and curing mode. Conversion is usually higher in cases where the cement is dual-cured, compared to self-cured.

Manipulation considerations can be found on the book's website http://evolve.elsevier.com/sakaguchi/restorative

Properties

Monomers released from resin cements are known to produce cytotoxic effects on connective tissue cells. Dual-cure resin cements show higher cytotoxicity at early setting stages when tested in self-cure mode, compared to specimens exposed to light-curing. After 7 days of incubation, Bis-GMA–based dual-cured cements are less cytotoxic than zinc polyacrylate, resin-modified glass ionomer, and resin cement containing 10-MDP monomer.

Mechanical properties of resin cements are defined by their filler content and degree of conversion reached by the organic matrix. As a rule of thumb, higher filler levels and higher conversion correspond to higher mechanical properties. Degree of conversion of dual-cure cements is between 50% and 73% in self-cure mode and 67% and 85% when light-cured. Compressive strength of dual- and light-cured resin composite cements has been reported from 180 to 300 MPa, therefore much higher than acid-base cements. Flexural strength is between 80 and 100 MPa, higher than the minimum value required by the ISO 4049 standard (50 MPa). Elastic modulus may vary significantly among commercial brands, between 4 and 10 GPa, but are comparable to other cements. The mechanical properties of dual-cure cements are slightly higher when the cement is only light-cured.

Film thicknesses measured according to ISO standards are between 13 and 20 µm, therefore within the maximum of 50 µm required by the ISO 4049. Water sorption and solubility of resin cements are much lower than that of resin-modified glass-ionomer cements. However, the cement line may become apparent after a prolonged period of clinical use because of discoloration. Shrinkage of resin cements varies between 2% and 5%.

Immediate shear bond strength of resin cements to dentin varies between 12 and 18 MPa. 10-MDP can bond to tooth structures, ceramics, and cast alloys by the reaction between its phosphate groups and calcium or with metal oxides. The integrity of the bonded interface is challenged by polymerization stress development. Polymerization stresses arise because of resin cement polymerization shrinkage, associated with the development of elastic behavior. In general, dual-cure cements develop higher polymerization stress values when light-cured because the curing reaction is faster than the self-cure reaction, allowing less time for viscous flow to accommodate the shrinkage before the resin composite reaches the vitrification stage. After the resin cement reaches the degree of conversion corresponding to the vitrification point of the organic matrix, all the shrinkage will contribute to stress build-up. When stresses at the interface surpass the bond strength of the adhesive layer to dentin or enamel, a contraction gap may form (Fig. 12.8).

Compomers (polyacid-modified resin composites) can be found on the book's website http://evolve.elsevier.com/sakaguchi/restorative

Self-Adhesive Resin Cements

Self-adhesive resin cements were developed with the aim to provide clinicians with a luting agent with a very simple application procedure, combining the advantages of glass ionomers (adhesion, fluoride release) with mechanical properties comparable to those of resin cements. Presented as two-paste or powder: liquid systems (Fig. 12.9), these materials are indicated for cementation of cast alloy single restorations and bridges, ceramic-metal crowns, and bridges, ceramic (except veneers), and indirect composite restorations. Good results are also obtained with luting of prefabricated posts and high-strength ceramics.

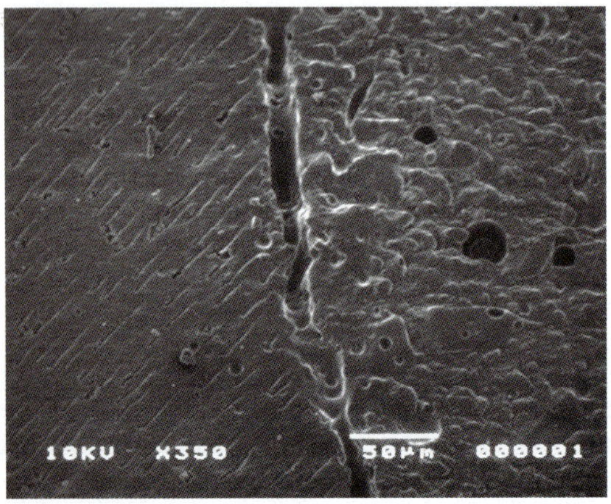

• **Fig. 12.8** Scanning electron microscope of an epoxy replica showing a contraction gap between dentin (*left*) and resin cement (*right*). (From Braga RR, Ferracane JL, Condon JR. Polymerization contraction stress in dual-cure cements and its effect on interfacial integrity of bonded inlays. J Dent. 2002;30(7–8):333–340. doi:10.1016/s0300-5712(02)00047-7.)

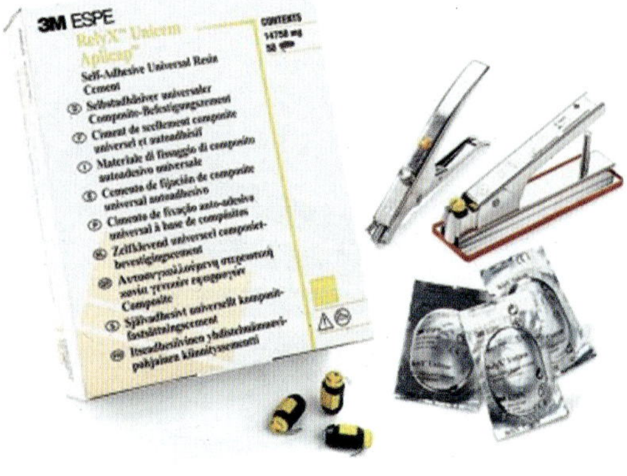

• **Fig. 12.9** Commercial examples of self-adhesive resin cements.

Composition

Formulations are proprietary and vary among manufacturers. Overall, two-paste materials contain multifunctional monomers with phosphoric acid groups, dimethacrylate resins, and initiators for both light-cured and self-cured reactions in one of the pastes. The other paste contains fluoroaluminosilicate, silanated barium glasses, or both, and silanated silica particles, initiators, and methacrylate monomers. The filler fraction is around 70% by mass (50% by volume).

Setting Reaction and Structure

The main curing mechanism is via free-radical polymerization, either self-activated or dual-cured. An initial low pH is necessary for the adhesion mechanism (described below). At later stages, acidity is neutralized in some cements by the reaction between phosphoric acid groups and the alkaline glass. The structure of the set material is mainly a cross-linked polymer, covalently bonded to filler particles by the silane layer. Some ionic bridging between carboxylic groups and ions released by the glass may also be present.

Manipulation considerations can be found on the book's website http://evolve.elsevier.com/sakaguchi/restorative

Properties

In terms of biocompatibility, self-adhesive resin cements present higher cytotoxicity than resin cements and acid-base cements. Cytotoxicity is reduced when cements are used in dual-cure mode. Their mechanical properties vary among commercial materials but, in general, are lower than those of conventional resin cements. Flexural strength is in the 50 to 100 MPa range and compressive strength is between 200 and 240 MPa. Values in the lower range are usually associated with the cement tested in self-cure mode, whereas higher values are obtained with light activation. Film thickness is between 15 and 20 µm. Bonding mechanism to the tooth structures is proposed to occur by micromechanical interlocking and chemical interaction between the acidic groups and the hydroxyapatite. The initial low pH makes the cement hydrophilic, allowing intimate contact with the moist dentin substrate. Shear bond strength to enamel varies from 3 to 15 MPa, intermediate between resin cements and glass ionomers. On dentin, some products have bond strengths comparable to resin cements, and these materials show good bond strength values to metal alloys and high-strength ceramics. The presence of unreacted acid groups increases water sorption, in comparison to conventional resin cements. Their fluoride content is low (around 10%) and its beneficial effects have not been clinically proven.

Resin Cements for Provisional Restorations

These provisional cements are paste-paste systems, which can be dual- or light-cured. They are useful for cementation of interim restorations in the aesthetic zone of the mouth because they are tooth-colored and fairly translucent. They are easy to clean, and some release fluoride. Resin cementation of provisional restorations is useful when the final cement will also be resin because there is no eugenol present to potentially impair polymerization of the final cement. Composite cements used for cementation of provisional restorations have a substantially lower compressive strength than composite cements used for permanent cementation (25 to 70 MPa and 180 to 265 MPa, respectively).

SELECTED PROBLEMS

Problem 1

A gold alloy casting seated properly before cementation but failed to seat when cemented with a glass-ionomer cement. What factors might have caused this difficulty, and how can it be corrected?

Solution

An excessive film thickness of glass-ionomer cement may result from (1) too high a powder/liquid ratio, (2) too long a time between completion of mixing and cementation, or (3) cement being placed on the tooth before being placed on the casting.

Problem 2

To obtain a root-cement-post and core unit that is bonded, what type of cement would be best to use and what are some pitfalls to avoid?

Solution

Dual- or self-cured resin cement with a compatible adhesive system is the best option for post-cementation. Light-cured resin cements may not completely polymerize at the apical end of the root. Many systems contain core build-up materials that are compatible with the cement. One type of adhesive cement forms strong bonds to alloy, ceramic, and tooth structure; however, it sets in anaerobic conditions. Therefore this type of cement should never be placed inside the root canal, but only on the post before seating.

Problem 3

A pressable, leucite-based ceramic crown was cemented with resin-modified glass-ionomer cement. Subsequently, the crown fractured and had to be replaced. What could have been done to prevent this failure?

Solution

Any leucite-based ceramic is etchable and also not as strong as alumina- or zirconia-based materials. Therefore, this restoration should have been etched with hydrofluoric acid gel, silanated, and then bonded with resin cement. The bonding process imparts strength to the entire restoration-tooth complex. Other all-ceramic materials such as zirconia, or alumina-based restorations are not etchable, but are much stronger, and therefore can be cemented with water-based cements.

Bibliography

Abo-Hamar SE, et al. Effect of temporary cements on the bond strength of ceramic luted to dentin. *Dent Mater.* 2005;21(9):794–803.

Wilson AD, Nicholson J. *Acid-Base Cements: Their Biomedical and Industrial Applications.* Cambridge University Press; 1993:398.

Berry EA 3rd, Powers JM. Bond strength of glass ionomers to coronal and radicular dentin. *Oper Dent.* 1994;19(4):122–126.

Bertolotti RL. Adhesion to porcelain and metal. *Dent Clin North Am.* 2007;51(2):433–451, ix–x.

Boeckh C, et al. Antibacterial activity of restorative dental biomaterials in vitro. *Caries Res.* 2002;36(2):101–107.

Braga RR, Ferracane JL, Condon JR. Polymerization contraction stress in dual-cure cements and its effect on interfacial integrity of bonded inlays. *J Dent.* 2002;30(7–8):333–340.

Brauer GM. New developments in zinc oxide-eugenol cement. *Ann Dent.* 1967;26(2):44–50.

Civjan S, Brauer GM. Physical properties of cements, based on zinc oxide, hydrogenated rosin, O-ethoxybenzoic acid, and eugenol. *J Dent Res.* 1964;43:281–299.

Davidson CL, Mjör IA. *Advances in Glass-Ionomer Cements 1999.* Quintessense; 1999.

Eisenburger M, Addy M, Rossbach A. Acidic solubility of luting cements. *J Dent.* 2003;31(2):137–142.

Farah JW, Powers JM. Adhesive resin cements. *Dent Advis.* 2005;22(8):1.

Farah JW, Powers JM. Self-adhesive resin cements and esthetic resin cements. *Dent Advis.* 2009;26(2):1.

Farah JW, Powers JM. Traditional crown and bridge cements. *Dent Advis.* 2006;23(2):1.

Fonseca RG, et al. Effect of metal primers on bond strength of resin cements to base metals. *J Prosthet Dent.* 2009;101(4):262–268.

Fujisawa S, Kadoma Y. Effect of phenolic compounds on the polymerization of methyl methacrylate. *Dent Mater.* 1992;8(5):324–326.

Furuchi M, et al. Effect of metal priming agents on bond strength of resin-modified glass ionomers joined to gold alloy. *Dent Mater J.* 2007;26(5):728–732.

He LH, Purton DG, Swain MV. A suitable base material for composite resin restorations: zinc oxide eugenol. *J Dent.* 2010;38(4):290–295.

Hembree JH Jr, George TA, Hembree ME. Film thickness of cements beneath complete crowns. *J Prosthet Dent.* 1978;39(5):533–535.

Irie M, Maruo Y, Nishigawa G, Suzuki K, Watts DC. Physical properties of dual-cured luting-agents correlated to early no interfacial-gap incidence with composite inlay restorations. *Dent Mater.* 2010;26(6):608–615.

Irie M, Suzuki K, Watts DC. Marginal and flexural integrity of three classes of luting cement, with early finishing and water storage. *Dent Mater.* 2004;20(1):3–11.

Jemt T, Stalblad PA, Oilo G. Adhesion of polycarboxylate-based dental cements to enamel: an in vivo study. *J Dent Res.* 1986;65(6):885–887.

Jivraj SA, Kim TH, Donovan TE. Selection of luting agents, part 1. *J Calif Dent Assoc.* 2006;34(2):149–160.

Johnson GH, et al. Retention of metal-ceramic crowns with contemporary dental cements. *J Am Dent Assoc.* 2009;140(9):1125–1136.

Jongsma LA, Kleverlaan CJ, Feilzer AJ. Influence of surface pretreatment of fiber posts on cement delamination. *Dent Mater.* 2010;26(9):901–907.

Kim TH, Jivraj SA, Donovan TE. Selection of luting agents: part 2. *J Calif Dent Assoc.* 2006;34(2):161–166.

Kious AR, Roberts HW, Brackett WW. Film thicknesses of recently introduced luting cements. *J Prosthet Dent.* 2009;101(3):189–192.

Knobloch LA, et al. Solubility and sorption of resin-based luting cements. *Oper Dent.* 2000;25(5):434–440.

Li Z, White S. Mechanical properties of dental luting cements. *J Prosthet Dent.* 1999;81(5):597–609.

Lööf J, et al. Mechanical property aspects of a biomineral based dental restorative system. *Key Eng Mater.* 2005;284–286:741–744.

Lööf J, et al. A comparative study of the bioactivity of three materials for dental applications. *Dent Mater.* 2008;24:653–659.

Mausner IK, Goldstein GR, Georgescu M. Effect of two dentinal desensitizing agents on retention of complete cast coping using four cements. *J Prosthet Dent.* 1996;75(2):129–134.
Mesu FP. Mechanical mixing of zinc oxide-eugenol cements. *J Prosthet Dent.* 1982;47(5):522–527.
Mojon P, et al. Early bond strength of luting cements to a precious alloy. *J Dent Res.* 1992;71(9):1633–1639.
Moura JS, et al. Effect of luting cement on dental biofilm composition and secondary caries around metallic restorations in situ. *Oper Dent.* 2004;29(5):509–514.
Nakamura T, Wakabayashi K, Kinuta S, Nishida H, Miyamae M, Yatani H. Mechanical properties of new self-adhesive resin-based cement. *J Prosthodont Res.* 2010;54(2):59–64.
Negm MM, Beech DR, Grant AA. An evaluation of mechanical and adhesive properties of polycarboxylate and glass ionomer cements. *J Oral Rehabil.* 1982;9(2):161–167.
Nicholson JW, Czarnecka B. The biocompatibility of resin-modified glass-ionomer cements for dentistry. *Dent Mater.* 2008;24(12):1702–1708.
Nicholson JW, Czarnecka B. Review paper: role of aluminum in glass-ionomer dental cements and its biological effects. *J Biomater Appl.* 2009;24(4):293–308.
Oilo G, Espevik S. Stress/strain behavior of some dental luting cements. *Acta Odontol Scand.* 1978;36(1):45–49.
Osborne JW, et al. A method for assessing the clinical solubility and disintegration of luting cements. *J Prosthet Dent.* 1978;40(4):413–417.
Peutzfeldt A. Dual-cure resin cements: in vitro wear and effect of quantity of remaining double bonds, filler volume, and light curing. *Acta Odontol Scand.* 1995;53(1):29–34.
Peutzfeldt A, Asmussen E. Influence of eugenol-containing temporary cement on bonding of self-etching adhesives to dentin. *J Adhes Dent.* 2006;8(1):31–34.
Piwowarczyk A, Lauer HC. Mechanical properties of luting cements after water storage. *Oper Dent.* 2003;28(5):535–542.
Piwowarczyk A, Lauer HC, Sorensen JA. In vitro shear bond strength of cementing agents to fixed prosthodontic restorative materials. *J Prosthet Dent.* 2004;92(3):265–273.
Piwowarczyk A, Lauer HC, Sorensen JA. The shear bond strength between luting cements and zirconia ceramics after two pre-treatments. *Oper Dent.* 2005;30(3):382–388.
Powis DR, Prosser HJ, Wilson AD. Long-term monitoring of microleakage of dental cements by radiochemical diffusion. *J Prosthet Dent.* 1988;59(6):651–657.
Radovic I, et al. Self-adhesive resin cements: a literature review. *J Adhes Dent.* 2008;10(4):251–258.
Robertello FJ, et al. Fluoride release of glass ionomer-based luting cements in vitro. *J Prosthet Dent.* 1999;82(2):172–176.
Schmid-Schwap M, et al. Cytotoxicity of four categories of dental cements. *Dent Mater.* 2009;25(3):360–368.
Schulman A, Vaidyanathan TK. Dental cements for luting and lining. *N Y J Dent.* 1977;47(5):142–146.
Shaw AJ, Carrick T, McCabe JF. Fluoride release from glass-ionomer and compomer restorative materials: 6-month data. *J Dent.* 1998;26(4):355–359.
Sidhu SK, Schmalz G. The biocompatibility of glass-ionomer cement materials. A status report for the American Journal of Dentistry. *Am J Dent.* 2001;14(6):387–396.
Smith D. The setting of zinc oxide/eugenol mixtures. *Br Dent J.* 1958;105(9):313–321.
Smith D. A new dental cement. *Br Dent J.* 1968;5:381–384.
Spinell T, Schedle A, Watts DC. Polymerization shrinkage kinetics of dimethacrylate resin-cements. *Dent Mater.* 2009;25(8):1058–1066.
Swartz ML, Phillips RW, Clark HE. Long-term F release from glass ionomer cements. *J Dent Res.* 1984;63(2):158–160.
Vrochari AD, Eliades G, Hellwig E, Wrbas KT. Water sorption and solubility of four self-etching, self-adhesive resin luting agents. *J Adhes Dent.* 2010;12(1):39–43.
White SN, Kipnis V. Effect of adhesive luting agents on the marginal seating of cast restorations. *J Prosthet Dent.* 1993;69(1):28–31.
White SN, Yu Z. Compressive and diametral tensile strengths of current adhesive luting agents. *J Prosthet Dent.* 1993;69(6):568–572.
Wiegand A, Buchalla W, Attin T. Review on fluoride-releasing restorative materials–fluoride release and uptake characteristics, antibacterial activity and influence on caries formation. *Dent Mater.* 2007;23(3):343–362.
Wilson AD, McLean JW. *Glass-Ionomer Cement.* Quintessence Books; 1988.
Wilson AD, Prosser HJ, Powis DM. Mechanism of adhesion of polyelectrolyte cements to hydroxyapatite. *J Dent Res.* 1983;62(5):590–592.

13

Technology

HONGSEOK AN

CHAPTER OUTLINE

Introduction

Computer-aided design and computer-aided manufacturing (CAD-CAM) technologies were introduced to dentistry almost 50 years ago but were not mainstream in restorative dentistry until recently. Currently, many CAD-CAM systems and workflows are available for the fabrication of various types of dental restorations and prostheses. The main advantages of digital workflows include improved quality control, efficiency, reproducibility, and access to newer materials.

The use of digital technologies has been rapidly embraced by clinicians and dental educators, but a lack of thorough understanding of the technology often leads to misuse. This chapter discusses the three main steps of a digital workflow, namely data acquisition, CAD, and CAM, and common technologies used for these steps.

Data Acquisition

Digital Scan File

CAD-CAM technologies can be used to design and fabricate dental restorations once the oral structures are digitized to a three-dimensional (3D) image format for computer processing. Therefore the first step of a digital workflow is digital scanning, which refers to the process of capturing in numerical format the raster images of a geometric object that can be viewed on a monitor (2D) or in a hologram (3D). In dentistry, digital scanning is achieved by capturing directly the optical image of the patient's anatomy (direct scanning) or indirectly of an impression or cast of the anatomy (indirect scanning).

Most dental CAD-CAM systems use their system-specific file type to store data but, at the same time, they allow the data to be imported and exported as a standard tessellation language (STL) file, a commonly used 3D data file type. STL files are composed of a point cloud that is interpreted by a series of triangles that represent the surface morphology of the scanned structure (Fig. 13.1). Typical resolutions of dental intraoral scanners range from 34 points/mm^2 to 80 points/mm^2, and higher resolution is generally considered desirable to maximize accuracy. However, a recent study conducted with four commercially available intraoral scanners found that there was no significant relationship between scanner resolution and accuracy, which implied that the resolution of current dental intraoral scanners is sufficient. When the same system is used for scanning and designing, a system-specific CAD file format may be preferred as it has the advantage of being able to fully utilize information in the scan file, such as shade matching, caries detection, prosthetic tooth detection, and motion capture.

Direct Scanning

Direct scanning, also called direct digitization, intraoral scanning, or digital impressioning, is made by directly scanning the patient's oral structures with a handheld optical scanning device designed for intraoral use (Fig. 13.2). Since its introduction in 1985, direct scanning has been used widely because it is accurate, convenient, time-efficient, straightforward to learn, and patient-friendly. It is useful especially when making scans for patients with a pronounced gag reflex, severe hypersensitivity, limited mouth opening, orthodontic brackets, mobile teeth, or severe undercuts.

Data Acquisition and Processing Principles

A 3D model of the object is built in three steps: image capturing, image registration, and image integration. In image capturing, the entire surface is sampled with multiple images to acquire a dense and accurate 3D image of the entire object. In image registration, all captured images are transformed into a common coordinate system. Once the set of multiple images is registered, the overlapped images must be integrated to generate a nonredundant surface model.

Image Capturing

Most intraoral scanners use laser or white light for image capturing. The light emitted by the scanning device is projected onto the object and reflected back to a sensor, where it is converted

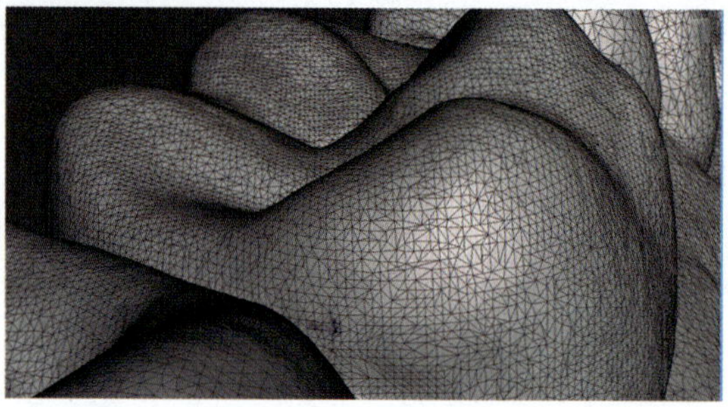

• **Fig. 13.1** STL file structure. Numerous data points are connected to form triangular meshes.

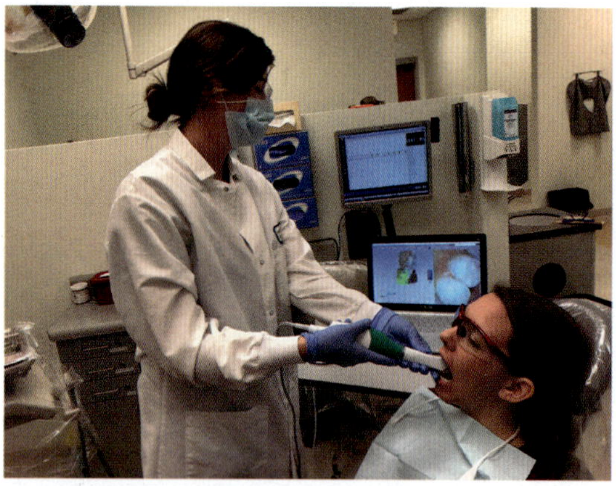

• **Fig. 13.2** Direct scanning (Emerald, Planmeca).

TABLE 13.1 Optical Image-Capturing Technologies Used by Different Intraoral Scanners

Image-capturing Technology	Scanner	Manufacturer
Confocal microscopy	iTero Element5	Align Technology
	CEREC Primescan	Dentsply Sirona
	Trios4	3Shape
Triangulation	CS3800	Carestream
	i500	Medit
	Emerald	Planmeca

to an electric signal that can be analyzed by a computer to create 3D images. Various optical image-capturing technologies are used by different intraoral scanners, including confocal microscopy, triangulation, optical coherence tomography, and active wave front sampling (Table 13.1). The most commonly used are confocal microscopy and active triangulation.

Image Registration and Integration

Intraoral scans are a compilation of multiple images that are partially superimposed to form a larger 3D image. Typical intraoral scanners capture 10 to 30 3D images per second, each covering an area of one to two teeth. 3D image reconstruction then requires matching corresponding distinct features within the two images through rotating and translating to correctly align and register them. Integration is the process of removing redundant data that is visible in both images and averaging out common points. As the scanning process progresses, 3D images are added to the integrated images and the reconstruction steps are repeated until the entire object is completed. The reconstructed image is typically further refined to reduce noise.

Accuracy and Influencing Factors

With current systems, the accuracy of direct scanning for a single-tooth or single-quadrant scan is suitable for fabrication of dental restorations and is comparable to that of polyvinyl siloxane impression materials. However, studies suggest that the accuracy of direct scanning of complete arches is less than that of conventional PVS impressions.

Factors Influencing Image-Capturing Accuracy

Inaccuracies in completed direct scans result from errors in the acquisition and registration steps. Reflections from various types of highly reflective restorative materials, such as polished metal, polished resin composite, or glazed ceramics, have been known to interfere with the scanning mechanism and increase errors. Most currently available powder-free systems are capable of direct scanning these material surfaces with clinically acceptable accuracy. However, in some situations, polished metal restorations may show clinically significant scanning discrepancies approaching 80 μm. Although powder application is not required for the most current intraoral scanners, it may still be beneficial for some systems when scanning highly polished metal restorations (Fig. 13.3).

Ambient conditions, such as temperature and light, may also impact scanning accuracy. It was reported that intraoral scans made at room temperature (15–24°C) were more accurate than scans made at higher temperatures (29°C). Studies also have found the best results are achieved under normal room light conditions (500–1000 lux), and that scanning under high illuminance ambient light decreased accuracy and increased scanning time.

Liquid on the tooth surface also negatively influences scanning accuracy due to light refraction. Therefore before direct scanning, it is highly advised to clean and dry the tooth surface, especially critical areas such as a tooth preparation finish line. Even with adequate moisture control, intraoral scanners only have a limited capability to capture subgingival finish lines, which can often be misrepresented, resulting in unacceptable marginal integrity for the restoration. Thus adequate gingival retraction must be achieved when scanning subgingival finish lines.

Factors Influencing Image Registration Accuracy

Even when individual image captures are accurate, errors during image registration can lower the accuracy of a 3D model generated from direct scanning (Fig. 13.4). Lack of sufficient morphological variations on the overlapping portion of two images may reduce reliability of the reconstructed image due to inability to correctly match them. This may especially be true when scanning edentulous areas where distinctive anatomies are lacking. In general, a mandibular edentulous arch is more difficult to scan directly compared with a maxillary edentulous arch due to the lack of distinguishable anatomies and the abundance of movable unattached mucosa. With advancements in direct scanning technology, recent in vitro studies have shown that the accuracy of direct scanning of edentulous arches may be suitable for the fabrication of removable dental prostheses. However, movement of peripheral mucosa during scanning can negatively influence scanning accuracy and it is not possible to perform border molding to capture the movable part of unattached mucosa with intraoral scanners. In addition, it has been reported that direct scanning accuracy decreases with the increased length of the scanned area due to the need to register

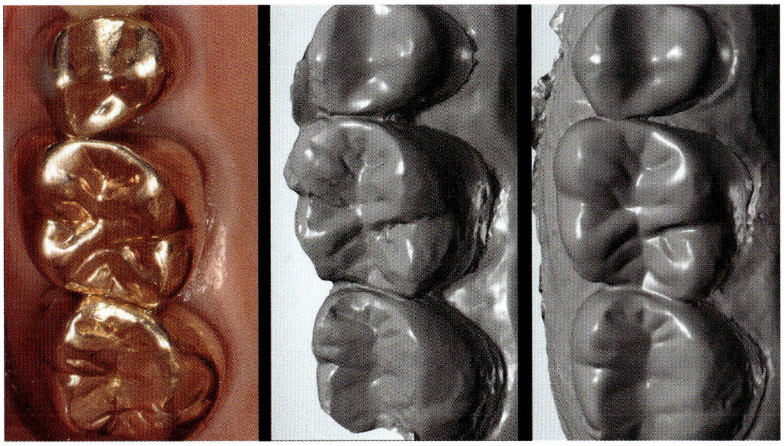

• **Fig. 13.3** Gold restorations (*left*) scanned with powder application (*middle*) and without powder application (*right*) (scanned with CEREC Omnicam).

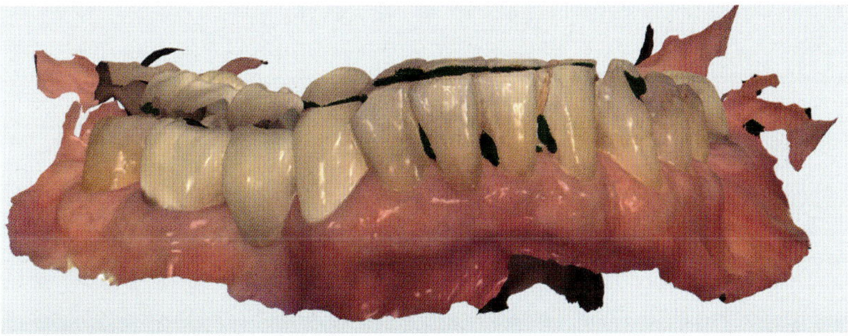

• **Fig. 13.4** Failed image reconstruction due to accumulated registration errors.

multiple images, which compounds the inaccuracies. Therefore clinical impression-making procedures for removable dental prostheses remain primarily analog.

Registration errors can be minimized when overlaps between registered images include larger areas and multiple distinctive 3D features. For example, occlusal surfaces are preferred as a starting point as they have more morphological variations compared with buccal or lingual surfaces. The optimal scanning strategy depends on scanning systems and clinical scenarios. While there is no one dominant scanning strategy that can be applied in all situations, scanning occlusal surfaces first followed by buccal and lingual surfaces seems to be a predictable scanning strategy that can minimize registration errors.

As intraoral scanners capture images at a constant rate, an increase in scanning speed or a decrease in scanner tip size may change the total number of registered 3D images and overlapped areas between images, potentially influencing the accuracy of the registration process. One recent study has shown that the use of a small scanner tip or fast scanning speed significantly lowers the accuracy of complete-arch scans.

Additional Features

Some intraoral scanners are equipped with various auxiliary tools that can support diagnostic or restorative procedures, such as diagnosis of dental caries and periodontal disease, tooth wear monitoring, occlusal analysis, shade matching, and jaw movement record.

Shade Matching

Some intraoral scanners have been updated to utilize their high-definition cameras to record tooth shades (Fig. 13.5). While convenient, recent studies have shown intraoral scanners at best serve as auxiliary tools because they are less accurate than conventional methods for shade matching. It is important to remember that translucency, texture, and surface characteristics all need to be considered to achieve excellent aesthetic outcomes.

Caries Detection

Some scanners recently have incorporated automated caries detection technologies using near-infrared transillumination or fluorescence methods, with studies showing promising outcomes in detecting occlusal and proximal caries. Accuracy can be improved by combining these technologies with traditional clinical and radiographic exams. If intraoral scanners can replace bitewing radiographs in the future, this would greatly minimize the use of radiation in dentistry.

Jaw Movement Record

With the recent advent of the dynamic jaw movement simulation technique known as a virtual articulator, various tools have been used to record and reproduce the patient's jaw movements (Fig. 13.6). The captured movements can be reproduced in the design software, facilitating restoration design and reducing occlusal errors in eccentric positions.

Indirect Scanning

While direct scanning is a great way to digitize oral structures, it is not indicated for all patients or available to all clinicians. One recent survey revealed that only 53% of the participant dentists used intraoral scanners. Indirect scanning can be achieved with

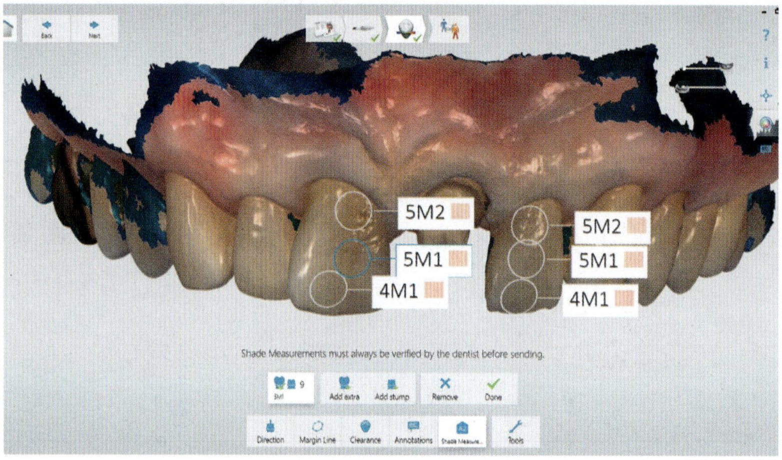

• **Fig. 13.5** Shade measurement (Trios3, 3Shape).

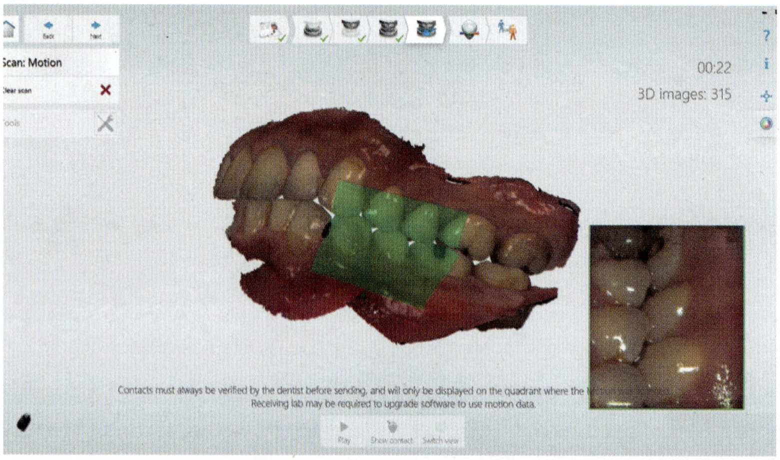

• **Fig. 13.6** Jaw movements record (Trios3, 3Shape).

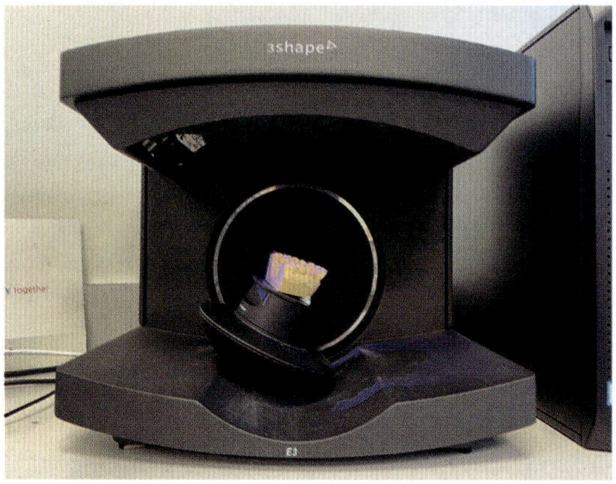

• **Fig. 13.7** Extraoral scanner (E3, 3Shape).

an extraoral scanner by optically scanning a conventionally made dental impression or a stone cast (Fig. 13.7).

Indirect Scanning Process

As with handheld intraoral scanners, stationary extraoral scanners also acquire 3D images of the object but utilize a different process for image reconstruction. The object is fixed on the scanning table and the movement of the light source is restricted. Some extraoral scanners support a high-quality mechanical control system, where the positions of the object and light source are precisely controlled by the computer during scanning. This means that the captured 3D images can be directly registered to the common coordinate system and then simply appended to each other without relying on matching the overlapping portion between images. For this reason, neither the presence of distinctive surface anatomies nor the length of the scanned area influences registration accuracy significantly.

Indirect digitization is most commonly achieved by scanning type IV or V dental stone casts made from polyvinyl siloxane or other types of dental impressions. One advantage of scanning stone is its matte surface, which eliminates the need for using contrast medium or powder. As the scanned object and the light source are controlled within the scanning system, the object can be scanned only from fixed angles. While most recent extraoral scanners are equipped with a precise motion control system that allows the object to be scanned from multiple angles, they still have restricted range of motion compared with intraoral scanners and this sometimes makes it difficult to obtain a clear scan of undercuts and interproximal areas. If critical areas such as tooth preparation finish lines are missed, a two-step scanning technique can be used to obtain an accurate scan of the missed areas. This two-step technique employs an initial scan with an extraoral scanner, followed by a second scan of individual teeth, which is then aligned to the initial scan to produce the complete virtual cast.

TABLE 13.2 Indications of Direct and Indirect Scanning

Direct Scanning	Indirect Scanning
• When adequate tissue retraction and saliva/bleeding control can be achieved predictably • Dental restorations with a supragingival or slightly subgingival finish line • Single-tooth or implant restorations, short-span tooth- or implant-supported fixed dental prostheses • Scans for diagnostic purposes, occlusal devices, surgical guides, or orthodontic treatments • Patients with a pronounced gag reflex, severe hypersensitivity, limited mouth opening, fixed orthodontic devices, mobile teeth, and other anatomical variations that make a conventional impression difficult	• When ideal tissue retraction and saliva/bleeding are challenging • Dental restoration with a deep subgingival finish line • Long-span or full-arch tooth- or implant-supported fixed dental prostheses • Removable dental prostheses • Any other types of dental restorations or prostheses when intraoral scanners are not available

Some extraoral scanners also provide the option of scanning conventional impressions, particularly those for complete dentures and triple tray impressions, without having to fabricate stone casts. The scanned image of the impression is then inverted to generate a virtual model. This approach has the advantage of being less time-consuming and labor-intensive, but it is not as popular as stone cast scanning because undercut areas are frequently missed and it is not possible to use two-step scanning technique. Scanning impressions can be more successful when the length of scanned areas is short and the depth of the impression is shallow. Second, stone casts are required in many cases to perform physical try-ins and adjustment of dental restorations. This makes the option of scanning impressions less attractive.

Factors Influencing Accuracy

Extraoral scanners typically have higher accuracy compared with intraoral scanners. However, the accuracy of virtual models generated by indirect scanning is not always more accurate than those generated by direct scanning because indirect digitization is the combined process of conventional impression taking, stone cast fabrication, and indirect scanning. Factors determining the accuracy of indirect digitization include the scanning system, type of impression material, impression technique, type of dental stone, and stone cast fabrication technique. Studies have concluded that indirect scanning is suitable for fabrication of dental restorations and prostheses, and is comparable to that of direct scanning when used for quadrant-arch scanning, but it is more reliable than direct scanning when used for complete arches. The digitization method, and direct or indirect scanning, should be carefully selected considering the type of restorations or prostheses, and other patient factors (Table 13.2).

Computer-Aided Design

Data Import

Once prepared teeth or other oral structures are successfully digitized, the digital image files are imported to the dental CAD-CAM software to design the dental prostheses. Most dental CAD-CAM systems have their own specific file format, commonly referred to as a "closed system." If the CAD program does not accept the file format of the scanned image, the scanned image file should be converted to a general 3D file format, such as *.stl or *.ply. While using a closed system has advantages of being efficient and preserving full data, it still has limitations in the potential expansion of workflows and in communication with other clinicians or technicians who are not equipped with the same system. For this reason, a closed system may be preferred when an efficient and repetitive execution of simple tasks is required (e.g., chairside design and milling of one-day restorations), whereas an open system may be preferred when more complex tasks are required (e.g., commercial laboratory).

Virtual Model Preparation

Once all necessary files are imported to create the virtual models, the design process begins. First, the virtual models should be examined by dentists or dental technicians to determine if they are suitable, especially focusing on the finish lines of prepared teeth. It is important to remember that many dental scanners automatically fill in missed areas to create a clean-looking virtual model. If the borders of the finish lines are not clearly visible, the images on the screen might not be an accurate representation of the actual finish lines on the prepared teeth, and the data should be rejected. Typical reasons for missed or distorted images around finish lines include inadequate gingival retraction, and presence of saliva or bleeding (Fig. 13.8A and B).

Unnecessary peripheries can be trimmed out to create smooth borders and some noncritical areas may be modified to create a cleaner and void-free virtual model (Fig. 13.9A). A path of insertion is then typically determined immediately before or after margin tracing to identify undercut areas. Many dental CAD programs automatically detect the optimal path of insertion, which may only be acceptable when the tooth preparation is ideal. Therefore a trained operator still must confirm and modify the path of insertion as necessary (Fig. 13.9B). The next step, margin tracing, is one of the most important steps in the virtual model preparation process (Fig. 13.9C). Many dental CAD programs provide the functionality to automatically detect the restoration margin, which is most successful when used on a properly trimmed stone model or a tooth with a supragingival finish line. In any case, the operator should always examine the margin tracing and manually correct it as necessary. Manual margin tracing can be more reliable when margins are partially obscured by surrounding gingival structures.

The last step of virtual model preparation is to determine the cement space, which is critically important in determining the marginal fit of the final restoration. While most dental CAD programs allow operators to set uniform cement space on the intaglio surface, the cement space on the margin is set in various ways, and the optimal cement space setting may vary depending on CAD-CAM systems, milling machines, materials, and cements.

Virtual Restoration Design

The dental restoration is then designed from the virtual model. Most dental CAD programs have tooth design libraries containing

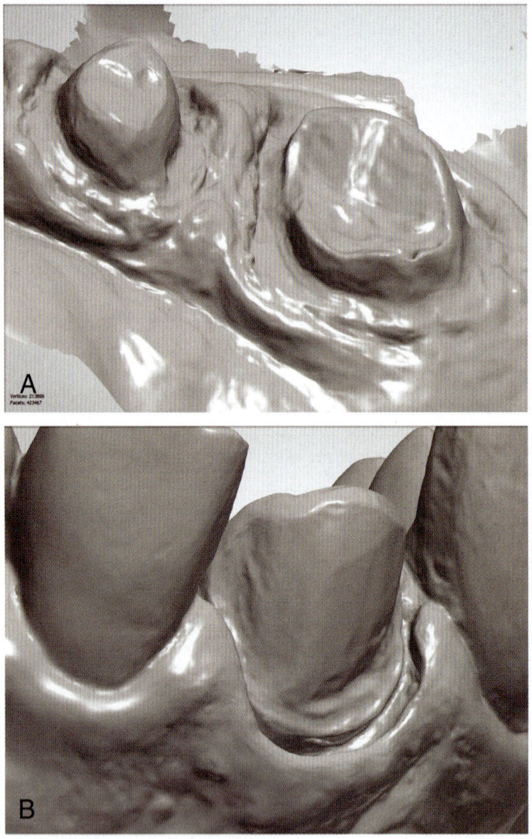

• **Fig. 13.8** Influence of gingival retraction and saliva control. (A) Unacceptable scan quality due to inadequate gingival retraction and saliva control. The finish lines of tooth preparation were distorted and transitioned indistinguishably to the surrounding gingival structures. Restorations fabricated with this scan may have poor marginal integrity. (B) Acceptable scan. As a result of adequate gingival retraction and saliva control, the finish line was accurately scanned.

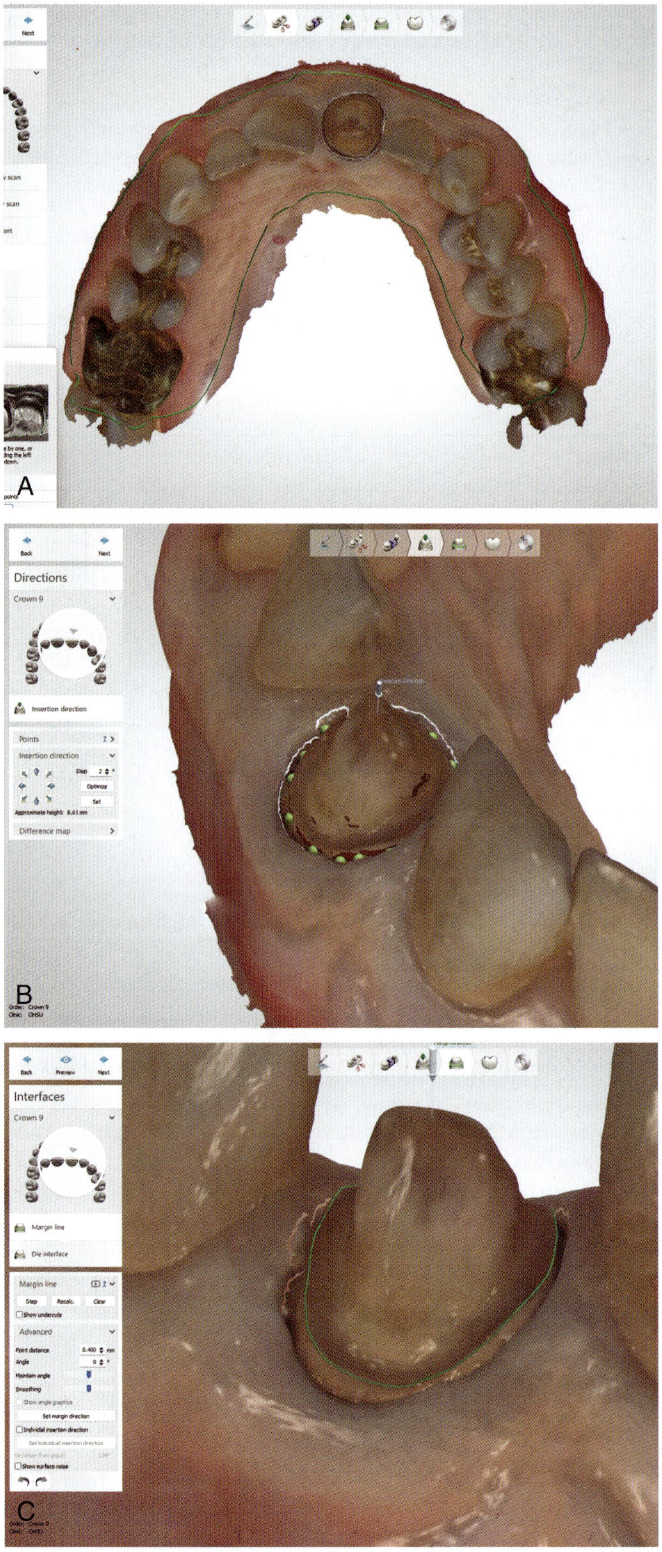

• **Fig. 13.9** Virtual model preparation steps. (A) Peripheral trimming. (B) Path of insertion. (C) Margin tracing.

different tooth forms (Fig. 13.10A). Once the preferred tooth form is selected, the CAD program typically offers a design proposal. Chairside design and milling systems usually provide only a few tooth forms to choose from but have a more optimized algorithm to calculate an adequate design proposal based on the selected tooth form and surrounding structures such as adjacent teeth (Fig. 13.10B). Studies suggest that the CAD program has sufficient accuracy in creating tooth morphology that is equivalent or superior to manually waxed tooth morphology for a partial or full crown. This approach makes the design process more efficient, especially for single-tooth restorations, even though careful examination and potential adjustments of the proposed design should still be made for each given clinical situation.

Laboratory dental CAD programs are designed to be used for a wider range of clinical applications, and therefore have a larger number of tooth form options, but may not provide advanced automatic design functionality. In any case, the proposed design should be examined and modified as necessary by a skilled operator using the tools provided on a 2D screen (Fig. 13.11A and B).

The use of other virtual images that serve as a design guide can be very helpful in creating the ideal design. For example, when preparing teeth with ideal contour and occlusion, the teeth can be scanned before preparation and the scanned images can be superimposed to the final digital impression to be used as a design guide. This technique is especially useful when designing dental prostheses for multiple teeth. A tooth on the contralateral side can also be a good design reference (mirror image), especially when used for central incisors (Fig. 13.12A and C).

When virtually designing frameworks for fixed dental prostheses that require ceramic veneering, it is recommended to design full-contour prostheses first unless there is a scanned image of a physical

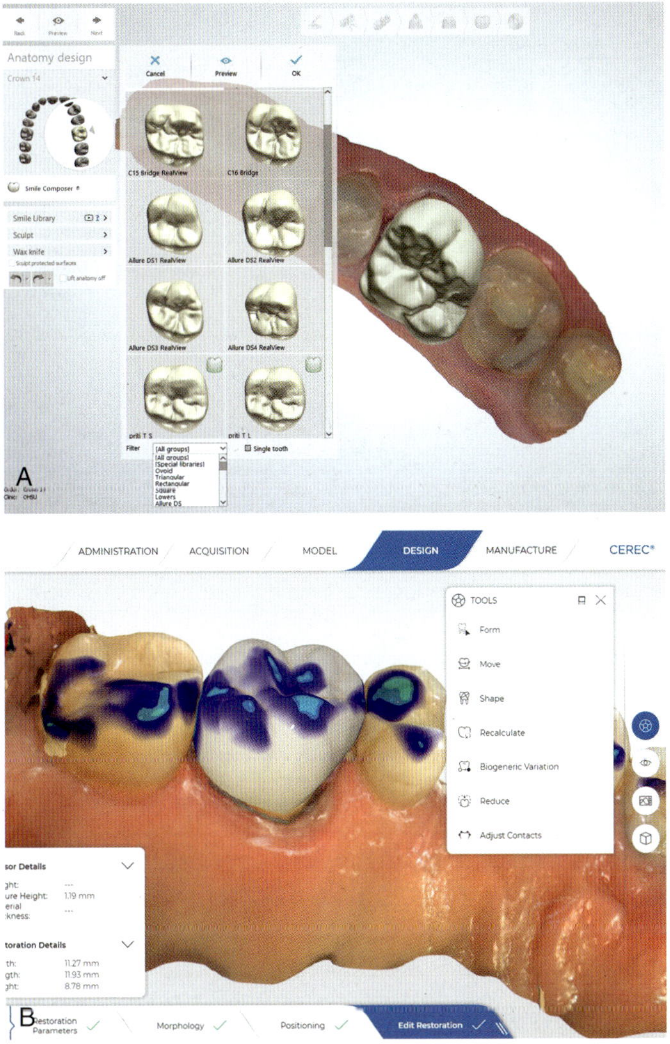

• **Fig. 13.10** Tooth design strategies. (A) Tooth form library. Some laboratory dental CAD programs provide tooth form libraries with a wide variety of selections. Significant design alterations are typically required to create ideal design. (B) Automatically design tooth form. Some chairside systems use the automatic design algorithm instead of tooth form libraries. Design alterations are still required to create ideal design.

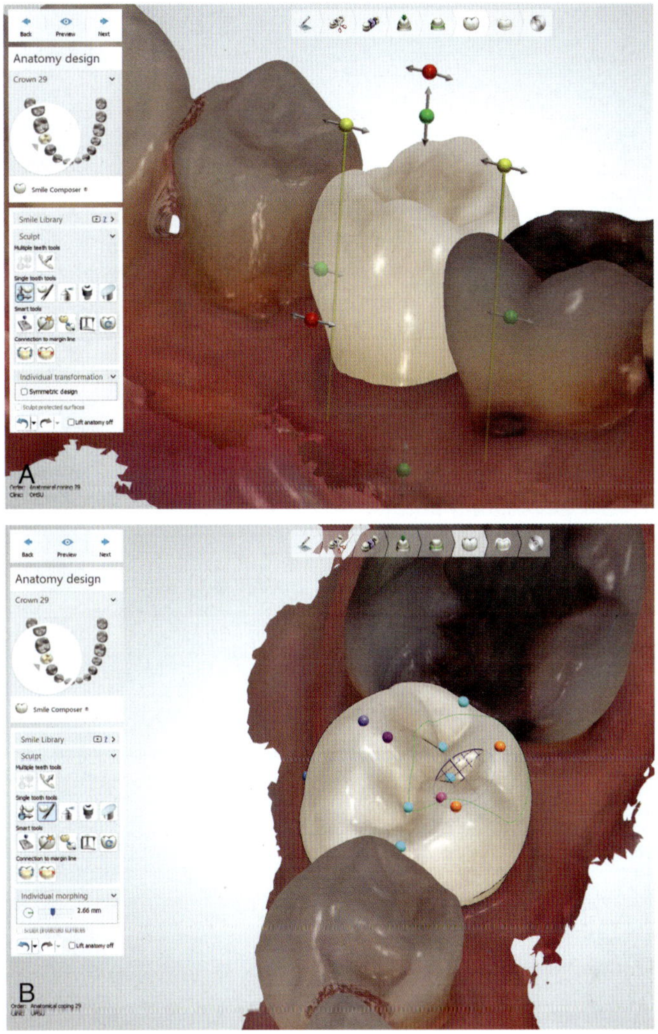

• **Fig. 13.11** Virtual design tools. (A) Restoration can be rotated, translated, and stretched. (B) Tooth contours can be modified to create ideal design.

model available to serve as a design guide. Then, the framework design can be completed by cutting back the full-contour design to create room for ceramic veneering. Some dental CAD programs provide an automated cut-back function (Fig. 13.13A). Manual cut-back using various design tools provided in the design program can also be used for some atypical designs or final adjustments of the framework. Predesigned frameworks can also be imported from the design library and modified as needed (Fig. 13.13B), though it is difficult to evaluate if the amount of cut-back is adequate. Scanned images of diagnostic models, interim prostheses, intraoral mock-ups, or other types of trial prostheses can be useful information when evaluating a framework design. This obviates the need for full-contour design and is especially helpful when designing a framework for a long-span prosthesis.

Virtual Simulation Technologies

Various types of virtual simulation technologies are available for diagnosis, treatment planning, design, and fabrication of dental restorations. As restoring proper function and aesthetics is the paramount goal in providing prosthodontic care to patients with damaged dentition, both aesthetics and occlusion should be considered essential components of virtual design. Many dental CAD programs are equipped with virtual simulation technology such as virtual aesthetic simulation and virtual articulator to assist in achieving these goals.

Virtual Aesthetic Simulation

Creating correct individual tooth size and establishing harmonious positional relationships between teeth and other facial components has been emphasized as a critical part of prosthodontic treatment planning. This facially generated treatment planning approach is especially important when migrated, malposed, damaged, or worn teeth need to be reoriented to the appropriate facial features. Determining position, inclination, and gingival levels of maxillary anterior teeth should be the first steps of comprehensive treatment planning because treatment should begin with a clear view of the aesthetic outcome. Many dental CAD programs are equipped with virtual aesthetic simulation technology, often called virtual smile design or digital smile design. Virtual smile design can be performed using 2D facial photos or 3D facial scans in combination with digital impressions. Virtual smile design helps clinicians make more predictable treatment plans by allowing them to visualize

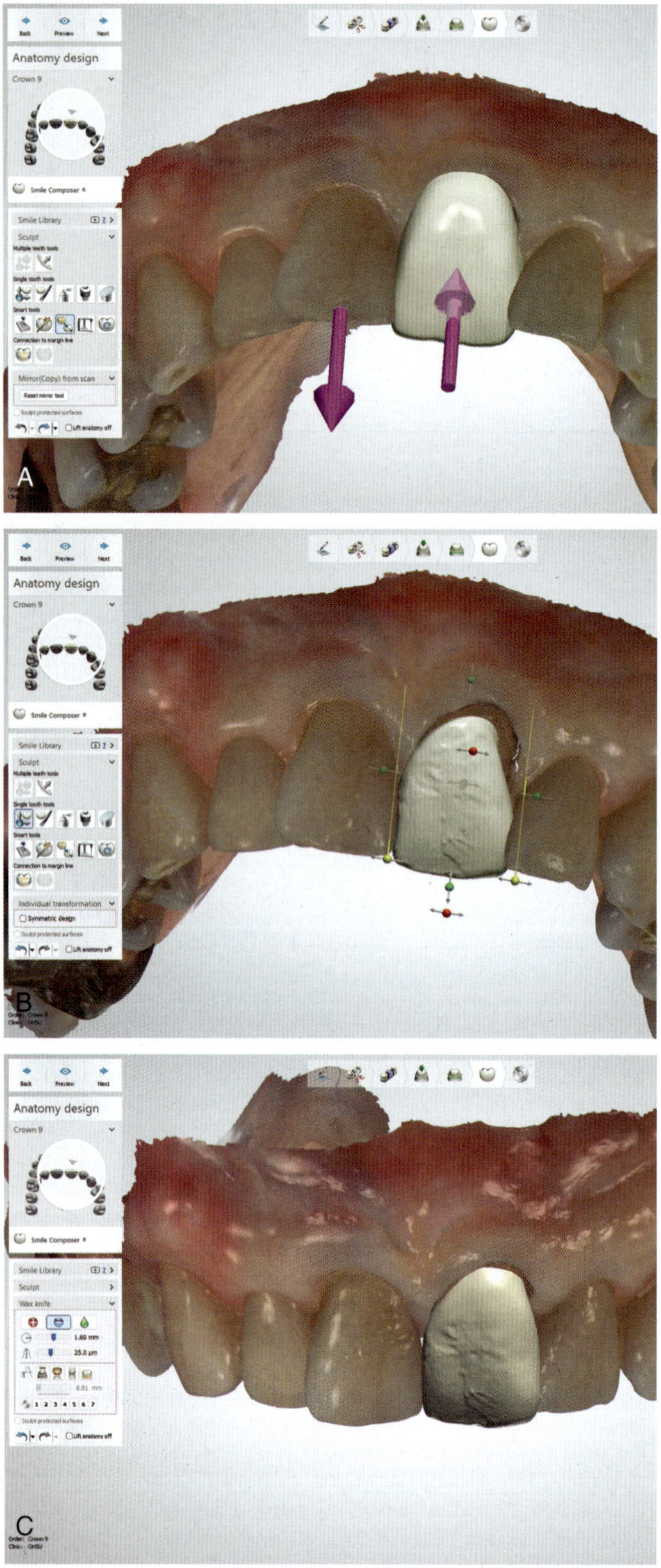

• **Fig. 13.12** Mirror image design. (A) Contralateral tooth is sampled to create a mirror image. (B) Sampled mirror image is modified to create ideal design. (C) Symmetric design is completed.

the aesthetic impact of restorative and surgical treatments from multiple angles before beginning the procedures. Recently available technology allows direct superimposition of scanned images of the patient's mouth to 2D facial photos of 3D facial scans. Then,

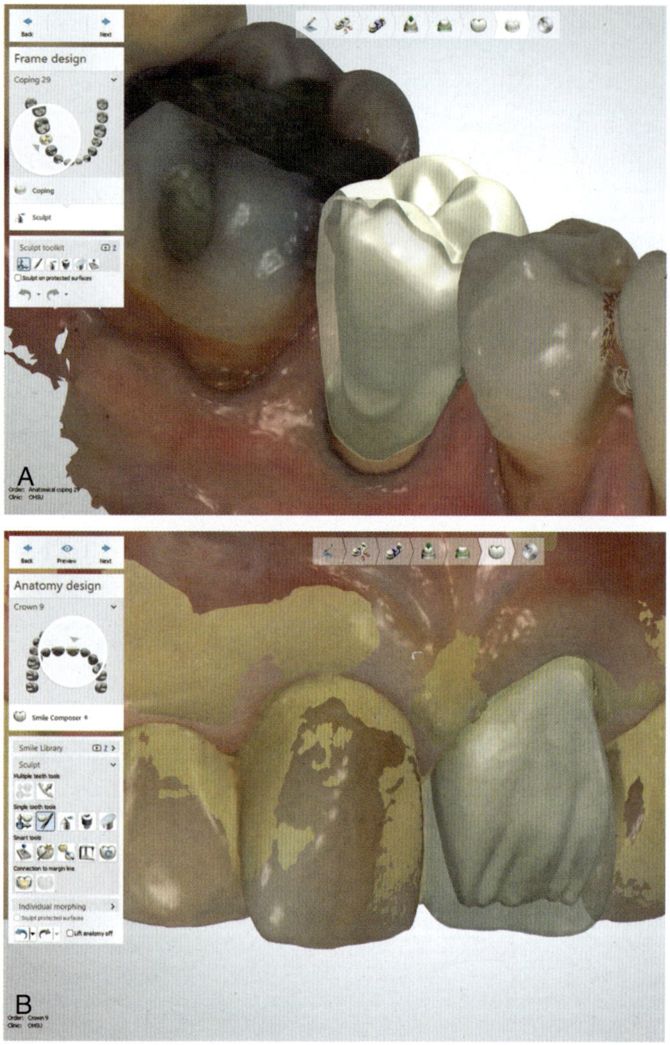

• **Fig. 13.13** Framework design. (A) Facial surface was cut back after full-contour design to create spaces for veneering ceramic. (B) Predesigned framework was used for the framework design. The scanned image of diagnostic wax-up was used to evaluate the space for veneering ceramic.

the proposed design can be transferred to a physical model with a higher accuracy using CAM. Virtual aesthetic simulation procedures are conducted in three steps: data collection, image alignment, and final design (Figs. 13.14A,B and 13.15A,B).

Virtual Mandibular Movement Simulation

Recently, a dynamic virtual articulator that is capable of replicating function of a traditional mechanical articulator has become available for many dental CAD systems. A virtual articulator is defined as a computer software tool that is capable of reproducing the inter-arch relationship and simulating eccentric mandibular movements (Fig. 13.16A–C).

Computer-Aided Manufacturing

Once the design step is completed, design files are transferred to the CAM software and hardware that converts the virtual design to a physical object. Various dental materials, including dental ceramics, polymers, and metal alloys, are used for fabrication of dental restorations using CAM, either with subtractive or additive manufacturing.

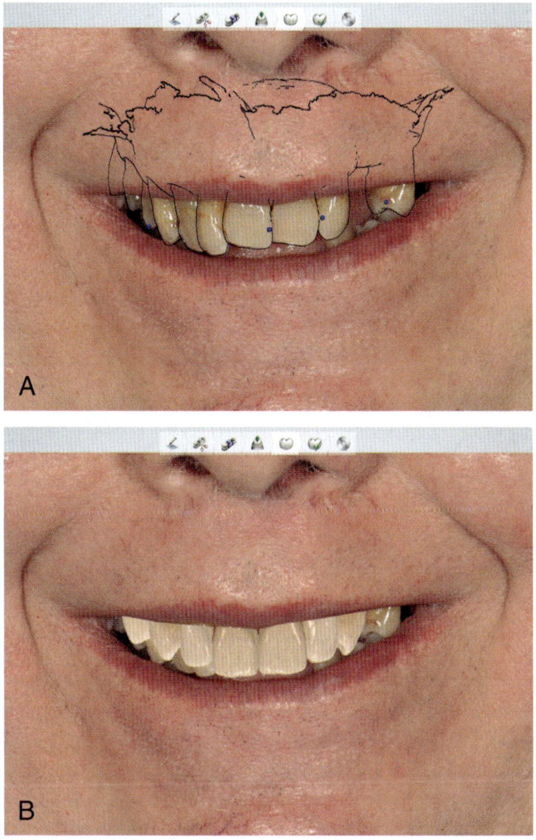

• **Fig. 13.14** Two-dimensional virtual aesthetic simulation. (A) Maxillary digital scan is aligned to the facial photo. (B) Aesthetic impact of the designed restorations is evaluated on the facial photo.

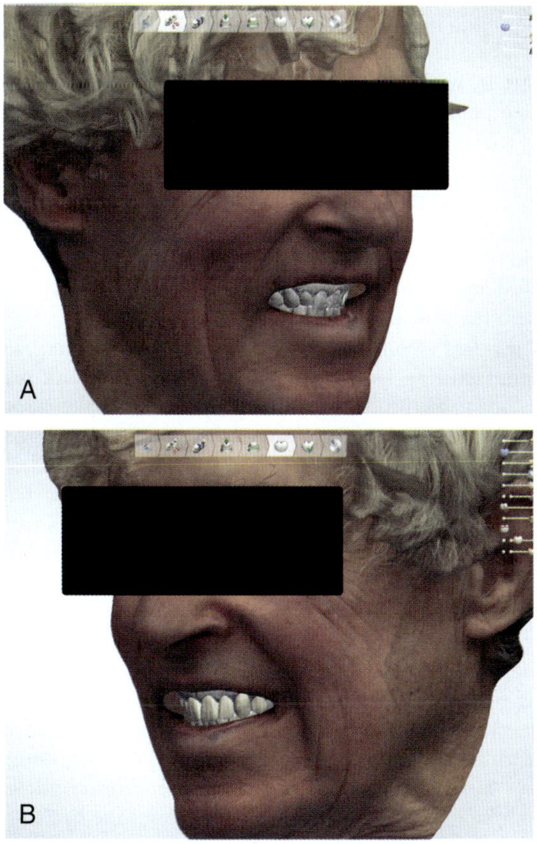

• **Fig. 13.15** Three-dimensional virtual aesthetic simulation. (A) Maxillary digital scan is aligned to the facial scan. (B) Aesthetic impact of the designed restorations is evaluated on the facial scan.

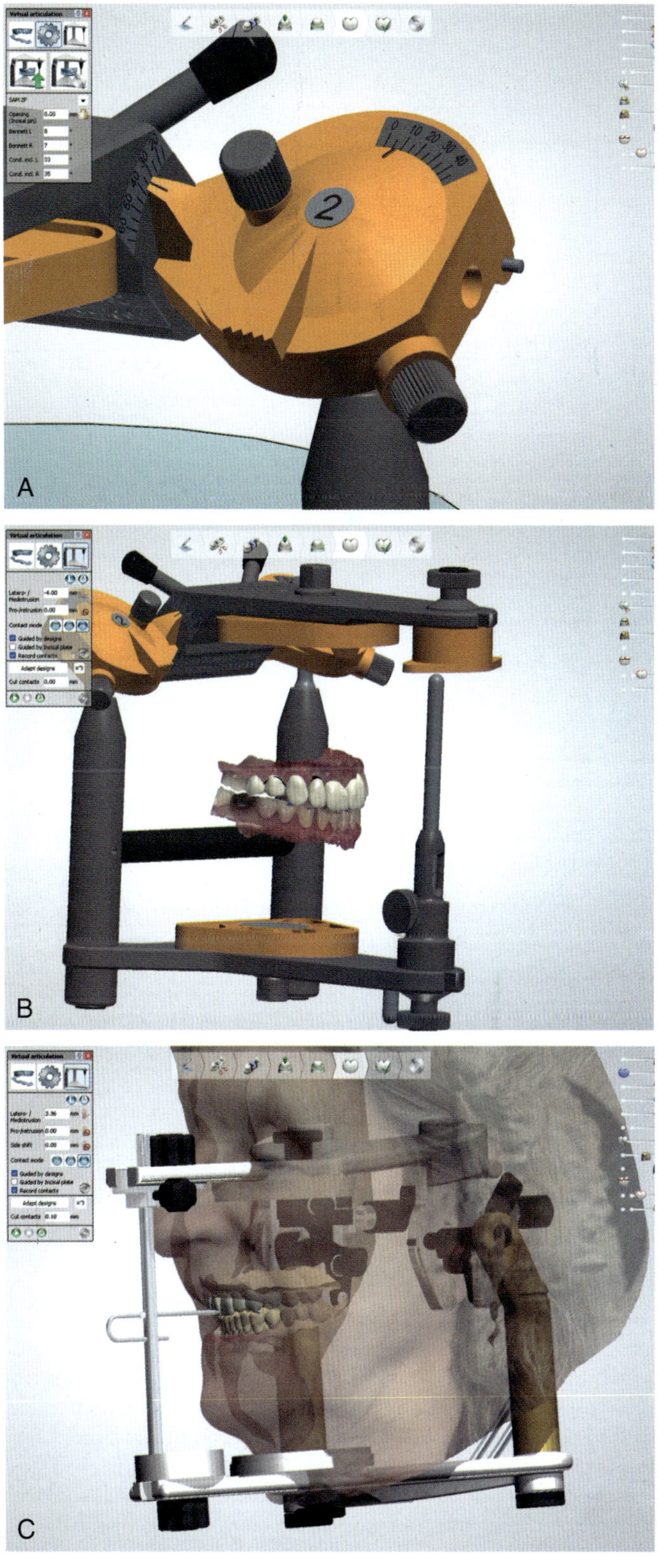

• **Fig. 13.16** Mathematically calculated virtual articulator. (A) Condylar elements can be adjusted. (B) Expected movements of patient's mandible are calculated based on the condylar element values. (C) Virtual patient. Combined aesthetic and functional (occlusal) simulation can make computer-aided design more predictable.

Subtractive Manufacturing

Subtractive manufacturing, also known as machining or milling, is a process in which a material is removed, typically by grinding, from a standard-shaped initial part (typically a block or puck)

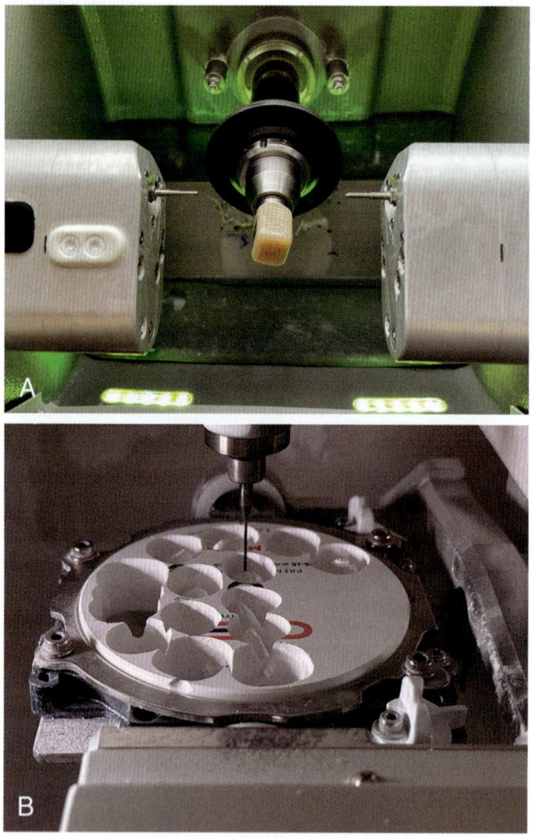

• **Fig. 13.17** Milling machines. (A) Four-axis milling machine (CEREC MC XL, Dentsply Sirona). (B) Five-axis milling machine (DWX-52D, Roland DGA).

to achieve the desired shape and dimensions. A milling machine, operated by a computer executing the sequences of commands, controls rotary milling tools to remove material precisely from the raw block until the desired shape and dimensions are achieved.

Milling Machines

The first dental milling machines allowed movements in three spatial directions (x-, y-, and z-axes) to produce reasonably accurate dental restorations with relatively simple anatomy. Most three-axis dental milling machines can turn the workpiece by 180 degrees, which allows the milling tools to be used for both intaglio and cameo surfaces of dental restorations. The advantages of three-axis milling machines include simplified control and lower cost. However, machinability at the bottom of the end mill is poor, and, sometimes, dental restorations with complex anatomy or undercuts cannot be milled accurately. In addition, the round-ended milling tools produce a cusp (milling mark) on the machined surface, which necessitates manual polishing after milling.

Currently, most commercially available chairside or laboratory milling machines use four-axis or five-axis milling (Fig. 13.17A and B). A four-axis milling machine functions similar to a three-axis machine, but, as the name indicates, it adds an axis of rotation (A-axis) to the standard X, Y, and Z linear movements. This extra rotational movement along the X-axis may be accomplished by moving the tool or the workpiece, making it easier to machine certain features, including undercuts. For advanced laboratory milling machines, another extra rotation movement along the Y-axis (B-axis) can be added as a fifth axis (Fig. 13.18), which not only facilitates the milling of complex anatomies but also yields smaller cusp heights at greater feeds than 3-axis milling. As a result, five-axis milling provides better surface finish with reduced production time. While milling machines with greater number of milling axes and additional movements are available, they are not commonly used in dentistry. Although the number of milling axes is not a primary factor that determines accuracy of milled restorations, some in vitro studies have shown that the use of five-axis milling machines may improve marginal fit of dental restorations.

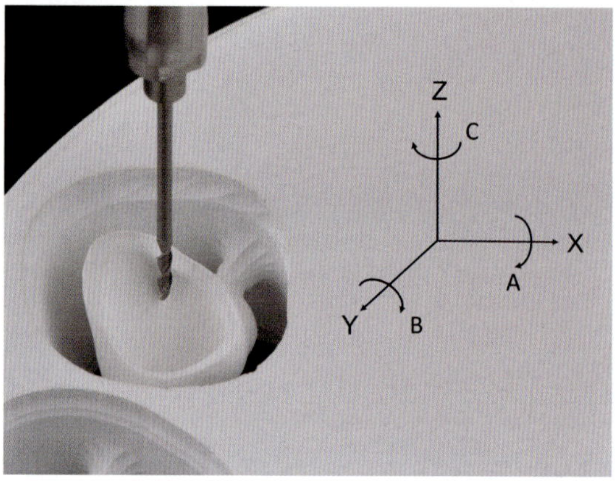

• **Fig. 13.18** Milling axes. Three linear axes (X-, Y-, Z-axes) and three rotational axes (A-, B-, C-). At least three linear axes are required for dental milling. In four-axis milling, one rotational axis is added to three linear axes. In five-axis milling, two different rotational axes (typically B- and C-axes, depending on the configuration of milling machines) are added to three linear axes.

Milling Tools

The first-generation dental milling machines used a lathe or disk-shaped milling tools and were able to fabricate simple restorations such as inlays or onlays, but restorations with complex geometries could not be milled until drill-shaped end mill cutters were introduced with flat or round ends (Fig. 13.19). Round-end or chamfer milling tools are most frequently used as they are optimized to generate smooth 3D curves while leaving the clean finish that is required for typical dental restorations. Important milling parameters for end milling include spindle speed, feed rate, tool diameter, and depth of cut (Fig. 13.20), which vary depending on the CAM system and material.

Due to the inability of a milling machine to reproduce negative shapes that are smaller than the milling tool diameter, subtractive manufacturing is suitable only for structures with relatively simple and smooth surface morphology. For example, complex or sharp structures such as irregular spikes, deep retentive grooves, or deep occlusal morphology cannot be accurately milled using a typical dental milling machine. If complex or sharp structures are present, the CAD-CAM software alters surface morphology of a design to allow for the diameter of the milling tool (milling tool diameter compensation). This typically results in overmilling around the sharp or irregular areas and is the most common cause of poor internal fit in milled restorations, frequently found around sharp incisal edges, line angles, or deep grooves (Fig. 13.21A–C). In order to prevent this issue, tooth preparation design for milled restorations should have simplified and rounded anatomy compared with tooth preparation design for conventional restorations.

Using milling tools with smaller diameters may allow more precise milling, but at the same time, increases the risk of milling tool wear and damage during the manufacturing process. Smaller milling tools also require higher spindle speeds. Because smaller

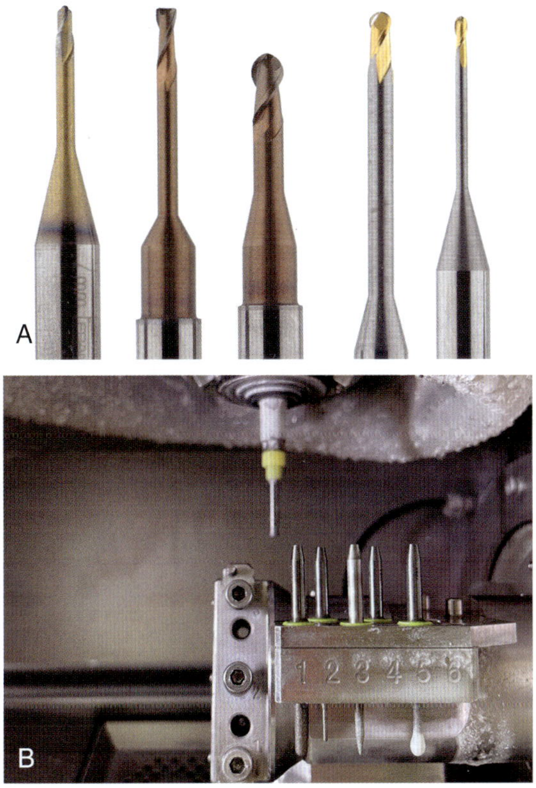

• **Fig. 13.19** Milling tools. (A) Carbide milling tools with various shapes and sizes are typically used for wax, resin-based polymers, partially sintered zirconia, and metal alloys. (B) Diamond-coated milling tools are used for glass ceramic materials. Milling tools for gross reduction (1), finishing (2), and occlusal anatomy (3).

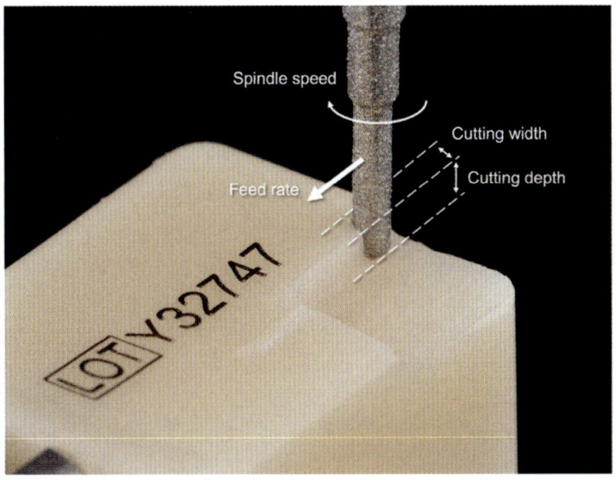

• **Fig. 13.20** Machining parameters.

tools have low stiffness, they may deform easily during the manufacturing process, which would negatively influence not only the quality and accuracy of milled restorations but also efficiency and economy of dental milling due to frequent replacement of milling tools. Loss of accuracy due to tool damage may be prevented by setting the depth of cut to a small value, but this makes milling slow and less efficient.

Considering both precision and efficiency, milling tools with 1.0 mm or greater diameter are commonly used for dentistry. While milling tools with smaller diameters (0.5–1.0 mm) are available for softer materials, such as resin or presintered zirconia, the use of milling tools smaller than 1.0 mm for hard ceramic materials does not seem practical. As the diameter and shape of milling tools vary depending on the system and material, clinicians should know the exact configurations of the milling tools and take them into consideration when preparing teeth.

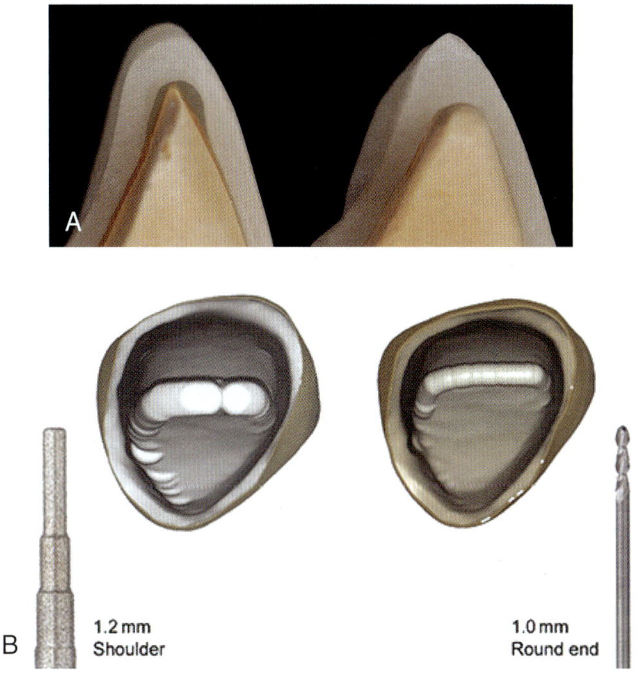

• **Fig. 13.21** Milling tool diameter compensation. (A) Overmilling around the sharp edge can result in poor internal adaptation of a milled restoration (*left*). Sharp edges should be rounded to prevent overmilling (*right*). (B) The result of milling tool diameter compensation depends on the shape and diameter of milling tools. A round-end tool with a smaller diameter can reduce the amount of overmilling.

Milling tools must be closely monitored during and after milling, and they should be replaced when necessary. While most dental milling systems provide a reliable milling tool monitoring system, visual inspection is still recommended (Fig. 13.22). Carbide milling tools with well-defined cutting edges are typically used for relatively soft dental materials such as wax, resin-based materials, and presintered zirconia. Since harder dental materials lead to greater tool wear, materials such as glass ceramics cannot be predictably milled using carbide milling tools, and instead diamond-coated milling tools with no cutting edges are commonly used.

Subtractive Manufacturing of Ceramic Materials

A wide range of dental ceramic materials are available for subtractive manufacturing (Table 13.3), with lithium disilicate ceramic and zirconia as the two most popular dental ceramic materials among dentists in the United States (Fig. 13.23).

Ceramic Milling Strategies

The main advantage of dental ceramic as a restorative material is its excellent aesthetics. On the other hand, a relatively high rate of mechanical complications, such as chipping or fracture, has been considered a limitation of dental ceramic materials. While the significant improvement in properties of ceramic materials has increased the longevity of such restorations, it has also made the manufacturing process more challenging. Machinability is the term referring to the ease with which a material can be cut or shaped while providing a satisfactory surface finish. A material

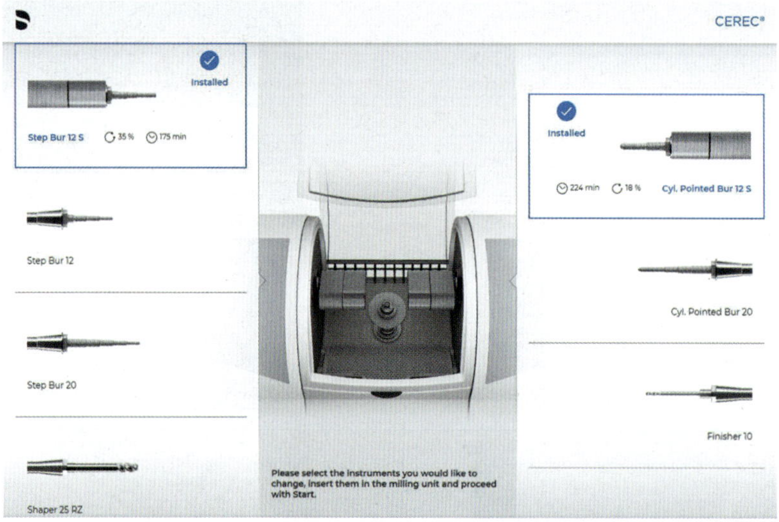

• **Fig. 13.22** Milling tool monitoring system (CEREC MC XL, Dentsply Sirona).

TABLE 13.3 **Examples of Currently Available Dental CAD-CAM Ceramic Products**

Material Group	Material	Brand Name	Manufacturer
Glass ceramic	Feldspathic glass ceramic	VITABLOCS Mark II	Vita Zahnfabrik
		CEREC Blocs	Dentsplay Sirona
	Leucite-reinforced glass ceramic	IPS Empress CAD	Ivoclar
High-strength glass ceramic	Lithium disilicate glass ceramic	IPS e.max CAD	Ivoclar
		CEREC Tessera	Dentsply Sirona
		Amber Mill	Haas
		GC Initial LiSi Block	GC
	Lithium silicate glass ceramic	Obsidian	Glidewell
	Zirconia-reinforced lithium silicate ceramic	Celtra Duo	Dentsply Sirona
		VITA Suprinity	Vita Zahnfabrik
Zirconia	Partially sintered zirconia	LAVA Plus, LAVA Aesthetic	3M
		CEREC MTL Zirconia	Dentsply Sirona
		Prettau	Zirkonzahn
		IPS e.max ZirCAD	Ivoclar
		VITA YZ	Vita Zahnfabrik
		Katana Zirconia	Kuraray Noritake
	Fully sintered zirconia	BruxZir NOW	Glidewell
Hybrid resin-ceramic	Nanoceramic resin	LAVA Ultimate	3M
		Cerasmart	GC
	Polymer-infiltrated ceramic network	VITA Enamic	Vita Zahnfabrik

with good machinability requires little power to cut, produces a smooth surface finish, and causes minimal tool wear or damage. Dental ceramic materials are brittle and hard, causing significant wear and damage on the milling tools. Worn or damaged milling tools can produce low-quality restorations. Since a high level of stress is anticipated during diamond grinding, most dental ceramic restorations, with the exception of presintered zirconia, are fabricated using the wet milling process, meaning that fluid (typically distilled water with some additives) is used to keep the surface temperature stable, lubricate the cutting surface, and eliminate debris from the milling tools. Both wet and dry milling may be used for presintered zirconia.

While diamond coating extends the lifetime of milling tools, it does not eliminate the risk of inducing surface damage such as micro-cracks and micro-chippings on the surface of the material. Glass-ceramic materials are especially sensitive to surface flaws, which can lead to strength degradation and premature failure of ceramic restorations.

To minimize these mechanical risks during milling, the hardness of the workpiece should be controlled below a certain level.

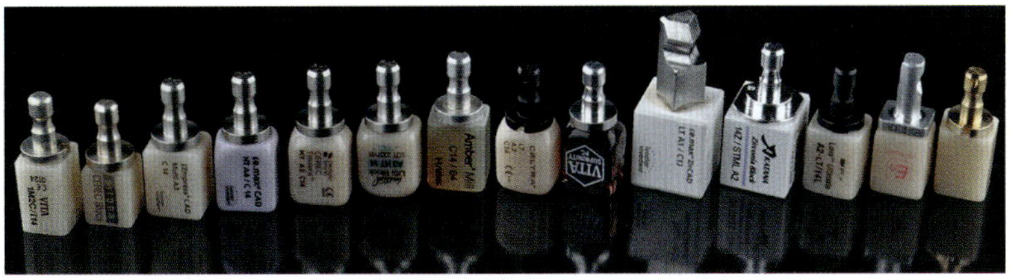

• **Fig. 13.23** Examples of commercially available ceramic materials for subtractive manufacturing. From the left to the right, VITABLOCS Mark II (feldspathic glass ceramic), CEREC Blocs (feldspathic glass ceramic), IPS Empress CAD (leucite-reinforced glass ceramic), IPS e.max CAD (lithium disilicate glass ceramic), CEREC Tessera (lithium disilicate glass ceramic), GC Initial LiSi Block (lithium disilicate glass ceramic), Amber Mill (lithium disilicate glass ceramic), Celtra Duo (zirconia-reinforced lithium silicate ceramic), VITA Suprinity (zirconia-reinforced lithium silicate ceramic), IPS e.max ZirCAD (partially sintered zirconia), Katana Zirconia (partially sintered zirconia), LAVA Ultimate (nanoceramic resin), VITA Enamic (polymer-infiltrated ceramic network), GC Cerasmart (nanoceramic resin).

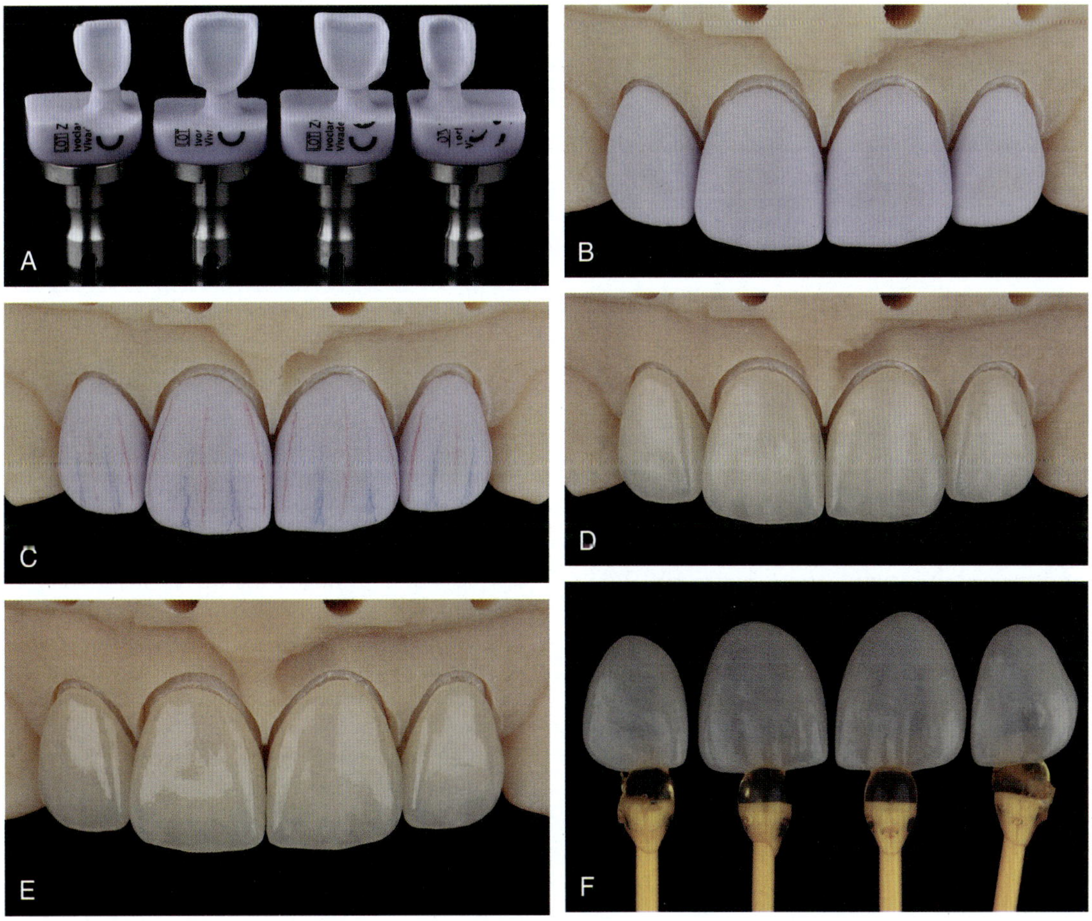

• **Fig. 13.24** Fabrication of monolithic lithium disilicate ceramic restoration. (A) Milled lithium disilicate restorations (IPS e.max CAD, Ivoclar). (B) Sprue removal and gross adjustment. (C) Detailed anatomy marking and manual adjustment. (D) External staining and crystallization. (E) Surface glazing. (F) Completed ceramic veneers.

For this reason, producing restorations from high-strength ceramic materials that are difficult to mill in their final state is usually accomplished by milling ceramic blocks purposely produced in a "soft" state, one in which the material has relatively low hardness. Once milling and contouring of the restoration are completed, the restoration is heat-treated and transformed into a product that has much higher hardness and strength. Both lithium disilicate ceramic and zirconia use this strategy.

When fabricating a lithium disilicate ceramic restoration, a precrystalized lithium disilicate block, often called blue state, is milled to achieve the desired shape and dimension. Precrystallized lithium disilicate ceramic, while having lower hardness than when it is crystallized to its final state, still has relatively high hardness compared with other dental materials and requires wet milling with diamond-coated milling tools. Once milling is completed, the object may be adjusted or recontoured if needed before it is fully crystallized by a heat treatment to produce enhanced physical and aesthetic properties (Fig. 13.24). The firing cycle for lithium disilicate ceramic restorations is relatively short and dimensional change during crystallization is known to be insignificant.

Although there are fully sintered zirconia products available for hard milling, most zirconia products are only partially sintered,

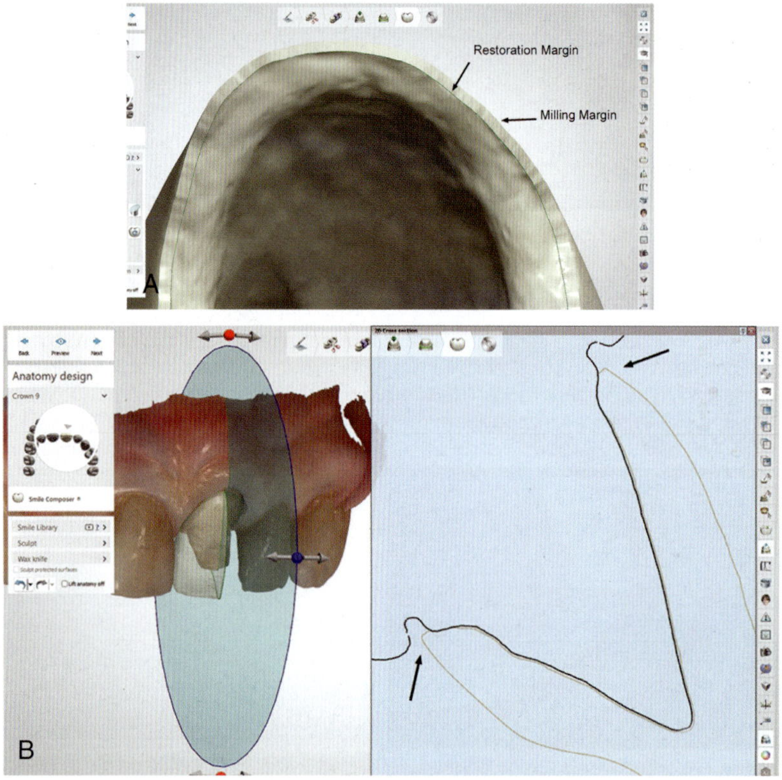

• **Fig. 13.25** Margin offset. (A) The milling margin is set 200 µm away from the actual restoration margin to avoid micro-chippings on the restoration margin. (B) The cervical area of the restoration is over-contoured to create the margin offset. Manual re-contouring is necessary after milling.

often called green state, and are "soft" enough to be fabricated by dry milling with regular carbide milling tools. After manual adjustment, milled zirconia restorations are subjected to a heat treatment for full sintering to produce a final product that has higher properties than glass ceramics (see Chapter 10). While most zirconia products have relatively long sintering times, fast-sintering zirconia recently has become available.

Zirconia undergoes approximately 20% of volumetric shrinkage during sintering, which is compensated by milling a presintered zirconia restoration 20% larger than the actual design. The ratio between the volume of presintered and fully sintered zirconia is called enlargement factor or enlargement coefficient and this number is unique to each zirconia product. The exact enlargement coefficient must be provided during restoration design to ensure accuracy of the final restoration. Although it is precisely calculated and compensated, this high sintering shrinkage of zirconia restorations can have a negative influence on the final accuracy of zirconia restorations. While long-span (>4 units) and curved configurations are known to be risk factors that can increase dimensional distortion during sintering, the final accuracy of zirconia restorations after sintering is known to be clinically acceptable in most short-span clinical cases.

Frequent micro-chippings on the restoration margin are still considered a limitation of milled glass-ceramic restorations, even those produced by soft milling. It was reported that 70% of CAD-CAM-generated lithium disilicate crowns had micro-chippings on their margins and the potential for marginal chipping increases with an acute marginal angle. In order to fabricate ceramic restoration with an intact margin, the CAD-CAM software modifies the restoration design around the margin and sets the milling margin slightly outside of the actual restoration margin (Fig. 13.25A). As materials with poor machinability require greater margin offset values in general, a relatively high margin offset value (typically 100–200 µm) is recommended for most glass-ceramic materials, including lithium disilicate ceramic. Presintered zirconia may be successfully fabricated with a lower margin offset value (~100 µm). At least 50–100 µm of margin offset is widely used even for materials with good machinability to compensate for material loss during postmilling contouring and finishing. This overcontoured area is then manually removed during postmilling finishing to achieve an adequate contouring and smooth finish (Fig. 13.25B). Diamond-impregnated silicone rotary instruments are recommended for margin finishing.

Considerations for Postmilling Processes

A monolithic ceramic restoration may be finished by either polishing or glazing. When a bilayered ceramic restoration is indicated, an extra layer of veneering ceramic may be applied on a milled monolithic ceramic framework.

The advantages of monolithic ceramic restorations include superior physical properties and high manufacturing efficiency. Most currently available ceramic materials used for subtractive manufacturing have superior physical properties compared with those of bilayered ceramics, and clinical studies have shown that monolithic restorations made of lithium disilicate or zirconia have a lower fracture rate. Inhomogeneous application of the veneer may introduce internal voids or other types of flaws, potentially compromising the structural integrity of the restoration.

To achieve more aesthetic outcomes, monolithic ceramic restorations may undergo additional firing cycles to be stained and glazed. When achieving an aesthetically pleasing outcome is not a

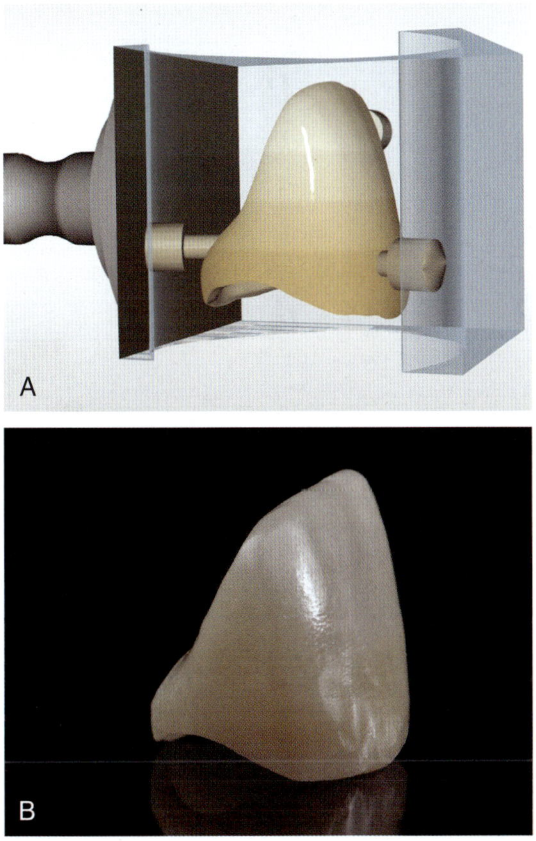

• **Fig. 13.26** Monolithic zirconia restoration fabricated from a multichromatic block. (A) The virtual design is positioned within the multichromatic block with four different shade/translucency levels to create restorations with vertical shade/translucency gradation. (B) The zirconia restoration is milled and sintered from a multichromatic zirconia block (Katana Zirconia STML). The incisal edge area has higher translucency and lighter shade. The cervical area shows lower translucency and darker shade. External staining can be added when desired.

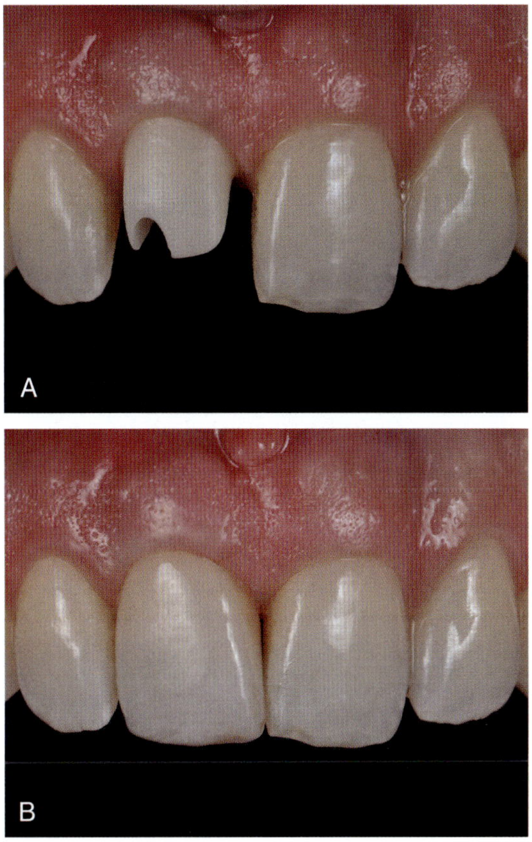

• **Fig. 13.27** Monolithic lithium disilicate ceramic restoration combined with a zirconia implant abutment. (A) Zirconia abutment with the desired base color was used. (B) Monolithic lithium disilicate ceramic restoration stained externally. An acceptable aesthetic outcome was achieved by using a monolithic restoration with external staining because the adjacent teeth had relatively simple color characteristics.

primary concern, monolithic restorations may be finished simply by polishing. Other than not requiring multiple firing cycles, polished lithium disilicate ceramic or zirconia restorations also have the advantage of being kind to the opposing dentition compared with glazed ones.

While preferred from a mechanical point of view, the greatest weakness of monolithic ceramic restorations is their limited ability to reproduce the complex optical characteristics of natural teeth. Although blocks with various translucencies and shades are available, monolithic restorations are innately monochromatic. Some ceramic products provide the option of using multichromatic blocks that are designed to have different translucencies and shades in different regions of the block, but shade variations that can be created by monolithic ceramic restorations are still limited (Fig. 13.26A and B). The aesthetic outcome of monolithic ceramic restorations can be considerably improved by external staining with subsequent glazing to protect the stain. CAD-CAM-generated ceramic frameworks should be fully heat-treated before applying veneering ceramics. The ceramic veneering process is highly technique-sensitive, and typically requires multiple firing cycles, though these should be kept to a minimum to prevent potential distortion and deterioration of aesthetic and mechanical properties of the framework.

The basic appearance of lithium disilicate ceramic or other CAD-CAM glass-ceramic materials is relatively close to that of natural teeth. Because ceramic blocks with a large variety of shades and translucencies are available, it is possible to achieve an acceptable aesthetic outcome without using veneering ceramics. The translucency of lithium disilicate ceramic blocks is mainly controlled by altering the volume and the size of crystals, with a reduced crystal size leading to an increased opacity. Studies show that these differences in composition to alter translucency generally do not affect the strength of the materials. Therefore monolithic restorations may be preferred for posterior teeth and some anterior teeth with relatively simple color characteristics, but facial veneering may be beneficial when complex intrinsic shading is required (Fig. 13.27A and B).

In contrast, the optical characteristics of zirconia do not resemble those of natural teeth. While external staining can be used to improve the aesthetic outcome, the inherent opaqueness of zirconia makes it difficult to reproduce a true tooth-like appearance. Translucency of zirconia can be enhanced by substituting some tetragonal zirconia grains with optically isotropic cubic zirconia particles, which is typically achieved by increasing the concentration of stabilizers such as yttria (see Chapter 10). However, zirconia with increased yttria concentration (4–6 mol%), so-called translucent zirconia, is still less translucent than lithium disilicate ceramic, and it has a significantly lower flexural strength compared with tetragonal zirconia. Thus translucent zirconia should be used with caution after carefully reviewing aesthetic and functional requirements of the restoration. Monolithic zirconia restorations are preferred in many cases due to their excellent

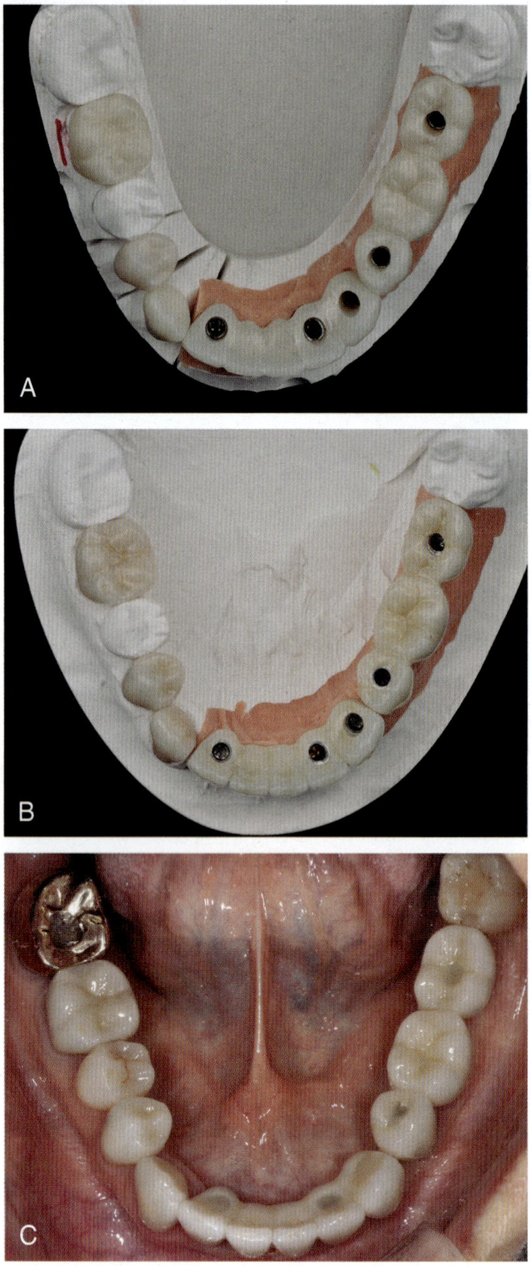

• **Fig. 13.28** Monolithic zirconia fixed dental prosthesis. (A) Fully sintered monolithic zirconia fixed dental prosthesis. (B) Externally stained and glazed. (C) 6 months follow-up.

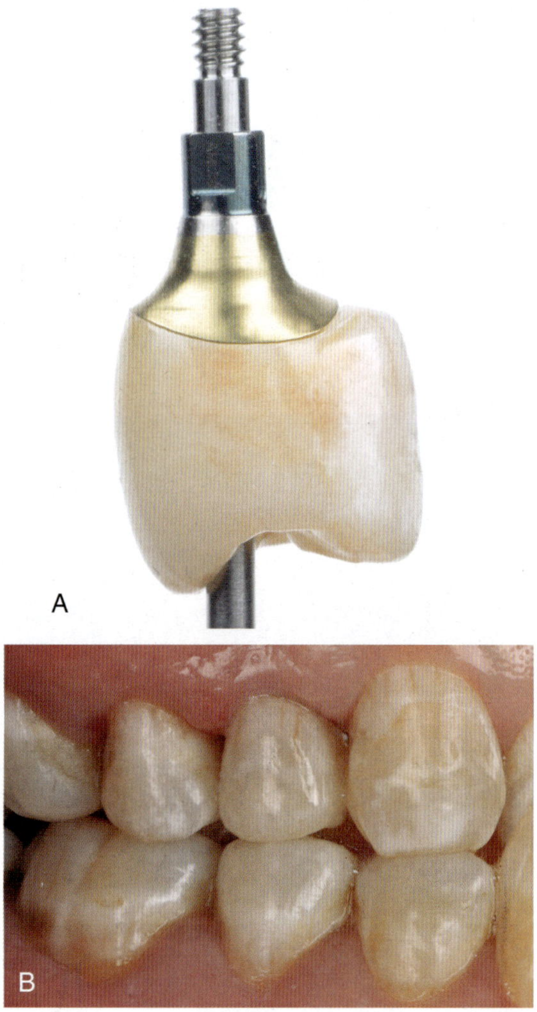

• **Fig. 13.29** Bilayered zirconia implant restoration. (A) In order to mask the dark metal color of the custom implant abutment, zirconia with low yttria concentration (3 mol%) was selected to fabricate the framework of the crown. The facial surface was minimally layered with veneering ceramic to achieve the desired aesthetic outcome. The occlusal and palatal surfaces were externally stained and glazed. (B) The dark metal color was masked effectively while successfully reproducing acceptable aesthetic on the facial surface.

mechanical properties, but bilayered restorations are still widely used when optimal aesthetic outcome is desired (Figs. 13.28A–C and 13.29A,B).

Subtractive Manufacturing of Other Materials

Wax

Some manufacturers provide machinable wax blocks to incorporate a digital workflow into a dental laboratory's fabrication of castable restorations as manual waxing is technique-sensitive, time-consuming, and labor-intensive. Machinable wax is harder than regular dental wax and is composed of acrylate polymers. When fabricating cast metal or heat-pressed ceramic restorations, the use of machinable wax blocks may improve efficiency by allowing clinicians to make an intraoral scan instead of a conventional impression and by allowing dental technicians to use CAD-CAM technologies to design and fabricate wax patterns to be used with conventional lost-wax casting techniques. The accuracy of ceramic or metal restorations fabricated using milled wax patterns has been shown to be acceptable, as long as the clinician understands that tooth preparation design for conventional cast restorations, such as sharp line angles and deep retention grooves, may not be accurately reproduced on the wax pattern due to milling tool diameter compensation.

Polymethyl Methacrylate (PMMA)

The excellent machinability of PMMA, available in a wide range of shades and translucencies, allows dry milling using carbide milling tools at a relatively low spindle speed. Although the chemical composition of machinable PMMA blanks is similar to that of traditional PMMA, physical properties such as flexural strength, wear resistance, and color stability, are superior to that of traditional PMMA due to the high degree of polymerization and

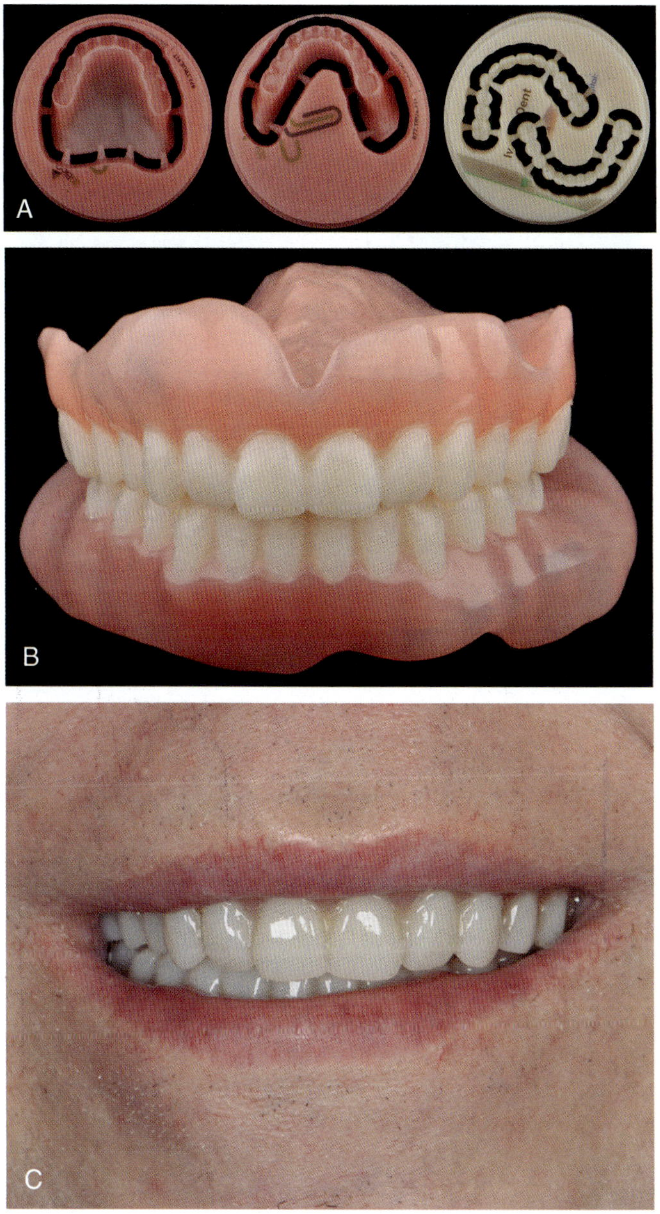

• **Fig. 13.30** Milled PMMA denture. (A) Milled denture bases and denture teeth. (B) Milled PMMA complete dentures. (C) Monochromatic appearance and limited embrasure spaces between denture teeth are still limitations.

highly dense and homogeneous structures achieved under well-controlled industrial manufacturing environments. PMMA is used to fabricate interim dental restorations or prostheses, removable dental prostheses, occlusal guards, and other intraoral devices (Fig. 13.30A–C). Because PMMA blanks are prepolymerized and free from processing shrinkage, the accuracy of milled PMMA prostheses is superior to those made by heat- or auto-polymerization methods.

Resin Composite, Hybrid Resin-Ceramic

Recently, traditional resin composite blocks have been replaced with hybrid resin-ceramic materials that reproduce tooth aesthetics very well (Fig. 13.31). These materials are created by either incorporating ceramic filler particles into a polymer matrix or infiltrating a continuous ceramic network with a polymer. As a result, mechanical properties including flexural strength, wear resistance,

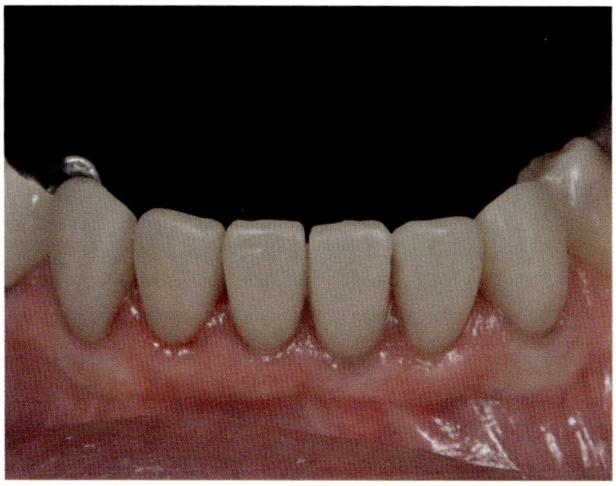

• **Fig. 13.31** Hybrid resin-ceramic crowns (#22–27, VITA Enamic).

and modulus of elasticity of these materials lay between those of resin composite and high-strength glass ceramic. This combination of low hardness coupled with high strength enables efficient milling with minimal micro-chippings and fabrication of restorations with a high resistance to sliding impact-induced cracking. Hybrid resin-ceramic materials are mainly used for indirect partial coverage restorations such as inlays or onlays, and outcomes from short-term clinical studies evaluating survival rates appear to be promising.

Metal Alloys

Various types of metal alloys including titanium, cobalt-chromium, and noble or high-noble gold alloys can be milled to fabricate dental restorations or prostheses, with milling of titanium alloys being the most common. The alloys are discussed in Chapter 9.

Additive Manufacturing

Additive manufacturing, often called 3D printing or rapid prototyping, is the process of sequentially joining materials to make objects from 3D model data, usually layer upon layer. It first appeared on the dental market in the early 1980s, and with the advancements in other digital technologies, it has now gained great popularity in dentistry (Table 13.4). Initially, additive manufacturing was developed for polymers, but the need for materials with enhanced properties has led researchers to develop applications for metals and ceramics.

Additive Manufacturing Technologies

The International Organization for Standardization (ISO) divides additive manufacturing processes into seven basic categories based on the fundamental parts of the machines' functionality (Table 13.5). The most commonly used additive manufacturing technology in dentistry is vat photopolymerization. Examples of all different types of 3D printers commercially available are shown in Table 13.6.

Stereolithography (SLA)

The SLA process uses an ultraviolet laser to selectively polymerize layers of UV-sensitive liquid monomer filled in a vat. Then, a "build" platform holding the object moves up or down vertically and the surface is recoated with liquid monomer followed by surface leveling, being ready for the next laser polymerization cycle. This process is repeated until the entire object is built layer-by-layer to completion.

There are two different approaches depending on the direction of the vertical movement during the manufacturing process:

TABLE 13.4 Advantages of Additive Manufacturing Compared With Subtractive Manufacturing

	Additive Manufacturing	Subtractive Manufacturing
Surface resolution	Surface resolution is determined by layer thickness, which represents the vertical accuracy.	The surface resolution is limited by the smallest tool diameter.
Material use	Additive manufacturing can save material. Waste material can be reused.	Material loss can reach 90%.
Production efficiency	A longer processing time is required, but multiple objects can be produced at the same time.	The processing time is shorter, but the number of objects that can be produced per machining operation is limited.
Shape complexity	Additive manufacturing is capable of producing complex geometries.	Suitable for relatively simple geometries. Shape complexity is limited by milling tools and axes.
Tool-related problems	No tool-related issues.	The tools used in subtractive manufacturing show signs of wear and damage after repeated use, which can lead to cracks or other flaws in the objects produced.

bottom-up or top-down. Most earlier SLA printers used the bottom-up approach, where the build platform lowers after polymerizing a layer to coat another layer of liquid monomer. One of the main limitations of this approach is that this requires a large vat of resin, which leads to large consumption of materials. When the top-down approach is used, the first layer is polymerized on the bottom of the vat and then lifted upward. Then, the gap between the first layer and the bottom is filled with liquid monomer, being ready for the next polymerization cycle. The unpolymerized liquid is removed by draining, allowing fabrication of the objects with a smaller vat and less material. For this reason, many latest-generation SLA printers use the top-down approach. The layer thickness varies depending on the printer model and its settings, but most SLA printers used in dentistry have a layer thickness ranging from 15 to 200 μm.

SLA was the first additive manufacturing technology introduced in dentistry and it is also the most popular one today. It is capable of producing objects with high accuracy and relatively smooth surface finish. The latest generation of SLA printers has become more affordable, making this technology even more popular and capable of being used with various resin-based polymer materials (Fig. 13.32A and B).

Digital Light Processing (DLP)

DLP is another type of SLA. The basic mechanisms are very similar, but the main difference is that DLP uses a projection of ultraviolet or visible light from a digital projector to flash a single image of the entire resin layer at once. This makes DLP faster than SLA. This is possible due to a digital micromirror device (DMD) chip, which is an array of micromirrors that redirect light from the UV source to project an image of the entire layer of the CAD

TABLE 13.5 Basic Categories of Additive Manufacturing Processes

Category	Definition	Manufacturing Process
Vat photopolymerization	Liquid photopolymer in a vat is selectively cured by light-activated polymerization.	• Stereolithography • Digital light processing • Continuous digital light processing • Liquid crystal display
Material jetting	Droplets of build material are selectively deposited.	• Material jetting • Nanoparticle jetting • Drop on demand
Binder jetting	A liquid bonding agent is selectively deposited to join powder materials.	• Binder jetting
Powder bed fusion	Thermal energy selectively fuses regions of a powder bed.	• Selective laser sintering • Direct metal laser sintering • Selective laser melting • Electron beam melting
Material extrusion	Material is selectively dispensed through a nozzle or orifice.	• Fused deposition modeling • Fused filament fabrication
Directed energy deposition	Focused thermal energy is used to fuse materials by melting as they are being deposited.	• Laser engineering net shape • Electron beam additive manufacturing
Sheet lamination	Sheets of material are bonded to form an object.	• Laminate object manufacturing

model. DLP is capable of producing small and complex objects with high accuracy, relatively smooth finish, and higher speed (Fig. 13.33A–C).

Continuous Digital Light Processing (CDLP)

Continuous digital light processing (CDLP) or continuous liquid interface production (CLIP) is a newly developed vat photopolymerization process. It is similar to DLP, but in contrast to the incremental build of DLP, CLIP involves a continuous build process that does not require detaching objects from the build platform. UV light is projected through the UV transparent and oxygen-permissible window. As the liquid resin starts polymerizing, the resin lying immediately above the window forms a thin oxygen-rich layer, called "dead zone," and does not polymerize. This dead zone enables continuous addition of new layers without having to detach the object from the window until the object is completely built. This results in high printing speed, precision, and continuous geometries along the z-axis (Fig. 13.34).

Material Jetting

Material jetting involves jetting small drops of material directly to the build platform from an array of nozzles, after which the

TABLE 13.6 Examples of Commercially Available 3D Printers for Dental Use

Manufacturer	3D Printer	Technology
3D Systems	NextDent 5100	Digital light processing
	ProX 800 for Dental	Stereolithography
	Projet MJP 2500 Plus	Material jetting
	DMP Dental 100	Direct metal laser sintering/ Selective laser melting
	DMP Flex 200	Direct metal laser sintering/ Selective laser melting
Ackuretta	Sol	Liquid crystal display
	DENTIQ	Liquid crystal display
Asiga	Max / Max X	Digital light processing
	Pro 4K UV	Digital light processing
Bego	Varseo X	Digital light processing
Carbon	L1	Continuous digital light processing (CLIP)
	M Series	Continuous digital light processing (CLIP)
DMG	3Delite	Digital light processing
	3Demax	Digital light processing
Envisiontec	D4K	Digital light processing
	Envision One	Continuous digital light processing
EOS	M290	Direct metal laser sintering/ Selective laser melting
	Formiga P110	Selective laser sintering
Forlabs	Form2	Stereolithography
	Form 3B+	Stereolithography
RapidShape	D30+ / D50+	Digital light processing
Shera	Sheraprint20/30/50	Digital light processing
SprintRay	Pro S Dental	Digital light processing
	MoonRay S	Digital light processing
Stratasys	J series	Material jetting
	Object30 Dental Prime	Material jetting

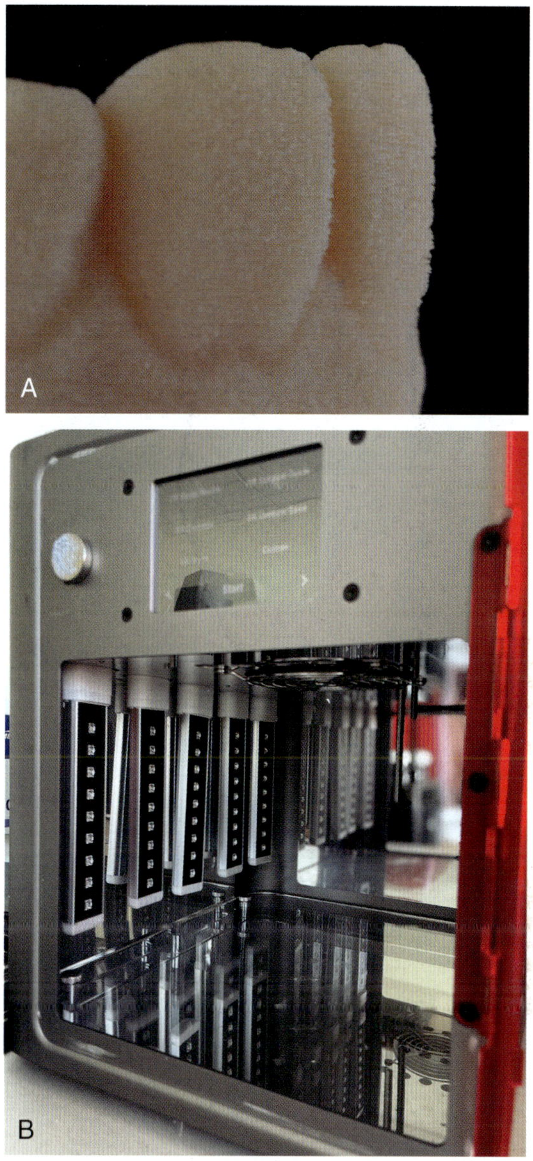

• **Fig. 13.32** Stereolithography. (A) Resin model printed using stereolithography. Rough surface texture due to the layer-by-layer manufacturing approach. The layers are perpendicular to the build orientation. (B) Post-processing (light curing) chamber.

material is immediately exposed to ultraviolet light for photopolymerization, producing objects in highly complex geometries at high resolution. In material jetting, small drops of material are loaded and immediately polymerized layer-by-layer. This enables printers to use different materials or colors for different layers. This multicolor printing is a special feature of material jetting technology and has great potential for applications when fabricating dental restorations or prostheses with color variations (Fig. 13.35A–C).

Selective Laser Sintering (SLS)

There are two types of SLS processes: indirect and direct. Indirect SLS uses polymers with low melting temperatures as binders, typically mixed with or coated on the high melting temperature primary powder. Direct SLS involves direct melting and consolidation of designated areas of the primary powder bed without binders, allowing fabrication of objects with high density. Direct SLS is typically used for metal powders and is also known as direct metal laser sintering (DMLS).

SLS is an additive manufacturing process of consolidating layers of powders of various materials using the heat of a laser beam. The fabrication chamber is filled with thermoplastic powder, and a laser beam is focused on the surface of the tightly compacted powder. The temperature of the fabrication chamber is maintained slightly below the melting point of the powder. A laser beam is focused on the surface of the thermoplastic powder to elevate the temperature and cause sintering. The object moves down by a layer thickness and another layer of powder is spread by the roller over the object. This process is repeated until the object is completely built. The particle size of the powder typically ranges from several micrometers to several hundred micrometers. The morphology and granulometry of the powder are known to be the main parameters influencing porosity of the printed object. CO_2, Nd:YAG and fiber lasers are commonly used for processing polymers, metals, and ceramics.

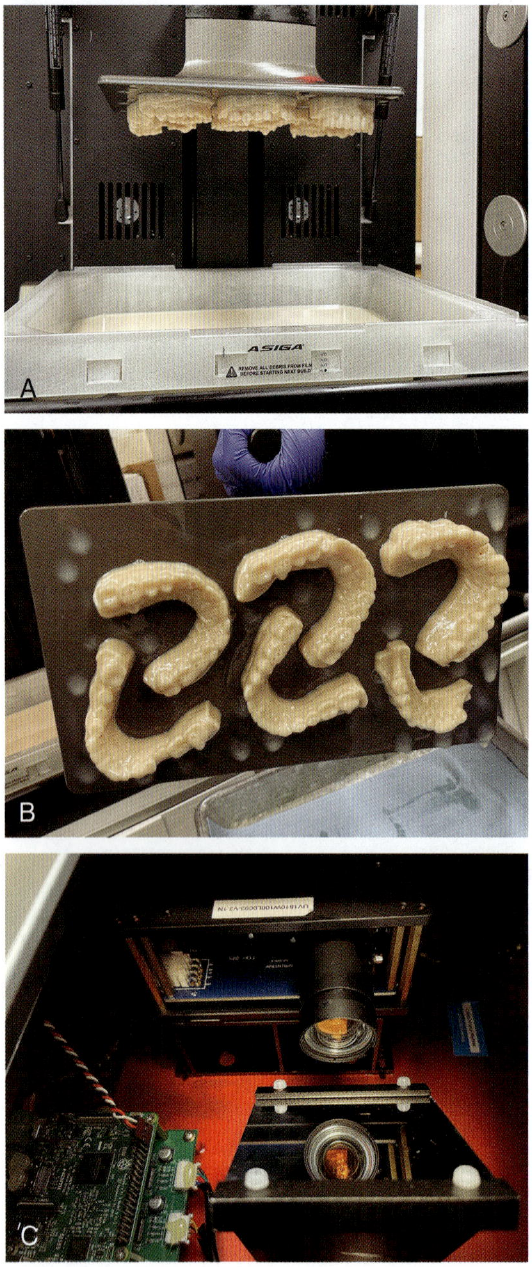

• **Fig. 13.33** Digital Light Processing (Pro 4K printer, ASIGA). (A) Liquid resin filled in a vat is polymerized layer-by-layer using DLP technology. (B) Efficiency of the manufacturing process can be enhanced by fabricating multiple models simultaneously. (C) Digital projector.

SLS is a relatively fast and economical manufacturing process. It is also capable of fabricating complex geometry, including overhangs and undercuts, as they can be supported by a solid powder bed. High accuracy and material versatility are also advantages of SLS. The major limitation of SLS, compared with vat polymerization technologies, is rough or porous surface finish, which typically requires manual finishing and polishing. The surface detail reproducibility of SLS is also not as great as that of SLA. SLS was developed for use with polymers but is now applied to ceramics and metals.

Selective Laser Melting (SLM)

SLM is typically used for additive manufacturing of metals and has become possible with the introduction of high-power

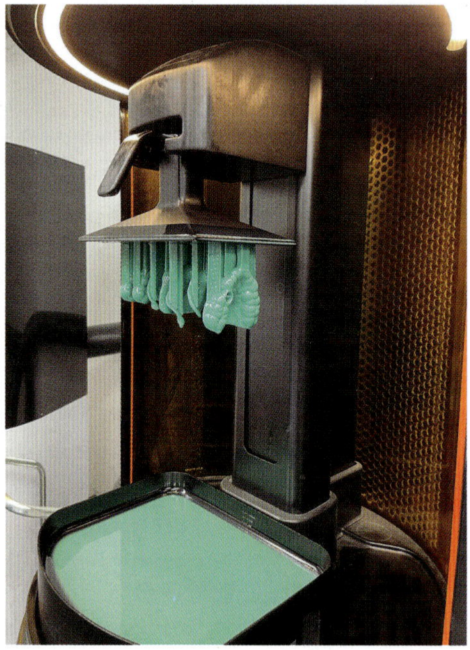

• **Fig. 13.34** Continuous liquid interface production (M2 Printer, Carbon).

lasers. A laser beam (most commonly Nd:YAG) is applied on the surface of the bed of densely compacted metal powder that does not contain binders. SLM is very similar to direct SLS, but SLM is done at higher laser power to achieve complete melting of the powders as opposed to partial melting. The fully molten metal powder is fused into a solid, similar to welding. The advantages of SLM include good part stability during fabrication, high accuracy, ability to produce complex geometry with negative angles and undercuts, and a wide range of material options, including high-noble, noble, and base metal alloys, the latter being predominantly titanium and Co-Cr for dental applications. As with SLS, poor surface finish is the main limitation of SLM (Fig. 13.36).

Additive Manufacturing of Polymer-Based Materials

Polymer Additive Manufacturing

Polymer-based resin materials are the most common option for additive manufacturing in dentistry to print various types of devices, including 3D models of dental arches and jaw bones, surgical templates, custom trays, interim dental restorations, removable dental prostheses, using SLA, DLP, CLIP, material jetting, material extrusion, or SLS. The polymers include PMMA, bisphenol A-glycidyl methacrylate (Bis-GMA), urethane dimethacrylate (UDMA), triethylene glycol dimethacrylate (TEGDMA), polyurethane, polylactic acid, acrylonitrile butadiene styrene, and polyetheretherketone (PEEK).

PMMA is frequently used for SLA or SLS to fabricate denture bases or occlusal guards. Although adding other materials such as PEEK, TiO_2, SiO_2, or Al_2O_3 can enhance its mechanical and biological properties to some degree, the mechanical properties of 3D-printed PMMA are slightly lower than that of milled PMMA. Various resin composite monomers, including bis-GMA, UDMA, and TEGDMA, have been used successfully for DLP and other additive manufacturing technologies, and potential clinical applications include interim restorations, dental casts, surgical guides, record bases, and custom trays.

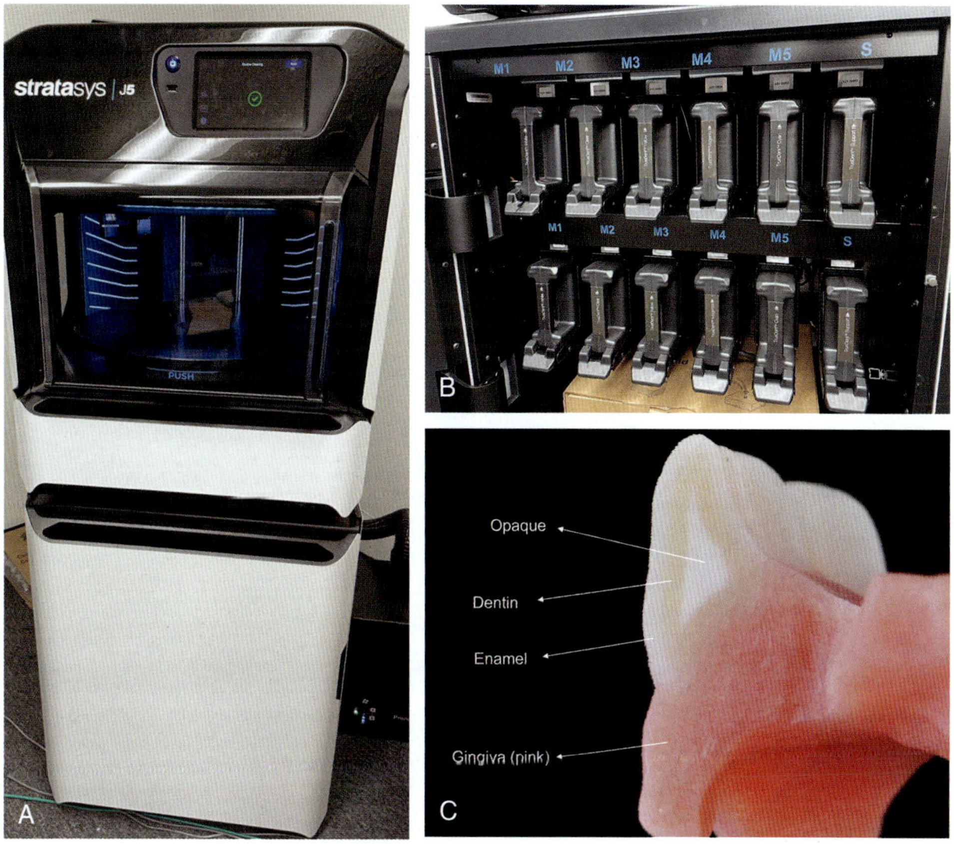

• **Fig. 13.35** Material jetting. (A) Material jetting printer (J5, Stratasys). Material is directly applied on the build platform. (B) Resin tanks with different color options. Some material jetting printers are capable of building an object using multiple colors. (C) Cross-section of an interim denture printed using material jetting. Material jetting technology allows multicolor printing.

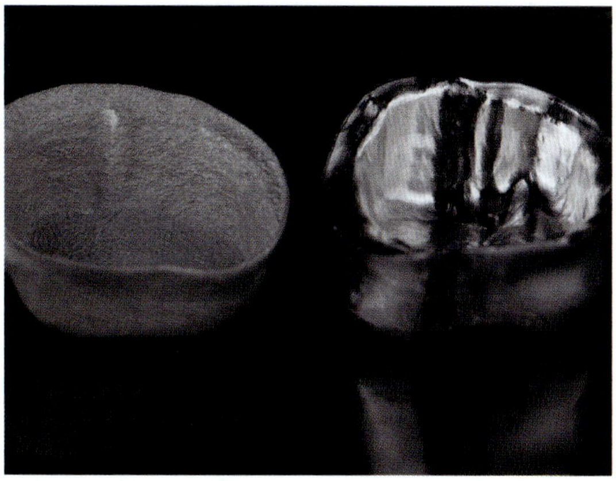

• **Fig. 13.36** Co-Cr metal coping fabricated by selective laser melting (*left*) and milling (*right*). Poor surface finish (porosity and roughness) is one of the main limitations of selective laser melting.

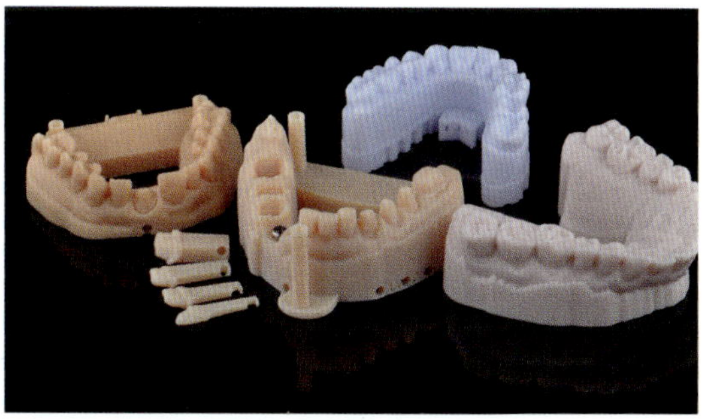

• **Fig. 13.37** 3D-printed models.

Clinical Application of 3D-printed Polymers

Generally, 3D-printed polymeric objects are not as dense as those fabricated with subtractive manufacturing technology, resulting in relatively lower mechanical properties and more porous surfaces. Some additive manufacturing processes also require postprocess light curing, which can lead to additional distortion of the printed objects. For this reason, clinical applications of 3D-printed polymeric materials are limited to devices that do not require high strength and longevity, such as 3D models, surgical templates, and interim prostheses. Recently, adjustment of components and addition of crosslinkers or photoinitiators have led to improvements in the mechanical properties of 3D-printed polymer materials to expand their use.

The most common use of 3D-printed polymers is fabrication of physical dental casts (Fig. 13.37), which are preferred by most dentists and dental technicians even when a digital workflow is used. Additive manufacturing by SLA, DLP, and material jetting can provide dental casts with acceptable accuracy at a reasonable cost.

SLA or DLP is typically used for fabrication of denture bases or occlusal guards (Figs. 13.38A,B and 13.39). The use of CAD-CAM technology for complete denture fabrication is increasing, but not yet mainstream. The flexural strength of 3D-printed denture base meets the ISO requirement (65MPa) but is significantly lower than that of milled or conventionally fabricated denture

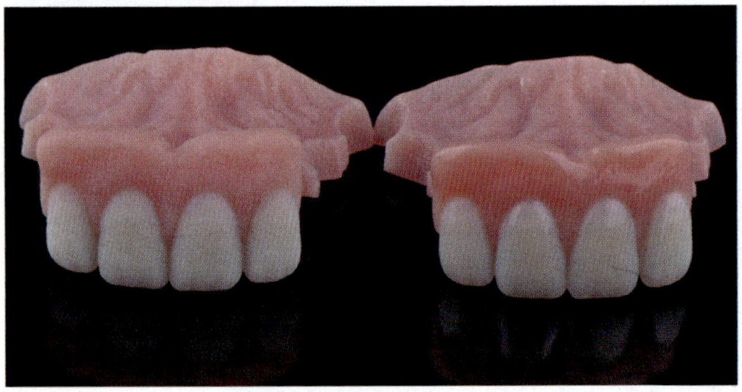

• **Fig. 13.38** 3D-printed interim removable dental prostheses. Before (*left*) and after (*right*) manual finishing.

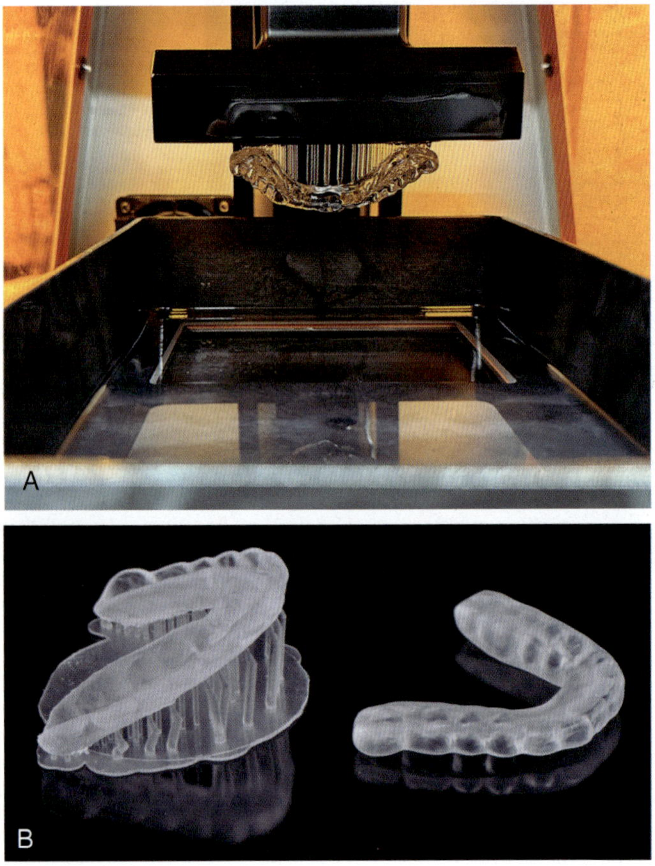

• **Fig. 13.39** 3D-printed occlusal guard. (A) Occlusal guard printed using continuous DLP. (B) Before (*left*) and after (*right*) manual finishing.

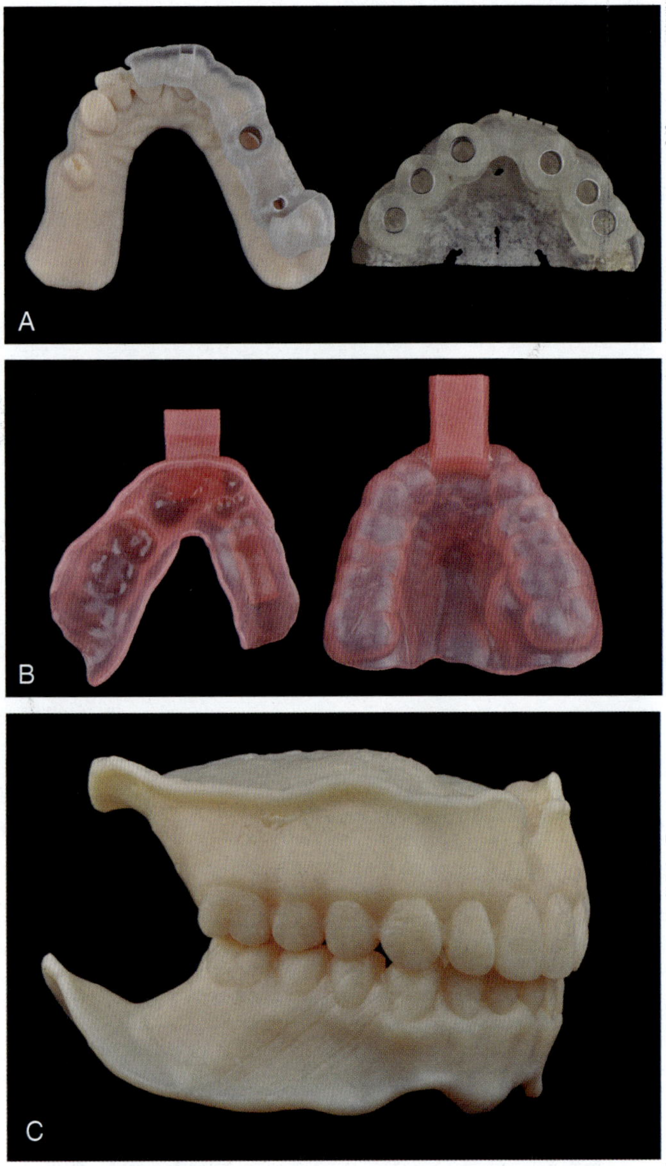

• **Fig. 13.40** Applications of 3D-printed polymers. (A) Tooth-borne implant surgical guide (*left*) and bone-borne implant surgical guide (*right*). (B) Custom impression trays. (C) Try-in dentures.

bases. Another potential limitation of 3D-printed polymers as a complete denture material is poor color stability, believed to be due in large part to increased water sorption and surface porosity. While printing angulation and layer thickness are known to be influencing factors, the accuracy of 3D-printed denture bases is slightly lower than for milled ones, though both are within clinically acceptable range. Reduced denture tooth bond strength as well as low adhesion to soft liners are also considered limitations of 3D-printed denture bases.

Occlusal guards should be strong enough to tolerate the stress generated by patients' parafunctional activities. Thus both fracture resistance and wear resistance are important criteria for clinical success when 3D-printed polymers are used for fabrication of occlusal guards. While the results from the studies are somewhat conflicting, it has been reported that the fracture resistance and wear resistance of 3D-printed occlusal guards are lower than those of milled occlusal guards. There are additional concerns about potential for increased monomer release and water sorption for 3D-printed occlusal guards.

Considering that criteria for interim restorations are not as rigorous as those for definitive restorations, 3D-printed resin composite appears to have adequate mechanical and surface properties for interim restorations. However, like many other 3D-printed resins, rough surface and potential for cytotoxicity remain concerns.

Various types of surgical templates, including implant surgical guides and bone regeneration scaffolds, removable dental prosthesis record bases, trial prostheses, and custom impression trays, are also common clinical applications of additive manufacturing of resin-based polymers (Fig. 13.40A–C). While almost all types of dental restorations or prostheses can be fabricated using both subtractive and additive manufacturing, clinicians should select manufacturing methods after carefully evaluating the properties

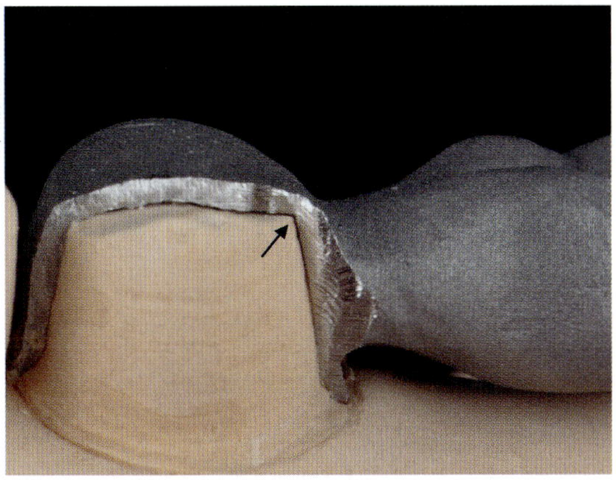

• **Fig. 13.41** Cross-section of the 3D-printed Co-Cr fixed dental prosthesis framework. Note that a clinically acceptable internal fit was achieved around the sharp edge. Additive manufacturing does not have the tool diameter compensation issue.

of materials as well as aesthetic and functional needs of the restorations. Many researchers and clinicians predict that the limitations of 3D-printed polymers will be overcome in the near future and the use of 3D-printed polymers in dentistry will continue to expand.

Additive Manufacturing of Metal Alloys

Metal Additive Manufacturing

Most metal restorations or prostheses are fabricated using the conventional lost-wax technique or subtractive manufacturing. However, the limitations of subtractive manufacturing, including milling tool diameter compensation, wear of milling tools, and waste of raw materials, especially for high-noble metal alloys, are driving the further development of additive manufacturing methods.

Powder bed fusion technologies, such as SLS and SLM, are used for additive manufacturing of metal alloys, but relatively poor surface finish and porosity are the main disadvantages. Surface finish can be improved by manual polish after processing, but porosity needs to be controlled as it is directly related to mechanical properties. While it is not possible to completely eliminate porosity, it can be reduced by optimizing processing parameters such as laser power, scanning velocity, hatch distance, powder particle size, and layer thickness. Full melting of the powder, as opposed to partial melting and sintering, minimizes the porosity and produces an almost completely dense material, which results in improved mechanical properties. For this reason, SLM is the most widely used technology for metal alloys in dentistry, including titanium, high-noble, noble, and base metal alloys, with Co-Cr being one of the most popular. 3D-printed Co-Cr alloys are used for the frameworks of fixed dental prostheses, removable dental prostheses, and implant-supported dental prostheses.

Clinical Applications of 3D-printed Metal Alloys

SLM-printed metal restorations have neither the distortion from metal shrinkage seen in the conventional lost-wax casting process nor the limitation from milling tool diameter in subtractive manufacturing (Fig. 13.41). Most often, Co-Cr alloys are used and studies have concluded that the accuracy of the 3D-printed frameworks is comparable or superior to that of milled or cast metal frameworks. SLM also allows fabrication of metal frameworks with less cost and time. However, the poor surface finish and porosity are still considered limitations. The typical rough surface seen in the 3D-printed metal restorations may not be a problem on the

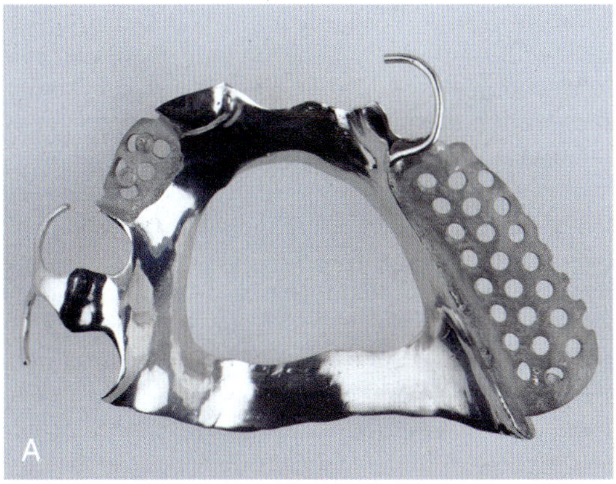

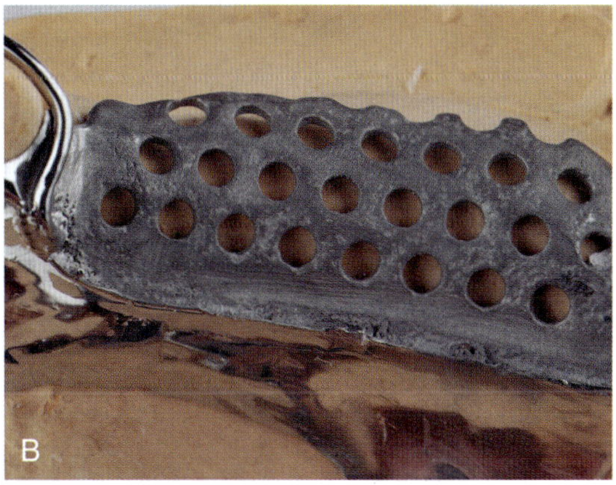

• **Fig. 13.42** Selective laser melting. (A) RPD framework fabricated using SLM technology. Manual finish is necessary to achieve adequate surface finish. (B) Note porosity around the internal line angle.

intaglio surface, but it requires a significant amount of manual adjustment and finish at the surface directly exposed to intraoral environments. Thus additive manufacturing is rarely used for full metal restorations covering occlusal and proximal surfaces. Since metal additive manufacturing is typically used for frameworks of metal-ceramic fixed dental prostheses, ceramic bond strength is another important parameter for clinical success. Multiple studies have shown that ceramic bond strength to 3D-printed Co-Cr alloys is acceptable. A recently published systematic review also concluded that manufacturing methods did not influence the ceramic bond strength of Co-Cr. 3D-printed Co-Cr frameworks have also been shown to have excellent strength, hardness, and corrosion resistance.

Additive manufacturing may be a more efficient process for larger metal objects such as frameworks for complete or partial removable dental prostheses (RPD) or complete-arch implant-supported prostheses (Fig. 13.42A and B). While there are some studies showing that the accuracy of RPD frameworks fabricated with SLM is slightly lower than that of conventionally fabricated RPD frameworks, a recently published review concluded that surface properties, strength, and accuracy of 3D-printed RPD frameworks are within the clinically acceptable range.

Additive Manufacturing of Dental Ceramics

Ceramic Additive Manufacturing

The high melting point of ceramic materials makes additive manufacturing quite complicated, so this technology is still in its infancy. Increased porosity and crack formation during the cooling process can weaken the ceramic resulting in compromised mechanical properties. While additive manufacturing has been attempted with various types of ceramic materials, including feldspathic porcelain and lithium disilicate glass ceramic, zirconia is the most widely investigated ceramic material for additive manufacturing.

SLA is the most commonly used additive manufacturing method for ceramics. When using indirect SLA, a thick ceramic suspension is prepared by mixing different components, including UV-polymerizable resin, photo-initiator, thickener, dispersant, and ceramic powder. Then, the SLA process is applied as usual. Highly concentrated resins are used as binders to create green-stage ceramic objects with high density and homogeneity. The 3D-printed ceramic object is subjected to postprinting processes to remove binders and fuse or sinter ceramic particles.

SLS (direct or indirect) or SLM processes can also be used for ceramic manufacturing. In indirect SLS, resin polymers are used as binders. The scanning laser melts the binder, which bonds ceramic particles together. After the binder is eliminated the ceramic object is further densified through sintering. In direct SLS, the scanning laser directly sinters the ceramic particles, but the high melting point of the ceramic requires very high temperature and long manufacturing time to achieve acceptable densities. Other ceramic additive manufacturing technologies include DLP, material jetting, sheet lamination, and material extrusion.

Clinical Applications of 3D-printed Ceramic

Most studies investigating 3D-printed ceramic restorations have focused on 3D-printed zirconia, typically fabricated using SLA or DLP. The accuracy and physical properties of different types of 3D-printed zirconia restorations, including single crowns, occlusal veneers, and fixed dental prostheses, are promising, though a recent meta-analysis concluded that both accuracy and flexural strength of 3D-printed zirconia were inferior to those of milled zirconia restorations. Thus, while 3D-printed ceramic restorations are not currently used in patient care, many researchers and clinicians predict that the limitations will be overcome in the near future.

Bibliography

Data Acquisition

Ahlholm P, Sipilä K, Vallittu P, Jakonen M, Kotiranta U. Digital versus conventional impressions in fixed prosthodontics: a review. *J Prosthodont.* 2018;27:35–41.

Akl MA, Mansour DE, Zheng F. The role of intraoral scanners in the shade matching process: a systematic review. *J Prosthodont.* 2023;32(3):196–203.

Al Hamad KQ, Al-Kaff FT. Trueness of intraoral scanning of edentulous arches: a comparative clinical study. *J Prosthodont.* 2023;32(1):26–31.

An H, Langas EE, Gill AS. Effect of scanning speed, scanning pattern, and tip size on the accuracy of intraoral digital scans. *J Prosthet Dent.* 2024;131(6):1160–1167.

An H, Mickesh GJ, Cho D, Sorensen JA. Effect of finish line location and saliva contamination on the accuracy of crown finish line scanning. *J Prosthodont.* 2024;33(1):86–94.

Arakida T, Kanazawa M, Iwaki M, Suzuki T, Minakuchi S. Evaluating the influence of ambient light on scanning trueness, precision, and time of intra oral scanner. *J Prosthodont Res.* 2018;62(3):324–329.

Atieh MA, Ritter AV, Ko CC, Duqum I. Accuracy evaluation of intraoral optical impressions: a clinical study using a reference appliance. *J Prosthet Dent.* 2017;118(3):400–405.

Bergevin R, Soucy M, Gagnon H, Laurendeau D. Towards a general multi-view registration technique. *IEEE Trans Pattern Anal Mach Intell.* 1996;18(5):540–547.

Chen Y, Medioni GG. Object modeling by registration of multiple range images. *Proceedings. 1991 IEEE International Conference on Robotics and Automation*; 1991;(3):2724–2729.

Chen Y, Zhai Z, Li H, et al. Influence of liquid on the tooth surface on the accuracy of intraoral scanners: an in vitro study. *J Prosthodont.* 2022;31(1):59–64.

Chochlidakis KM, Papaspyridakos P, Geminiani A, Chen CJ, Feng IJ, Ercoli C. Digital versus conventional impressions for fixed prosthodontics: a systematic review and meta-analysis. *J Prosthet Dent.* 2016;116:184–190. e12.

Ender A, Attin T, Mehl A. In vivo precision of conventional and digital methods of obtaining complete-arch dental impressions. *J Prosthet Dent.* 2016;115(3):313–320.

Ender A, Mehl A. Influence of scanning strategies on the accuracy of digital intraoral scanning systems. *Int J Comput Dent.* 2013;16(1):11–21.

Flügge TV, Att W, Metzger MC, Nelson K. Precision of dental implant digitization using intraoral scanners. *Int J Prosthodont.* 2016;29(3):277–283.

Gavounelis NA, Gogola CC, Halazonetis DJ. The Effect of scanning strategy on intraoral scanner's accuracy. *Dent J (Basel).* 2022;10(7):123.

Giménez B, Özcan M, Martínez-Rus F, Pradíes G. Accuracy of a digital impression system based on parallel confocal laser technology for implants with consideration of operator experience and implant angulation and depth. *IJOMI.* 2014;29(4):853–862.

Güth JF, Runkel C, Beuer F, Stimmelmayr M, Edelhoff D, Keul C. Accuracy of five intraoral scanners compared to indirect digitalization. *Clin Oral Investig.* 2016;21:1445–1455.

Jacob HB, Wyatt GD. Buschang PH. Reliability and validity of intraoral and extraoral scanners. *Prog Orthod.* 2015;16:38.

Kamgar-Parsi B, Jones JL, Rosefeld A. Registration of multiple overlapping range images: scenes without disintictive features. *IEEE Transactions on Pattern Analysis and Machine Intelligence.* 1991;13(9):857–871.

Kim JE, Amelya A, Shin Y, Shim JS. Accuracy of intraoral digital impressions using an artificial landmark. *J Prosthet Dent.* 2017;117(6):755–761.

Knechtle N, Wiedemeier D, Mehl A, Ender A. Accuracy of digital complete-arch, multi-implant scans made in the edentulous jaw with gingival movement simulation: an in vitro study. *J Prosthet Dent.* 2022;128(3):468–478.

Kontis P, Güth JF, Schubert O, Keul C. Accuracy of intraoral scans of edentulous jaws with different generations of intraoral scanners compared to laboratory scans. *J Adv Prosthodont.* 2021;13(5):316–326.

Kuhr F, Schmidt A, Rehmann P, Wöstmann B. A new method for assessing the accuracy of full arch impressions in patients. *J Dent.* 2016;55:68–74.

Kurz M, Attin T, Mehl A. Influence of material surface on the scanning error of a powder-free 3D measuring system. *Clin Oral Investig.* 2015;19(8):2035–2043.

Latham J, Ludlow M, Mennito A, Kelly A, Evans Z, Renne W. Effect of scan pattern on complete-arch scans with 4 digital scanners. *J Prosthet Dent.* 2020;123(1):85–95.

Lee SJ, Gallucci GO. Digital vs. conventional implant impressions: efficiency outcomes. *Clin Oral Implants Res.* 2013;24(1):111–115.

Li L, Chen H, Li W, Wang Y, Sun Y. Design of wear facets of mandibular first molar crowns by using patient-specific motion with an intraoral scanner: a clinical study. *J Prosthet Dent.* 2023;129(5):710–717.

Logozzo S, Zanetti EM, Franceschini G, Kilpelä A, Mäkynen A. Recent advances in dental optics—part I: 3D intraoral scanners for restorative dentistry. *Opt Lasers Eng.* 2014;54:203–221.

Mada SK, Smith ML, Smith LN, Midha PS. Overview of passive and active vision techniques for hand-held 3D data acquisition. *Proc SPIE.* 2003;4877:16–27.

Medina-Sotomayor P, Pascual-Moscardó A, Camps I. Relationship between resolution and accuracy of four intraoral scanners in complete-arch impressions. *J Clin Exp Dent.* 2018;10(4):e361–e366.

Metzger Z, Colson DG, Bown P, Weihard T, Baresel I, Nolting T. Reflected near-infrared light versus bite-wing radiography for the detection of proximal caries: a multicenter prospective clinical study conducted in private practices. *J Dent.* 2022;116:103861.

Michou S, Benetti AR, Vannahme C, Hermannsson PG, Bakhshandeh A, Ekstrand KR. Development of a fluorescence-based caries scoring system for an intraoral scanner: an in vitro study. *Caries Res.* 2020;54(4):324–335.

Michou S, Lambach MS, Ntovas P, et al. Automated caries detection in vivo using a 3D intraoral scanner. *Sci Rep.* 2021;11(1):21276.

Michou S, Vannahme C, Bakhshandeh A, Ekstrand KR, Benetti AR. Intraoral scanner featuring transillumination for proximal caries detection. An in vitro validation study on permanent posterior teeth. *J Dent.* 2022;116:103841.

Müller P, Ender A, Joda T, Katsoulis J. Impact of digital intraoral scan strategies on the impression accuracy using the TRIOS Pod scanner. *Quintessence Int.* 2016;47(4):343–349.

Passos L, Meiga S, Brigagão V, Street A. Impact of different scanning strategies on the accuracy of two current intraoral scanning systems in complete-arch impressions: an in vitro study. *Int J Comput Dent.* 2019;22(4):307–319.

Patzelt SB, Vonau S, Stampf S, Att W. Assessing the feasibility and accuracy of digitizing edentulous jaws. *J Am Dent Assoc.* 2013;144(8):914–920.

Revilla León M, Gohil A, Barmak AB, et al. Influence of ambient temperature changes on intraoral scanning accuracy. *J Prosthet Dent.* 2023;130(5):755–760.

Revilla-León M, Subramanian SG, Özcan M, Krishnamurthy VR. Clinical study of the influence of ambient light scanning conditions on the accuracy (Trueness and Precision) of an intraoral scanner. *J Prosthodont.* 2019;29(2):107–113.

Revilla-León M, Young K, Sicilia E, Cho SH, Kois JC. Influence of definitive and interim restorative materials and surface finishing on the scanning accuracy of an intraoral scanner. *J Dent.* 2022;120:104114.

Schepke U, Meijer HJ, Kerdijk W, Cune MS. Digital versus analog complete-arch impressions for single-unit premolar implant crowns: operating time and patient preference. *J Prosthet Dent.* 2015;114(3):403–406. e1.

Schimmel M, Akino N, Srinivasan M, Wittneben JG, Yilmaz B, Abou-Ayash S. Accuracy of intraoral scanning in completely and partially edentulous maxillary and mandibular jaws: an in vitro analysis. *Clin Oral Investig.* 2021;25(4):1839–1847.

Tabatabaian F, Namdari M, Mahshid M, Vora SR, Mirabbasi S. Accuracy and precision of intraoral scanners for shade matching: a systematic review. *J Prosthet Dent.* 2022;S0022–3913(22)00565 0.

Tapie L, Lebon N, Mawussi B, Fron-Chabouis H, Duret F, Attal JP. Understanding dental CAD/CAM for restorations—accuracy from a mechanical engineering viewpoint. *Int J Comput Dent.* 2015;18(4):343–367.

Ferro KJ, Morgano SM, Driscoll CF, Freilich MA, Guckes AD, Knoernschild KL, McGarry TJ, eds. The glossary of prosthodontic terms: ninth edition. *J Prosthet Dent.* 2017;117(5S):e1–e105.

Ting-Shu S, Jian S. Intraoral digital impression technique: a review. *J Prosthodont.* 2015;24(4):313–321.

Tsirogiannis P, Reissmann DR, Heydecke G. Evaluation of the marginal fit of single-unit, complete-coverage ceramic restorations fabricated after digital and conventional impressions: a systematic review and meta-analysis. *J Prosthet Dent.* 2016;116:328–335.e2.

Valenti M, Schmitz JH. A reverse digital workflow by using an interim restoration scan and patient-specific motion with an intraoral scanner. *J Prosthet Dent.* 2021;126(1):19–23.

Wismeijer D, Mans R, van Genuchten M, Reijers HA. Patients' preferences when comparing analogue implant impressions using a polyether impression material versus digital impressions (Intraoral Scan) of dental implants. *Clin Oral Implants Res.* 2014;25(10):1113–1118.

Computer-Aided Design

An H, Fischer CM, Miller SE, Al-Bitar KM, Luepke PG. A fully digital workflow to achieve predictable esthetic and functional outcomes: a case series. *Int J Periodontics Restorative Dent.* 2022;42(2):165–174.

Coachman C, Georg R, Bohner L, Rigo LC, Sesma N. Chairside 3D digital design and trial restoration workflow. *J Prosthet Dent.* 2020;124(5):514–520.

Galibourg A, Brenes C. Virtual smile design tip: from 2D to 3D design with free software. *J Prosthet Dent.* 2019;121(5):863–864.

Gül Amuk N, Karsli E, Kurt G. Comparison of dental measurements between conventional plaster models, digital models obtained by impression scanning and plaster model scanning. *Int Orthod.* 2019;17(1):151–158.

Hmaidouch R, Neumann P, Mueller WD. Influence of preparation form, luting space setting and cement type on the marginal and internal fit of CAD/CAM crown copings. *Int J Comput Dent.* 2011;14(3):219–226.

Iwai T, Komine F, Kobayashi K, Saito A, Matsumura H. Influence of convergence angle and cement space on adaptation of zirconium dioxide ceramic copings. *Acta Odontol Scand.* 2008;66(4):214–218.

Juntavee N, Millstein PL. Effect of surface roughness and cement space on crown retention. *J Prosthet Dent.* 1992;68(3):482–486.

Kale E, Seker E, Yilmaz B, Özcelik TB. Effect of cement space on the marginal fit of CAD-CAM-fabricated monolithic zirconia crowns. *J Prosthet Dent.* 2016;116(6):890–895.

Kollmuss M, Jakob FM, Kirchner HG, Ilie N, Hickel R, Huth KC. Comparison of biogenerically reconstructed and waxed-up complete occlusal surfaces with respect to the original tooth morphology. *Clin Oral Investig.* 2013;17(3):851–857.

Lee Y-C, Lee C, Shim J-S, et al. Comparison between occlusal errors of single posterior crowns adjusted using patient specific motion or conventional methods. *Appl Sci.* 2020;10(24):9140.

Lin WS, Harris BT, Phasuk K, Llop DR, Morton D. Integrating a facial scan, virtual smile design, and 3D virtual patient for treatment with CAD-CAM ceramic veneers: a clinical report. *J Prosthet Dent.* 2018;119(2):200–205.

Litzenburger AP, Hickel R, Richter MJ, Mehl AC, Probst FA. Fully automatic CAD design of the occlusal morphology of partial crowns compared to dental technicians' design. *Clin Oral Investig.* 2013;17(2):491–496.

Quaas S, Loos R, Rudolph H, Luthardt RG. Randomized controlled trial comparing direct intraoral digitization and extraoral digitization after impression taking. *Int J Prosthodont.* 2015;28(1):30–32.

Revilla-Leon M, Frazier K, da Costa JB, et al. Intraoral scanners: an American Dental Association Clinical Evaluators Panel survey. *J Am Dent Assoc.* 2021;152(8):669–670. e2.

Spear FM, Kokich VG. A multidisciplinary approach to esthetic dentistry. *Dent Clin North Am.* 2007;51(2):487–505, x–xi.

Wesemann C, Muallah J, Mah J, Bumann A. Accuracy and efficiency of full-arch digitalization and 3D printing: a comparison between desktop model scanners, an intraoral scanner, a CBCT model scan, and stereolithographic 3D printing. *Quintessence Int.* 2017;48(1):41–50.

Zimmermann M, Mehl A. Virtual smile design systems: a current review. *Int J Comput Dent.* 2015;18(4):303–317.

Computer-Aided Manufacturing—Subtractive

Abdulmajeed AA, Donovan TE, Cooper LF, Walter R, Sulaiman TA. Fracture of layered zirconia restorations at 5 years: a dental laboratory survey. *J Prosthet Dent.* 2017;118(3):353–356.

Al-Dwairi ZN, Tahboub KY, Baba NZ, Goodacre CJ, Özcan M. A comparison of the surface properties of CAD/CAM and conventional polymethylmethacrylate (PMMA). *J Prosthodont.* 2019;28(4):452–457.

Al-Dwairi ZN, Tahboub KY, Baba NZ, Goodacre CJ. A comparison of the flexural and impact strengths and flexural modulus of CAD/CAM and conventional heat-cured polymethyl methacrylate (PMMA). *J Prosthodont.* 2020;29(4):341–349.

Angeletaki F, Gkogkos A, Papazoglou E, Kloukos D. Direct versus indirect inlay/onlay composite restorations in posterior teeth. A systematic review and meta-analysis. *J Dent.* 2016;53:12–21.

Arslan M, Murat S, Alp G, Zaimoglu A. Evaluation of flexural strength and surface properties of prepolymerized CAD/CAM PMMA-based polymers used for digital 3D complete dentures. *Int J Comput Dent.* 2018;21(1):31–40.

Awada A, Nathanson D. Mechanical properties of resin-ceramic CAD/CAM restorative materials. *J Prosthet Dent.* 2015;114(4):587–593.

Beuer F, Neumeier P, Naumann M. Marginal fit of 14-unit zirconia fixed dental prosthesis retainers. *J Oral Rehabil.* 2009;36(2):142–149.

Bousnaki M, Chatziparaskeva M, Bakopoulou A, Pissiotis A, Koidis P. Variables affecting the fit of zirconia fixed partial dentures: a systematic review. *J Prosthet Dent.* 2020;123(5):686–692.

Campanelli de Morais D, de Oliveira Abu-Izze F, Rivoli Rossi N, et al. Effect of consecutive firings on the optical and mechanical properties of silicate and lithium disilicate based glass-ceramics. *J Prosthodont.* 2021;30(9):776–782.

Ceylan G, Emir F, Doğdu C, Demirel M, Özcan M. Effect of repeated millings on the surface integrity of diamond burs and roughness of different CAD/CAM materials. *Clin Oral Investig.* 2022;26(8):5325–5337.

Chen XP, Xiang ZX, Song XF, Yin L. Machinability: zirconia-reinforced lithium silicate glass ceramic versus lithium disilicate glass ceramic. *J Mech Behav Biomed Mater.* 2020;101:103435.

Cho HD, Jun YT, Yang MY. Five axis CNC milling for effective machining of sculptured surfaces. *Int J Prod Res.* 1993;31(11):2559–2573.

Cho JH, Yoon HI, Han JS, Kim DJ. Trueness of the inner surface of monolithic crowns fabricated by milling of a fully sintered (Y, Nb)-TZP block in chairside CAD-CAM system for single-visit dentistry. *Materials (Basel).* 2019;12(19):3253.

Corazza PH, de Castro HL, Feitosa SA, Kimpara ET, Della Bona A. Influence of CAD-CAM diamond bur deterioration on surface roughness and maximum failure load of Y-TZP-based restorations. *Am J Dent.* 2015;28(2):95–99.

Edelhoff D, Beuer F, Schweiger J, Brix O, Stimmelmayr M, Guth JF. CAD/CAM-generated high-density polymer restorations for the pretreatment of complex cases: a case report. *Quintessence Int.* 2012;43(6):457–467.

Fabian Fonzar R, Carrabba M, Sedda M, Ferrari M, Goracci C, Vichi A. Flexural resistance of heat-pressed and CAD-CAM lithium disilicate with different translucencies. *Dent Mater.* 2017;33(1):63–70.

Fathi HM, Al-Masoody AH, El-Ghezawi N, Johnson A. The accuracy of fit of crowns made from wax patterns produced conventionally (Hand Formed) and via CAD/CAM technology. *Eur J Prosthodont Restor Dent.* 2016;24(1):10–17.

Giannetopoulos S, van Noort R, Tsitrou E. Evaluation of the marginal integrity of ceramic copings with different marginal angles using two different CAD/CAM systems. *J Dent.* 2010;38(12):980–986.

Gold SA, Ferracane JL, da Costa J. Effect of crystallization firing on marginal gap of CAD/CAM fabricated lithium disilicate crowns. *J Prosthodont.* 2018;27(1):63–66.

Goodacre CJ, Bernal G, Rungcharassaeng K, Kan JY. Clinical complications in fixed prosthodontics. *J Prosthet Dent.* 2003;90(1):31–41.

Gosavi SS, Gosavi SY, Alla RK. Titanium: a miracle metal in dentistry. *Trends Biomater Artif Organs.* 2013;27(1):42–46.

Güth JF, Almeida E, Silva JS, Ramberger M, Beuer F, Edelhoff D. Treatment concept with CAD/CAM-fabricated high-density polymer temporary restorations. *J Esthet Restor Dent.* 2012;24(5):310–318.

Hamza TA, Ezzat HA, El-Hossary MM, Katamish HA, Shokry TE, Rosenstiel SF. Accuracy of ceramic restorations made with two CAD/CAM systems. *J Prosthet Dent.* 2013;109(2):83–87.

Hamza TA, Sherif RM. In vitro evaluation of marginal discrepancy of monolithic zirconia restorations fabricated with different CAD-CAM systems. *J Prosthet Dent.* 2017;117(6):762–766.

Harada K, Raigrodski AJ, Chung KH, Flinn BD, Dogan S, Mancl LA. A comparative evaluation of the translucency of zirconias and lithium disilicate for monolithic restorations. *J Prosthet Dent.* 2016;116(2):257–263.

Hey J, Beuer F, Bensel T, Boeckler AF. Single crowns with CAD/CAM-fabricated copings from titanium: 6-year clinical results. *J Prosthet Dent.* 2014;112(2):150–154.

Hmaidouch R, Neumann P, Mueller WD. Influence of preparation form, luting space setting and cement type on the marginal and internal fit of CAD/CAM crown copings. *Int J Comput Dent.* 2011;14(3):219–226.

Homsy FR, Özcan M, Khoury M, Majzoub ZAK. Comparison of fit accuracy of pressed lithium disilicate inlays fabricated from wax or resin patterns with conventional and CAD-CAM technologies. *J Prosthet Dent.* 2018;120(4):530–536.

Kelvin Khng KY, Ettinger RL, Armstrong SR, Lindquist T, Gratton DG, Qian F. In vitro evaluation of the marginal integrity of CAD/CAM interim crowns. *J Prosthet Dent.* 2016;115(5):617–623.

Khorasani AM, Yazdi MRS, Safizadeh MS. Analysis of machining parameters effects on surface roughness: a review. *Int J Comput Mater Sci Surf Eng.* 2012;5(1):68–84.

Kino H, Imada T, Ogawa K, Nakagawa H, Kojima H. An experimental investigation on micro end milling with high-speed up cut milling for hardened die steel. *Materials (Basel).* 2020;13(21):4745.

Komine F, Gerds T, Witkowski S, Strub JR. Influence of framework configuration on the marginal adaptation of zirconium dioxide ceramic anterior four-unit frameworks. *Acta Odontol Scand.* 2005;63(6):361–366.

Lalande D, Hodd JA, Brousseau JS, Ramos V, Dunham D, Rueggeberg F. Marginal discrepancy dimensions of single unit metal crowns fabricated by using CAD-CAM-milled acrylate resin polymer blocks or a conventional waxing technique. *J Prosthet Dent.* 2018;119(6):948–953.

Lawson NC, Bansal R, Burgess JO. Wear, strength, modulus and hardness of CAD/CAM restorative materials. *Dent Mater.* 2016;32(11):e275–e283.

Lawson NC, Janyavula S, Syklawer S, McLaren EA, Burgess JO. Wear of enamel opposing zirconia and lithium disilicate after adjustment, polishing and glazing. *J Dent.* 2014;42(12):1586–1591.

Lebon N, Tapie L, Vennat E, Mawussi B. Influence of CAD/CAM tool and material on tool wear and roughness of dental prostheses after milling. *J Prosthet Dent.* 2015;114(2):236–247.

Lin MT, Sy-Muñoz J, Muñoz CA, Goodacre CJ, Naylor WP. The effect of tooth preparation form on the fit of Procera copings. *Int J Prosthodont.* 1998;11(6):580–590.

Lu T, Peng L, Xiong F, et al. A 3-year clinical evaluation of endodontically treated posterior teeth restored with two different materials using the CEREC AC chair-side system. *J Prosthet Dent.* 2018;119(3):363–368.

Makhija SK, Lawson NC, Gilbert GH, et al. Dentist material selection for single-unit crowns: findings from the National Dental Practice-Based Research Network. *J Dent.* 2016;55:40–47.

Matzinger M, Hahnel S, Preis V, Rosentritt M. Polishing effects and wear performance of chairside CAD/CAM materials. *Clin Oral Investig.* 2019;23(2):725–737.

Mörmann WH. The evolution of the CEREC system. *J Am Dent Assoc.* 2006;137(Suppl):7S–13S.

Ozdogan A, Ozdemir H. Effects of multiple firing processes on the mechanical properties of lithium disilicate glass-ceramics produced by two different production techniques. *J Prosthet Dent.* 2021;125(3):527.e1–527.e7.

Papadiochou S, Pissiotis AL. Marginal adaptation and CAD-CAM technology: a systematic review of restorative material and fabrication techniques. *J Prosthet Dent.* 2018;119(4):545–551.

Papia E, Arnoldsson P, Baudinova A, Jimbo R, Vult VON Steyern P. Cast, milled and EBM-manufactured titanium, differences in porcelain shear bond strength. *Dent Mater J.* 2018;37(2):214–221.

Rayyan MM, Aboushelib M, Sayed NM, Ibrahim A, Jimbo R. Comparison of interim restorations fabricated by CAD/CAM with those fabricated manually. *J Prosthet Dent.* 2015;114(3):414–419.

Reich S, Kappe K, Teschner H, Schmitt J. Clinical fit of four-unit zirconia posterior fixed dental prostheses. *Eur J Oral Sci.* 2008;116(6):579–584.

Roperto RC, Oliveira MP, Porto TS, Ferreira LA, Melo LS. Akkus A. Can tooth preparation design affect the fit of CAD/CAM restorations? *Compend Contin Educ Dent.* 2017;38(3):e13–e17.

Ruse ND, Sadoun MJ. Resin-composite blocks for dental CAD/CAM applications. *J Dent Res.* 2014;93(12):1232–1234.

Spitznagel FA, Scholz KJ, Strub JR, Vach K, Gierthmuehlen PC. Polymer-infiltrated ceramic CAD/CAM inlays and partial coverage restorations: 3-year results of a prospective clinical study over 5 years. *Clin Oral Investig.* 2018;22(5):1973–1983.

Sriram S, Shrankari V, Chacko Y. Computer aided designing/computer aided manufacturing in dentistry (CAD/CAM)—a review. *Int Curr Res Rev.* 2018;10(20):20–24.

Steinmassl O, Dumfahrt H, Grunert I, Steinmassl PA. CAD/CAM produces dentures with improved fit. *Clin Oral Investig.* 2018;22(8):2829–2835.

Sulaiman TA, Abdulmajeed AA, Donovan TE, Cooper LF, Walter R. Fracture rate of monolithic zirconia restorations up to 5 years: a dental laboratory survey. *J Prosthet Dent.* 2016;116(3):436–439.

Sulaiman TA, Delgado AJ, Donovan TE. Survival rate of lithium disilicate restorations at 4 years: a retrospective study. *J Prosthet Dent.* 2015;114(3):364–366.

Svanborg P. A systematic review on the accuracy of zirconia crowns and fixed dental prostheses. *Biomater Investig Dent.* 2020;7(1):9–15.

Swain MV, Coldea A, Bilkhair A, Guess PC. Interpenetrating network ceramic-resin composite dental restorative materials. *Dent Mater.* 2016;32(1):34–42.

Tinschert J, Natt G, Mautsch W, Spiekermann H, Anusavice KJ. Marginal fit of alumina-and zirconia-based fixed partial dentures produced by a CAD/CAM system. *Oper Dent.* 2001;26(4):367–374.

Tsitrou EA, Northeast SE, van Noort R. Brittleness index of machinable dental materials and its relation to the marginal chipping factor. *J Dent.* 2007;35(12):897–902.

Wiedenmann F, Böhm D, Eichberger M, Edelhoff D, Stawarczyk B. Influence of different surface treatments on two-body wear and fracture load of monolithic CAD/CAM ceramics. *Clin Oral Investig.* 2020;24(9):3049–3060.

Wu X, Liu Y, Zhou X, Mou A. Automatic identification of tool wear based on convolutional neural network in face milling process. *Sensors (Basel).* 2019;19(18):3817.

Yan J, Kaizer MR, Zhang Y. Load-bearing capacity of lithium disilicate and ultra-translucent zirconias. *J Mech Behav Biomed Mater.* 2018;88:170–175.

Yao J, Li J, Wang Y, Huang H. Comparison of the flexural strength and marginal accuracy of traditional and CAD/CAM interim materials before and after thermal cycling. *J Prosthet Dent.* 2014;112(3):649–657.

Zhang F, Inokoshi M, Batuk M, et al. Strength, toughness and aging stability of highly-translucent Y-TZP ceramics for dental restorations. *Dent Mater.* 2016;32(12):e327–e337.

Zhang Y. Making yttria-stabilized tetragonal zirconia translucent. *Dent Mater.* 2014;30(10):1195–1203.

Computer-Aided Manufacturing—Additive

Al Hamad KQ, Al-Rashdan BA, Ayyad JQ, et al. Additive manufacturing of dental ceramics: a systematic review and meta-analysis. *J Prosthodont.* 2022;31(8):e67–e86.

Al Jabbari YS, Koutsoukis T, Barmpagadaki X, Zinelis S. Metallurgical and interfacial characterization of PFM Co-Cr dental alloys fabricated via casting, milling or selective laser melting. *Dent Mater.* 2014;30(4):e79–e88.

Al Maaz A, Thompson GA, Drago C, An H, Berzins D. Effect of finish line design and metal alloy on the marginal and internal gaps of selective laser melting printed copings. *J Prosthet Dent.* 2019;122(2):143–151.

Alammar A, Kois JC, Revilla-León M, Att W. Additive manufacturing technologies: current status and future perspectives. *J Prosthodont.* 2022;31(S1):4–12.

Alamo L, Cassiano FB, Bordini EAF, et al. An organotypic model of oral mucosa cells for the biological assessment of 3D-printed resins for interim restorations. *J Prosthet Dent.* 2024;132(1):251–259.

Balkenhol M, Köhler H, Orbach K, Wöstmann B. Fracture toughness of cross-linked and non-cross-linked temporary crown and fixed partial denture materials. *Dent Mater.* 2009;25(7):917–928.

Berli C, Thieringer FM, Sharma N, et al. Comparing the mechanical properties of pressed, milled, and 3D-printed resins for occlusal devices. *J Prosthet Dent.* 2020;124(6):780–786.

Brown GB, Currier GF, Kadioglu O, Kierl JP. Accuracy of 3-dimensional printed dental models reconstructed from digital intraoral impressions. *Am J Orthod Dentofacial Orthop.* 2018;154(5):733–739.

Chen SG, Yang J, Jia YG, Lu B, Ren L. TiO2 and PEEK reinforced 3D printing PMMA composite resin for dental denture base applications. *Nanomaterials (Basel).* 2019;9(7):1049.

Cho SH, Schaefer O, Thompson GA. Guentsch A. Comparison of accuracy and reproducibility of casts made by digital and conventional methods. *J Prosthet Dent.* 2015;113(4):310–315.

Doreau F, Chaput C, Chartier T. Stereolithography for manufacturing ceramic parts. *Adv Eng Mater.* 2000;2:493–496.

Dupin S, Lame O, Barrès C, Charmeau JY. Microstructural origin of physical and mechanical properties of polyamide 12 processed by laser sintering. *Eur Polym J.* 2012;48(9):1611–1621.

Goodacre BJ, Goodacre CJ. Additive manufacturing for complete denture fabrication: a narrative review. *J Prosthodont.* 2022;31(S1):47–51.

Gruber S, Kamnoedboon P, Özcan M, Srinivasan M. CAD/CAM complete denture resins: an in vitro evaluation of color stability. *J Prosthodont.* 2021;30(5):430–439.

Grymak A, Aarts JM, Ma S, Waddell JN, Choi JJE. Wear behavior of occlusal splint materials manufactured by various methods: a systematic review. *J Prosthodont.* 2022;31(6):472–487.

Grymak A, Waddell JN, Aarts JM, Ma S, Choi JJE. Evaluation of wear behaviour of various occlusal splint materials and manufacturing processes. *J Mech Behav Biomed Mater.* 2022;126:105053.

Hada T, Kanazawa M, Iwaki M, et al. Effect of printing direction on the accuracy of 3D-printed dentures using stereolithography technology. *Materials (Basel).* 2020;13(15):3405.

Hazeveld A, Huddleston Slater JJ, Ren Y. Accuracy and reproducibility of dental replica models reconstructed by different rapid prototyping techniques. *Am J Orthod Dentofacial Orthop.* 2014;145(1):108–115.

Huettig F, Kustermann A, Kuscu E, Geis-Gerstorfer J, Spintzyk S. Polishability and wear resistance of splint material for oral appliances produced with conventional, subtractive, and additive manufacturing. *J Mech Behav Biomed Mater.* 2017;75:175–179.

ISO 17296-2:2015(E). *Additive Manufacturing—General Principles—Part 2: Overview of Process Categories and Feedstock.* International Organization for Standardization; 2021.

ISO/ASTM 52900:2021(E). *Additive Manufacturing—General Principles—Fundamentals and Vocaburary.* International Organization for Standardization; 2021.

Jin MC, Yoon HI, Yeo IS, Kim SH, Han JS. The effect of build angle on the tissue surface adaptation of maxillary and mandibular complete denture bases manufactured by digital light processing. *J Prosthet Dent.* 2020;123(3):473–482.

Kalberer N, Mehl A, Schimmel M, Müller F, Srinivasan M. CAD-CAM milled versus rapidly prototyped (3D-printed) complete dentures: an in vitro evaluation of trueness. *J Prosthet Dent.* 2019;121(4):637–643.

Kasperovich G, Haubrich J, Gussone J, Requena G. Correlation between porosity and processing parameters in TiAl6V4 produced by selective laser melting. *Mater Des.* 2016;105:160–170.

Kessler A, Hickel R, Reymus M. 3D printing in dentistry-state of the art. *Oper Dent.* 2020;45(1):30–40.

Khanlar LN, Salazar Rios A, Tahmaseb A, Zandinejad A. Additive manufacturing of zirconia ceramic and its application in clinical dentistry: a review. *Dent J (Basel).* 2021;9(9):104.

Khorsandi D, Fahimipour A, Abasian P, et al. 3D and 4D printing in dentistry and maxillofacial surgery: printing techniques, materials, and applications. *Acta Biomater.* 2021;122:26–49.

Kim KB, Kim JH, Kim WC, Kim JH. Three-dimensional evaluation of gaps associated with fixed dental prostheses fabricated with new technologies. *J Prosthet Dent.* 2014;112(6):1432–1436.

Koutsoukis T, Zinelis S, Eliades G, Al-Wazzan K, Rifaiy MA, Al Jabbari YS. Selective laser melting technique of Co-Cr dental alloys: a review of structure and properties and comparative analysis with other available techniques. *J Prosthodont.* 2015;24(4):303–312.

Kozak J, Zakrzewski T, Witt M, Dębowska-Wąsak M. Selected problems of additive manufacturing using SLS/SLM processes. *Trans Aerosp Res.* 2021;1(262):24–44.

Kruth JP, Mercelis P, Van Vaerenbergh J, Froyen L, Rombouts M. Binding mechanism in selective laser sintering and selective laser melting. *Rapid Prototyp J.* 2005;11(1):26–36.

Lanza R, Langer R, Vacanti JP, Atala A. *Principles of Tissue Engineering.* 5th ed.. Elsevier; 2020:1391–1415.

Li J, Chen C, Liao J, et al. Bond strengths of porcelain to cobalt-chromium alloys made by casting, milling, and selective laser melting. *J Prosthet Dent*. 2017;118(1):69–75.

Lin CH, Lin YM, Lai YL, Lee SY. Mechanical properties, accuracy, and cytotoxicity of UV-polymerized 3D printing resins composed of Bis-EMA, UDMA, and TEGDMA. *J Prosthet Dent*. 2020;123(2):349–354.

Lutz AM, Hampe R, Roos M, Lümkemann N, Eichberger M, Stawarczyk B. Fracture resistance and 2-body wear of 3-dimensional-printed occlusal devices. *J Prosthet Dent*. 2019;121(1):166–172.

Mangano FG, Admakin O, Bonacina M, Biaggini F, Farronato D, Lerner H. Accuracy of 6 desktop 3D printers in dentistry: a comparative in vitro study. *Eur J Prosthodont Restor Dent*. 2020;28(2):75–85.

Mazzoli A. Selective laser sintering in biomedical engineering. *Med Biol Eng Comput*. 2013;51(3):245–256.

Muehlemann E, Özcan M. Accuracy of removable partial denture frameworks fabricated using conventional and digital technologies. *Eur J Prosthodont Restor Dent*. 2022;30(2):76–86.

Ortega NM, Revilla-León M, Ortega R, Gómez-Polo C, Barmak AB. Gómez-Polo M. Comparison of surface roughness of additively manufactured implant-supported interim crowns fabricated with different print orientations. *J Prosthodont*. 2024;33(2):141–148.

Örtorp A, Jönsson D, Mouhsen A. Vult von Steyern P. The fit of cobalt-chromium three-unit fixed dental prostheses fabricated with four different techniques: a comparative in vitro study. *Dent Mater*. 2011;27(4):356–363.

Pouzada AS. *Design and Manufacturing of Plastics Products: Integrating Traditional Methods with Additive Manufacturing*. Elsevier; 2021:381–456.

Prpić V, Schauperl Z, Ćatić A, Dulčić N, Čimić S. Comparison of mechanical properties of 3D-printed, CAD/CAM, and conventional denture base materials. *J Prosthodont*. 2020;29(6):524–528.

Revilla-León M, Ceballos L, Martínez-Klemm I, Özcan M. Discrepancy of complete-arch titanium frameworks manufactured using selective laser melting and electron beam melting additive manufacturing technologies. *J Prosthet Dent*. 2018;120(6):942–947.

Revilla-León M, Gómez-Polo M, Park SH, Barmak AB, Özcan M. Adhesion of veneering porcelain to cobalt-chromium dental alloys processed with casting, milling, and additive manufacturing methods: a systematic review and meta-analysis. *J Prosthet Dent*. 2022;128(4):575–588.

Revilla-León M, Meyer MJ, Zandinejad A, Özcan M. Additive manufacturing technologies for processing zirconia in dental applications. *Int J Comput Dent*. 2020;23(1):27–37.

Revilla-León M, Özcan M. Additive manufacturing technologies used for processing polymers: current status and potential application in prosthetic dentistry. *J Prosthodont*. 2019;28(2):146–158.

Reyes-Sevilla M, Kuijs RH, Werner A, Kleverlaan CJ, Lobbezoo F. Comparison of wear between occlusal splint materials and resin composite materials. *J Oral Rehabil*. 2018;45(7):539–544.

Rungrojwittayakul O, Kan JY, Shiozaki K, et al. Accuracy of 3D printed models created by two technologies of printers with different designs of model base. *J Prosthodont*. 2020;29(2):124–128.

Schweiger J, Edelhoff D, Güth JF. 3D Printing in digital prosthetic dentistry: an overview of recent developments in additive manufacturing. *J Clin Med*. 2021;10(9):2010.

Scotti CK, Velo MMAC, Rizzante FAP, Nascimento TRL, Mondelli RFL, Bombonatti JFS. Physical and surface properties of a 3D-printed composite resin for a digital workflow. *J Prosthet Dent*. 2020;124(5):614.e1–614.e5.

Simoneti DM, Pereira-Cenci T, Dos Santos MBF. Comparison of material properties and biofilm formation in interim single crowns obtained by 3D printing and conventional methods. *J Prosthet Dent*. 2022;127(1):168–172.

Takaichi A, Suyalatu Nakamoto T, et al. Microstructures and mechanical properties of Co-29Cr-6Mo alloy fabricated by selective laser melting process for dental applications. *J Mech Behav Biomed Mater*. 2013;21:67–76.

Tamac E, Toksavul S, Toman M. Clinical marginal and internal adaptation of CAD/CAM milling, laser sintering, and cast metal ceramic crowns. *J Prosthet Dent*. 2014;112(4):909–913.

Tigmeanu CV, Ardelean LC, Rusu LC, Negrutiu ML. Additive manufactured polymers in dentistry, current state-of-the-art and future perspectives—a review. *Polymers (Basel)*. 2022;14(17):3658.

Tzeng JJ, Yang TS, Lee WF, Chen H, Chang HM. Mechanical properties and biocompatibility of urethane acrylate-based 3D-printed denture base resin. *Polymers (Basel)*. 2021;13(5):822.

Wang H, Feng Q, Li N, Xu S. Evaluation of metal-ceramic bond characteristics of three dental Co-Cr alloys prepared with different fabrication techniques. *J Prosthet Dent*. 2016;116(6):916–923.

Wedekind L, Güth JF, Schweiger J, et al. Elution behavior of a 3D-printed, milled and conventional resin-based occlusal splint material. *Dent Mater*. 2021;37(4):701–710.

Whitaker M. The history of 3D printing in healthcare. *Bull R Coll Surg Engl*. 2014;96(7):228–229.

Xiang N, Xin XZ, Chen J, Wei B. Metal-ceramic bond strength of Co-Cr alloy fabricated by selective laser melting. *J Dent*. 2012;40(6):453–457.

Xin XZ, Chen J, Xiang N, Gong Y, Wei B. Surface characteristics and corrosion properties of selective laser melted Co-Cr dental alloy after porcelain firing. *Dent Mater*. 2014;30(3):263–270.

Yoon HI, Hwang HJ, Ohkubo C, Han JS, Park EJ. Evaluation of the trueness and tissue surface adaptation of CAD-CAM mandibular denture bases manufactured using digital light processing. *J Prosthet Dent*. 2018;120(6):919–926.

You SM, You SG, Kang SY, Bae SY, Kim JH. Evaluation of the accuracy (trueness and precision) of a maxillary trial denture according to the layer thickness: an in vitro study. *J Prosthet Dent*. 2021;125(1):139–145.

Yunizar MF, Watanabe M, Ichikawa T. Current development status of additive manufacturing technologies for fabricating removable partial denture frameworks: a literature review. *Int J Comput Dent*. 2022;25(1):57–70.

14

Dental and Orofacial Implants

JASON ALAN GRIGGS

CHAPTER OUTLINE

The practice of restorative dentistry seeks to replace the form and function of missing tooth structures. It was therefore expected that dentistry would follow orthopedic medicine in the use of implants to anchor prosthetic devices, and that has happened. Global dental implant sales are expected to reach over $9.62 billion by 2030 at a compounded annual growth rate of 9.8%. In 2022 North America exhibited the largest market share, followed by Europe and the Asia-Pacific region. The Asia-Pacific region is expected to see the highest growth rate between 2023 and 2030.

Dental implants are fixtures that serve as replacements for the root of a missing natural tooth. Implants may be placed in the mandible or maxilla. When properly designed and placed, dental implants integrate with bone over time and serve as an anchor for dental prostheses. Dental implants are used to replace a single missing tooth or many teeth or to support a complete removable denture.

Worldwide, modern single-tooth implants have a success rate of nearly 95% survival at 15 years. Implants are permanent devices that are surgically anchored in the oral cavity and often provide significant advantages over other fixed or removable prosthodontic options. Implants are often more conservative than traditional fixed partial dentures because they save tooth structure by eliminating the need for reduction of adjacent abutment teeth and they support the maintenance of healthy bone in the region. Implants also increase the stability of overdentures, resulting in bite forces similar to that of patients who retain their natural dentition.

Classification

Historically, dental implants have been classified according to their design. This design was in turn based on the way in which they are surgically implanted. The three types of implants commonly used for the past 40 years are the subperiosteal implant, the transosteal implant, and the endosseous implant (Table 14.1). More recently, zygomatic implants have been used in case of a severely atrophic or missing maxilla.

Endosseous Implant

Endosseous implants are by far the most common type of implant placed today. Implants are placed directly into the mandible or maxilla (Fig. 14.1). A pilot hole is drilled into the alveolar or basal bone beneath (in cases in which the alveolar bone has been partially or completely resorbed), and the implant body is inserted into this site. The top of the implant is positioned so that it either protrudes slightly through the cortical plate or is flush with the surface of the bone. Typically, a superstructure containing a prosthetic tooth or teeth connects to the implant body through an abutment that is screwed into the body directly through the mucosa.

Osseointegration and Biointegration

A major issue for implant design is the development of a device made from materials that are physically and biologically compatible with alveolar bone. Ideally, bone should integrate with the device and remodel the bone structure around it, rather than responding to it as a foreign substance by encapsulating it with fibrous tissue. Under optimum circumstances, bone differentiation occurs directly adjacent to the material (osseointegration). Ideally this osseointegration provides a stable bone-implant connection that can support a dental prosthesis and transfer applied loads without concentrating stresses at the critical interface between bone and the implant.

Osseointegration is formally defined as the close approximation of bone to an implant material (Fig. 14.2). To achieve osseointegration, the bone must be viable, the space between the bone and implant must be less than 10 nm and contain no fibrous tissue, and the bone–implant interface must be able to survive loading by

TABLE 14.1 Implant Design Classification Scheme

Implant Design	Contact With Bone	Composition	Location Used
Subperiosteal	Directly on bone surface under the gingival tissues; no bone penetration	Co-Cr-Mo (Vitallium)	Maxilla and mandible
Transosteal	Completely through the bone, penetrating the cortical wall twice	Titanium or Ti alloy	Mandible only
Endosteal	Within the bone, penetrating the cortical wall once	Titanium or Ti alloy	Maxilla and mandible

a dental prosthesis by remaining intact. In current practice, osseointegration is an absolute requirement for the successful implant-supported dental prosthesis. To achieve osseointegration between an implant and bone, a number of factors must be correct. The bone must be prepared in a way that does not cause necrosis or inflammation. The implant must be allowed to heal for a time without a load unless initial stability of the implant (as measured using vibration resonance in a magnetic field) is sufficient to prevent micromotion. Finally, the proper material must be implanted, because not all materials will promote osseointegration.

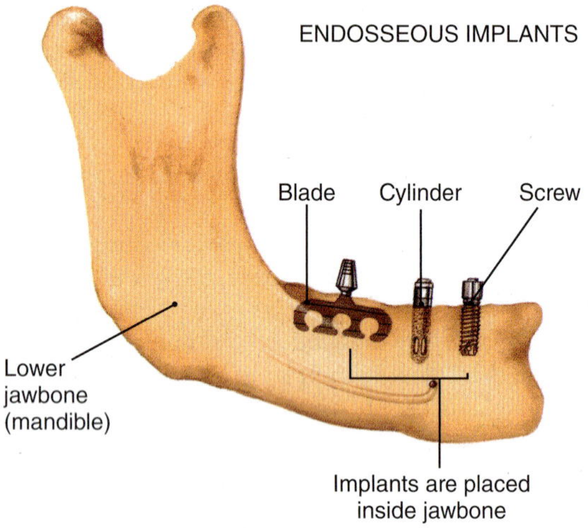

• **Fig. 14.1** Endosteal implant design. Shown here are three different endosseous implant designs. Notice that all of the designs are implanted directly within the bone. Although the blade design has fallen out of use, the press-fit (cylinder) and screw-shaped versions continue to be the most widely placed implant designs in use today.

In recent years, various surface configurations have been proposed as means of improving the cohesiveness of the implant–tissue interface, maximizing load transfer, minimizing relative motion between the implant and tissue, minimizing fibrous integration and loosening, and lengthening the service life of the construct. Because of the necessity of developing a stable interface before loading, effort has been placed on developing materials and methods to accelerate tissue apposition to the implant surface. Surface-roughened implants and ceramic coatings have been implemented into clinical practice. Other techniques include electrical stimulation, bone grafting, and the use of growth factors and other tissue engineering approaches described in Chapter 16.

The application of bioactive ceramics as implant materials was traditionally limited to their use as bone bonding and augmentation materials. There has been interest in coating titanium alloys with bioactive materials to promote an implant-bone connection. Bioactive ceramic materials are more than just biocompatible. The use of the term *bioactive* implies that they have the ability to elicit a favorable tissue response when implanted in vivo. These ceramics form a direct chemical bond with natural tissues and are most often designed with high solubility to bioresorb or biodegrade,

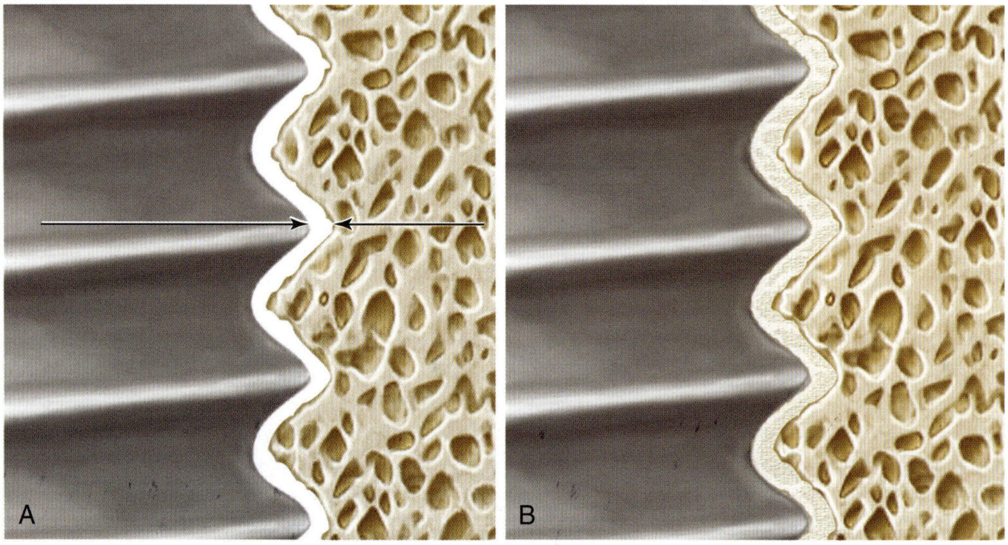

• **Fig. 14.2** Osseointegration and biointegration. (A) In osseointegration, the implant material *(left)* and the bone *(right)* closely approximate one another. This approximation must be closer than 10 nm *(arrows)*. In the intervening space, there can be no fibrous tissue. (B) In biointegration, the implant and bone are fused and continuous with one another. Osseointegration commonly occurs with titanium alloys, whereas biointegration occurs with ceramics and ceramic-coated metallic implants.

in order to be replaced over time by natural tissues. Commonly implanted dental ceramics include calcium phosphates with various calcium-to-phosphorus ratios (e.g., hydroxyapatite [HA] and tricalcium phosphate), bioactive glasses (mixtures of SiO_2, CaO, P_2O_5, and sometimes Na_2O, and MgO), and glass ceramics.

Important examples of bioactive glasses and glass-ceramics include Bioglass (a glass containing a mixture of silica, phosphate, calcia, and soda); Ceravital (which has a lower alkali oxide concentration compared to Bioglass); Biogran (which has a different physical conformation compared to Bioglass); and A-W glass ceramic (a glass-ceramic–containing crystalline oxyapatite and fluorapatite [$Ca_{10}\{PO_4\}_6\{O,F_2\}$] and β-wollastonite [$SiO_2CaO$] in a MgO-CaO-$SiO_2$ glassy matrix). In addition, many other glass and glass-ceramic compositions, based on recently developed sol-gel synthesis methods, are being developed. Calcium phosphate ceramics vary in composition, depending on processing-induced physical and chemical changes. Among this group are the apatite ceramics. Of particular interest is HA, which is the synthetic version of the inorganic phase found in teeth and is similar to the inorganic phase found in bone (hydroxycarbonate apatite). For this reason, it is the bioactive ceramic material that has been most extensively investigated.

The impetus for using synthetic HA as a biomaterial stems from the perceived advantage of using a material similar to the mineral phase in natural tissues to replace them. Because of this similarity, better tissue bonding is expected. Additional perceived advantages of HA and other bioactive ceramics include low thermal conductivity, elastic properties similar to those of bone, control of in vivo degradation rates through control of material properties, and the possibility of the ceramic functioning as a barrier to metallic corrosion products when it is coated onto a metal substrate.

However, temperature-induced phase transformations while processing HA provoke considerable changes in its in vitro dissolution rate and the altered structure changes the biological reaction to the material, which becomes more or less bioactive, respectively, with vitrification and crystallization. Given the multitude of chemical compositions and structures resulting from processing bioactive ceramics and the resultant fact that pure HA is rarely used, the broader term *calcium phosphate ceramics* has been proposed in lieu of the more specific term HA. Each individual calcium phosphate ceramic is then defined by its own unique set of chemical and physical properties.

Although calcium phosphate ceramics are too brittle and too stiff to serve as stand-alone dental implants for prosthetic tooth replacement, there has been continuing interest in using a thin (50 to 75 µm) layer of ceramic materials to coat the surface of metallic implants. This provides the beneficial osseointegration characteristics of the ceramic combined with the high strength of the metallic alloy. Most manufacturers provide implants coated with calcium phosphate ceramic for use in sites where poor bone quality exists. A major limitation in using this concept in all clinical situations, however, has revolved around the inability to predict and maintain the bond strength of the coating to the metal. When the bioactive ceramic material resorbs in vivo, an unpredictable change occurs in the implant–bone interface, and implant micromotion and loosening may occur. This makes the long-term stability of these implants uncertain.

If successful, the ceramic coating becomes completely fused with the surrounding bone. In this case, the interface is called *biointegration* rather than osseointegration, and there is no intervening space between the bone and the implant (see Fig. 14.2). A number of ceramic coatings have been used in this manner.

Typically, these coatings have been applied to the surface of an implant via a plasma-spray deposition process. This results in a complex mixture of HA, tricalcium phosphate, and tetracalcium phosphate in the coating, rather than a recapitulation of the starting powder mixture. Physical properties of importance to the functionality of calcium phosphate ceramics include powder particle size, particle shape, pore size, pore shape, pore-size distribution, specific surface area, phases present, crystal structure, crystal size, grain size, density, coating thickness, hardness, and surface roughness.

The long-term integrity of the ceramic coating in vivo is not known, but evidence indicates that these coatings will resorb over time. In addition, results of ex vivo pushout tests indicate that the ceramic–metal bond fails before the ceramic–tissue bond and is the weak link in the system. Thus the weak ceramic–metal bond and the integrity of that interface over a lengthy service life of functional loading suggests reason for concern.

Factors Affecting the Endosteal Implant

Geometry

Two primary objectives influence a patient's decision to pursue dental implant treatment: aesthetics and function. To fulfill these objectives over an extended period, a dental implant must be capable of withstanding the occlusal forces generated in the oral environment and in turn transfer this load to the supporting tissues. Not only must loads be transferred, but they should also be of an appropriate direction and magnitude so tissue viability is maintained. In this respect, the implant principally acts to minimize and distribute the biomechanical forces. The forces are characterized by their magnitude, duration, and type. The ability to transfer force largely depends on attaining interfacial fixation. The interface between the implant and bone must stabilize in as short a time as possible postoperatively, and once stable, must remain so throughout its service life. Designing an "optimal" implant that meets all the foregoing objectives requires the integration of material, physical, chemical, mechanical, biological, and economic factors.

Magnitude of the Force

The amount of load applied during normal chewing varies greatly, depending on the specific patient, the location in the arch, and the state of their dentition. Bite force values reported in the literature range from about 40 to 1250 N. The magnitude of force is greatest in the molar region because this area acts like the hinge of a lever (Fig. 14.3). The incisor region, in comparison, experiences about 10% of the magnitude seen in the posterior segment. This difference in load borne by the teeth and supporting bone dictates differences in mechanical requirements between anterior and posterior implants. Since stress depends not only on the applied load but also on the area over which this load is distributed, the loss of some teeth by a patient will greatly increase the stresses applied to the remaining teeth and implants in partially edentulous patients.

A prime requirement for any dental implant is adequate supporting bone height, width, and density. It is well established that bone grows in response to strain, and the presence of an excessive magnitude of stress applied to the bone will result in resorption or loss of bone. However, in the absence of a critical minimum level of strain for normal bone maintenance, the bone will also resorb. Therefore if the patient has been edentulous for a prolonged time,

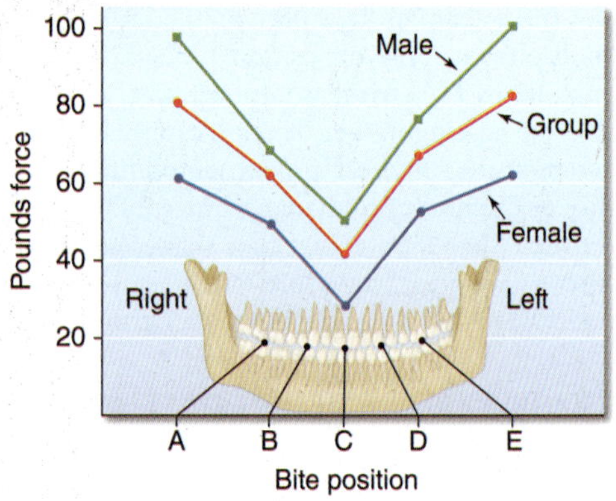

• **Fig. 14.3** Mean adult bite force at different positions in the jaw. (From Rugh SD, Solberg WK. The measurement of human oral forces. Behav Res Methods Instrum. 1972;4(3):125.)

the underlying bone will have resorbed and become less dense. It is common to place implants preferentially in the anterior mandible because this region has the greatest trabecular bone density when compared with the premolar or molar regions in both dentate and edentulous patients. When planning implant treatment, careful consideration must be given to the load distribution.

A great majority of the materials considered to be biocompatible are not suitable for use as implants, because their ultimate strength is not high enough to withstand the forces to which they are subjected during normal function. However, in order to survive and continue to function effectively, it is not only the ultimate strength, but also the modulus of elasticity (or stiffness) of the material that must be considered. Unless the bone experiences at least 1000 microstrains on a routine basis, it will begin to resorb. Most ceramic materials are extremely stiff; for example, polycrystalline aluminum oxide has a modulus of elasticity of ≈372 GPa. This stiffness is too high to transfer an adequate amount of an applied force to the bone. Instead, the stiffer implant material will carry a disproportionate amount of the load, causing stress shielding of the bone. By contrast, titanium has a modulus of elasticity of ≈100 GPa; still too high to be ideal, but much closer to that of bone (≈20 GPa). It will permit normal physiological loading of the bone.

Duration of the Force

When considering repetitive loading such as that occurring during mastication, it is more appropriate to consider the endurance limit of a material rather than its ultimate strength. The endurance limit is the highest amount of stress to which a material may be repeatedly subjected without failing. This limit is typically only about half of the ultimate strength of the material.

The tooth root-form implant is designed to be loaded parallel to the long axis and is vulnerable to fatigue failure from cyclic bending loads. These bending loads often result from premature contact, bruxism, inappropriate occlusal schemes, and the use of angled abutments. Off-axis loading should be avoided in design of the implant superstructure.

Type of Force

An implant experiences three types of loads in function: tensile forces, compressive forces, and shear forces. As discussed, a well-designed implant transfers and distributes these forces to the supporting bone. Bone is composed of both inorganic and organic constituents, and the inorganic components render it strongest when loaded in compression. Bone is about 30% weaker when placed in tension and nearly 70% weaker when subjected to shear forces. Therefore occlusion is a crucial consideration in designing the implant loading.

Smooth-sided cylindrical implant designs place the interface between the implant and the bone in nearly pure shear, the weakest possible loading scenario. These implant designs rely either on microscopic texturing of the implant body to offer some mechanical interlocking and provide retention, or on a coating. If the coating on these fails or resorbs, bone loss usually results from the lack of load transfer.

By contrast, screw-shaped implants have threads to engage the bone in compression and transfer the applied load. The thread designs have been extensively researched to provide a minimum of shear forces and maximal compression to the bone. This allows for the most favorable bone response. A number of recent thread designs have been introduced that use rounded thread tips (to reduce shear forces at the tip), changes in the thread angle (to maximize compression), two or more thread profiles on the same implant (which will cut at different locations in the osteotomy, thereby increasing the contact area), and/or a reduced thread height accompanied by an increased thread pitch (spreading the implant loading over a greater contact area while simultaneously increasing the strength of the implant body).

The concept of osseointegration around cylindrical or screw-shaped implants represents a situation of bone ongrowth. An alternative method of implant fixation is based on bone tissue ingrowth into roughened or three-dimensional porous surface layers. Such designs incorporating sintered beads or a sintered wire mesh are typical of orthopedic implants. Recently, implants with porous metal bodies have been developed and marketed. These new designs incorporate macroscale porosity or porous cellular structures, resembling cancellous bone. This results in a modulus of elasticity close to that of bone, thereby reducing the resulting stress shielding. Such retention systems have been shown to have higher bone/metal shear strength than other types of fixation. Increased interfacial shear strength results in a better stress transfer from the implant to the surrounding bone, a more uniform stress distribution between the implant and bone, and lower stresses in the implant. In principle, the result of a stronger interfacial bond is a decreased propensity for implant loosening. The theoretical progression of macroscale surface effects from the lowest implant/tissue shear strength to the highest is as follows: smooth, textured, screw threaded, plasma sprayed, and porous coated, porous body design.

Implant Diameter

An increase in implant length or diameter increases the total surface area of the implant. As a consequence, the area for distribution of the occlusal forces is increased and the stress on the bone is decreased. The bending fracture resistance (and hence rigidity) of the implant increases greatly as the implant width increases and is related to the implant radius raised to the fourth power. This dramatic increase can be deleterious if the diameter chosen causes stress shielding by reducing bone strain to subphysiologic levels.

Implant Length

As with increases in the width, increases in implant length also increase the surface area and reduce the bone stress. However, careful consideration of the bone quality is advised. In the highly dense type of bone usually found in the anterior mandible, overheating of the bone while drilling is a major cause of future failure. Preparation of an extra-long implant site tends to increase heating in this type of bone. Any immediate stability advantages provided by this long implant are transitory because once the implant osseointegrates, the apical region of the implant receives minimal stress transfer. Most of the stresses are still concentrated around the upper cortical plate through which the implant emerges. Conversely, in regions of poor bone quality, typically found in the posterior mandible and maxilla, anatomical considerations dictate the length of implant placed.

Surfaces and Biocompatibility

In analyzing an implant/tissue system, three aspects are important: (1) the individual constituents, namely the implant materials and tissues; (2) the effect of the implant and its breakdown products on the local and systemic tissues; and (3) the interfacial zone between the implant and tissue. Regarding the ultrastructure of the implant–tissue interface, it is important to understand that, although this zone is relatively thin (on the order of 0.1 nm), the constituents of the zone (heterogeneous metallic oxide, proteinaceous layer, and connective tissue) have a substantial effect on the maintenance of interfacial integrity. Furthermore, interfacial integrity depends on material, mechanical, chemical, surface, biological, and local environmental factors, all of which change as functions of time in vivo. Thus implant success is a function of biomaterial and biomechanical factors, as well as of surgical techniques, tissue healing, and a patient's overall medical and dental status.

Ion Release

Implant materials may corrode or wear, leading to the generation of particulate debris, which may in turn elicit both local and systemic biological responses. Metals are more susceptible to electrochemical degradation than are ceramics. Therefore a fundamental criterion when choosing a metallic implant material is that it must *not* elicit significant adverse biological response. Titanium alloys are well tolerated by the body because of their passive oxide layers. The main elemental ingredients, as well as the minor alloying constituents, are endured by the body when exposed in trace amounts. However, larger amounts of any metal cannot be tolerated, and minimizing mechanical and chemical breakdown of implant materials is a primary objective.

Titanium and other implant metals are in their passive state under typical physiological conditions, and breakdown of passivity should not occur. Both commercially pure titanium (CP Ti) and the titanium alloy Ti-6Al-4V possess excellent corrosion resistance for a full range of oxide states and pH levels. It is the extremely coherent, conformal oxide layer and the fact that titanium repassivates almost instantaneously through surface-controlled oxidation kinetics that renders titanium so corrosion resistant. The low dissolution rate and near chemical inertness of titanium dissolution products allow the bone to thrive and therefore osseointegrate with titanium. Transfixing screws that connect the implant abutment to the implant body are often made of 316 L stainless steel, which has self-passivating properties similar to those of titanium and its alloys.

Surfaces

Analysis of the implant surface is necessary to ensure a twofold requirement. First, implant materials must not adversely affect local tissues, organ systems, or organ functions. Second, the in vivo environment must not degrade the implant and compromise its long-term function. The interface zone between an implant and the surrounding tissue is therefore the most important entity in defining the biological response to the implant and the response of the implant to the body.

The success of any implant depends on its bulk and surface properties, the site of implantation, tissue trauma during surgery, and motion at the implant-tissue interface. Surface analysis in implantology therefore aids in material characterization, determining structural and composition changes occurring during processing, identifying biologically induced surface reactions, and analyzing environmental effects on the interfaces.

The surface of a material is always different in chemical composition, form, and structure from the bulk material because the atomic bonding at the surface is fundamentally different from that in the bulk. The surface of a metal can be considered an abrupt cessation of the orderly stacking of atoms below. As such the coordination number of these atoms differs and hence their physical and chemical properties are different from atoms deeper in the bulk, arising from their molecular arrangement, surface reactions, and potential contamination with other species. These differences may lead to changes in the interaction of the implant surface with the biological system.

In this regard, interface chemistry is primarily determined by the properties of the metal oxide and less so by the metal itself. Little or no similarity is found between the properties of the metal and the properties of the oxide, but the adsorption and desorption phenomena can still be influenced by the properties of the underlying metal. Characterization of surface composition, binding state, form, and function are important in the analysis of implant surfaces and implant-tissue interfaces.

Surface Alterations

In efforts to improve the in vivo performance of dental implants, considerable research continues to be conducted to investigate the effects of macro-, micro-, and nanoscale surface features on osseointegration. Many of these research reports are contradictory; for example, Ti and HA surfaces are highly cytocompatible, yet particles of these materials of a certain size cause cell death in culture. Therefore few absolutes have been identified, but some overarching guiding principles have slowly emerged. The first of these is that cells in vitro (and possibly in vivo) undergo contact guidance on the implant surface. In other words, cells grow preferentially in and along nanometer- to micrometer-sized grooves and ridge patterns on the surface of an implant. These minute grooves influence cell behavior by causing the cells to align themselves in the direction of the groove and migrate guided by the surface grooves (Fig. 14.4). Interestingly, very deep nanoscale grooves enhance cell guidance, while increasingly wider grooves decrease this effect. Furthermore, modification of the implant surface to incorporate these micro- and nanoscale surface features on top of macrotexturing increases the bone–implant contact area and the biomechanical interaction between implant and anchoring bone, especially in the immediate term after implantation. Cell shape, proliferation rate, and differentiation rate also depend on the texture of the implant surface to a great extent.

Nanometer-scale surface textures, smaller than the cell itself, particularly influence nonguided cell adhesion, migration, and proliferation on the surface of implants. This scale of feature is similar to the size and topography of proteins normally found in the extracellular matrix of bone. It is likely that it is the influence

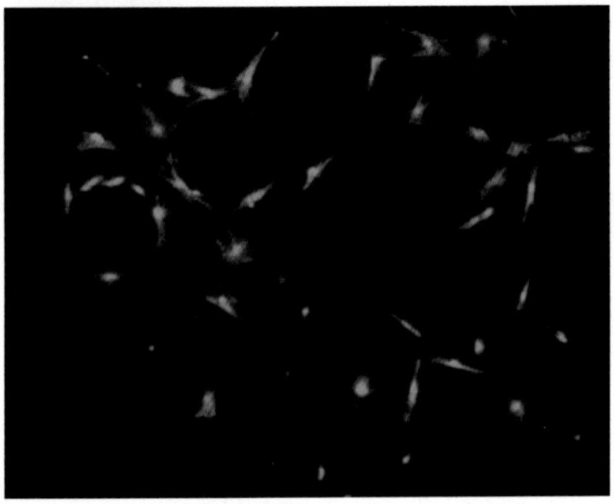

• **Fig. 14.4** Light microscope image of cells grown on a patterned surface. Notice the contact guidance of the cells provided by the surface texture. (Courtesy John C. Mitchell, Midwestern University College of Dental Medicine-Arizona, Glendale, AZ.)

of these features on serum protein adsorption that facilitates cell interaction with the implant surface. An adsorbed protein layer on the surface permits effective cell integrin interaction with the underlining topography. Those proteins that have dimensions similar to the nanoscale textural features will not have their three-dimensional conformation changed by adsorption to the surface, while surface features smaller or larger than the proteins tend to alter protein conformation and activity during adsorption. However, conclusive evidence of the mechanism by which topographic effects are recognized by focal adhesions, and how this information is transferred and interpreted by the cells, remains an area of intense investigation.

A second principle is that varying the macroscale surface texture of an implant material significantly affects the interface between the implant and bone in vivo. In general, rough-surfaced implants exhibit greater shear bond strengths to bone than corresponding smooth-surfaced implants. Upon microscopic examination, rough implants exhibit apparent direct bone apposition, whereas smooth implants exhibit various degrees of fibrous tissue encapsulation. Because this direct bone apposition is the method by which dental implants are retained in the jaw, they appear to be significantly affected by macroscale surface texture. Not all surface roughness, however, has the same desirable effects. The exact dimensions or degree of roughness that is optimal remains ambiguous.

A third defining principle is that the molecular events that occur in cells when they encounter the surface of a material likely dominate all subsequent cell interactions with that material. These interactions are highly specific, mediated by proteins at the surface of the material and the cell, and are extremely dynamic in nature. Osteoblasts use integrin receptors to bind to specific surface-adsorbed proteins, and these proteins change over time and maturity of the cell. These attachment proteins may be present in physiologic serum, or they may be expressed directly by the cells themselves. As a result of these interactions, transmembrane integrin receptors will alert the cell of the nature of its substrate and modify its attachment to the material. Therefore fundamental properties of materials such as pH, pI, surface charge, zeta potential, wettability, and van der Waal's forces may play significant roles in cell-material interaction.

As a result of these observations, during the last 30 years, implant surfaces have been greatly changed. While machined surfaces were the norm, now surfaces that are prepared by grit blasting, followed by either acid etching or coating to enhance the topography and/or remove embedded grit particles, dominate the marketplace. The resulting microscale retentive features not only roughen the implant surface, creating a greater implant-bone contact area but also play a role in activation of key biochemical sequences that ultimately accelerate the wound healing process and encourage osteogenesis.

It is quite clear that the chemistry of the implant surface plays a significant role in osseointegration and anchorage of the implant within the bone. This remains an area of intense commercial research. A surface modification technique that incorporates grit blasting, followed by acid etching with a solution that results in fluoride ions deposited on the implant surface, has been brought to the market. This preparation procedure results in a surface with varied chemical formulas within the surface oxide layer. This fluoride-containing surface has been shown to enhance gene expression and lead to enhanced osteogenesis.

Other new technologies to alter surfaces are also emerging on the market. These methods hold the promise to simultaneously alter an implant oxide layer thickness, chemistry, and/or structure. Additional surface treatments being explored include chemical surface hydroxylation to enhance the hydrophilicity of the implant surface and laser micromachining to create micro- and nano-structured surface roughness in hard-to-reach areas such as inside implant threads. Finally, other techniques such as electrochemical anodization processes can grow thick porous oxide layers with varied chemistries while creating microscale open pores on the surface. Integrating phosphorus into the growing anodization oxide layer has even been shown to promote early molecular adhesion on the implant surface. There is a growing awareness that the type of metallic oxide at the implant surface dictates cellular and protein binding onto that surface. Comprehension of this phenomenon is moving these surface technologies rapidly forward. However, these new surface oxides are continually altered by the inward diffusion of oxygen, and by hydroxide formation and the outward diffusion of metallic ions. Thus an ideal, single-oxide stoichiometry rarely exists.

Surface Coatings

The use of an additional surface coating treatment warrants additional discussion. Calcium phosphate–based coatings have traditionally been the most heavily investigated. These materials are commonly applied to the implant surface as a plasma-spray coating. In this high-temperature process, a 20- to 50-µm thick layer of material is deposited onto the roughened implant surface and allowed to cool. These coatings rely on relatively weak mechanical interlocking between the coating and the roughened surface to maintain adhesion to the metallic surface. Furthermore, the rapid cooling of the molten ceramic sprayed onto the surface produces uncontrollable crystallinity changes within the material and results in large-scale cracking of the coating. Although research studies have noted enhanced bioactivity with these types of coatings, their use has been limited in the dental profession because the coating ultimately provides additional interfaces that may undergo stress-induced failure that leads to uncertainty as to their service life, as discussed previously.

Another coating approach under investigation involves the attachment of biological mediators to the implant surface. In particular, the immobilization of short peptide sequences onto the implant surface has been demonstrated to influence cell response in vitro. Cell integrins, which bind to specific short peptide sequences, are responsible for these cell responses. In particular, the tripeptide sequence L-arginine, glycine, and L-aspartic acid (RGD) plays an important role in cell adhesion and is present in many extracellular matrix proteins, including fibrin, collagen, vitronectin, fibronectin, and osteopontin. The covalent bonding of recombinant forms of these sequences, via silane chemistry, onto an implant surface may stimulate mesenchymal cell attachment and provoke osteoblast proliferation and differentiation at the site. Additional peptide sequences under investigation include the following: YIGSR, IKVAV, KRSR (to improve cell adhesion), and FHRRIKA (to increase osteoblast mineralization).

In addition to small peptide sequences, the use of entire recombinant proteins on the implant surface has been investigated. The use of immobilized cytokine growth factors such as bone morphogenetic protein, transforming growth factor-β, fibroblast growth factor, vascular endothelial growth factor, and platelet-derived growth factor have been shown to positively increase the regeneration of tissues around an implant. However, the homogeneous coating of the implant surfaces and the release of these proteins into the surrounding tissues are rather unpredictable and uncontrolled with respect to both duration and dosage. Although further research is needed to illuminate these unresolved issues, this treatment holds promise as a future therapy.

Implant Materials and Processing

In general, two basic classes of materials (ceramics and metals) are used as implants, either alone or in hybrid fashion. Metallic implant materials are largely titanium based: either CP Ti or Ti-6Al-4V. However, it is essential to note that synergistic relationships between processing, composition, structure, and properties of the bulk metals and their surface oxides effectively leave more than two metals. Casting, forging, and machining, to form near-net-shaped end products, alter the bulk microstructure, surface chemistry, and properties. Similarly, densification of ceramics and deposition of ceramic and metal coatings by hot isostatic pressing or sintering can change bulk and surface composition, structure, and properties. Thus the many material processing sequences necessary to yield the end-stage dental implant have a strong influence on the properties and functionality of the implant, primarily through temperature and pressure effects.

Metallic dental implants are almost exclusively titanium-based alloys, although cobalt-based alloys have been used historically and experimentally in dentistry. The attributes of titanium, namely corrosion resistance and high strength, are discussed in Chapter 9.

The initial rationale for using ceramics in dentistry was based on their relative biological inertness as compared with that of metals. Ceramics are fully oxidized materials and therefore chemically stable and less likely to elicit an adverse biological response than are metals, which oxidize only at their surface. As discussed previously, a greater emphasis recently has been placed on bioactive and bioresorbable ceramics, materials that not only elicit normal tissue formation, but may also form an intimate bond with bone tissue and even be replaced by tissue over time.

Challenges and the Future

Although there is no consensus regarding methods of evaluating dental implants and which criteria are most important, clinical evaluations have generally shown that dental implants are successful in about 95% of cases within 5 years after implantation. Despite advances in the synthesis and processing of materials, surgical techniques, and clinical protocols, clinical failures occur at rates of approximately 2% to 5% per year. Causes of failure and current problems with dental implants include (1) early loosening from a lack of initial osseointegration; (2) late loosening, or loss of osseointegration; (3) bone resorption; (4) infection; (5) fracture of the implant or abutment; and (6) delamination of the coating from the bulk implant in the case of coated implants. The most common failure mechanism is alveolar crest resorption due to overloading. This inevitably leads to progressive peri-implant lesions, decreased areas of supporting tissues, and ultimately implant loosening. Aseptic failures are most often the cumulative result of more than one of the aforementioned factors.

Changes in implant materials and design will be accomplished by groups composed of academic dental researchers and implant manufacturers. They will continue to perform careful, multi-institutional clinical trials and prospective studies of compatibility, stress shielding, and bone loading among other factors. These three areas in particular present a major motivation for change in implant materials. Although very biocompatible, the current alloys suffer from a large elastic modulus mismatch with the supporting bone. Research work is underway to create composite materials (fiber-reinforced PEKK, polyether ketone ketone) that are biologically compatible and have the same modulus of elasticity as bone. Similar moduli will result in a stress distribution that more closely mimics that seen physiologically. In addition, the work being performed to investigate implant texture effects is likely to reveal additional fundamental principles that will incrementally improve implant designs.

However, in spite of these new research directions, the future of implant dentistry lies in the hands of the restorative dentist. After an implant has been placed and healed, it is the restorative dentist who is responsible for designing and delivering the restoration or prosthesis to the patient. Patient satisfaction with the function and aesthetics of the implant-supported prosthesis defines the success, or failure, of an implant case. Implants are in the mainstream of routine dental care in many countries. Their clinical success justifies the offering of implants along with more traditional therapies of fixed and removable partial prostheses for restoring edentulous spaces.

Bibliography

Albrektsson T, Branemark PI, Hansson HA, et al. Osseointegrated titanium implants: requirements for ensuring a long-lasting, direct bone-to-implant anchorage in man. *Acta Orthop Scand.* 1981;52:155.

Alqurashi H, Khurshid Z, Syed AUY, et al. Polyetherketoneketone (PEKK): an emerging biomaterial for oral implants and dental prostheses. *J Advanced Res.* 2021;28:87.

Ameen AP, Short RD, Johns R, et al. The surface analysis of implant materials. 1. The surface composition of a titanium dental implant material. *Clin Oral Implants Res.* 1993;4:144.

Aparicio C, Gil FJ, Fonseca C, et al. Corrosion behaviour of commercially pure titanium shot blasted with different materials and sizes of shot particles for dental implant applications. *Biomaterials.* 2003;24:263.

Arvidson K, Fartash B, Moberg LE, et al. In vitro and in vivo experimental studies on single crystal sapphire dental implants. *Clin Oral Implants Res.* 1991;2:47.

Baschong W, Suetterlin R, Hefti A, et al. Confocal laser scanning microscopy and scanning electron microscopy of tissue Ti-implant interfaces. *Micron.* 2001;32:33.

Berglundh T, Abrahamsson I, Lang NP, et al. De novo alveolar bone formation adjacent to endosseous implants. *Clin Oral Implants Res.* 2003;14:251.

Block MS, Kent JN. Sinus augmentation for dental implants: the use of autogenous bone. *J Oral Maxillofac Surg.* 1997;55:1281.

Boggan RS, Strong JT, Misch CE, et al. Influence of hex geometry and prosthetic table width on static and fatigue strength of dental implants. *J Prosthet Dent.* 1999;82:436.

Botticelli D, Berglundh T, Lindhe J. The influence of a biomaterial on the closure of a marginal hard tissue defect adjacent to implants: an experimental study in the dog. *Clin Oral Implants Res.* 2004;15:285.

Branemark PI, Adell R, Breine U, et al. Intra-osseous anchorage of dental prostheses. I. Experimental studies. *Scand J Plast Reconstr Surg.* 1969;3:81.

Branemark PI, Albrektsson T. Titanium implants permanently penetrating human skin. *Scand J Plast Reconstr Surg.* 1982;16:17.

Bucci-Sabattini V, Cassinelli C, Coelho PG, et al. Effect of titanium implant surface nanoroughness and calcium phosphate low impregnation on bone cell activity in vitro. *Oral Surg Oral Med Oral Pathol Oral Radiol Endod.* 2010;109(2):217.

Catledge SA, Fries MD, Vohra YK, et al. Nanostructured ceramics for biomedical implants. *J Nanosci Nanotechnol.* 2002;2:293.

Clark P, Connolly P, Curtis ASG, et al. Cell guidance by ultrafine topography in vitro. *J Cell Sci.* 1991;99(1):73.

Cook SD, Dalton JE. Biocompatibility and biofunctionality of implanted materials. *Alpha Omegan.* 1992;85:41.

Cook SD, Klawitter JJ, Weinstein AM. A model for the implant-bone interface characteristics of porous dental implants. *J Dent Res.* 1982;61:1006.

Cook SD, Weinstein AM, Klawitter JJ, et al. Quantitative histologic evaluation of LTI carbon, carbon-coated aluminum oxide and uncoated aluminum oxide dental implants. *J Biomed Mater Res.* 1983;17:519.

Cooper LF, Masuda T, Yliheikkila PK, et al. Generalizations regarding the process and phenomenon of osseointegration. Part II. In vitro studies. *Int J Oral Maxillofac Implants.* 1998;13:163.

Curtis ASG, Gadegaard N, Dalby MJ, et al. Cells react to nanoscale order and symmetry in their surroundings. *IEEE Trans Nanobiosci.* 2004;3(1):61.

Dalby MJ, Yarwood SJ, Riehle MO, et al. Increasing fibroblast response to materials using nanotopography: morphological and genetic measurements of cell response to 13-nm-high polymer demixed islands. *Exp Cell Res.* 2002;276(1):1.

de Lavos-Valereto IC, Deboni MC, Azambuja Jr. N, et al. Evaluation of the titanium Ti-6Al-7Nb alloy with and without plasma-sprayed hydroxyapatite coating on growth and viability of cultured osteoblast-like cells. *J Periodontol.* 2002;73:900.

De Maeztu MA, Alava JI, Gay-Escoda C. Ion implantation: surface treatment for improving the bone integration of titanium and Ti6Al4V dental implants. *Clin Oral Implants Res.* 2003;14:57.

Den Braber ET, De Ruijter JE, Smits HTJ, et al. Quantitative analysis of cell proliferation and orientation on substrata with uniform parallel surface micro-grooves. *Biomat.* 1996;17(11):1093.

Denissen HW, Klein CP, Visch LL, et al. Behavior of calcium phosphate coatings with different chemistries in bone. *Int J Prosthodont.* 1996;9:142.

Dubruille JH, Viguier E, Le Naour G, et al. Evaluation of combinations of titanium, zirconia, and alumina implants with 2 bone fillers in the dog. *Int J Oral Maxillofac Implants.* 1999;14:271.

Elias CN, Meirelles L. Improving osseointegration of dental implants. *Expert Rev Med Devices.* 2010;7(2):241.

Fontijn-Tekamp FA, Slagter AP, van Hof MA, et al. Bite forces with mandibular implant-retained overdentures. *J Dent Res.* 1998;77(10):1832.

Galgut PN, Waite IM, Brookshaw JD, et al. A 4-year controlled clinical study into the use of a ceramic hydroxylapatite implant material for the treatment of periodontal bone defects. *J Clin Periodontol.* 1992;19:570.

Galgut PN, Waite IM, Tinkler SM. Histological investigation of the tissue response to hydroxyapatite used as an implant material in periodontal treatment. *Clin Mater.* 1990;6:105.

Gatti AM, Zaffe D, Poli GP, et al. The evaluation of the interface between bone and a bioceramic dental implant. *J Biomed Mater Res.* 1987;21:1005.

Giannoni P, Muraglia A, Giordano C, et al. Osteogenic differentiation of human mesenchymal stromal cells on surface-modified titanium alloys for orthopedic and dental implants. *Int J Artif Organs.* 2009;32(11):811.

Gineste L, Gineste M, Ranz X, et al. Degradation of hydroxylapatite, fluorapatite, and fluorhydroxyapatite coatings of dental implants in dogs. *J Biomed Mater Res.* 1998;48:224.

Glantz PO. The choice of alloplastic materials for oral implants: does it really matter. *Int J Prosthodont.* 1998;11:402.

Grand View Research. *Dental implants market size, share & trends analysis report by implant type (Zirconium, Titanium), by region (North America, Europe, Asia Pacific, Latin America, MEA), and segment forecasts, 2023 –2030*; 2022:1 GVR-1-68038-566-3.

Guy SC, McQuade MJ, Scheidt MJ, et al. In vitro attachment of human gingival fibroblasts to endosseous implant materials. *J Periodontol.* 1993;64:542.

Haas R, Donath K, Fodinger M, et al. Bovine hydroxyapatite for maxillary sinus grafting: comparative histomorphometric findings in sheep. *Clin Oral Implants Res.* 1998;9:107.

Hall EE, Meffert RM, Hermann JS, et al. Comparison of bioactive glass to demineralized freeze-dried bone allograft in the treatment of intrabony defects around implants in the canine mandible. *J Periodontol.* 1999;70:526.

Haman JD, Scripa RN, Rigsbee JM, et al. Production of thin calcium phosphate coatings from glass source materials. *J Mater Sci Mater Med.* 2002;13:175.

Hatano N, Shimizu Y, Ooya K. A clinical long-term radiographic evaluation of graft height changes after maxillary sinus floor augmentation with a 2:1 autogenous bone/xenograft mixture and simultaneous placement of dental implants. *Clin Oral Implants Res.* 2004;15:339.

Hedia HS, Mahmoud NA. Design optimization of functionally graded dental implant. *Biomed Mater Eng.* 2004;14:133.

Hobkirk JA. Endosseous implants: the host-implant surface. *Ann Acad Med Singapore.* 1986;15:403.

Hodosh M, Shklar G. A polymethacrylate-silica composite material for dental implants. *J Biomed Mater Res.* 1977;11:893.

Holden CM, Bernard GW. Ultrastructural in vitro characterization of a porous hydroxyapatite/bone cell interface. *J Oral Implantol.* 1990;16:86.

Hovgaard MB, Rechendorff K, Chevallier J, et al. Fibronectin adsorption on tantalum: the influence of nanoroughness. *J Phys Chem B.* 2008;112(28):8241.

Hucke EE, Fuys RA, Craig RG. Glassy carbon: a potential dental implant material. *J Biomed Mater Res.* 1973;7:263.

Hurson S. Threaded implant design criteria. *Int J Dent Symp.* 1994;2:38.

Jarcho M. Retrospective analysis of hydroxyapatite development for oral implant applications. *Dent Clin North Am.* 1992;36:19.

Jokstad A, Braegger U, Brunski JB, et al. Quality of dental implants. *Int Dent J.* 2003;53:409.

Kamel I. A porous and potentially tough dental implant material. *J Dent Res.* 1976;55:1143.

Karoussis IK, Bragger U, Salvi GE, et al. Effect of implant design on survival and success rates of titanium oral implants: a 10-year prospective cohort study of the ITI Dental Implant System. *Clin Oral Implants Res.* 2004;15:8.

Kasemo B, Gold J. Implant surfaces and interface processes. *Adv Dent Res.* 1999;13:8.

Kay JF. Calcium phosphate coatings for dental implants. Current status and future potential. *Dent Clin North Am.* 1992;36:1.

Kikuchi S, Takebe J. Characterization of the surface deposition on anodized-hydrothermally treated commercially pure titanium after immersion in simulated body fluid. *J Prosthodont Res.* 2010;54(2):70.

Klinger A, Tadir A, Halabi A, et al. The effect of surface processing of titanium implants on the behavior of human osteoblast-like Saos-2 cells. *Clin Implant Dent Relat Res.* 2011;13:64.

Kohal RJ, Bachle M, Emmerich D, et al. Hard tissue reaction to dual acid-etched titanium implants: influence of plaque accumulation. A histological study in humans. *Clin Oral Implants Res.* 2003;14:381.

Kohal RJ, Weng D, Bachle M, et al. Loaded custom-made zirconia and titanium implants show similar osseointegration: an animal experiment. *J Periodontol.* 2004;75:1262.

Kohn DH. Overview of factors important in implant design. *J Oral Implantol.* 1992;18:204.

Kononen M, Hormia M, Kivilahti J, et al. Effect of surface processing on the attachment, orientation, and proliferation of human gingival fibroblasts on titanium. *J Biomed Mater Res*. 1992;26:1325.

Krennmair G, Seemann R, Schmidinger S, et al. Clinical outcome of root-shaped dental implants of various diameters: 5-year results. *Int J Oral Maxillofac Implants*. 2010;25:357.

Lacefield WR. Current status of ceramic coatings for dental implants. *Implant Dent*. 1998;7:315.

Lemons JE. Dental implant biomaterials. *J Am Dent Assoc*. 1990;121:716.

Linder L, Albrektsson T, Branemark PI, et al. Electron microscopic analysis of the bone-titanium interface. *Acta Orthop Scand*. 1983;54:45.

Liu J, Jin T, Chang S, et al. The effect of novel fluorapatite surfaces on osteoblast-like cell adhesion, growth, and mineralization. *Tissue Eng Part A*. 2010;16(9):2977.

Lord MS, Foss M, Besenbacher F. Influence of nanoscale surface topography on protein adsorption and cellular response. *Nano Today*. 2010;5(1):66.

Lutz R, Srour S, Nonhoff J, et al. Biofunctionalization of titanium implants with a biomimetic active peptide (P-15) promotes early osseointegration. *Clin Oral Implants Res*. 2010;21(7):726.

Massaro C, Rotolo P, De Riccardis F, et al. Comparative investigation of the surface properties of commercial titanium dental implants. Part I: chemical composition. *J Mater Sci Mater Med*. 2002;13:535.

Meyer U, Wiesmann HP, Fillies T, et al. Early tissue reaction at the interface of immediately loaded dental implants. *Int J Oral Maxillofac Implants*. 2003;18:489.

Morris HF, Ochi S. Hydroxyapatite-coated implants: a case for their use. *J Oral Maxillofac Surg*. 1998;56:1303.

Mueller WD, Gross U, Fritz T, et al. Evaluation of the interface between bone and titanium surfaces being blasted by aluminium oxide or bioceramic particles. *Clin Oral Implants Res*. 2003;14:349.

Muller-Mai C, Schmitz HJ, Strunz V, et al. Tissues at the surface of the new composite material titanium/glass-ceramic for replacement of bone and teeth. *J Biomed Mater Res*. 1989;23:1149.

Najjar TA, Lerdrit W, Parsons JR. Enhanced osseointegration of hydroxylapatite implant material. *Oral Surg Oral Med Oral Pathol*. 1991;71:9.

O'Neal RB, Sauk JJ, Somerman MJ. Biological requirements for material integration. *J Oral Implantol*. 1992;18:243.

Omar O, Svensson S, Lennerås M, et al. In vivo gene expression at anodically oxidized versus machined titanium implants. *J Biomed Mater Res*. 2010;92:1552.

Pelaez-Vargas A, Gallego-Perez D, Ferrell N, et al. Early spreading and propagation of human bone marrow stem cells on isotropic and anisotropic topographies of silica thin films produced via microstamping. *Microsc Microanal*. 2010;22:1–7.

Piattelli A, Scarano A, Piattelli M, et al. Histologic aspects of the bone and soft tissues surrounding three titanium non-submerged plasma-sprayed implants retrieved at autopsy: a case report. *J Periodontol*. 1997;68:694.

Piattelli M, Scarano A, Paolantonio M, et al. Bone response to machined and resorbable blast material titanium implants: an experimental study in rabbits. *J Oral Implantol*. 2002;28:2.

Piddock V. Production of bioceramic surfaces with controlled porosity. *Int J Prosthodont*. 1991;4:58.

Puleo DA, Nanci A. Understanding and controlling the bone-implant interface. *Biomaterials*. 1999;20:2311.

Quaranta A, Iezzi G, Scarano A, et al. A histomorphometric study of nanothickness and plasma-sprayed calcium-phosphorous-coated implant surfaces in rabbit bone. *J Periodontol*. 2010;81(4):556.

Rahal MD, Branemark PI, Osmond DG. Response of bone marrow to titanium implants: osseointegration and the establishment of a bone marrow-titanium interface in mice. *Int J Oral Maxillofac Implants*. 1993;8:573.

Rechendorff K, Hovgaard MB, Foss M, et al. Enhancement of protein adsorption induced by surface roughness. *Langmuir*. 2006;22(26):10885.

Roberts WE. Bone dynamics of osseointegration, ankylosis, and tooth movement. *J Indiana Dent Assoc*. 1999;78:24.

Rugh SD, Solberg WK. The measurement of human oral forces. *Behav Res Meth Instrum*. 1972;4:125.

Ruhling A, Hellweg A, Kocher T, et al. Removal of HA and TPS implant coatings and fibroblast attachment on exposed surfaces. *Clin Oral Implants Res*. 2001;12:301.

Rupprecht S, Bloch A, Rosiwal S, et al. Examination of the bone-metal interface of titanium implants coated by the microwave plasma chemical vapor deposition method. *Int J Oral Maxillofac Implants*. 2002;17:778.

Scarano A, Pecora G, Piattelli M, et al. Osseointegration in a sinus augmented with bovine porous bone mineral: histological results in an implant retrieved 4 years after insertion. A case report. *J Periodontol*. 2004;75:1161.

Schlegel AK, Donath K. BIO-OSS—a resorbable bone substitute. *J Long Term Eff Med Implants*. 1998;8:201.

Schwarz MS. Mechanical complications of dental implants. *Clin Oral Implants Res*. 2000;11:156.

Smith DC. Dental implants: materials and design considerations. *Int J Prosthodont*. 1993;6:106.

Stanford CM, Brand RA. Toward an understanding of implant occlusion and strain adaptive bone modeling and remodeling. *J Prosthet Dent*. 1999;81:553.

Steflik DE, Corpe RS, Young TR, et al. The biologic tissue responses to uncoated and coated implanted biomaterials. *Adv Dent Res*. 1999;13:27.

Steflik DE, McKinney Jr RV, Koth DL, et al. The biomaterial-tissue interface: a morphological study utilizing conventional and alternative ultrastructural modalities. *Scan Electron Microsc*. 1984;2:547.

Steinemann SG. Titanium—the material of choice. *Periodontol 2000*. 1998;17:7.

Sullivan DY, Sherwood RL, Mai TN. Preliminary results of a multicenter study evaluating a chemically enhanced surface for machined commercially pure titanium implants. *J Prosthet Dent*. 1997;78:379.

Sun L, Berndt CC, Gross KA, et al. Material fundamentals and clinical performance of plasma-sprayed hydroxyapatite coatings: a review. *J Biomed Mater Res*. 2001;58:570.

Svanborg LM, Andersson M, Wennerberg A. Surface characterization of commercial oral implants on the nanometer level. *J Biomed Mater Res B Appl Biomater*. 2010;92(2):462.

Tamura Y, Yokoyama A, Watari F, et al. Surface properties and biocompatibility of nitrided titanium for abrasion resistant implant materials. *Dent Mater J*. 2002;21:355.

Taylor TD, Laney WR. *Dental Implants: Are They For Me?* 2nd ed. Quintessence Publishing Co; 1993.

Triplett RG, Frohberg U, Sykaras N, et al. Implant materials, design, and surface topographies: their influence on osseointegration of dental implants. *J Long Term Eff Med Implants*. 2003;13:485.

Ungvári K, Pelsöczi IK, Kormos B, et al. Effects on titanium implant surfaces of chemical agents used for the treatment of peri-implantitis. *J Biomed Mater Res B Appl Biomater*. 2010;94(1):222.

Variola F, Brunski JB, Orsini G, et al. Nanoscale surface modifications of medically relevant metals: state-of-the art and perspectives. *Nanoscale*. 2011;3(2):335.

Vercaigne S, Wolke JG, Naert I, et al. Bone healing capacity of titanium plasma-sprayed and hydroxylapatite-coated oral implants. *Clin Oral Implants Res*. 1998;9:261.

Vlacic-Zischke J, Hamlet SM, Friis T, et al. The influence of surface microroughness and hydrophilicity of titanium on the up-regulation of TGFβ/BMP signaling in osteoblasts. *Biomaterials*. 2011;32(3):665–671.

Wagner WC. A brief introduction to advanced surface modification technologies. *J Oral Implantol*. 1992;18:231.

Wataha JC. Materials for endosseous dental implants. *J Oral Rehabil*. 1996;23:79.

Weinlaender M. Bone growth around dental implants. *Dent Clin North Am*. 1991;35:585.

Wennerberg A, Albrektsson T. On implant surfaces: a review of current knowledge and opinions. *Int J Oral Maxillofac Implants*. 2010;25(1):63.

Yang JY, Ting YC, Lai JY, et al. Quantitative analysis of osteoblast-like cells (MG63) morphology on nanogrooved substrata with various groove and ridge dimensions. *J Biomed Mater Res A*. 2009;90(3):629.

15
Tissue Engineering

JOHN C. MITCHELL

CHAPTER OUTLINE

Tissue engineering is a term coined at a meeting sponsored by the National Institutes of Health in 1987. This discipline is a rapidly developing multidisciplinary branch of science that combines many of the basic principles of biology, medicine, and engineering. The primary goal of tissue engineering is the restoration, maintenance, or enhancement of tissue and organ function.

In addition to having therapeutic applications, in which a particular organ is custom grown to replace a failing or missing body part, tissue engineering has diagnostic applications in which tissues are fabricated in vitro and used for in vitro biocompatibility testing of compounds. Examples include application in drug metabolism and uptake, toxicity, or pathogenicity. Tissue engineering research therefore translates fundamental knowledge in physics, chemistry, and biology into materials, devices, and strategies. It also integrates biomaterials, cell biology, and stem cell research; engineering characteristics of three-dimensional structures and mass transport issues; biomechanical characteristics of native and replacement tissues, biomolecules, and growth factors; and bioinformatics to support gene/protein expression and analysis.

Tissue engineering as a discipline grew out of the pressing need for replacement tissues and organs. During 2022 in the United States alone over 41,939 solid organs (heart, lung, intestine, kidney, pancreas, and liver) were transplanted. More than three-quarters of those organs came from deceased donors. Meanwhile, during this same period, 62,589 new potential recipients were added to the waiting list and nearly 5500 patients died while waiting for a transplant (Box 15.1). Clearly the demand for organs greatly exceeds the supply. Enthusiasm for tissue engineering comes from the promise of making transplants easier and more common. In dentistry, the disciplines of periodontology and oral and maxillofacial surgery often use bone tissue transplant materials to repair defects.

Today there are four primary classes of tissue/organ transplants: autograft, allograft, xenograft, and alloplast (Box 15.2).

Autograft

An autograft is a tissue or organ that is transferred from one location to another within a single individual (Fig. 15.1). It is common to transplant tissues such as hair, blood, and even limited amounts of skin and bone. These tissues regenerate to some extent, repairing the void left after their removal. This method of transplantation avoids immunologic complications and is considered the "gold standard" for success.

Allograft

Allografts are tissues or organs that are transplanted from one individual to another within the same species (Fig. 15.2). Routinely, tissues and organs are removed from living and deceased donors and transferred to a different recipient. Blood, bone, skin, corneas, ligaments, and tendons are routinely collected in banks and frozen, to be used in future surgical procedures.

Xenograft

The Center for Biologics Evaluation and Research (CBER) is the branch of the Food and Drug Administration (FDA) that oversees and regulates human tissue transplants. They define xenotransplants as "transplantation, implantation, or infusion into a human recipient of either (a) live cells, tissues, or organs from a nonhuman animal source or (b) human body fluids, cells, tissues, or organs that have had ex vivo contact with live nonhuman animal cells, tissues, or organs." This therapeutic regimen has been used experimentally to treat neurodegenerative disorders, liver failure, and diabetes when compatible human materials are not widely available.

Xenografts are now common in dentistry. One example is Bio-Oss (a product derived from cow bone) that is used to augment defects in the maxilla and mandible (Fig. 15.3).

• BOX 15.1 Summary of Transplant Data, United States

Candidate Waiting List as of May 9 2023[a]

All	114,178
All—added in 2022	62,589
Kidney	96,061
Pancreas	837
Kidney/pancreas	2020
Liver	10,601
Intestine	205
Heart	3402
Lung	1002
Heart/lung	34
Removed from list due to death, 2022	6037

Transplants Performed in 2022[a]

Total	41,307
Deceased donor	34,843
Living donor	6464

Median Waiting Times for Liver Transplant

Type O blood 2003-2006	1195 days (3.3 years)
Type O blood 2007-2010	1055 days (2.9 years)
Type O blood 2011-2014	1638 days (4.5 years)

[a]Based on data from the Organ Procurement and Transplantation Network, U.S. Department of Health & Human Services (http://optn.transplant.hrsa.gov/).

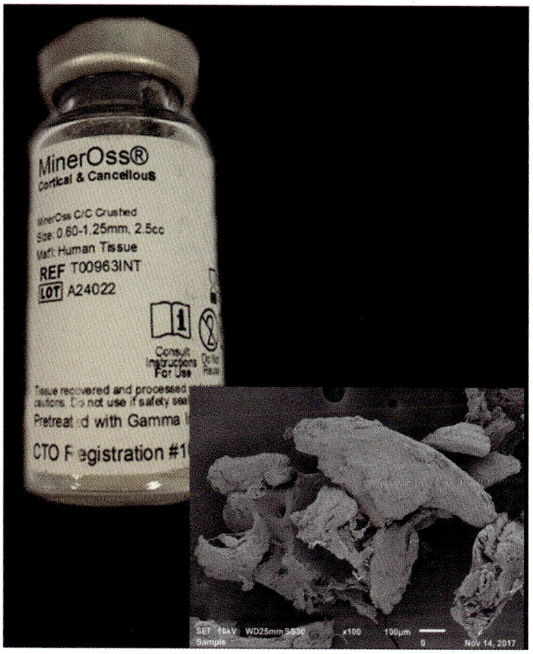

• **Fig. 15.2** Freeze-dried bone allograft is harvested from humans and sold in sterilized vials in both demineralized and nondemineralized form (original magnification ×100 for inset image). (Courtesy Lydia P. Mitchell, Midwestern University College of Dental Medicine-Arizona, Glendale, AZ.)

• BOX 15.2 Sources of Tissue for Grafting

Autograft: The patient's own tissue
Allograft: Human source other than the patient (could be cadaveric)
Xenograft: Tissue from a different species
Alloplast: Synthetic origin

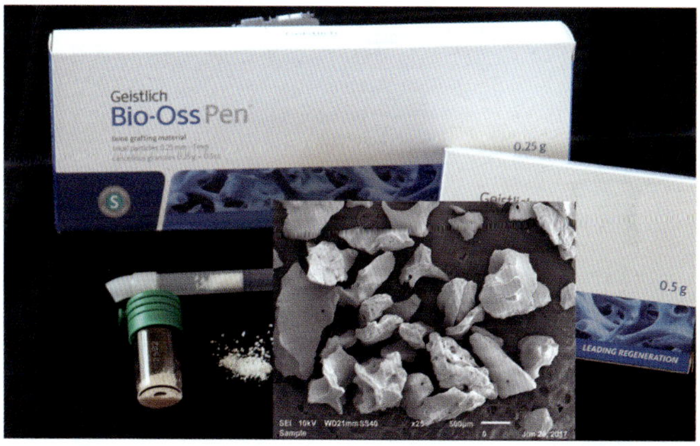

• **Fig. 15.3** Bio-Oss is a porous bone mineral matrix xenograft prepared from bovine sources that has been sterilized by gamma ionizing radiation. Note the large pores visible (original magnification ×25 for inset image). (Courtesy John C. Mitchell, Midwestern University College of Dental Medicine-Arizona, Glendale, AZ.)

Alloplasts

Alloplasts are the newest type of grafting materials. These grafts are fabricated completely from synthetic materials, making them quite different from the other three types of grafts because no living component is used. Alloplastic materials, such as dental implants, are becoming increasingly common in dentistry. Dental implants fabricated from metals and ceramics are considered routine restorative treatments in many countries. These materials integrate with bone and help restore function for the patient and have excellent long-term success.

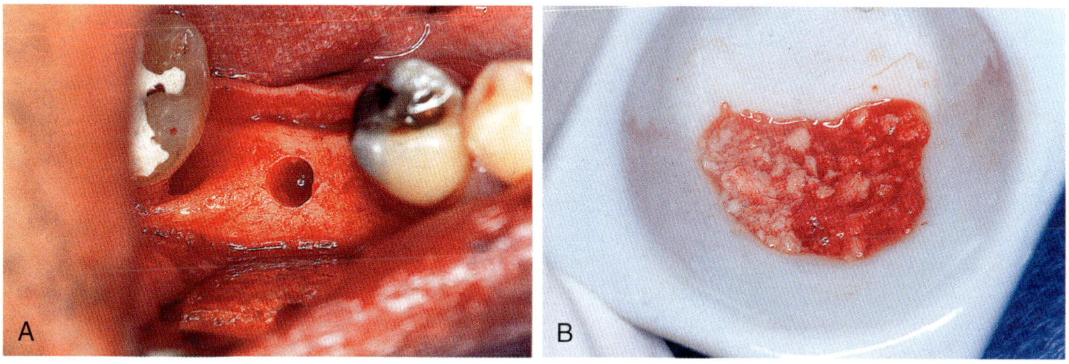

• **Fig. 15.1** Autograft bone (B) is harvested (A) from the patient into whom it will be reimplanted. (From Newman MG, Takei HH, Klokkevold PR, et al. *Carranza's Clinical Periodontology*. 11th ed. Saunders; 2012.)

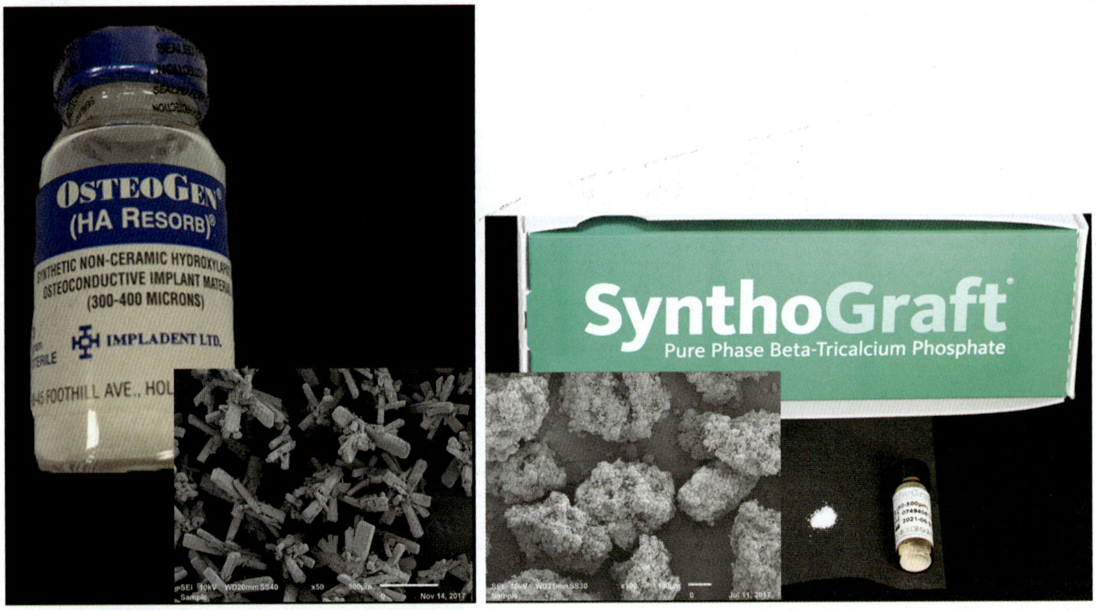

• **Fig. 15.4** OsteoGen *(left)* is a highly crystalline osteoconductive, bioactive, and resorbable bone graft material that is a biphasic mixture of β-tricalcium phosphate and hydroxylapatite. The Ca:P ratio is designed to mimic that of human bone (original magnification x50 for inset image); SynthoGraft *(right)* is a popular pure, single-phase β-tricalcium phosphate alloplast that is resorbable and has nanometer-scale porosity (original magnification ×100 for inset image). (Courtesy John C. Mitchell, Midwestern University College of Dental Medicine-Arizona, Glendale, AZ.)

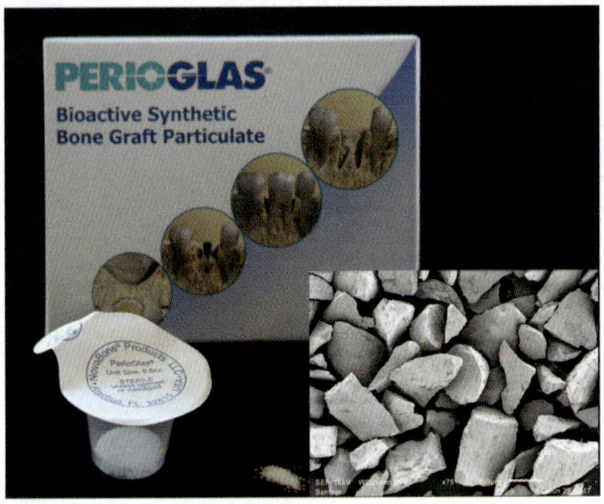

• **Fig. 15.5** Bioactive glasses are receiving increased attention because of their surface bioactivity. Shown here is PerioGlas (original magnification ×75 for inset image). (Courtesy John C. Mitchell, Midwestern University College of Dental Medicine-Arizona, Glendale, AZ.)

Bone grafting alloplasts are also common (Figs. 15.4 and 15.5). Autograft bone placed in the reconstruction of craniofacial structures can be augmented with ceramic and bioactive glasses. These alloplasts are available in nearly unlimited quantities with no adverse immunological reaction. An important benefit is that they do not pose the risk of transmitting disease from one individual to another.

Strategies for Tissue Engineering

Tissue engineering began with the concept of using biomaterials and cells to assist the body in healing itself. As the discipline matured, its goal shifted to developing logical strategies for optimizing new tissue formation through the judicious selection of conditions that will enhance the performance of tissue progenitors in a graft site, ultimately encouraging the production of a desired tissue or organ. Several strategies are now available for developing new organs and tissues (Box 15.3).

• BOX 15.3 Strategies for Tissue Engineering

Injection of cells: Undifferentiated cells (usually not from the patient) are injected directly into the vicinity of injury.

Guided tissue regeneration: Undesired cells are excluded from repopulating a defect or injury site by placing a physical barrier to prevent their migration. Desirable cells are able to enter the site from the surrounding tissue.

Cell induction: Growth and differentiation factors are injected (or implanted with a time-release substrate) within the injury or defect site. Circulating cells are induced to differentiate and populate the site with a desirable phenotype. Alternatively, gene vectors are injected and cause the growth/differentiation factors to be produced endogenously.

Cells in a scaffold matrix: Preformed scaffolds are seeded with cells from a patient. This construct is grown in vitro to expand the number of cells and to allow the cells to begin to produce a matrix. After a suitable growth interval, the construct is implanted back into the patient. As the cells grow and develop into tissues, the scaffold slowly resorbs, leaving no trace of its former presence.

Injection of Cells

With the cell injection method, disaggregated cells at an undifferentiated stage of development are injected into the recipient. Considerable research has been conducted into the use of this method to combat systemic diseases such as Alzheimer's and Parkinson's disease, as well as juvenile-onset diabetes and multiple sclerosis. It also holds potential for treating damaged nerve and muscle sites. Commonly referred to as *stem cells*, the injected cells are more

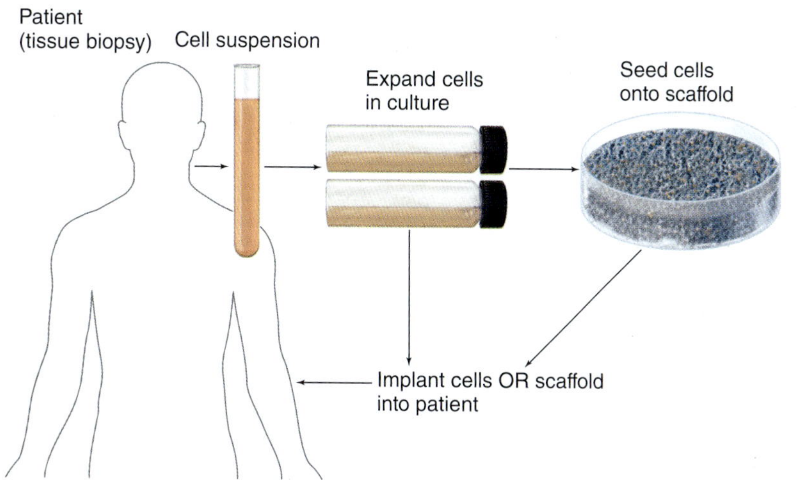

• **Fig. 15.6** Cell injection therapy. May involve the use of scaffold into which the cells are expanded, or they may be directly injected into their target site without a substrate.

appropriately termed *undifferentiated* or *progenitor cells* (see later discussion in the section on Stem Cells). These cells are capable of forming new tissue with one or more phenotypes. As a therapeutic regimen, the cells are injected into the vicinity of the site in which they are intended to propagate. They migrate to the area of injury and begin to replicate and replace the lost tissue or produce a desired compound such as insulin (Fig. 15.6). This strategy has already been successful in regenerating small areas of cartilage in temporomandibular joints.

Guided Tissue Regeneration

Guided tissue regeneration (GTR) is a surgical procedure for regenerating tissue by enhancing the opportunity for one cell type to populate an area while providing contact guidance to the developing cells. The desired cell types can then populate an area without competition because unwanted cell types are excluded. In the laboratory, this method has been successful in creating a biodegradable polymer conduit through which nerve cell regeneration and reconnection can occur. GTR is commonly used in periodontal treatment to regenerate lost periodontal tissues such as the bone, periodontal ligament (PDL), and connective tissue attachment that supports the teeth. The procedure involves placement of a membrane under the mucosa and over the residual bone (Fig. 15.7). The barrier helps exclude the faster-growing epithelium and gingival connective tissues during the postsurgical healing phase, allowing the slower-growing PDL and bone cells to migrate into the protected areas.

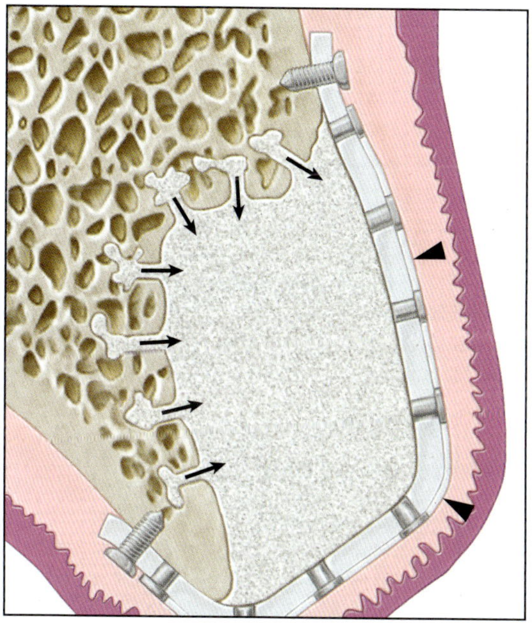

• **Fig. 15.7** Guided bone regeneration (GBR). GBR is being used to isolate the site being regenerated from the overlying tissues by means of a titanium-reinforced membrane barrier *(arrowheads)*. The newly forming bone may be augmented by the addition of particulate grafting material. The barrier is securely attached to the margins of the defect to prevent displacement during healing. Notice that decortication of the underlying bone bed allows invasion of the site by osteogenic precursor cells from the bloodstream and surrounding bone.

Cell Induction

In the last decade, there has been explosive growth in understanding the role of cytokines, developmental proteins, and growth factors in molecular biology. Many of these growth factors are available as recombinant human lyophilized proteins. There have been tremendous advances in administering various mixtures of these growth factors directly to tissues to induce them down a particular differentiation lineage. Often these growth and differentiation factors can be simply injected into a target site. This technique, as a tissue-engineering regimen, targets local connective tissue progenitors already present in the region where new tissues are desired and induces those cells to generate the desired tissue. Some of the injected proteins may serve as mitogens to recruit cells to migrate into the area, where other growth factors cause them to differentiate. Alternatively, they can be delivered by a substrate that releases them over time.

Gene therapy can be used with cell induction methods. In this application, a gene sequence that encodes for production of a specific growth factor or therapeutic compound is inserted wholly into the genome of the recipient cell. Insertion is achieved by a carrier, called a *vector*, to deliver the therapeutic gene to the patient's target cells. The most common vector is a genetically altered virus that has been modified to carry human DNA. Because viruses have evolved a way of encapsulating and delivering their genes to

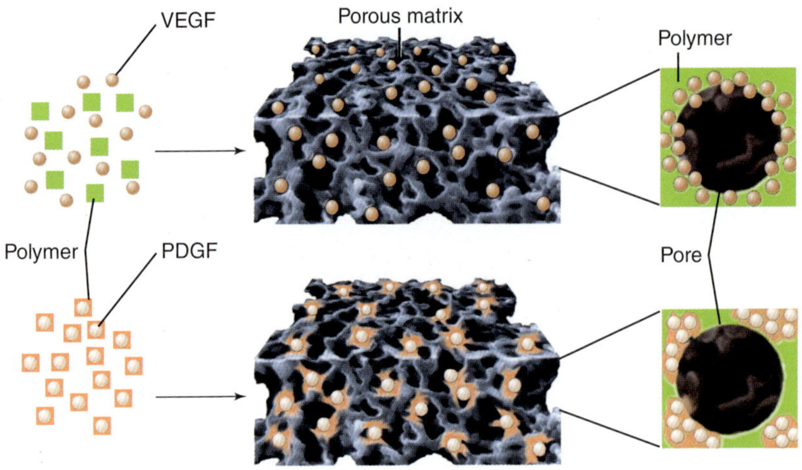

• **Fig. 15.8** Scaffold systems. These systems may serve as delivery substrates for various therapeutic compounds, in addition to providing the cells with a suitable surface on which to grow. Multiple factors may even be delivered with different release profiles by varying the method in which they are incorporated into the substrate. In this example, vascular endothelial growth factor *(VEGF)* is incorporated largely near the surface of the scaffold and is subject to rapid release in vivo. In contrast, the preencapsulated platelet-derived growth factor *(PDGF)* is more uniformly incorporated throughout the scaffold and is subject to release regulated by the degradation of the matrix polymer. (Modified from Richardson TP, Peters MC, Ennett AB, et al. Polymeric system for dual growth factor delivery. *Nat. Biotechnol.* 2001;19(11):1029–1034.)

human cells, they can be manipulated to insert these therapeutic genes into the recipient cells. Therefore vectors are injected into a site along with an initial bolus of the therapeutic compound, and the vectors then upload their genes into resident cells. After incorporating this DNA into their genome, the newly transfected cells begin to replicate the desired growth factor endogenously. This method promotes continuous protein production at the site long after the initially injected growth factors diffuse from their target tissues or degrade enzymatically.

Cells Within Scaffold Matrices

Three-dimensional porous scaffolds can be used with cells to provide many of the advantages of the aforementioned methods. These preformed scaffolds are usually made of bioresorbable materials. The scaffolds promote new tissue formation by providing a surface and void volume that encourages attachment, migration, proliferation, and the desired differentiation of connective tissue progenitors throughout the region where new tissue is required. Typically the scaffold is seeded with progenitor cells that are allowed to attach and proliferate in vitro. The cell constructs are often grown in a nutrient media supplemented with growth factors necessary for cell and tissue development. During the growth phase, a static or dynamic mechanical load may be applied to the construct, stimulating the cells to align in response to the load. The aligned cells tend to produce a highly organized extracellular matrix (ECM) that results in improved tissue structure and function. After a suitable time in vitro, the entire construct is then implanted in vivo, where the tissue must continue to develop while forming a connection with the existing vascular system. The scaffold gradually degrades until it is completely replaced by new tissues. As the scaffold degrades, the developing tissues gradually experience a higher fraction of the loads on the tissue and ultimately begin to function as native tissues.

The scaffold can therefore serve a dual function, as both a rigid substrate for cell growth and as a delivery vehicle for the release of therapeutic regulatory compounds in vivo. The release of bioactive molecules that are attached to the scaffold surface or encapsulated within the scaffold matrix can change the function of connective tissue progenitor cells (activation, proliferation, migration, differentiation, or survival) to create new or enhanced tissues (Fig. 15.8). There are several critical variables in design and function of the scaffold. Variables include the composition of the scaffold; its three-dimensional architecture; surface chemistry; mechanical properties; and the physical, chemical, and biological environment in the area surrounding the scaffold during its functional lifetime, which is often determined by its degradation characteristic. All cells require access to metabolic molecules (oxygen, glucose, and amino acids) and removal of cellular waste products (carbon dioxide, nitrogen compounds, and salts) in order to survive. There also must be a balance between consumption and delivery of these molecules if cells are to thrive. The design of the scaffold must accommodate these issues. Eventually a rich blood supply will perform these tasks, but such a circulatory system takes time to mature.

Patients who receive allogeneous tissue and organ transplants are often treated with immunosuppressive drugs for their lifetime to prevent rejection of the grafted tissue. These drugs can have a multitude of severe side effects, including headaches, nausea, weight gain, and increased susceptibility to infection. The ideal source of cells for tissue-engineering therapies is from the patient. Autograft tissue eliminates the potential for adverse immunological reactions. However, autograft tissues usually require an additional surgical site and the associated expense, discomfort, and healing time.

Stem Cells

Stem cells are particular cells within the body that are unspecialized, and capable of division and self-renewal prior to differentiation into a specialized cell type. They are commonly used in tissue-engineering therapies because they are not terminally differentiated and can migrate within the body to sites requiring repair

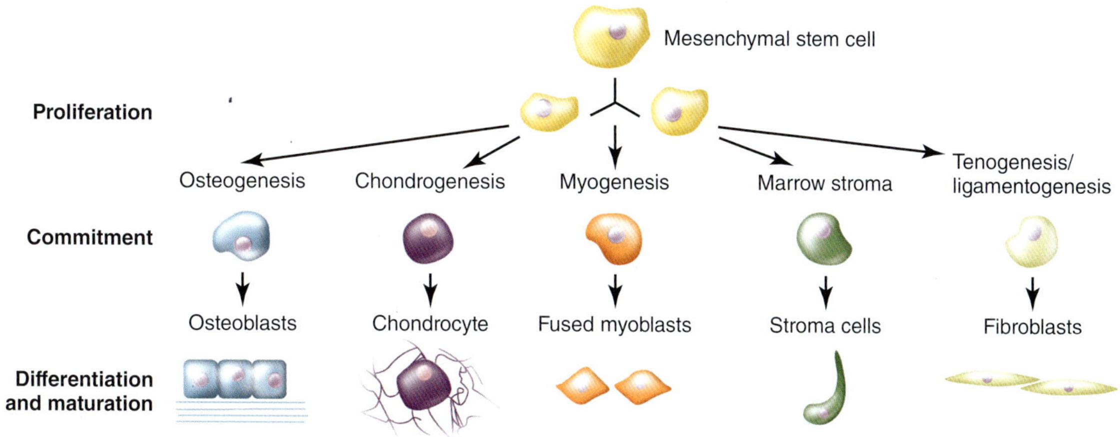

• **Fig. 15.9** Differentiation pathways of mesenchymal cells. A circulating mesenchymal cell may become one of any of the cell types shown here. The pathway down which it travels is influenced by both local and systemic factors.

or replacement. Stem cells are able to produce progeny cells with multiple phenotypes. There are different types of stem cells within the body: totipotent cells are single cells that can divide to generate any cell type, including extraembryonic tissues; pluripotent cells can become any of the over 200 types of cells in the body, but they lack the capability to generate extraembryonic tissues such as a placenta; multipotent cells are capable of forming one of a number of specific tissue types; oligopotent cells can take on only two or at most three different functions; and finally a unipotent cell can divide and migrate, but is restricted to forming only a single cell or tissue type.

Until very recently most stem cell researchers worked with only two types of cells: embryonic stem cells (which are pluripotent) and somatic or "adult" stem cells (usually considered to be multipotent progenitor cells). Besides their origin, there are important differences between these stem cell types. For example, adult mesenchymal stem cells (MSCs) have been shown to be capable only of transdifferentiation into neural tissue, cartilage, bone, and fat. Therefore these "adult" cells were thought to be restricted to developing into one of only a limited number of cell types. MSCs are found in small numbers in bone marrow and are also found circulating in the bloodstream. Isolating these cells from mature skeletal tissues is difficult, and routine methods to multiply them in vitro have not yet been perfected. Embryonic stem cells, by contrast, can be grown relatively easily in culture. Because a large number of cells are needed for successful stem cell replacement therapy, the choice of cell type is important.

Despite being easier to culture, embryonic stem cells are prone to immunogenic rejection. This is a significant drawback. By contrast, adult stem cells, and tissues derived from them, are less likely to induce rejection because the origin of the cells is the patient. In that case, the patient's own cells could be multiplied in culture, induced to differentiate into the specific cell type needed, and then reimplanted.

Recently, five additional stem cell types have been identified within dental tissues. These mesenchymal-derived cell populations include (1) *d*ental *p*ulp *s*tem *c*ells from permanent human teeth (DPSCs), (2) *s*tem cells from the pulp of *h*uman *e*xfoliated *d*eciduous teeth (SHEDs), (3) *periodo*ntal *l*igament *s*tem *c*ells (PDLSCs), (4) *s*tem *c*ells from *a*pical *p*apilla (SCAPs) and (5) *d*ental *f*ollicle *p*rogenitor *c*ells (DFPCs). Each of these populations has specific advantages and drawbacks for replacing lost tissues.

Compared to bone-derived MSCs, DPSC and SHED cells appear to have greater proliferative capabilities while maintaining the ability to produce the same range of progeny (Fig. 15.9). These cells have proven to be multipotent and provide for regeneration of odontoblasts, osteoblasts, chondrocytes, myocytes, neurons, and adipocytes. When implanted in vivo, these cells have shown the ability to generate an ectopic dentin-pulp complex.

Periodontal ligament stem cells are another highly promising stem cell population for tissue regeneration and have been shown to differentiate into osteoblasts, cementoblasts, adipocytes, and chondrocytes. However, the scarcity of human PDLSCs severely limits their application for tissue regeneration in periodontal therapy.

Stem cells isolated from the apical papilla of immature permanent teeth (SCAPs), along with progenitor cells arising from the *dental follicle* (DFPCs) have also been demonstrated to differentiate into osteoblasts, adipocytes, chondrocytes, and neuronal cells. However, similar to PDLSCs, these cell types suffer from difficulties in acquisition. Also, when harvested, cells from these regions have a highly heterogeneous cell population, presenting highly varied phenotypes and differentiation capabilities. A better understanding of ways to identify subpopulations of these cells will be needed to use them in therapeutic situations.

Even more recently, culture conditions and viral vectors were found in which differentiated adult cells can be "reprogrammed" to take on an embryonic stem cell–like state. The development of these technological advances led to receipt of the 2012 Noble Prize for Physiology or Medicine "for the discovery that mature cells can be reprogrammed to become pluripotent." These new types of stem cells are called *induced pluripotent stem cells* (iPSCs). They are capable of generating cells that have the characteristics of all three germ layers and can differentiate into many different tissue types: for example, neural tissues, cardiac tissues, liver tissues, pancreatic tissues, or even blood cells. Because these cells and tissues are patient derived, immunogenic rejection is unlikely. To reduce the potential of cancer development from viral vectors during reprogramming, nonviral delivery methods are being researched heavily, mostly involving various types of material nanoparticles as the new delivery systems.

Compared to other tissues, cells from dental-derived tissues are readily obtainable and easy to harvest. They can be obtained from gingival tissues and the oral mucosa by swiping with a cotton swab, or by removal of pulpal tissues from extracted permanent or deciduous teeth. Thus these iPSC types currently hold the greatest promise for future success with stem cell therapies.

An interesting facet of iPSC technology has emerged in the last few years: epigenetic memory of these cells seems to preferentially differentiate them back to their original cell type. This might provide an advantage in the differentiation of cells into hard tissues but could also be a shortcoming in the ability to repair other tissues. For this reason, DPSC-derived iPSCs have been mainly chosen as the starting cells for most oral tissue repair (bone, blood vessels, periodontium, nerve, and teeth).

Research into stem cell differentiation has led to significant discoveries, but the ultimate cause of differentiation remains unclear. Left in a cell culture plate alone, several tissue types will result from a single group of stem cells. However, with suitably timed administration of the appropriate growth factors, a single cell type emerges and begins to organize into a tissue. The fate of a cell is also controlled by changes in the migration, proliferation, differentiation, or survival of its progeny. Transplanted stem cells may even fuse with existing cells in a body and assume the characteristics of that tissue. Tactile stimulus or other factors to upregulate or downregulate genes to initiate these changes are being studied.

Biomaterials and Scaffolds

Three types of biomaterials have been studied as scaffolds and carrier systems: (1) natural (or biological) materials, (2) ceramic or glass materials, and (3) polymeric materials. Each type has advantages and disadvantages in particular locations and tissues to be regenerated. All scaffolds must be nontoxic and nonimmunogenic, biodegradable, sterilizable, able to withstand mechanical loads, sufficiently porous to permit migration and growth of cells into their interior, and be supportive of a new fractal circulatory system to promote the exchange of metabolic constituents.

Biological Materials

Natural materials such as collagen, lyophilized bone (both allogenous and xenogenous), and coral have been used as tissue engineering substrates. Collagen has been extensively tested as a scaffold for bone regeneration. One of the first materials used for bone tissue engineering was the insoluble collagenous matrix obtained after extraction of the bone matrix with various chemical agents. This collagenous matrix, with freeze-dried bone, formed new endochondral bone when used with growth factors in vivo. Coral, based on calcium carbonate, is strikingly similar to the structure of alveolar bone. When coral is treated with phosphoric acids, the resulting calcium phosphate is very strong and biocompatible. Many patients prefer nonbiological implantable substrates because of the high potential for viral, prion, and disease transmission from biological materials.

Ceramic and Glass Materials

Three decades of research have shown that certain types of glasses, glass ceramics, and pure ceramics can bond tightly with living bone tissue. Hydroxylapatite, the major inorganic (ceramic) constituent of bone, was one of the first alloplastic materials used as a bone augmentation scaffold. Ceramic and glass-ceramic materials are generally biocompatible and perform adequately when biomechanical loads are applied. Their use as scaffolds is limited because of their long degradation times in vivo and lack of native porosity.

Some of these limitations might be overcome in the near future with recent advances in sol-gel synthesis methods for nanoporous and nanoparticulate glasses. These newer materials are more bioactive and resorbable than materials fabricated by "melt-derived" processes. In general, the sol-gel process converts a colloidal liquid, *sol,* into a solid *gel* of particles with liquid entrapped in pores. The starting precursors are usually metal-organic compounds, or alkoxides $M(OR)_n$, in which M is a metal network former and R is an alkyl group. These liquid precursors are mixed and hydrolyzed. This forms silanol groups that condense to create an interconnected network of siloxane bonds, with water and alcohols as by-products. Precise control of the synthesis and drying steps results in a final glassy solid with a very large degree of interconnected mesoporosity (pore diameters in the range of 2 to 50 nm) and a high specific surface area. This nanoporous glass is an outstanding matrix for entrapping and adsorbing cytokines and drugs, for example. As the glassy matrix resorbs, these compounds are released in an activated form.

In addition, these bioactive glasses chemically bond to both hard and soft tissues, and they stimulate the formation of new bone in vivo. Bioactive glasses exchange ions with surrounding fluids within seconds of immersion into the body or media. In brief, the processes on the glass surface are characterized by this rapid ion exchange, followed by dissolution of the glass network and reprecipitation and growth of a silica gel layer on the surface, which in turn precipitates a calcium-deficient carbonate apatite (hydroxyl carbonate apatite [HCA]) layer onto its surface. This layer reorganizes and quickly results in the formation of a crystalline HCA layer on the glass surface. As these layers are forming and growing outward from the surface, extracellular proteins become entrapped in the growing layers and invoke subsequent cellular reactions including cell attachment and colonization, proliferation, and differentiation into relevant progenitor cells (Fig. 15.10).

The interaction of bioactive glasses with living tissue, in particular forming strong chemical bonds to a tissue, is referred to as *bioreactivity* or *bioactivity*. It is now believed that a biologically induced active apatite surface layer must form at the interface between the material and the bone to create a material bond with the bone. In addition, the ionic species released from the reacting glasses upregulate at least seven families of genes found in mesenchymal cells and osteoblasts.

Polymeric Materials

Polymers are by far the most common materials used for tissue-engineering scaffolds. Polylactic acid and polyglycolic acid (and copolymers of these two) as well as polycaprolactone are common examples. These polymers are metabolized in vivo, and their acidic degradation products are easily removed from the body. They can easily be cast into a mesh or other desired shape or can simply be extruded as fibers that are used to loosely pack an anatomically designed mold. The same material from which the scaffold is designed can be used to encapsulate growth factors to provide a timed release of the protein as the capsule degrades. Polymers often release acidic and toxic products when they degrade, creating inflammation around the implantation site. Their survival time in the body is difficult to control, and they become stiffer as they degrade.

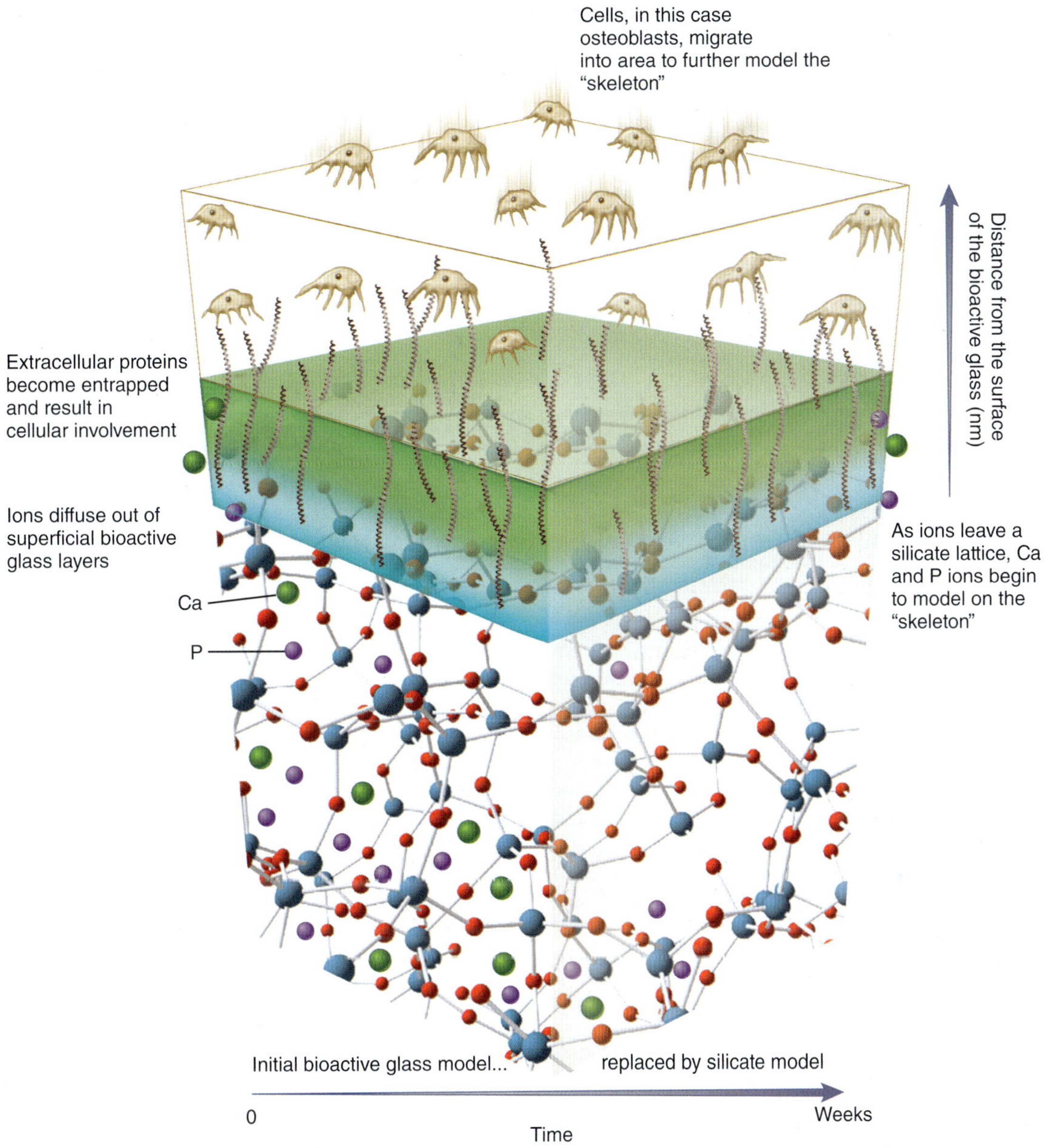

• **Fig. 15.10** The in vivo reactions that occur when a bioactive glass is implanted. *Ca*, Calcium *(green)*; *P*, phosphorus *(purple)*.

Protein-Based Hydrogels

Recently, protein-based hydrogels have been widely investigated as natural ECM analogs for use as tissue engineering scaffolds. These materials are highly biocompatible and have excellent biological properties such as enzyme degradation in response to matrix metalloproteinases (MMPs) and provide a degree of control over cellular adhesion, proliferation, migration, and differentiation. Matrigel®, a gelatinous protein mixture derived from mouse tumors, was one of the first successful in vitro hydrogel tissue engineering scaffolds. However, due to its origin from tumors, it is unsuitable for clinical application.

Gelatin methacryloyl (GelMA) is now the most popular hydrogel alternative to Matrigel®. GelMA is a synthetic gelatin-based material that also displays biocompatibility, low immunogenicity, low cost, easy availability, controlled degradation from MMP cleavage, and controllable cell adhesion due to incorporation of arginine-glycine-aspartic acid (RGD) sequences. For use as a scaffold in different body locations, the mechanical properties of GelMA are variable, and controlled by altering the degree of methacryloyl functionalization within the construct. Furthermore, due to their high water content, cells and growth factors are easily incorporated and immobilized within the hydrogel, allowing for easy transplantation.

Cell Culture Methods

Cells can be grown as a monolayer (or sheet) on a polystyrene growth plate treated to optimize cell attachment and proliferation. Culturing cells on three-dimensional scaffolds for later implantation is more difficult. Scaffolds thicker than 1 mm often produce

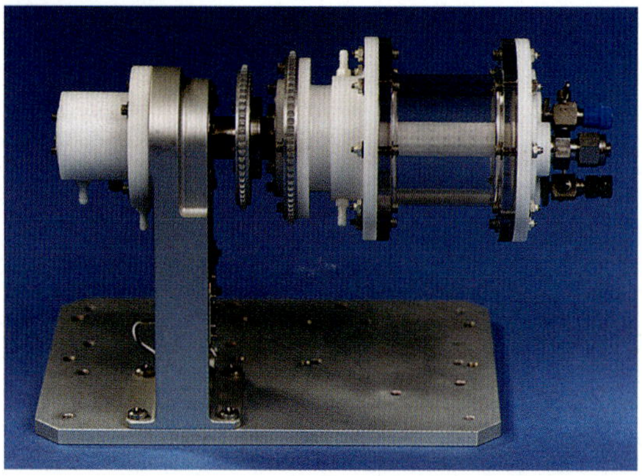

• **Fig. 15.11** Image of National Aeronautics and Space Administration (NASA) bioreactor. (Courtesy NASA/Johnson Space Center, Houston, TX.)

a shell of viable cells and new ECM surrounding a necrotic core. Some type of perfusion bioreactor system (Fig. 15.11) must be used to mimic the mass transport in vivo environment more closely. Alternatively, the tissues can be fabricated in a well-vascularized region, in vivo. This allows a circulatory system to develop along with the cells.

Optimal culture conditions for tissue-engineering scaffolds require high seeding efficiency to minimize growth time and homogeneous cell distribution in the scaffolds to ensure a uniform, organized tissue. Mechanical loads can improve tissue organization if they are applied to the developing cells as the cells begin to embed themselves within their ECM. Physiological loads are continually applied to natural tissues during development and use, so some loads applied in vitro begin to prepare the cells and tissues for implantation. Early loading aligns the cells into a stronger, more organized matrix, which in turn creates improved tissue function.

Tissue-Engineered Dental Tissues

Substantial research has been done to develop methods for regenerating tooth structure and its supporting tissues. The FDA has already approved two commercially available tissue-engineered living skin products. It is probable that tissue-engineered bone and cartilage might soon follow.

Two approaches are being used to fabricate PDL. The first harvests existing PDL cells from the patient. The cells are grown and expanded in vitro (Fig. 15.12). They are then cultured as a monolayer without any substrate. Once the layer is continuous, with tight intercellular junctions, the sheet of cells is released from the culture plate and placed in situ on the tooth surface to repair the periodontal defect.

The second approach is a cell and scaffold method in which cells are again harvested from the PDL of the patient. The cells are then seeded onto a three-dimensional polymer matrix. This is grown in vitro and eventually implanted back into the patient's periodontal defect (Fig. 15.13).

Another oral tissue being targeted by considerable research is a tissue-engineered salivary gland. The technique uses human parotid cells grown in vitro to develop an orally implantable, functioning, fluid-secreting tissue.

Finally, the most exciting target for tissue engineering is the whole tooth. Several research groups have announced that they succeeded in growing primitive teeth using tissue-engineering methods. One group created a tooth-shaped porous scaffold of bioresorbable polymer and seeded it with individual cells taken from a tooth bud. This cell-seeded construct was implanted into the omentum of a rat to provide fluid and nutrient transfer during growth and development. A mixture of cell types from the tooth bud migrated to the appropriate region during growth and differentiated to form pulp tissue, dentin, and enamel in the correct anatomical relationships and ratios. Another group successfully used DPSCs, and epithelial cells harvested from donor pigs. DPSCs were grown, expanded, and differentiated into odontoblasts and osteoblasts. The cells were combined onto scaffolds composed of gelatin-chondroitin-hyaluronan, and implanted into pig alveolar sockets, after tooth germ resection. Seven of eight animals developed teeth containing enamel-like crowns, dentin, cementum, root, and pulp structures. Although these early experiments have produced partial teeth, they have shown that the concept will work in vivo to create entire teeth de novo.

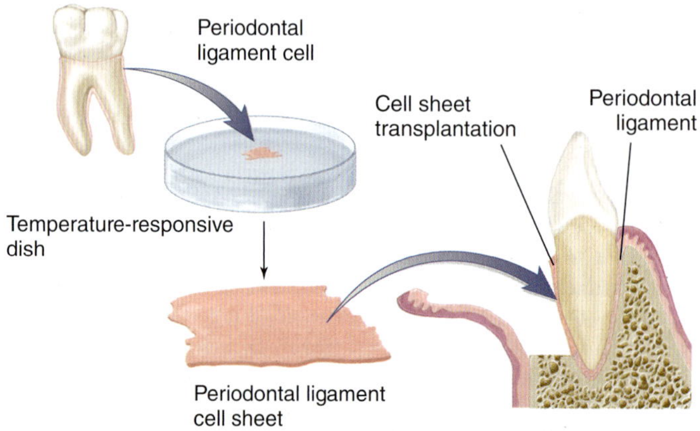

• **Fig. 15.12** One method of periodontal ligament engineering under development. Periodontal cells are extracted from a patient's tooth and grown on temperature-responsive culture plates in vitro. Upon lowering the temperature on these cultures, the confluent layer of cells spontaneously lifts off of the plate as a sheet of cells with intact cell junctions. These sheets are then implanted with various treatments to attempt regeneration of the periodontal tissues. (Modified from Yamato M, Okano T. Cell sheet engineering. *Mater. Today.* 2004;7(5):42–47.)

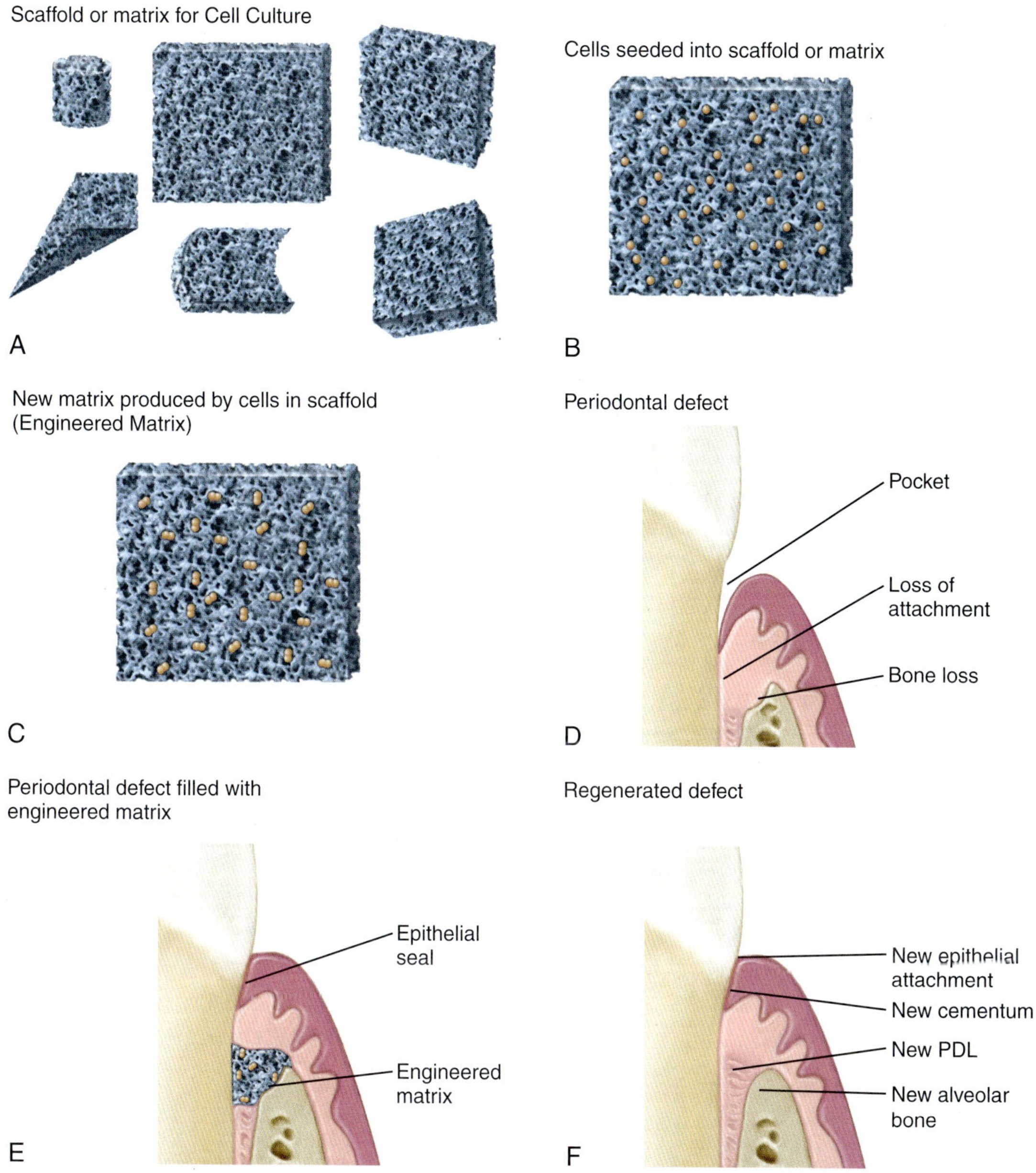

• **Fig. 15.13** A more classical approach to periodontal tissue regeneration being developed. (A) The support scaffold is developed and shaped to the desired geometry. (B) In this method, cells are again harvested from the patient's periodontal ligament (*PDL*) and seeded into a scaffold, where they are expanded in vitro. (C) The cells are allowed to grow for a time to allow synthesis of an appropriate matrix for implantation. (D) A periodontal defect is shown. (E) The tissue-engineered matrix is implanted into the defect site, leading to a regenerative response. (F) In this method, the fully regenerated periodontal defect is expected to be indistinguishable from other sites in the patient's mouth. (Modified from Bartold PM, McCulloch CA, Narayanan AS, et al. Tissue engineering: a new paradigm for periodontal regeneration based on molecular and cell biology. *Periodontol 2000.* 2000;24:253–269.)

Bibliography

Abukawa H, Terai H, Hannouche D, et al. Formation of a mandibular condyle in vitro by tissue engineering. *J Oral Maxillofac Surg.* 2003;61:94.

Aframian DJ, David R, Ben-Bassat H, et al. Characterization of murine autologous salivary gland graft cells: a model for use with an artificial salivary gland. *Tissue Eng.* 2004;10:914.

Agrawal CM, Ray RB. Biodegradable polymeric scaffolds for musculoskeletal tissue engineering. *J Biomed Mater Res.* 2001;55:141.

Almany L, Seliktar D. Biosynthetic hydrogel scaffolds made from fibrinogen and polyethylene glycol for 3D cell cultures. *Biomaterials.* 2005;26:2467.

Al-Salihi KA, Samsudin AR. Bone marrow mesenchymal stem cells differentiation and proliferation on the surface of coral implant. *Med J Malaysia.* 2004;59:45.

Alsberg E, Hill EE, Mooney DJ. Craniofacial tissue engineering. *Crit Rev Oral Biol Med.* 2001;12:64.

Altman GH, Diaz F, Jakuba C, et al. Silk-based biomaterials. *Biomaterials.* 2003;24:401.

Angelini L, Eleuteri E, Coppola M. *Surgery in Italy. Arch Surg.* 2001;136:1318.
Anusaksathien O, Giannobile WV. Growth factor delivery to re-engineer periodontal tissues. *Curr Pharm Biotechnol.* 2002;3:129.
Auger FA, Berthod F, Moulin V, et al. Tissue-engineered skin substitutes: from in vitro constructs to in vivo applications. *Biotechnol Appl Biochem.* 2004;39:263.
Badylak SF. Xenogeneic extracellular matrix as a scaffold for tissue reconstruction. *Transpl Immunol.* 2004;12:367.
Bartold PM, McCulloch CA, Narayanan AS, et al. Tissue engineering: a new paradigm for periodontal regeneration based on molecular and cell biology. *Periodontology.* 2000;24:253.
Baum BJ, Mooney DJ. The impact of tissue engineering on dentistry. *J Am Dent Assoc.* 2000;131:309.
Baum BJ. Prospects for re-engineering salivary glands. *Adv Dent Res.* 2000;14:84.
Beele H. Artificial skin: past, present and future. *Int J Artif Organs.* 2002;25:163.
Bhishagratna KL. An English Translation of the Sushruta Samhita. *Chowkhamba Sanskrit Series Office.* 1963:352–356.
Blum JS, Barry MA, Mikos AG. Bone regeneration through transplantation of genetically modified cells. *Clin Plast Surg.* 2003;30:611.
Bohl KS, Shon J, Rutherford B, et al. Role of synthetic extracellular matrix in development of engineered dental pulp. *J Biomater Sci Polym Ed.* 1998;9:749.
Bonassar LJ, Vacanti CA. Tissue engineering: the first decade and beyond. *J Cell Biochem Suppl.* 1998;30:297.
Buckley MJ, Agarwal S, Gassner R. Tissue engineering and dentistry. *Clin Plast Surg.* 1999;26:657.
Cao X, Deng W, Qu R, et al. Non-viral co-delivery of the four Yamanaka factors for generation of human induced pluripotent stem cells via calcium phosphate nanocomposite particles. *Adv Funct Mater.* 2013;23(43):5403–5411.
Chai Y, Slavkin HC. Prospects for tooth regeneration in the 21st century: a perspective. *Microsc Res Tech.* 2003;60:469.
Chen FM, Jin Y. Periodontal tissue engineering and regeneration: current approaches and expanding opportunities. *Tissue Eng Part B Rev.* 2010;16(2):219–255.
Chen S, Tomov ML, Ning L, et al. Extrusion-based 3D bioprinting of adhesive tissue engineering scaffolds using hybrid functionalized hydrogel bioinks. *Adv Biol (Weinh).* 2023;7:e2300124. https://doi.org/10.1002/adbi.202300124.
Cordeiro MM, Dong Z, Kaneko T, et al. Dental pulp tissue engineering with stem cells from exfoliated deciduous teeth. *J Endod.* 2008;34:962–969.
Dard M, Sewing A, Meyer J, et al. Tools for tissue engineering of mineralized oral structures. *Clin Oral Investig.* 2000;4:126.
Demarco FF, Casagrande L, Zhang Z, et al. Effects of morphogen and scaffold porogen on the differentiation of dental pulp stem cells. *J Endod.* 2010;36(11):1805–1811.
Deporter D. Surgical site development in the partially edentulous patient. In: Zarb G, Lekholm U, Albrektsson T, et al., eds. *Aging, Osteoporosis and Dental Implants.* Quintessence Publishing Co; 2002.
Di Silvio L, Gurav N, Sambrook R. The fundamentals of tissue engineering: new scaffolds. *Med J Malaysia.* 2004;59:89.
Du C, Moradian-Oldak J. Tooth regeneration: challenges and opportunities for biomedical material research. *Biomed Mater.* 2006;1(1):R10–R17.
Duailibi MT, Duailibi SE, Young CS, et al. Bioengineered teeth from cultured rat tooth bud cells. *J Dent Res.* 2004;83:523.
Duan X, Tu Q, Zhang J, et al. Application of induced pluripotent stem (iPS) cells in periodontal tissue regeneration. *J Cell Physiol.* 2011;226(1):150–157.
Earthman JC, Sheets CG, Paquette JM, et al. Tissue engineering in dentistry. *Clin Plast Surg.* 2003;30:621.
Giannobile WV. What does the future hold for periodontal tissue engineering? *Int J Periodontics Restorative Dent.* 2002;22:6.
Goldberg M, Smith AJ. Cells and extracellular matrices of dentin and pulp: a biological basis for repair and tissue engineering. *Crit Rev Oral Biol Med.* 2004;15:13.
Gosain AK, Persing JA. Biomaterials in the face: benefits and risks. *J Craniofac Surg.* 1999;10:404.
Gronthos S, Mankani M, Brahim J, et al. Postnatal human dental pulp stem cells (DPSCs) in vitro and in vivo. *Proc Natl Acad Sci U S A.* 2000;97(25):13625–13630.
Gunatillake PA, Adhikari R. Biodegradable synthetic polymers for tissue engineering. *Eur Cell Mater.* 2003;20:1.
Guo L, Li J, Qiao X, et al. Comparison of odontogenic differentiation of human dental follicle cells and human dental papilla cells. *PLoS One.* 2013;8(4):e62332.
Hadlock TA, Vacanti JP, Cheney ML. Tissue engineering in facial plastic and reconstructive surgery. *Facial Plast Surg.* 1998;14:197.
Hidalgo C, Méndez-Ruette M, Zavala G, et al. A novel porous hydrogel based on hybrid gelation for injectable and tough scaffold implantation and tissue engineering applications. *Biomed Mater.* 2023;18(4). https://doi.org/10.1088/1748-605X/acd499.
Hollister SJ, Maddox RD, Taboas JM. Optimal design and fabrication of scaffolds to mimic tissue properties and satisfy biological constraints. *Biomaterials.* 2002;23:4095.
Hubbell JA. Biomaterials in tissue engineering. *Biotechnology.* 1995;13:565–576.
Ikeda H, Sumita Y, Ikeda M, et al. Engineering bone formation from human dental pulp- and periodontal ligament-derived cells. *Ann Biomed Eng.* 2011;39(1):26–34.
Jin Q, Anusaksathien O, Webb SA, et al. Engineering of tooth-supporting structures by delivery of PDGF gene therapy vectors. *Mol Ther.* 2004;9:519.
Jin QM, Zhao M, Webb SA, et al. Cementum engineering with three-dimensional polymer scaffolds. *J Biomed Mater Res A.* 2003;67:54.
Kaigler D, Mooney D. Tissue engineering's impact on dentistry. *J Dent Educ.* 2001;65:456.
Kang J, Fan W, Deng Q, He H, Huang F. Stem cells from the apical papilla: a promising source for stem cell-based therapy. *Biomed Res Int.* 2019;2019:6104738. doi: 10.1155/2019/6104738.
Kim YS, Min KS, Jeong DH, et al. Effects of fibroblast growth factor-2 on the expression and regulation of chemokines in human dental pulp cells. *J Endod.* 2010;36(11):1824–1830.
Krebsbach PH, Robey PG. Dental and skeletal stem cells: potential cellular therapeutics for craniofacial regeneration. *J Dent Educ.* 2002;66:766.
Kuboki Y, Sasaki M, Saito A, et al. Regeneration of periodontal ligament and cementum by BMP-applied tissue engineering. *Eur J Oral Sci.* 1998;106:197.
Lalan S, Pomerantseva I, Vacanti JP. Tissue engineering and its potential impact on surgery. *World J Surg.* 2001;25:1458.
Langer R. Tissue engineering. *Mol Ther.* 2001;1:12.
Lavik E, Langer R. Tissue engineering: current state and perspectives. *Appl Microbiol Biotechnol.* 2004;65:1.
Lee CH, Kim J-H, Lee HJ, et al. The generation of iPS cells using non-viral magnetic nanoparticle based transfection. *Biomaterials.* 2011;32(28):6683–6691.
Lee KY, Mooney DJ. Hydrogels for tissue engineering. *Chem Rev.* 1869;101:2001.
LeGeros RZ. Properties of osteoconductive biomaterials: calcium phosphates. *Clin Orthop.* 2002;395:81.
Lenza RF, Jones JR, Vasconcelos WL, et al. In vitro release kinetics of proteins from bioactive foams. *J Biomed Mater Res A.* 2003;1:121.
Letic-Gavrilovic A, Todorovic L, Abe K. Oral tissue engineering of complex tooth structures on biodegradable DLPLG/beta-TCP scaffolds. *Adv Exp Med Biol.* 2004;553:267.
Lindroos B, Maenpaa K, Ylikomi T, et al. Characterisation of human dental stem cells and buccal mucosa fibroblasts. *Biochem Biophys Res Commun.* 2008;368(2):329–335.
MacNeil RL, Somerman MJ. Development and regeneration of the periodontium: parallels and contrasts. *Periodontol.* 1999;2000(19):8–20.
Malhotra N, Kundabala M, Acharya S. Current strategies and applications of tissue engineering in dentistry—a review part 2. *Dent Update.* 2009;36(10):639–642, 644–646.

Mantesso A, Sharpe P. Dental stem cells for tooth regeneration and repair. *Expert Opin Biol Ther*. 2009;9(9):1143–1154.

Matalova E, Fleischmannova J, Sharpe PT, et al. Tooth agenesis: from molecular genetics to molecular dentistry. *J Dent Res*. 2008;87(7):617–623.

Mitalipov S, Wolf D. Totipotency, pluripotency and nuclear reprogramming. *Adv Biochem Eng Biotechnol*. 2009;114:185–199.

Miura M, Gronthos S, Zhao M, et al. SHED: stem cells from human exfoliated deciduous teeth. *Proc Natl Acad Sci U S A*. 2003;100:5807.

Miyoshi K, Tsuji D, Kudoh K, et al. Generation of human induced pluripotent stem cells from oral mucosa. *J Biosci Bioeng*. 2010;110(3):345–350.

Murphy WL, Mooney DJ. Controlled delivery of inductive proteins, plasmid DNA and cells from tissue engineering matrices. *J Periodontal Res*. 1999;34:413.

Murray PE, Garcia-Godoy F. Stem cell responses in tooth regeneration. *Stem Cells Dev*. 2004;13:255.

Nakahara T, Nakamura T, Kobayashi E, et al. In situ tissue engineering of periodontal tissues by seeding with periodontal ligament-derived cells. *Tissue Eng*. 2004;10:537.

Nakashima M, Reddi AH. The application of bone morphogenetic proteins to dental tissue engineering. *Nat Biotechnol*. 2003;21:1025.

Newman MG, Takei HH, Klokkevold PR, et al. *Carranza's Clinical Periodontology*. 11th ed. Saunders; 2012.

Nör JE. Tooth regeneration in operative dentistry. *Oper Dent*. 2006;31(6):633–642.

Ohazama A, Modino SA, Miletich I, et al. Stem-cell-based tissue engineering of murine teeth. *J Dent Res*. 2004;83:518.

Ohgushi H, Miyake J, Tateishi T. Mesenchymal stem cells and bioceramics: strategies to regenerate the skeleton. *Novartis Found Symp*. 2003;249:118.

Otsu K, Kumakami-Sakano M, Fujiwara N, et al. Stem cell sources for tooth regeneration: current status and future prospects. *Front Physiol*. 2014;5:36.

Pappalardo S, Carlino V, Brutto D, et al. How do biomaterials affect the biological activities and responses of cells? An in vitro study. *Minerva Stomatol*. 2010;59(9):445–464.

Pradeep AR, Karthikeyan BV. Tissue engineering: prospect for regenerating periodontal tissues. *Indian J Dent Res*. 2003;14:224.

Ratner BD. Replacing and renewing: synthetic materials, biomimetics, and tissue engineering in implant dentistry. *J Dent Educ*. 2001;65:1340.

Ratner D. Skin grafting from here to there. *Dermatol Clin*. 1998;16:75.

Richardson T, Peters M, Ennett A, et al. Polymeric system for dual growth factor delivery. *Nature Biotech*. 2001;19:1029.

Ripamonti U, Reddi AH. Tissue engineering, morphogenesis, and regeneration of the periodontal tissues by bone morphogenetic proteins. *Crit Rev Oral Biol Med*. 1997;8:154.

Saber SE. Tissue engineering in endodontics. *J Oral Sci*. 2009;51(4):495–507.

Saito MT, Silvério KG, Casati MZ, et al. Tooth-derived stem cells: update and perspectives. *World J Stem Cells*. 2015;7(2):399–407.

Salgado AJ, Coutinho OP, Reis RL. Bone tissue engineering: state of the art and future trends. *Macromol Biosci*. 2004;9:743.

Saltzman WM, Olbricht WL. Building drug delivery into tissue engineering. *Nat Rev Drug Discov*. 2002;1:177.

Schmelzeisen R, Schimming R, Sittinger M. Soft tissue and hard tissue engineering in oral and maxillofacial surgery. *Ann R Australas Coll Dent Surg*. 2002;16:50.

Seo B-M, Miura M, Gronthos S, et al. Investigation of multipotent postnatal stem cells from human periodontal ligament. *Lancet*. 2004;364(9429):149–155.

Seong JM, Kim BC, Park JH, et al. Stem cells in bone tissue engineering. *Biomed Mater*. 2010;5(6):062001.

Shin H, Jo S, Mikos AG. Biomimetic materials for tissue engineering. *Biomaterials*. 2003;24:4353.

Smith AJ, Lesot H. Induction and regulation of crown dentinogenesis—embryonic events as a template for dental tissue repair. *Crit Rev Oral Biol Med*. 2001;12:425–437.

Smith AJ. Tooth tissue engineering and regeneration—a translational vision. *J Dent Res*. 2004;83:517.

Stock UA, Vacanti JP. Tissue engineering: current state and prospects. *Annu Rev Med*. 2001;52:443.

Tatullo M, Marrelli M, Shakesheff KM, White LJ. Dental pulp stem cells: function, isolation and applications in regenerative medicine. *J Tissue Eng Regen Med*. 2015;9:1205–1216.

Thesleff I, Tummers M. Stem cells and tissue engineering: prospects for regenerating tissues in dental practice. *Med Princ Pract*. 2003;12:43.

Tomokiyo A, Wada N, Maeda H. Periodontal ligament stem cells: regenerative potency in periodontium. *Stem Cells Dev*. 2019;28(15):974–985. doi: 10.1089/scd.2019.0031.

Ueda M, Tohnai I, Nakai H. Tissue engineering research in oral implant surgery. *Artif Organs*. 2001;25:164.

Ulloa-Montoya F, Verfaillie CM, Hu WS. Culture systems for pluripotent stem cells. *J Biosci Bioeng*. 2005;100:12–27.

Vacanti CA, Vacanti JP. The science of tissue engineering. *Orthop Clin North Am*. 2000;31:351.

Vacanti JP, Langer R. Tissue engineering: the design and fabrication of living replacement devices for surgical reconstruction and transplantation. *Lancet*. 1999;354:SI32.

Vunjak-Novakovic G. The fundamentals of tissue engineering: scaffolds and bioreactors. *Novartis Found Symp*. 2003;249:34.

Whitaker MJ, Quirk RA, Howdle SM, et al. Growth factor release from tissue engineering scaffolds. *J Pharm Pharmacol*. 2001;53:1427.

Xiao S, Zhao T, Wang J, et al. Gelatin methacrylate (GelMA)-based hydrogels for cell transplantation: an effective strategy for tissue engineering. *Stem Cell Rev Rep*. 2019;15(5):664–679. https://doi.org/10.1007/s12015-019-09893-4.

Xu HH, Zhao L, Weir MD. Stem cell-calcium phosphate constructs for bone engineering. *J Dent Res*. 2010;89(12):1482–1488.

Xue Y, Dånmark S, Xing Z, et al. Growth and differentiation of bone marrow stromal cells on biodegradable polymer scaffolds: an in vitro study. *J Biomed Mater Res A*. 2010;95(4):1244–1251.

Yamato M, Okano T. Cell sheet engineering. *Mater Today*. 2004;7:42.

Yannas IV. Synthesis of tissues and organs. *Chembiochem*. 2004;5:26.

Young CS, Terada S, Vacanti JP, et al. Tissue engineering of complex tooth structures on biodegradable polymer scaffolds. *J Dent Res*. 2002;81:695.

Zaky SH, Cancedda R. Engineering craniofacial structures: facing the challenge. *J Dent Res*. 2009;88(12):1077–1091.

Zhao M, Jin Q, Berry JE, et al. Cementoblast delivery for periodontal tissue engineering. *J Periodontol*. 2004;75:154.

Zhu K, Li J, Lai H, Yang C, Guo C, Wang C. Reprogramming fibroblasts to pluripotency using arginine-terminated polyamidoamine nanoparticles based non-viral gene delivery system. *Int J Nanomed*. 2014;9(1):5837–5847.

Zhu W, Liang M. Periodontal ligament stem cells: current status, concerns, and future prospects. *Stem Cells Int*. 2015;2015.972313.

Websites

The Nobel Prize in Physiology or Medicine 2012. 2012. Accessed April 4, 2016. http://www.nobelprize.org/nobel_prizes/medicine/laureates/2012/.

US Department of Health and Human Services. Organ procurement and transplantation network. Accessed November 15, 2017. http://optn.transplant.hrsa.gov/.

US Food and Drug Administration. Vaccines, blood and biologics: tissue and tissue products. 2016. Accessed November 15, 2017. http://www.fda.gov/BiologicsBloodVaccines/TissueTissueProducts/default.htm.

Appendix A

Conversion of Units

This appendix presents several tables that will assist the reader in converting units.

Table of Weights and Measures

Lengths

1 millimeter (mm)	= 0.001 meter	= 0.03937 inch
1 centimeter (cm)	= 0.01 meter	= 0.3937 inch
1 meter (m)		= 39.37 inches
1 yard (yd)	= 0.9144 meter	= 36 inches
1 inch (in)	= 2.54 centimeters	= 25.4 millimeters
1 micrometer (µm)	= 0.001 millimeter	= 0.00003937 inch
1 micrometer (µm)	= 10,000 Angstrom units	
1 Angstrom unit (Å)	= 0.1 nanometer	= 3.937×10^{-9} inch
1 nanometer (nm)	= 0.001 micrometer	= 10 Angstrom units

Weights

1 milligram (mg)	= 0.001 gram	= 0.015 grain
1 gram (g)	= 0.0022 pound	= 15.432 grains
1 gram (g)	= 0.035 ounce	
1 kilogram (kg)	= 1000 grams	= 2.2046 pounds
1 ounce (oz)	= 28.35 grams	
1 pound (lb)	= 453.59 grams	= 16 ounces
1 pennyweight (Troy dwt)	= 1.555 grams	= 24 grains
1 grain (gr)	= 0.0648 gram	

Forces

1 newton (N)	= 0.2248 pound force	= 0.102 kilogram force = 100,000 dynes
1 dyne (d)	= 0.00102 gram force	

Capacity (Liquid)

1 milliliter (mL)	= 1 cubic centimeter	= 0.0021 pint
1 liter (L)	= 1000 cubic centimeters	= 1.057 quarts
1 quart (qt)	= 0.946 liter	= 32 ounces
1 ounce (oz)	= 29.6 milliliters	
1 cubic foot (cu ft)	= 28.32 liters	

Area

sq in (in^2)	sq ft (ft^2)	sq mm (mm^2)	sq cm (cm^2)
1	0.00694	645.16	6.4516
144	1	92,903	929.03
0.00155	0.000011	1	0.01
0.155	0.0011	100	1

Volume

cu in (in^3)	cu mm (mm^3)	cu cm (cc, cm^3)
1	16,387	16.387
0.0000610	1	0.001
0.0610	1000	1

Conversion Tables

Conversion Factors (Linear)

	Millimeters (mm)	Centimeters (cm)	Inches (in)
1 Angstrom unit (Å)	0.0000001	0.00000001	0.000000003937
1 nanometer (nm)	0.000001	0.0000001	0.00000003937
1 micrometer (µm)	0.001	0.0001	0.00003937

Conversion Factors (Force per Area)

To change kilograms force per square centimeter (kgf/cm^2) to pounds force per square inch (lbf/in^2), multiply by 14.223 ($1\ kgf/cm^2 = 14.223\ lbf/in^2$).

To change kilograms force per square centimeter (kgf/cm^2) to megapascals (MPa), multiply by 0.0981 ($1\ kgf/cm^2 = 0.0981$ MPa). NOTE: $1\ MN/m^2 = 1$ MPa.

To change kilograms force per square millimeters (kgf/mm^2) to gigapascals (GPa), multiply by 0.00981.

To change pounds force per square inch (lbf/in^2) to megapascals (MPa), multiply by 0.00689.

To change meganewtons force per square meter (MN/m^2) to pounds force per square inch (lbf/in^2), multiply by 145 ($1\ MN/m^2 = 145\ lb/m^2$).

To change meganewtons per square meter (MN/m^2) to gigapascals (GPa), divide by 1000.

Conversion of Thermometer Scales

Temperature Fahrenheit (°F) = (9/5 temperature Celsius) + 32°
Temperature Celsius (°C) = 5/9 (temperature Fahrenheit − 32°)

Conversion Factors (Miscellaneous)

1 foot-pound (ft-lb) = 13,826 gram-centimeters = 1.356 newton-meters
1 radian = 57.3 degrees
1 watt = 14.3 calories/minute

Conversion of Exponentials to Decimals

Exponential no.	Decimal no.
1×10^{-5} (or 10^{-5})	0.00001
1×10^{-3}	0.001
1×10^{-1}	0.1
1×10^{0} (or 10^{0})	1
1×10^{1}	10
1×10^{4}	10,000
1×10^{7} (or 10^{7})	10,000,000

Comparative Table of Troy, Avoirdupois, and Metric Weights

Grain	Troy (dwt)	Troy (oz)	Avoirdupois (oz)	Avoirdupois (lb)	Gram (g)
1	0.042	0.002	0.00228	0.00014	0.065
24	1	0.05	0.0548	0.0034	1.555
480	20	1	1.097	0.0686	31.10
437.5	18.23	0.91	1	0.063	28.35
7000	291.67	14.58	16	1	453.59
15.43	0.64	0.032	0.035	0.0022	1

Prefixes and Symbols for Exponential Numbers

Factor	Prefix	Symbol
10^{18}	exa	E
10^{15}	peta	P
10^{12}	tera	T
10^{9}	giga	G
10^{6}	mega	M
10^{3}	kilo	k
10^{2}	hecto	h
10	deca	da
10^{-1}	deci	d
10^{-2}	centi	c
10^{-3}	milli	m
10^{-6}	micro	μ
10^{-9}	nano	n
10^{-12}	pico	p
10^{-15}	femto	f
10^{-18}	atto	a

Index

Note: Page numbers followed by "*f*" indicate figures, "*t*" indicate tables, and "*b*" indicate boxes.